T0201522

Coalitions and Partnerships
in Community Health

Coalitions and Partnerships in Community Health

Frances Dunn Butterfoss

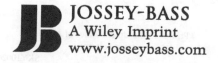

JOSSEY-BASS
A Wiley Imprint
www.josseybass.com

Published by Jossey-Bass
A Wiley Imprint
989 Market Street, San Francisco, CA 94103-1741   www.josseybass.com

Jossey-Bass books and products are available through most bookstores. To contact Jossey-Bass directly call our Customer Care Department within the U.S. at 800-956-7739, outside the U.S. at 317-572-3986, or fax 317-572-4002.

Jossey-Bass also publishes its books in a variety of electronic formats. Some content that appears in print may not be available in electronic books.

Credits are on page 579

Library of Congress Cataloging-in-Publication Data

Butterfoss, Frances Dunn.
    Coalitions and partnerships in community health / Frances Dunn Butterfoss.
        p. ; cm.
    Includes bibliographical references.
    ISBN-13: 978-0-7879-8785-5 (alk. paper)
    ISBN-10: 0-7879-8785-9 (alk. paper)
    1. Community health services. 2. Coalitions. 3. Medical cooperation.
    4. Medical partnership. I. Title.
        [DNLM: 1. Health Care Coalitions—organization & administration.
    2. Community Health Planning—organization & administration. 3. Public
Health. WA 546.1 B9877c 2007]
    RA427.B95 2007
    362.12—dc22   2007002209

Printed in the United States of America
FIRST EDITION

HB Printing   SKY10026483_042121

CONTENTS

Preface   xvii

Acknowledgments   xxiii

About the Author   xxv

PART I: MAKING THE CASE FOR COALITIONS AND PARTNERSHIPS   1

1 Historical Perspective of Coalitions   3

Cooperation and Settlement in Early America   3

The Development of Associations   4

Community Organizing for Social Change: Trade Unions, Settlement Houses,
and Neighborhood and Community Development   5

Social Work Approach   6

Political Activist Approach   7

Neighborhood-Maintenance, or Community-Development, Approach   8

Contemporary Efforts and Models of Social Action Community Organizing   10

Contemporary Roots of Coalitions and Partnerships for Health Promotion   12

Community Development   12

Citizen Participation   12

Empowerment   13

Community Capacity   14

Community Competence   15

Social Capital   15

Coalitions: A Public Health Strategy to Build Capable, Competent Communities   16
The Rise of Coalitions (1990–2006)   17
    Alcohol, Tobacco, and Other Drug Abuse Prevention   17
    Immunization Promotion   19
    Oral Health Promotion   19
    Teen Pregnancy Prevention   20
    Injury Prevention   20
    HIV/AIDS Prevention   20
    Promoting Health Insurance   21
    Prevention of Chronic Disease: Cardiovascular Disease, Cancer,
        and Diabetes   21
    Asthma   22
    Multiple Health Issue Coalitions: Turning Point Initiative   23
    Racial and Ethnic Approaches to Community Health (REACH) 2010   23
    Steps to a HealthierUS   24
Summary   24
Questions for Review   25

2 Principles of Collaboration and Partnering:
   Coalitions Defined   26

Defining Collaboration   26
Intensity and Levels of Collaborative Work   27
What's in a Name?   29
Models of Collaboration   30
What Makes a Coalition a Coalition?   31
Types of Coalitions   32
How Community Coalitions Differ from Other Types of Coalitions   34
    Community Coalitions   34
    State Coalitions   34
    Regional or National Coalitions   36
Competing Coalitions   36
Coalition Spotlight: Changing with the Times—The Consortium
    for Infant and Child Health (CINCH)   37
Summary   38
Questions for Review   38

3 Why Coalitions?   49

Why Coalitions Form   49
The Importance of Community Context   51
Benefits of a Coalition Approach   53
Challenges of a Coalition Approach   55
Applying Democratic Principles to Coalition Building   57

When Coalitions Are Not the Solution   58
To Be or Not to Be? Should Coalitions Ever Disband?   59
Summary   60
Questions for Review   60

4 **The Community Coalition Action Theory (CCAT)   61**

The Community Coalition Action Theory (CCAT): Origin and Roots   62
Coalition Frameworks and Models   62
  Community Organization and Development Model   62
  Framework for Partnerships for Community Development   63
  Framework of Organizational Viability   64
  Community Coalition Model   65
  Work Group on Health Promotion and Community Development Model   67
  The Collaboration Framework   68
  Typology of Community Organization and Community Building   69
  The Conceptual Framework for Coalition Assessment   69
  Model of Community Health Governance   69
Community Coalition Action Theory: Assumptions and Constructs   71
  Outline of the CCAT Theory   71
  Empirical Support for the CCAT Theory   76
  Stages of Development   76
  Community Context   77
  Lead Agency or Convener Group   77
  Coalition Membership   78
  Coalition Operations and Processes   78
  Leadership and Staffing   80
  Coalition Structures   81
  Pooled Member and External Resources   81
  Member Engagement   82
  Assessment and Planning   82
  Implementation of Strategies   83
  Community Change Outcomes   83
  Health and Social Outcomes   83
  Community Capacity   84
Application of CCAT: Consortium for the Immunization
  of Norfolk's Children (CINCH)   84
  Stages of Development   85
  Community Context   85
  Lead Agency or Convener Group   85
  Coalition Membership   86
  Coalition Operations and Processes   86
  Leadership and Staffing   86

     Coalition Structures 87
     Pooled Member and External Resources 87
     Member Engagement 87
     Assessment and Planning 87
     Implementation of Strategies 88
     Community Change and Health Outcomes 88
     Community Capacity 88
  Strengths and Limitations of the Theory, or Model 89
  Future Directions 90
  Summary 91
  Questions for Review 91

PART II: BUILDING EFFECTIVE COALITIONS AND PARTNERSHIPS 93

5 Lead Agency, Coalition Staff, and Leadership 95

  Who Is the Lead Agency? 96
     Types of Lead Agencies 96
     The Role of Lead Agencies 97
     What Makes a Good Lead Agency? 97
  Coalition Staff 98
  Staff Roles 99
  Coalition Leadership 108
     Collaborative, or Transformational, Leaders 109
     Leadership Recruitment 117
     Leadership Styles 118
     Leadership Traits, Skills, and Roles 121
  Team Leadership 126
  Training, Technical Assistance, and Orientation 126
     Training 127
     Technical Assistance 128
     Trainers' and Technical-Assistance Consultants' Roles, Responsibilities,
       and Characteristics 129
     Coalition Roles, Responsibilities, and Characteristics 129
     Building and Sustaining Technical-Assistance
       Consultant–Coalition Relationships 129
     Training and Technical Assistance Venues 130
  Summary 134
  Questions for Review 135
  Resources 135

6 Coalition Membership and Teamwork   138

Member Organizations versus Individual Members   138
Categories of Membership   139
Member Characteristics, Capacities, and Skills   140
Member Responsibilities   142
Member Roles   144
Member Recruitment   144
  Investing in Recruitment   *148*
  Building Member Diversity   *149*
Member Retention   158
Does Size Matter?   162
Building Effective Teams and Work Groups   163
  Stages of Team Development   *164*
  Traits of Teams and Work Groups   *165*
  Team and Work Group Roles   *174*
Building Community Ownership of the Coalition   175
Summary   176
Questions for Review   177
Resources   177
  Organizations   *177*
  Publications   *179*

7 Essential Coalition Processes   181

Communication   182
  The Communication Process   *183*
  Miscommunication   *185*
  Communication Channels   *185*
  Features of Effective Group Communication   *186*
Problem Solving   190
Effective Decision Making   195
  Decision-Making Styles   *196*
    Techniques for Building Majority-Rule Decisions   199
    Techniques for Building Consensus   199
  Prioritizing   *200*
    Multi-Voting   201
    Zero to Ten Rating   201
    Ethical Decision Making   202
Resolving Conflict   203
  Types of Conflict   *204*

General Conflict Resolution Strategies 207

Conflict Management Skills 208

Turfism 212

Types of Turf Issues That Coalitions Face 213

Avoiding and Resolving Turf Battles 213

Effective Turf Management Tips 215

Coalition Spotlight: Virginians for a Healthy Future 216

Summary 217

Questions for Review 218

Resources 219

General 219

Decision Making 219

Conflict Resolution 219

8 Coalition Infrastructure 222

Formalized Rules and Procedures 223

Coalition Vision and Mission Statements 223

SWOT Analysis 224

Vision Statements 224

Mission Statements 225

Slogans or Bylines 225

Roles and Job Descriptions 225

Organizational Charts 227

Steering Committees and Governance 229

Work Groups and Subgroups 230

Bylaws and Guidelines for Operations 231

Coalition Meetings 240

Meeting Basics 241

Timing of Meetings 242

Ground Rules 243

Meeting Process 244

Meeting Roles 244

Common Meeting Challenges 245

Agenda 249

Minutes 250

Parliamentary Procedure 250

Coalition Spotlight: Conducting Empowering Meetings 255

Summary 256

Questions for Review 256

Resources 256

PART III: SUSTAINING EFFECTIVE COALITIONS AND PARTNERSHIPS 259

9 Marketing the Coalition and Its Agenda 261

Marketing or Promoting the Coalition 262
Developing an Effective Organizational Message 262
Developing a Business Plan 265
Coalition Branding: Logo and Name 267
Promotional Materials 267
  Brochures 268
  Newsletters 270
  Websites 273
  Coalition Spokespersons 275
Summary 276
Questions for Review 276
Resources 277

10 Funding, Resource Development, and Sustainability 278

Sources of Coalition Funds 279
Sustainability 279
Social Enterprise 280
Social Entrepreneurs 281
Funding Characteristics 281
To Incorporate or Not? 282
Developing the Coalition Budget 285
Steps in the Budgeting Process 287
Fund-Raising 290
  The Resource Development Team 292
  The Resource Development Plan 293
  Resource Planning Steps 293
Obtaining Corporate, Foundation, and Government Grants 298
  Identifying and Researching Grant Funding Sources 299
  Contacting the Funder 301
  Building Support for the Grant Proposal 301
  Requests for Proposals 302
  Proposal Timelines 303
  Writing a Grant Proposal 303
  Reviewing Process for Competitive Grant Applications 304
  Letters of Intent 305
  The Grant Application 305

Dealing with Rejection 309

Improving Competitive Applications 310

Coalition Spotlight: Arkansas Oral Health Coalition 314

Summary 316

Questions for Review 316

Resources 316

PART IV: COALITIONS AND PARTNERSHIPS IN ACTION 319

11 Community Assessment 321

Choosing Coalition Issue(s) That Resonate with the Community 322

Framing the Issue to Build Support 323

Impact of the Issue on the Coalition 326

Priority Populations 326

Involving the Priority Population in the Work 327

An Asset-Based Approach to Community Assessments 328

Benefits and Challenges of Conducting Assessments 330

Conducting the Assessment 331

Determining the Assessment's Purpose and Scope 332

Defining the Assessment's Goals and Objectives 332

Selecting the Approach and Methods for Collecting Data 332

Designing and Pilot-Testing the Instruments and Procedures 347

Preparing a Timeline and Budget 348

Collecting the Data 348

Analyzing the Data 348

Preparing and Disseminating the Findings 349

Evaluating the Assessment's Merit and Worth 351

Coalitions and Assessments: Issues and Lessons Learned 351

Coalition Spotlight: Community Assessment with the Metropolitan Boston
Haitian HIV Prevention Coalition 352

Summary 352

Questions for Review 353

Resources 353

12 Coalitions and Planning 356

Public Health Planning Models 357

Getting To Outcomes: Methods and Tools for Planning, Evaluation
and Accountability (GTO) 359

The Strategic Planning Process 361

Evaluating Strategic and Action Plans and the Planning Process 371

Coalition Spotlight: Strategic Planning with the Decade
of Hope Coalition in Dulce, New Mexico 379

Summary   389

Questions for Review   390

Resources   390

13 Coalition Activities and Interventions   391

Phases of Program Implementation   392

Selecting and Implementing Projects   392

  The Project Team   394

  Assessing Promising Practices and Interventions   395

  Characteristics of Successful Interventions   399

  Implementing Community-Based Strategies   401

  Levels of Intervention   401

  Replicating Community-Based Strategies   402

  Types of Intervention Strategies   403

Social Marketing   407

  Essential Elements of Social Marketing   407

  Features of Social Marketing   408

  Creating a Social Marketing Plan   409

Media Advocacy   411

  How Does Media Advocacy Work?   412

  Media Advocacy Strategies   413

  Interview Basics   416

  Developing an Advocacy Strategy   417

  The Advocacy Team   418

Coalition Spotlight: Media Advocacy with Los Angeles County Alcohol,

  Tobacco, and Drug Policy Coalition   419

Legal and Ethical Issues in Community Interventions   421

  Liability   422

  Confidentiality   422

  Informed Consent   423

  Disclosure   424

  Competence   424

  Conflict of Interest   424

Coalition Spotlight: Comprehensive Community Interventions—Injury

  Free Coalition for Kids of Philadelphia   425

Summary   426

Questions for Review   427

Resources   428

  Examples of Social Marketing Campaigns   428

  Other Social Marketing and Media Advocacy Resources   428

  Ethics Websites   431

14 **Evaluating Coalitions and Partnerships** 433

Evaluation Paradigms 435
Coalition Evaluation: Promoting Self-Reflection and Improvement 436
Key Concepts and Levels of Coalition Evaluation 437
   Key Terms of Coalition Evaluation 438
   Ecological Levels of Outcomes 439
   Levels of Coalition Evaluation 440
Evaluation Frameworks and Models 442
   *Kansas University Work Group's Framework for Participatory Evaluation
      of Community Initiatives* 443
   CDC's Framework for Program Evaluation in Public Health 444
   The Kellogg Foundation's Steps to Program Evaluation 446
Evaluation Steps 447
Coalition Measures 470
   Level 1. Measures of Coalition Infrastructure, Function, and Processes 470
   Level 2. Measures of Coalition Programs and Interventions 474
   Level 3. Measures of Health Status and Community Change Outcomes 475
Coalition Evaluation Instruments 476
Challenges of Evaluating Community-Based Initiatives 486
The Challenges of Coalition Evaluation 487
Solving the Coalition Evaluation Dilemma 490
Coalition Spotlight: The California Coalition for Childhood Immunization 492
Summary 493
Questions for Review 493
Resources 494
   General Evaluation Instruments 494
   Other Resources 497

15 **Coalitions and Partnerships: Their Promise and Future** 501

Reflections on the Power of Working in Partnership 501
Lessons Learned from Coalition Evaluations 502
Summing Up: Factors That Promote Coalition Success 505
Implications and Future Research 507

References 511

Name Index 553

Subject Index 561

*To Tom and our children, Jennifer, Ryan,
and Adam, for always believing in me*

PREFACE

Although coalitions and partnerships successfully bring people together, expand resources, and focus on a problem of community concern better than any single group or agency could do alone, not every coalition is successful and not every coalition has achieved results without having its members incur costs related to their participation. To maximize the likelihood of coalition success, this book will provide an in-depth, analytical, practical approach to building, sustaining, and nurturing these complex organizations. Butterfoss and Kegler's Community Coalition Action Theory provides a theoretical foundation that orients the book toward action-oriented partnerships. These focus on preventing or ameliorating a community-defined problem by analyzing the problem; gathering data and assessing need; developing an action plan with solutions; implementing these solutions; reaching community-level outcomes, such as health behavior changes; and creating social change.

Several practitioner-focused manuals and workbooks exist in the literature, but they tend to provide quick, easy-to-digest snapshots of how coalition work should be approached and managed. To date, no comprehensive text that meets the broader needs of the public-health community, including researchers, academics, and practitioners, is available.

Coalitions and Partnerships in Community Health is a one-stop shop for the tools needed to be successful in collaborative work. It includes rich research and practice-based approaches to the work of building, sustaining, and evaluating community coalitions. Each chapter includes practical approaches to the issues, recommendations for action, resources for further study, and examples from actual coalition work. It is equally useful for the seasoned professional who wishes to expand his or her knowledge of these collaborative processes, and for the novice just starting out. The text has two important primary audiences: (1) faculty and students in the health and human services professions for courses in Community Building/ Development; Community Organizing; Assessment and Planning; Program Implementation and Evaluation; Participatory Research and Evaluation; and (2) health and human services practitioners working in community settings such as public health agencies and nonprofit/for-profit agencies that focus on prevention and disease management (including immunization, chronic disease—for example, asthma, cardiovascular disease, arthritis, cancer, Human Immuno-Deficiency Virus/Acquired Immuno-Defiency Syndrome (HIV/AIDS)—substance and alcohol abuse prevention, injury, oral health, mental health, violence, and crime prevention).

I have over fifteen years of experience in building, leading, managing, and evaluating local, regional, state, and national coalitions formed to address a wide variety of public health and social issues. Throughout this period, I have trained hundreds of coalition members and leaders on how best to use coalitions and partnerships to accomplish desired health and community outcomes. Thus, this book is based on extensive research and field experience that will bring to life the issues inherent in building effective partnerships. I opted for a single-author approach to this work because I believe that is the best way to convey my philosophy concerning this important community work. I envision this text as an unfolding story about how coalitions and partnerships are born, nurtured, struggle to maintain their independence, and either learn how to be effective or disband. I hope you enjoy reading it as much as I did writing it.

The four parts of the text are: (I) Making the Case for Coalitions and Partnerships (Chapters 1–4), (II) Building Effective Coalitions and Partnerships (Chapters 5–8), (III) Sustaining Effective Coalitions and Partnerships (Chapters 9–10), and (IV) Coalitions and Partnerships in Action (Chapters 11–14). Part IV follows the classic public health planning model: Community Assessment, Planning, Implementation, and Evaluation. Finally, Chapter 15 contains considerations about the promise and future of coalitions and partnerships.

PART I: MAKING THE CASE FOR COALITIONS AND PARTNERSHIPS

In Part I, the foundation for coalitions and partnerships will be laid. Chapter One explores the rich history of cooperation and collaboration that resulted in the formation of associations and collaboratives of all types. It traces the roots of community organizing for social change and the subsequent development of trade unions, settlement houses, and neighborhood and community organizations. Then it explores the contemporary roots of coalitions and partnerships for health promotion by looking at the key concepts of community and citizen participation, empowerment, community capacity, and social capital. The chapter concludes with a brief look at the various efforts that have promoted coalitions as a public health strategy to build capable, competent communities.

Chapter Two focuses on the principles of collaboration and partnering. It begins by defining collaboration, including the levels and intensity of collaborative work and the various names, definitions, and models of different collaborative efforts. Then it explores what makes a coalition a unique kind of collaborative organization and highlights the types of coalitions that have been built.

Chapter Three gets to the heart of the text by questioning why coalitions are formed in the first place. The importance of community context is explained, as well as the benefits and challenges inherent in using a coalition approach. The realities of partnering are exposed by revealing situations where coalitions are not the best or only solution.

Chapter Four presents various coalition frameworks and models. The Open Systems Model developed by Katz and Kahn (1978) and Prestby and Wandersman's Framework of Organizational Viability (1985) suggest environmentally attuned components of organizational functioning: resource acquisition, maintenance subsystem or structure, production subsystem (actions or activities), and external goal attainment. The work of community coalitions for preventing alcohol, tobacco, and other drug abuse (ATOD) led to evaluation-based community coalition models by Butterfoss, Goodman, and Wandersman (1993) and Francisco, Paine, and Fawcett (1993). Collaboration-based models have also been instrumental in developing coalition theory, especially the *Collaboration Framework* of the National Network for Collaboration (1996), Minkler's Community Organizing and Community Building Typology (2005), and Braithwaite and colleagues' Community Organization and Development Model (COD) (1989) for developing effective community coalition boards in a culturally competent context. Sofaer's Conceptual Framework for Coalition Assessment (2001) and Lasker's Model of Community Health Governance (2003) are also featured. The chapter centers on Butterfoss and Kegler's Community Coalition Action Theory (CCAT) (2002) by describing its origin and roots, constructs and assumptions, and empirical support. The theory is then applied to an actual community coalition to illustrate its utility. The chapter concludes with a discussion of the strengths and limitations as well as the future directions of the theory.

PART II: BUILDING EFFECTIVE COALITIONS AND PARTNERSHIPS

Part II delves into the actual work of building these unique partnerships. Chapter Five explores the engine behind every coalition and partnership—the lead agency, staff, and leaders that are developed from the active membership. It covers the role, function, and desirable traits that each of these actors should possess to inspire and support its members to participate, grow, and succeed. The concepts of collaborative and transformative leadership help to convince the reader that these organizations must serve as catalysts to be effective.

If Chapter Five covers the coalition's engine, then Chapter Six is its fuel. Coalition members are the heart of the coalition—its lifeblood. If they aren't happy and fulfilled, learning and gaining new skills that are transferable, then the coalition is doing them a disservice. The chapter covers desirable member characteristics, capacities and skills, roles, and responsibilities. It focuses on recruiting and retaining for every coalition an engaged, diverse membership that represents its community and makes the organization culturally competent. Furthermore, information is provided to help this engaged citizenry to build effective teams and community ownership of the coalition.

Chapter Seven focuses on the essential coalition procedures that can make or break a partnership. Effective methods for improving communication, decision making, and problem-solving methods and skills are provided. The tough issues of turfism and conflict are investigated; strategies to cope with both are invaluable for any coalition.

Chapter Eight is a nuts-and-bolts chapter that focuses on the rudiments of coalition structure and governance. From developing the coalition's vision and mission, to creating guidelines and bylaws, this is a how-to chapter. The basics of topics from meeting management to creating viable governing groups are explored in depth.

PART III: SUSTAINING EFFECTIVE COALITIONS AND PARTNERSHIPS

Building effective partnerships is one thing, but sustaining them beyond a typical three-year funding period is quite another. This section gives the reader tools to do just that. Chapter Nine focuses on the idea of marketing the coalition and its activities to its priority community, funders, potential partners and supporters, and the community at large. The keys to effective marketing that promote the coalition's goals are presented, with tools for creating promotional materials and a business-like approach to the work.

Chapter Ten covers the topic often of highest concern in the entire field of collaborative work—resources! How to develop a mindset for sustainability by convening the coalition leadership into a Resource Development Team that creates a plan for sustainability is not a new issue, but it is not often tackled. The steps for conducting a resource assessment and setting realistic fund-raising goals to arrive at a diversified, stable economic base for the coalition are explored. The intricacies of budgeting and obtaining competitive federal foundation grants are essential for survival.

PART IV: COALITIONS AND PARTNERSHIPS IN ACTION

In Part IV, we get down to the real work of the coalition—why it exists in the first place. Chapter Eleven provides a comprehensive look at assessment, from choosing or framing the health issue to generate support, to involving the community in the work. Using an asset-based approach to assessment, the reader is guided through the steps of assessment with detailed coverage of methods of community-based data collection, analysis, and reporting. The use of mixed methods and qualitative approaches is highlighted here.

Chapter Twelve focuses on Coalitions and Planning. The planning models that have served public-health efforts well are presented here. The elements and procedures for developing strategic plans to guide long-range work and action plans that guide program implementation also are covered in detail.

Chapter Thirteen focuses on the activities and strategies that coalitions and partnerships are most likely to pursue in the community setting. From selecting promising practices using a teamwork approach, to deciding on which levels of intervention are needed, this chapter is invaluable for the researcher and practitioner. Next, the elements of social marketing are presented, with an emphasis on a marketing plan that helps members of the priority audience and community adopt change strategies for better health. Finally, media advocacy, advocacy approaches, strategies, and tips are highlighted. Because much of coalition work is focused on legislative and environmental change, this approach is essential to understanding and using it strategically. The complex issues behind replication of programs and the legal and ethical considerations that are faced in this work are also considered.

Chapter Fourteen is nearest to my heart because it is the culmination of all the efforts and experience of coalition members, leaders, and staff in this work. Evaluation causes the most angst for the coalition; it reveals whether the organization and its programs work well. After highlighting the various evaluation frameworks that have a self-reflection-and-improvement approach, the challenges of coalition evaluation are explored. The various paradigms and concepts of participatory and coalition evaluation are presented, and a step-by-step look at how this type of evaluation can be accomplished in a community setting is revealed. Most important, the chapter provides extensive examples of specific short-, intermediate-, and long-term process and outcome measures, and an extensive resource list of instruments and websites that can jump-start an evaluation. Numerous instruments for assessing the coalition and its programs are included in the appendices.

Chapter Fifteen is a reflection on the promise that coalitions have demonstrated, according to the findings of an esteemed, creative, daring cadre of evaluators, researchers, and practitioners. The factors that promote success, suggestions for future research, and the promise of what is yet to come complete this work.

ACKNOWLEDGMENTS

Writing this book was a labor of love that provided me an opportunity to share with others a small portion of what I have learned in my years of working in partnership with communities. I hesitate to name names for fear of excluding someone, so I apologize to any persons I have failed to acknowledge and thank.

First, I want to acknowledge the Consortium for Infant and Child Health and Project Immunize Virginia for allowing me to test ideas, theories, and interventions. Our volunteer members and leaders, so giving of themselves, are an incredible force in shaping community and policy change; through them, I have learned much of what is written here. Most especially, thanks to Mohammed Achter and Margaret Davies, the first of a long line of superb Coalition Chairs; and Pat Louis, Amy Paulson, Clint Crews, and Sarah Nasca, equally brave Coalition Coordinators.

Also, my thanks goes to Eastern Virginia Medical School Department Chairs Arno Zaritsky and Don Lewis, Valerie Stallings at the Norfolk Department of Public Health, and James Farrell at the Virginia Department of Health for providing financial and other support for our coalitions over the years. I so appreciate Ardythe Morrow's faith in and encouragement of my coalition vision long before it was popular and the tireless efforts of other colleagues at the Center for Pediatric Research, Eastern Virginia Medical School, Children's Hospital of The King's Daughters, and Old Dominion University, including DeWitt Webster, Tricia Daniels, Nancy Stromann, Clare Houseman, Richardeen Benjamin, Jan Teagle, and Ann Campbell.

I have also learned from those I have trained or to whom I have provided technical assistance on building, sustaining, and evaluating their coalitions. From the Bahamas and Virgin Islands, to North Dakota, Mississippi, and Pennsylvania, I have been enriched by your stories, struggles, and perseverance. You have welcomed me into your coalitions, offices, homes, and hearts, and I am very grateful. My gratitude is also offered to Pat Bakalian, Annemarie Beardsworth, Jim Bender, Carol Cowden, Debbie McCune Davis, Vicki Evans, Rich Greenaway, Kathy Gustafson, and many others from the Immunization Coalition Conference posse.

If it were not for the influence and inspiration of Bob Goodman and Abe Wandersman at the University of South Carolina, I may never have started research with coalitions—I thank them for their wisdom and guidance. Many other colleagues have helped shape my ideas; some I know only through their work, while others have actively collaborated with me: Adrienne Paine Andrews, Bill Berkowitz, David Chavis, Matt Chinman, Noreen Clark, Larry Cohen, Frank Dukes, Diane Dunet, Eugenia Eng, Stephen Fawcett, Paul Florin, Vince Francisco, and Amy Friedmann, Linda Jo Doctor and other Allies partners, Larry Green, Sue Heitzman, Pam Imm, Barbara Israel, Gillian Kaye, Michelle Kegler, Marsh Kreuter, Roz Lasker, Renee Lavinghouse, Paul Mattesich, Ken McLeroy, Meredith Minkler, Roger Mitchell, Edith Parker, Beth Rosenthal, Shoshanna Sofaer, Alan Steckler, John Stevenson, Nina Wallerstein, Elia Weiss, and Tom Wolff. I also thank Elaine Auld and Eleanor Dixon-Terry at the Society for Public Health Education (SOPHE) for their inspiration and support.

Finally, I must thank Andy Pasternak and Seth Schwartz at Jossey-Bass for helping bring this project to fruition. For three years, Andy asked me to submit a proposal for this book. His nudging and encouragement made me finally realize that I must write it. Seth, Liah Rose, Sheri Gilbert, and Jill Pellerin took on the Herculean task of turning my manuscript into a published work.

ABOUT THE AUTHOR

Frances Dunn Butterfoss holds the EVMS Foundation Professorship in the Department of Pediatrics at Eastern Virginia Medical School (EVMS) in Norfolk, Virginia. She is also the director of the Division of Behavioral Research and Community Health. Dr. Butterfoss is the founding director and a current board member of CINCH, a community child health partnership, and PIV, a state immunization coalition. These coalitions promote immunizations, access to insurance and health care, asthma management, obesity and injury prevention, and data-driven health assessment and research. She teaches in the EVMS/Old Dominion University Master's in Public Health program and serves on its curriculum committee. A former director of the National Immunization Coalition Training Institute (1995–1998), she provides consultation and training across the country on how to develop, sustain, and evaluate coalitions for health promotion and disease prevention. Dr. Butterfoss has received research support from many federal and foundation grants and has published widely in professional journals and textbooks. Fran is an Associate Editor of *Health Promotion Practice* and past President of the Society for Public Health Education (SOPHE). Her awards include SOPHE's Health Education Mentor (2002), EVMS' Woman in Medicine and Science Professional Achievement (2004), YWCA of South Hampton Roads' Woman of Distinction (2006), and Norman B. Arnold Alumni Award (2006). She completed undergraduate and master's degrees from the University of Pennsylvania and her doctorate in health promotion and education from the Arnold School of Public Health at the University of South Carolina. She lives in Yorktown, Virginia, with her husband, Thomas Butterfoss. They have three wonderful children, and one granddaughter.

*Coalitions and Partnerships
in Community Health*

PART ONE

MAKING THE CASE FOR COALITIONS AND PARTNERSHIPS

CHAPTER ONE

Historical Perspective of Coalitions

Americans of all ages, all stations of life, and all types of disposition are forever forming associations. . . . In democratic countries, knowledge of how to combine is the mother of all other forms of knowledge; on its progress depends that of all others.
—Alexis de Tocqueville, 1835, from Heffner, 2001

The concept of building coalitions to improve the human condition is hardly new. The collaborative work essential to the success of modern coalitions in promoting health and preventing disease has existed since the beginning of human history. This chapter outlines an abbreviated chronicle of the key approaches and notable individuals who shaped the ideals of community participation, community organizing, and community development. Unless we give credit to these foundations, we will not share the rich understanding of the roots that make working within coalitions an effective strategy for improving health.

COOPERATION AND SETTLEMENT IN EARLY AMERICA

When early indigenous people first recognized that hunting and gathering could be improved by working together in groups to increase their store of food, the ideologies of cooperation and collaboration were born. The tasks were usually divided along gender lines, with males being responsible for hunting and providing shelter and protection, while women focused on planting, gathering, homemaking, and child-rearing. People understood the necessity of matching tasks to skill sets and relying on cooperation. Even when people began to live in settlements, environments were often harsh and demanded that people band together for survival.

As we approach the celebration of the 400th anniversary of America's settlement in Jamestown, Virginia, in 1607, archeological findings indicate that these early pioneers relied on each other and indigenous Indian tribes, such as the Powhatan, to procure food and shelter. Those first years (1609–1610), called the "starving time," brought untold hardships from weather, insects, lack of potable water, disease, and the unfulfilled promise of needed supplies from England.[1] As in modern-day community relations, conflicts emerged and "the Indians whose succor spared Jamestown more than once had cause to regret their generosity" (Billings, 1990, p. 5). They became embroiled in a losing struggle to maintain their cultural identity, setting the stage for tragic conflicts involving Native American–white relations for three centuries. Similar scenarios were repeated throughout the settlement of the United States, with a pattern of interdependence and cooperation among people to share resources and skills. However, that cooperative spirit was also characterized by conflict, as competition for resources arose. These early forays into cooperation gave way to more formal collaborative efforts in the form of associations, explored next here.

THE DEVELOPMENT OF ASSOCIATIONS

As the pioneering spirit and character of the new United States emerged in the next century, Benjamin Franklin came to believe that people who cooperated and volunteered together could accomplish great things. The ultimate networker, in 1727, he organized a group of friends to engage in a structured discussion group called the Junto, whose members were drawn from diverse backgrounds and occupations (for example, printers, cabinet-makers, cobblers, merchants). They shared a spirit of inquisitiveness and a desire to improve themselves and their community. As their leader, Franklin insisted that their discussions and debates be "conducted in the sincere spirit of inquiry after truth, without fondness for dispute or desire of victory . . ." (Franklin, 1868, p. 60). Friday evening meetings were organized around a series of questions that served as a springboard for community action.

Always aware of his civic duty and mindful of the "greater good," Franklin used the Junto to help establish a volunteer firefighting association, mutual insurance companies, a public hospital, a network of night watchmen to improve security, and a circulating library. The Library Company, American Philosophical Society, and Pennsylvania Hospital still exist today (Independence Hall Association, 2005; Twin Cities Public Television, 2002). Later in his life, Franklin actively worked for the independence of America. He was elected to the Second Continental Congress, helped draft and signed the Declaration of Independence, and served as ambassador to the Court of Louis XVI in France, which led to the Treaty of Paris (1783). In his late seventies, he served as delegate to the Constitutional Convention and signed the Constitution. His last public act was to write an antislavery treatise in 1789.

Perhaps due to Franklin's influence, the French political thinker and historian Alexis de Tocqueville became fascinated with America's democratic system and its associations. De Tocqueville was convinced that democracy balanced liberty with equality, and community with concern for the individual. He wrote two volumes of *Democracy in America* after an eighteen-month visit to that country in 1831–32 to study its penal system. In writing *On the Use Which the Americans Make of Associations in Civil Life,* he expressed the idea that *association,* or the coming together of people for a common purpose, would bind Americans to an ideal of nation larger than selfish desires, a *civil society* (Heffner, 2001). According to de Tocqueville, powerful individuals were more rare under conditions of equality in democratic societies; therefore, independent citizens needed to form associations in order to have influence (Brogan, 2005).

The power of the association has reached its highest degree in America. Associations are made for the purposes of trade and for political, literary, and religious interests. It is never by recourse to a higher authority that one seeks success, but by an appeal to individual powers working in concert [p. 12].

De Tocqueville observed that Americans continually formed associations of every type to combat individualism and circulate new ideas (Cosentino, 1989).

Americans of all ages, all stations of life, and all types of disposition are forever forming associations. . . . In democratic countries knowledge of how to combine is the mother of all other forms of knowledge; on its progress depends that of all others [p. 112].

De Tocqueville also correctly predicted that democracy would increase, and its rights and privileges would eventually be granted to women, Native Americans, and Africans (Brogan, 2005).

John McKnight (1995), known for his asset-based community development work, credits de Tocqueville with recognizing that both formal and informal associations provide the context for citizens to participate in their communities. De Tocqueville identified three steps in citizen problem solving: (1) Groups of citizens decide they have the power to identify a problem. (2) They decide they have the power to solve the problem. (3) They decide they themselves will become the key actors in implementing the solution. This process emphasizes the strengths, assets, and capacities of local citizens, and can only take place when community members are involved in local decision-making activities. In their landmark text, Kretzmann and McKnight (1993) elaborate further on the types of civic skills and social capital necessary to "build communities from the inside out" (p. 2). The following section illustrates how far-reaching that involvement can be when citizens engage in collaborative efforts to further social justice and community change.

COMMUNITY ORGANIZING FOR SOCIAL CHANGE: TRADE UNIONS, SETTLEMENT HOUSES, AND NEIGHBORHOOD AND COMMUNITY DEVELOPMENT

Succeeding generations of Americans continued to struggle for democracy and equality. "Americans have a history of organizing for social, economic, and political justice" (Bobo, Kendall, and Max, 2001, p. 4). In the 1800s, community-organizing movements began, focused on improving Americans' health and quality of life. Feminists Lucretia Mott and Susan B. Anthony and abolitionists Frederick Douglass, William Lloyd Garrison, Sojourner Truth, and Harriet Tubman all worked with a vision toward the greater good.

Community organizing is a process by which disempowered people—most often with low to moderate incomes—are brought together to act in their common self-interest, while seeking the ideals of participatory democracy (Delgado, 1993). Community organizing encompasses many philosophies, approaches, issues, and constituencies in both rural and urban settings. It enables ordinary people to work for change and can have significant impact at the block, neighborhood, community, city, regional, state, and national levels (Fisher and Romanofsky, 1981). Three dominant approaches toward community organizing have emerged in the twentieth century: social work, political activism, and neighborhood maintenance–community development (Fisher, 1994).

Social Work Approach

The *social work approach* envisions community as a social organism with certain needs that must be coordinated to help the neighborhood remain viable. Community is built by gathering together existing social services, and lobbying for and delivering needed social resources. The organizer then promotes consensus and either enables the community to harness its resources or advocates on behalf of the community to obtain more services.

This approach was used in the social settlement movement in industrial cities of the East and Midwest in the first two decades of the twentieth century. Social settlements were "houses" set up in working-class neighborhoods by educated middle-class citizens to combat problems of poverty, housing, child labor, and tuberculosis. Input or support was not solicited from the people or communities they served. Philanthropic resources were offered in terms of education (classes in English and vocational skills), social services (legal and employment assistance, medical care and child care, recreational programs, and public baths), or lobbying (labor reform and public schools). For example, Hull House was founded by Jane Addams in Chicago in 1889 and offered services to more than 2,000 people per week.

> *So far as Settlement can discern and bring to local consciousness*
> *neighborhood needs which are common needs, and can give vigorous help*
> *to the municipal measures through which such needs shall be met,*
> *it fulfills its most valuable function.*
> —Addams, 1912, p. 320

Eventually, reformers like Florence Kelley, Julia Lathrop, and others who directed their efforts to the root causes of poverty joined Addams. They recruited trade unions, churches, benefit societies, social clubs, and individuals to lobby the Illinois legislature to protect immigrants from exploitation, limit the working ages and hours of women and children, mandate schooling for children, recognize labor unions, and provide for sanitation and industrial safety.

In the 1920s and 1930s, labor militants like Eugene V. Debs created unemployment councils to raise demands for public relief. This working-class movement used a range of tactics, including local and national demonstrations, hunger marches, and petition drives. It supported community-based tenant organizations to fight evictions, farmers' unions to fight foreclosures, veterans' committees to demand bonuses, cultural associations among immigrants and artists, sharecroppers' unions among southern blacks, and in-plant organizing committees (Parachini and Covington, 2001).

The legacy of Eugene V. Debs and these early organizers led to the Social Security Act, New Deal programs, organizing across the working class, and forming associations like the Congress of Industrial Organizations (CIO) that ensured the right to organize, minimum wage, and the eight-hour workday for all (Bobo, Kendall, and Max, 2001).

Political Activist Approach

The *political activist approach* views the community as a political entity, not a social organism. The neighborhood is seen as a potential power base that can keep power, get more power, or build alternative institutions apart from powerful ones that already exist. The organizer's role here is to help the community understand and mobilize around a problem in terms of power. The political activist approach uses less consensus building than does the social work approach, because the neighborhood may be put into conflict with individuals, groups, or institutions that stand to lose power. This type of community organizing is also called *social action organizing* (Burghardt, 1987; Rothman and Tropman, 1995). Fisher describes these efforts as "grassroots based, conflict oriented, with a focus on direct action, and geared to organizing the disadvantaged or aggrieved to take action on their own behalf" (Fisher and others, 2005, p. 51).

One cannot talk about the political activist approach without referencing the soul of community organizing, Saul Alinsky, who emerged as an organizer in the late 1930s. Influenced by the militant labor movement of his time, in 1938, Alinksy organized the Back of the Yards Neighborhood Council (BYNC) in a working-class, ethnic neighborhood next to the slaughterhouses in Chicago. By building a strong coalition of the union, Roman Catholic parishes, small businesses, voluntary associations, and residents, BYNC got jobs and services from corporations, the political machine, and the federal government. BYNC eventually won victories on numerous issues such as child welfare, public school improvement, and neighborhood stabilization.

BYNC successes led to the formation of the Industrial Areas Foundation, which was backed by the Archdiocese of Chicago, the Congress of Industrial Organizations, and Marshall Fields and was the base of operations for Alinsky for the rest of his life. His collaboration with Fred Ross led to the formation of the Community Service Organization for Mexican American Workers in California, which trained César Chávez to lead the United Farm Workers Union.

In the late 1950s, Alinsky broadened his base of support from Chicago to Catholic dioceses and mainline Protestant denominations all over the county, to support urban reform and fight racism. Alinsky (1972) emphasized several tenets of community organizing, namely:

- Organizations should encourage democratic decision making and indigenous leadership.
- Organizations should be open to all members of the community—the more diverse the organization, the stronger.
- Community organizing depends on gaining the support of traditional community leaders and existing organizations.
- Organizations must be geared to meeting people's self-interests, however they define those interests. Let the people decide, no matter what they decide.
- Based on the beliefs of the emancipationist Frederick Douglass, power concedes nothing without a fight. Organizations should use conflict strategies to yield the greatest gains.
- Organizations should fight for concrete victories, because winning builds organization.

Many other political activist organizations emerged in the 1960s out of the civil rights and student movements, such as Students for a Democratic Society and the Black Panthers. Although similar to the Alinsky model in stressing the need for democratic practices and confronting power with power, they emphasized fundamental social change, without great concern for building stable organizations. As a result, many did not last long; some dissolved on their own, and others were purposefully infiltrated and dismantled. Poor urban neighborhoods in the 1990s experienced persistent poverty and had fewer of the social institutions formed by Alinsky-style organizing that had helped them in the past. Most recent activist organizing occurs based on communities of identity—communities of color, gender, sexual orientation, ethnicity, or race (Fisher, 1994).

Neighborhood-Maintenance, or Community-Development, Approach

The *neighborhood-maintenance, or community-development, approach* aims to maintain or improve the physical and commercial value of the neighborhood or community, and not to accumulate power. First coined by the United Nations in 1955, *community development* was designed to create conditions of economic and social progress for the whole community, with its active participation and the fullest possible reliance on the community's initiative (Brager, Sprecht, and Torczyner, 1987). This approach is based on the assumptions that communities can develop the capacity to deal with their own problems; people should participate in making, adjusting, and controlling the major changes taking place in their communities; and changes in community systems that are self-imposed or self-developed have a meaning and permanence that imposed changes do not (Butterfoss and Kegler, 2002).

The neighborhood associations that emerged out of the suburban sprawl of the 1950s were essentially civic organizations developed by homeowners themselves to enforce deed restrictions in their neighborhoods. They functioned as improvement associations to supply services and lobby city hall for street repairs, park development, schools, and traffic signs. In some cases, they were used to prevent racial integration and panic selling. Most often, these types of organizations use peer pressure to maintain property. Sometimes they work with local officials or institutions to apply pressure to obtain services, and occasionally they take a more activist approach when they learn that they can achieve their goals only through confrontational or political means (Delgado, 1993).

However, the community development approach usually deemphasizes dissent and confrontation—these organizations see themselves as proactive consensus builders. The approach attempts to move toward community economic development and building community partnerships with local economic and political powers. In particular, nonprofit community development corporations that serve low-income communities, are governed by community-based boards, and develop businesses or housing developments have proliferated (Parachini and Covington, 2001).

In summary, Fisher and Romanofsky (1981) grouped community-organizing activities in the United States into four historical periods:

1890–1920. The bigness and disorganization of cities during this period of rapid industrialization and immigration was dealt with by organizing immigrant neighborhoods into "efficient, democratic, and, of course, enlightened units within the metropolis" (Fisher and Romanofsky, 1981, p. xii). Because reformers mostly built community through settlement houses and other service mechanisms, the dominant approach was social work.

1920–1940. Community organizing was established as a subdiscipline of social work. During the Great Depression, little was written about community organizing. Most organizations had a national orientation because the economic problems that the nation faced did not seem to be amenable to change at the neighborhood or community level.

1940–1960. Saul Alinsky's political activist approach fueled a new interest in community organizing from the social work perspective. Civil rights efforts and government involvement in reshaping cities and neighborhoods through postwar urban renewal programs aligned well with Alinsky's community movements. He promoted new awareness of community organizing among academics, who trained a generation of organizers like César Chávez.

1960–1980. Neighborhood organizing became widespread in the 1960s. In the early 1970s, activists and theorists such as Kurt Lewin informed organizations, movements, and strategies until the end of the century, in response to federal antipoverty programs and upheavals in cities. Lofquist's prevention model (1983) focused on strengths and assets of community members and associations. Building on an assets approach, civic associations and neighborhood block clubs were formed across the country to foster community spirit, civic duty, and social unity.

CONTEMPORARY EFFORTS AND MODELS OF SOCIAL ACTION COMMUNITY ORGANIZING

From the 1980s until today, community organizing has involved three basic approaches: campaigns, grassroots organizing, and coalition building. *Campaigns* are an effort to organize the community for a short-lived purpose, such as public awareness of a health or social issue, voter identification and turnout, or recruitment for public health screening and immunizations.

In *grassroots organizing*, community groups are built from scratch, and leadership is developed where none existed before—in other words, the unorganized are organized. The southern civil rights movement in the United States and national liberation struggles in the southern hemisphere serve as important models for community-based grassroots organizing oriented to self-determination and sharing the political liberties and material affluence of societies that have exploited people of color (Fisher, 2005). Fisher emphasizes that a key lesson learned from the struggles endured by people of color is that "if oppressed people—often illiterate, rural peasants with few resources—could mobilize, take risks, and make history, then people of other oppressed or threatened constituencies can, with sufficient organization and leadership, do the same" (p. 57).

Coalition building efforts seek to unite existing groups, such as churches, schools, and civic associations, to pursue a common agenda more effectively. Because coalitions often rely on existing leadership, they are sometimes derisively called *grass tips organizing* (Grohol, 2005). Powerful, multi-organizational groups and coalitions with track records have the potential to become significant long-term change agents. These groups have become increasingly sophisticated in "attracting allies, developing community cohesion, and marshalling power, not only locally but also on regional, state, and national levels" (Parachini and Covington, 2001, p. 9). This kind of organizing is based in geographic communities or communities of interest; is decentralized according to sectors and identity groups; has democratic processes and goals; and is funded most often by voluntary sources (Fisher, 2005).

Several models and typologies of community organization exist; for detail on the subject, readers are referred to Minkler's seminal text, *Community Organizing and Community Building for Health* (2005, pp. 26–133).The most well-known model is Rothman's (2001) typology of locality development, social planning, and social action.

Locality development is process-oriented and emphasizes consensus and cooperation aimed at building group identity and sense of community. *Social planning* is task-oriented and uses an outside consultant to help with problem solving. *Social action* combines the two models and focuses on increasing the community's skill at problem solving to achieve power and specific change (Rothman, 2001). Most organizers use a mixture of two or more of these models. For example, the Planned Action toward Community Health (PATCH) public health initiative mixed social planning and locality development models (Bracht, Kingsbury, and Rissel, 1999).

Some researchers and practitioners have recently found this typology to be limited because locality development discourages organizing that is not geographically based;

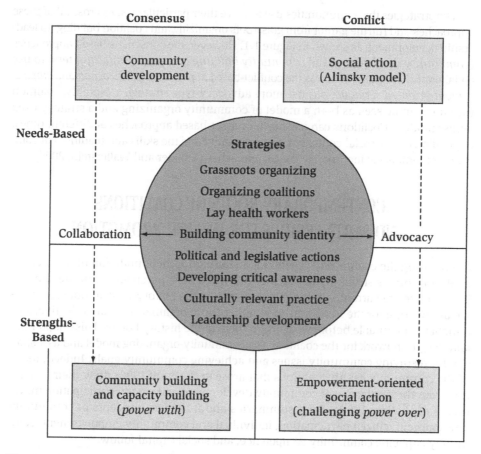

Figure 1.1 Community organization and community-building typology.

Source: Minkler & Wallerstein, 2005, p. 33. From *Community Organizing and Community Building for Health,* 2nd ed., edited by Meredith Minkler. Copyright © 2005 by Rutgers, the State University. Reprinted by permission of Rutgers University Press.

social planning relies on outside experts and not on building community capacity for planning and problem solving; and the model is problem-based, not strength-based, and organizer-centered rather than community-centered (Himmelman, 1992; Kaye and Wolff, 1995; LaBonte, 1994; Minkler and Wallerstein, 2003a).

Newer models of collaborative empowerment and community building have emerged over the past decade to complement the classic organizing approaches described earlier. These models are community-centered and emphasize community strengths, development of shared goals, and equitable power relationships.

Minkler's and Wallerstein's (2005) typology of community organization and community building, shown here in Figure 1.1, incorporates the classic need-based models (consensus-building *community development* and conflict-based *social action*) with the newer asset-based models (consensus-building *community and capacity building* and conflict-based, empowerment-based *social action*).

The strategies that communities use to solve their particular issues cross all of these approaches and run the gamut from grassroots organizing and coalition building, to leadership development, as shown in Figure 1.1. However, the consensus-based approaches (*community development* and *community building or capacity building*) tend to use collaborative strategies, whereas the conflict-based approaches (*social action* and *empowerment-oriented social action*) use more advocacy-type strategies. Notably, coalition building can be seen as both a model of community organizing and a strategy used across models. Coalitions can use need- or asset-based approaches at different times, depending on the social context of the community and the skills and readiness of community members to incorporate these approaches (Minkler and Wallerstein, 2005).

CONTEMPORARY ROOTS OF COALITIONS AND PARTNERSHIPS FOR HEALTH PROMOTION

In searching the community-organizing literature for the foundation of the modern coalition, one is struck by the lack of recent historic perspective on the subject. Because we are currently in the midst of writing the history on coalitions, perhaps we are waiting for the verdict as to whether these organizations are effective, sustainable, and durable before we consign them to the history books. This chapter has laid the groundwork for the coalition as a community-organizing model and as a strategy for resolving community issues and achieving community goals. Indeed, many of the community health coalitions that arose in the early 1990s drew their inspiration from the resurgence of community development and citizen participation movements of the late 1980s. Brief summaries about the key concepts of community development, citizen participation, individual and community empowerment, community capacity, community competence, and social capital follow.

Community Development

Coined by the United Nations in 1955, community development was designed to create conditions of economic and social progress for the whole community, with its active participation and the fullest possible reliance on the community's initiative (Brager, Sprecht, and Torczyner, 1987). This approach is based on several assumptions, namely that communities can develop capacity to deal with their own problems; people should participate in making, adjusting, or controlling the major changes taking place in their communities; and changes in community living that are self-imposed or self-developed have a meaning and permanence that imposed changes do not. Additional assumptions underlying community approaches to problem solving are that holistic approaches can deal successfully with problems where fragmented approaches cannot; democracy requires cooperative participation and action in the affairs of the community; and people must learn the skills that make this possible.

Citizen Participation

Several research studies in the early 1990s focused on *citizen participation*. The Neighborhood Participation Project examined the process of citizen participation through a systematic study of block organizations in a Nashville neighborhood (Florin and Wandersman, 1990; Prestby and others, 1990; Prestby and Wandersman, 1985; Giamartino and Wandersman, 1983). *Community participation* is broadly defined as the process of involving people in the institutions or decisions that affect their lives (Checkoway, 1989). Closely related, *citizen participation* is the mobilization of citizens for the purpose of undertaking activities to improve the conditions in the community.

Community-participation researchers posed questions similar to those used in coalition research: Who participates, who does not, and why? What are the effects of citizen participation in block organizations? What are the characteristics of organizations that are active and successful versus those which are inactive? (Florin and Wandersman, 1990). Research questions asked in the Block Booster Project in New York City also helped shape the coalition research agenda (Perkins and others, 1990). The study suggested that aspects of a community's social and physical environment are more important indicators for participation in block associations than demographic attributes (years of residence, race, income, and home ownership) or crime-related problems, perceptions, or fears.

Perkins, Brown, and Taylor (1996) investigated resident survey data and observational ratings of the physical environment to determine the predictors of participation in neighborhoods in Baltimore, New York City, and Salt Lake City. In all three cities, informal neighboring and involvement in community organizations (for example, faith-based groups) consistently predicted participation, suggesting that people who are more involved in helping their neighbors are generally more involved in grassroots community issues.

Arnstein (1969) posited that citizen participation is a categorical term for *citizen power* (p. 216) and a method enabling citizens to bring about social reform that permits them to share in society's benefits. She offers a typology of citizen participation in the form of an eight-rung ladder. The bottom two rungs (manipulation and theory) are both regarded as "nonparticipation." At these levels, citizens are arranged on advisory committees or boards to educate them and get their support or to involve them in activities that are not likely to lead to change. Rungs three (informing), four (consultation), and five (placation) are presented as different "degrees of tokenism." Here, citizens have varying ability to express opinions and concerns, but no power to make decisions. The top three rungs (partnership, delegated power, and citizen control) are all regarded as degrees of "citizen power."

Empowerment

Empowerment is an often overused term that refers to a community's capacity to identify problems and solutions or to achieve equity (Cottrell, 1983; Rappaport, 1984). The accepted, broad public health definition of empowerment is the "process by which individuals, communities, and organizations gain mastery over their lives in the context of changing their social and political environments to improve equity and the quality of life" (Minkler and Wallerstein, 2005, p. 34).

A resurgence of interest in community empowerment fueled the formation of community coalitions in the 1990s (Israel, Checkoway, Schultz, and Zimmerman, 1994;

LaBonte, 1994; Zimmerman and Rappaport, 1988). Zimmerman (2000) notes that empowerment can be used at the individual, organizational, or community level, and it is at the heart of citizen participation and control. Empowerment involves challenging power through community organizing and advocacy, and expanding power by strengthening community networks and organizations (Minkler and Wallerstein, 2005). Organizational empowerment speaks to coalitions because it involves both the process of change as well as its outcomes (for example, increasing community participation, achieving goals, attracting resources) (Zimmerman, 2000).

Nine factors that influence community empowerment are participation, leadership, problem assessment, organizational structures, resource mobilization, linkages to other individuals and organizations, inquisitiveness, program management, and the role of outside agents (Israel, Schultz, Parker, and Becker, 1998, pp. 180–181).

Unlike the block organizations referred to earlier, some coalition members may be characterized as "interested citizens" (or volunteers), although many represent organizations. Thus research and conceptual work done in the field of interorganizational relations is also relevant to coalition history. Much of the early research on interorganizational relations focused on the formation of collaborative relationships in an effort to understand why organizations join collaborative alliances (Gray and Wood, 1991; Berlin, Barnett, Mischke, and Ocasio, 2000; Provan and Milward, 1995).

Gray and Wood (1991) discuss several perspectives that help to inform interorganizational collaboration. For example, resource dependence theory posits that acquiring resources and reducing uncertainty are the primary forces underlying collaboration (Sharfman, Gray, and Yan, 1991; Mizruchi and Galaskiewicz, 1994). Institutional theory suggests that organizations adjust to institutional directives and norms in an attempt to achieve legitimacy (Gray and Wood, 1991; Gulati, 1995). Political science emphasizes the negotiation of potential conflict through coalitions and power distribution within coalitions (Bazzoli and others, 1997).

Community Capacity

Community coalitions have been recognized as a promising strategy for building capacity and competence among member organizations and, ultimately, in the communities they serve (Chavis, 2001; Kegler, Steckler, McLeroy, and Malek, 1998b). *Community capacity* is defined as the "characteristics of communities that affect their ability to identify, mobilize, and address social and public health problems" (Goodman and others, 1998, p. 259). Dimensions of community capacity that coalitions can impact either positively or negatively include citizen participation and leadership, skills, resources, social and organizational networks, sense of community, understanding of community history, community power, community values, and critical reflection (Goodman and others, 1998).

Collaborative capacity refers to the conditions needed to promote effective collaboration and build sustainable community change (Goodman and others, 1998). Collaborative capacity is needed at four levels in the coalition: within members, within member relationships, within the organizational structure, and within the programs that coalitions sponsor (Foster-Fishman and others, 2001).

An emphasis on capacity is helpful, because a coalition's ability to promote change is dynamic (depending on the coalition's membership, focus, and stage of development), adjustable (enhanced by technical assistance and training efforts), and transferable (the capacity developed within one coalition experience can carry over to other community-based efforts) (Foster-Fishman and others, 2001, p. 242). Crisp and colleagues (2000) identified partnership and coalition development as one of four distinct approaches to building capacity, arguing that two-way communication between groups not previously working together can result in more resources for planning and implementation.

Community Competence

The term *community competence* was developed by Cottrell (1983) to define how a well-functioning community behaves. Competence is similar to empowerment and is achieved when various parts of the community collaborate to identify its problems and needs, reach working consensus on goals and priorities, agree on ways and means to implement those goals, and collaborate effectively (Eng and Parker, 1994, p. 199).

The dimensions of community competence are commitment, participation, self-other awareness and clarity of situational differences, conflict containment and accommodation, management of relations within society, skills for facilitating participant interaction and decision making, articulateness, and communication (Eng and Parker, 1994). Community competence has been described as skillful application of community capacity (Goodman and others, 1998). Associated increases in community capacity and competence should contribute to future successful community problem-solving efforts (Goodman and others, 1998).

Social Capital

Finally, one last concept is integral to our discussion of community participation and organizational relations. *Social capital* is a term that describes the features that enhance coordination and cooperation within and among organizations, just as physical capital and human capital are tools that enhance individual productivity in society. In Robert Putnam's well-known work *Bowling Alone: America's Declining Social Capital*, he defines *social capital* as "the relationships and structures within a community, such as civic participation, networks, norms of reciprocity, and trust, that promote cooperation for mutual benefit" (Putnam, 1995, p. 66).

In essence, social capital is a bonding relationship between community members that results from their participation, trust, and reciprocity (Putnam, 1995; Minkler and Wallerstein, 2005). Putnam asserts that in the last thirty years, Americans have participated less in the political process and in organized religion. They have reduced their membership in unions and civic, fraternal, school service, and voluntary organizations. Finally, bowling in organized leagues decreased by 40 percent from 1980 to 1993, while the total number of bowlers increased by 10 percent during that same time (Putnam, 1995).

Even though Americans are more involved in tertiary and nonprofit organizations (that do not require face-to-face contact with other members or attendance at meetings), associational membership has declined by at least 25 percent during the last quarter century. This trend appears to be related to women moving into the work force, increased mobility of the population, demographic changes (for example, fewer marriages, more divorces, fewer children), and pursuit of more individual leisure activities (for example, televisions, VCRs, video games) (Putnam, 1995). Restoring civic engagement and trust, then, is a key task that coalitions and partnerships must address if they are to survive.

The remainder of this chapter will chronicle the emergence and proliferation of community coalitions and partnerships as strategies not only to build communities but also to improve the health outcomes among their residents.

COALITIONS: A PUBLIC HEALTH STRATEGY TO BUILD CAPABLE, COMPETENT COMMUNITIES

The rise of coalitions as a prominent health promotion strategy parallels the growth of community-wide health promotion over the past three decades. This growth is partially due to the widespread dissemination of strategies employed in the National Heart, Lung, and Blood Institute's community demonstration projects (Mittelmark, 1999). These projects, which include the Stanford Three Community and Five City Projects, and the Minnesota and Pawtucket Heart Health Programs, used community advisory boards to plan and implement community-wide cardiovascular disease prevention strategies (Shea and Basch, 1990; Carlaw, Mittelmark, Bracht, and Luepker, 1984; Mittelmark and others, 1986; Lefebvre, Lasater, Carleton, and Peterson, 1987; Farquahr, Fortmann, Flora, and others, 1990). Although these groups were not technically *coalitions,* they employed some of the same processes and strategies that coalitions currently use. Additionally, the Centers for Disease Control and Prevention (CDC) advocated forming community coalitions in the Planned Approach to Community Health, which was widely adopted by state and local health departments in the late 1980s and early 1990s (Kreuter, 1992; Green and Kreuter, 1992).

In contrast to traditional, individual-focused behavior change efforts, community approaches—including those that build coalitions—attempt to alleviate community problems by organizing the community to bring about change. These community-wide approaches recognize that behaviors are inextricably tied to the environment (Milio, 1989; Thompson and Kinney, 1990; Stokols, 1992; Tesh, 1988). No single approach for community change is as effective as a broad-based coalition effort that provides the means for multiple strategies and involves key community individuals (McLeroy and others, 1994). The general focus of community organizing for health promotion is on changing systems, rules, social norms, or laws, ultimately to change the social acceptability of certain behaviors. The venue for community organizing is often the policy arena and often involves community-elected officials, businesses, community groups, media, and local and state legislatures to create positive community change.

Community coalitions have the potential to involve multiple sectors of the community and to conduct multiple interventions that focus on both individuals and their environments. The pooling of resources and the mobilization of talents and diverse approaches inherent in a successful coalition approach make it a logical strategy for disease prevention based on a social-ecological model that acknowledges the significance of the environment on health.

Finally, how well community coalitions develop the *capacity* of communities to address future critical health issues is vital. Community coalitions are a promising strategy for building capacity and competence among member organizations and, ultimately, in the communities they serve (Chavis, 2001; Kegler, Steckler, McLeroy, and Malek, 1998b).

THE RISE OF COALITIONS (1990–2006)

The proliferation of local, state, and national coalitions during the past sixteen years is remarkable. Health coalitions have been developed for health promotion, disease prevention, and access to care and treatment. Primarily, these coalitions are single-issue focused, although recently newer coalitions for reducing health disparities and chronic disease focus on multiple issues. Most of the coalitions are grass roots and community-based, but the logic of developing state and even federal counterparts takes advantage of the synergy created when collaboration across populations occurs. The international community is also involved in coalition building for cardiovascular disease, HIV/AIDS, immunization, and injury prevention, among other issues. The following summary of coalition development during this period is not all-inclusive but rather provides a snapshot of health coalition initiatives that are most visible and well funded.

Alcohol, Tobacco, and Other Drug Abuse Prevention

From 1990 until the present, coalitions continue to be used as an organizing strategy and process for change in public health. As the crack-cocaine outbreak of the late 1980s affected cities across America, citizens came together to form the kind of community coalitions familiar today (DrugStrategies, 2001). The first national meeting of community coalitions occurred in 1990, and the Community Anti-Drug Coalitions of America (CADCA) emerged as the voice for these grassroots coalitions (Birkby, 2003). The private sector and federal government rapidly became involved in contributing significant financial support and technical assistance for these groups. From 1990 to 2002, the Robert Wood Johnson Foundation (RWJF) contributed over $72 million to fund fifteen communities (between 100,000 to 250,000 residents) in eleven states to develop *community partnerships* in the Fighting Back initiative, which sought to prevent alcohol and other drug abuse among youth (Thompson, Spickard, and Dixon, 2001; Robert Wood Johnson Foundation, 2002).

The large number of communities that submitted proposals to the RWJF initiative spurred the Center for Substance Abuse Prevention to provide $375 million to fund 251 community partnerships in 1990–91 (Birkby, 2003). The John S. and James L. Knight Foundation funded eleven antidrug coalitions in their Community Initiatives program. Later, politicians adopted the Drug Free Communities Act and provided long-term support to reduce substance abuse in youth (DrugStrategies, 2001).

Evaluations of these health promotion coalitions have yielded a wide range of results. Some have been successful organizations, whereas others have disappeared; some have produced measurable changes in attitudes and community policies, whereas others appear to have had little effect (DrugStrategies, 2001).

During the same period, health advocates became concerned about the high rate of tobacco use. In 1988, the National Cancer Institute (NCI) launched the Community Intervention Trial for Smoking Cessation (COMMIT), a community-based smoking intervention trial in eleven pairs of matched communities. Then, in partnership with the American Cancer Society, NCI provided $128 million to fund the American Stop Smoking Intervention Study (ASSIST), the largest government-funded demonstration project to help states develop effective strategies to reduce smoking. From 1993 to 1999, ASSIST funded seventeen state health departments to use state and local coalitions to plan and implement programs to promote smoke-free environments, counter tobacco advertising and promotion, limit youths' tobacco access and availability, and increase tobacco prices by raising excise taxes. Study results showed that ASSIST states had a greater decrease in adult smoking prevalence than non-ASSIST states, and states that approved more tobacco control policies had larger decreases in per capita cigarette consumption (National Cancer Institute, 2003).

In 1993, the CDC launched its Imperatives to Prevent and Control Tobacco Use (IMPACT) program with cooperative agreements to the thirty-three states that did not receive ASSIST funding. In 1997, the federal government spent about $46 million for tobacco control efforts (The Advocacy Institute, 1998). At the state level, tobacco excise tax increases, dedicated in part to tobacco control, created large antitobacco efforts in some states. For example, California spent over $132 million in 1996 on tobacco control programs that included educational programs, cessation efforts, support for community coalitions, and a statewide media campaign.

Private efforts, such as the SmokeLess States initiative funded by the Robert Wood Johnson Foundation in 1994, provided additional resources to state-level coalitions working to reduce tobacco use. Over time, RWJF spent $110 million to expand the SmokeLess States program to fund at least some activities in thirty-one states and two cities; nine states were also funded by the SmokeLess States National Program Office (NPO) to assist in developing plans for comprehensive tobacco programs. Finally, individual state settlements with tobacco companies and the 1998 Master Settlement Agreement (MSA) between tobacco companies and the remaining states provided new revenues to states (Robert Wood Johnson Foundation, 2005b). Some states have committed some or a significant share of these funds to comprehensive tobacco control programs (U.S. Department of Health and Human Services [USDHHS], 2000).

Although greater funding has reduced tobacco use, little is known about the relative impact of subcomponents of these tobacco control programs, such as state and community coalition interventions (Farrelly, Pechacek, and Chaloupka, 2001). SmokeLess States focused most on reducing tobacco use by strengthening tobacco control legislation and regulation with major impact. For example, thirteen of the sixteen states that raised tobacco excise taxes since 1994 were SmokeLess States. Similarly, a disproportionate number of new local clean indoor air ordinances were adopted in SmokeLess States. Moreover, of the thirty-nine states that committed settlement funds to tobacco control programs, thirty are SmokeLess States, with average funding levels nearly five times those of the other nine states (ImpactTeen, 2005).

Immunization Promotion

Likewise, in response to the 1989–1991 measles epidemic that resulted in 55,000 reported cases and 123 deaths, the former first ladies of the United States and Arkansas, Rosalynn Carter and Betty Bumpers, founded Every Child by Two (ECBT) in 1991. To promote timely immunization of all American children by age two, ECBT supports statewide immunization efforts in developing public and private partnerships, collaborative activities with managed care organizations, school-based sites for preschool immunizations, education of health care providers, immunization registries, and global eradication of polio and measles (Every Child by Two, 2005). In 1993, President Clinton was prompted to support the Childhood Immunization Initiative, which established coalition development in all states, twenty-nine large urban areas, and seven territories as one of its major goals (Centers for Disease Control and Prevention, 1993). The Horizons project was funded by the Health Care Financing Administration (HCFA) as a collaborative venture between professional review organizations and nine historically black colleges and universities in eight southern states. Its goal was to increase vaccine coverage rates among older black populations by providing vaccines in nontraditional community settings, such as shopping malls, senior citizen centers, voting sites, and parks (Centers for Disease Control and Prevention, 2000c).

Many of these coalitions, still active in their communities, promote similar goals to ECBT and advocate for policy change at the state level. National-level partnerships to improve immunization rates across the age span include the Hepatitis B Coalition, the Immunization Action Coalition, and the National Partnership for Immunization. These groups bring together health care professionals, state coalitions, advocacy groups, and vaccine companies to promote immunization awareness, education, and access to and delivery of vaccines to the general public.

Oral Health Promotion

Wide-scale building of oral health coalitions in the United States is relatively recent. These coalitions have developed in response to the lack of fluoridated water in nearly 30 percent of medium to large metropolitan areas; the high rates of caries among children and adults of low income; and the need to create statewide plans to improve oral health knowledge, prevention of oral cancers, and dental sealants for children. In 2003, the Surgeon General issued the first Oral Health Call to Action, which brought these issues to national attention (U.S. Department of Health and Human Services, 2003).

After two years of discussion, the National Oral Health Partnership was launched in 2005, with funding from major partners such as Oral Health America, the American Dental Association, the American Dental Hygienists Association, and Delta Dental (insurer). The Oral Health Division of the CDC funds active oral health programs in fifteen states to promote state planning, sealant programs, and the development of state oral health coalitions. Illinois, California, and Kentucky have the largest coalitions, with Kentucky's being the oldest (established in 1989) (Oral Health America, 2001). Currently, coalitions exist in eighteen states, with funding from insurers, dental product and other business corporations, grants, and the CDC. Thirteen states also have health care coalitions that address oral health issues.

Teen Pregnancy Prevention

Most reviews of the adolescent pregnancy prevention literature find serious program shortcomings and conclude that broad-based, community-wide, comprehensive interventions focused on prevention are the best approach (Brindis, 1991; Carnegie Corporation, 1989; Dryfoos, 1990; Moore and others, 1995; Santelli and Beilenson, 1992). Community partnerships have often been promoted to coordinate these community efforts (Edwards and Stern, 1998). The National Strategy to Prevent Teen Pregnancy was initiated by USDHHS in 1997 in response to a call from Congress for a strategy to reduce teen pregnancies and to assure that at least 25 percent of U.S. communities have teen pregnancy prevention programs in place (Edwards and Stern, 1998). Since then, multiple efforts have continued to mobilize communities to prevent adolescent pregnancy: The CDC provides $6.5 million to thirteen community partnerships in eleven states to develop comprehensive programs; the California Wellness Foundation provided $60 million to California partnerships; the Annie E. Casey Foundation committed $5 million to five communities; and the Colorado Trust in Colorado and the Flinn Foundation in Arizona provided millions of dollars of support for similar efforts (Gallagher and Drisko, 2000).

Injury Prevention

Safe Kids USA was founded in 1987 by Children's National Medical Center, with support from the Johnson & Johnson Corporation to prevent accidental injury, a leading killer of children aged fourteen and under. In 2005, the nearly twenty-year-old National Safe Kids USA joined with the international Safe Kids movement to become Safe Kids Worldwide (Safe Kids, 2005). More than 450 coalitions in all fifty states and sixteen countries bring together safety and health experts, educators, corporations, governments, foundations, and volunteers to educate and protect families. Creating national awareness and promoting sound research, child safety laws and regulations, and lifesaving devices (for example, child safety seats, helmets, smoke alarms) are goals that are accomplished by empowering local communities to build grassroots coalitions.

HIV/AIDS Prevention

The Ryan White Care Act mainly covered access to treatment and nondiscriminatory provision of services for HIV/AIDS. However, from 1993 to 1998, the CDC directed states and localities receiving HIV prevention funds to conduct community planning efforts that involved communities and especially persons living with HIV and AIDS. Many of these communities also established coalitions that included persons living with either HIV or AIDS or both to ensure that their concerns were heard. In 2002, USDHHS's Health Resource and Services Administration (HRSA) funded $10 million to plan and expand community-based HIV/AIDS care. This funding covers fifty-eight one-year planning grants, twenty-nine capacity-building grants to develop or enhance care, and twelve community-based dental partnership grants.

Although these grants are not directed only to coalition building, many communities have formed durable partnerships around this critical prevention issue (HRSA, 2002). The Minority Community Health Coalition Demonstration Program was developed in 1999 as part of the Minority HIV/AIDS Initiative to address the epidemic in minority communities. The program is intended to demonstrate the effectiveness of community coalitions involving nontraditional partners to develop an integrated response to the HIV/AIDS crisis through community dialogue and interaction; to address sociocultural, linguistic, and other barriers to HIV/AIDS treatment in order to increase the number of people who seek and accept services; and to develop and conduct HIV/AIDS education and outreach for hardly reached populations. Currently funded by the Office of Minority Health (OMH) of the USDHHS, the seventeen grants are administered by community-based, minority-serving organizations that work in a coalition setting with at least two other partners. Notable national partnerships include AIDS Action; AIDS Alliance for Children, Youth and Families; AIDS Treatment Activists Coalition; AIDS Vaccine Advocacy Coalition; Communities Advocating Emergency AIDS Relief Coalition (CAEAR); and the Community HIV/AIDS Mobilization Project Office of Minority Health, 2003.

In Africa, the growth of coalitions and networks for HIV/AIDS advocacy has accelerated in the past ten years, following various United Nations global conferences and conventions. Coalitions that operate at national, regional, and subregional levels include Society of Women Against AIDS in Africa (SWAA), with chapters in many African countries; the AIDS NGO Network of East Africa (ANNEA); and Persons Living with HIV/AIDS (PLWHA). Although many of these coalitions exist, the presence or absence of funding to support one or two key individuals determines whether the local coalition is an active, effective tool for advocacy (Opubor, Egero, and Mensah-Kumah, 2000).

Promoting Health Insurance

In 1997, Congress designated funds for the State Children's Health Insurance Program (SCHIP) or Medicaid to provide health care coverage to children in working families with modest incomes. Although since 1972 the Robert Wood Johnson Foundation has sought to expand health insurance coverage as part of its mission to improve health and health care for all Americans, the foundation helped make both the new SCHIP and Medicaid programs easier for families to use and understand through their Covering Kids and Families (CKF) initiative, begun in 2001.

The cornerstones of the CKF initiative are the statewide and local coalitions in every state that work with public officials, health professionals, businesses, social service agencies, and faith-based and other organizations. The goals of these coalitions are to simplify enrollment and renewal processes for Medicaid and SCHIP programs to make them more family-friendly; make administrative procedures more efficient; and conduct outreach programs to identify, enroll, and retain eligible children. Programs for adults and pregnant women were recently added (Robert Wood Johnson Foundation, 2005a).

Prevention of Chronic Disease: Cardiovascular Disease, Cancer, and Diabetes

Despite the fact that cardiovascular disease is the leading cause of death in every state, the CDC currently funds only eight programs (through state health departments) to help prevent and control heart disease, stroke, and other cardiovascular disease. States often partner with the American Heart Association and other site agencies to supplement funding for this important issue. CDC's Comprehensive Cancer Control program has existed since 1998 and funds forty-nine states (excluding Idaho), five tribal health agencies, and six territories to establish broad-based coalitions, assess the burden of cancer, develop plans and priorities for prevention and control, and implement these plans. The American Cancer Society and numerous foundations are major partners in these efforts. The National Alliance of State Prostate Cancer Coalitions (NASPCC) formed in 2005 to represent state coalitions made up of cancer survivors and community and family members. NASPCC aims to raise the national awareness and priority of prostate cancer throughout the United States.

CDC's Diabetes and Control Program funds states in a manner similar to those programs for cardiovascular disease and cancer. Coalition building is recommended at state and community levels. Under CDC's National Program to Promote Diabetes Education Strategies in Minority Communities, eight national organizations were funded to build coalitions to improve education and access to diabetes treatment. Funded organizations include the Black Women's Health Imperative, National Alliance for Hispanic Health, National Medical Association, Papa Ola Lokani (Asian Pacific Islander group), and Khmer Health Advocates (Cambodian).

Asthma

The alarm for asthma officially sounded in 1998, when the CDC reported that childhood asthma had reached epidemic proportions, with the number of cases increasing 160 percent for children under five and 74 percent for children five to fourteen years old from 1980 to 1994 (Mannino and others, 1998). Because asthma does not have a single etiology, the focus of effective management is control and prevention. Inner-city communities have responded to this challenge by forming broad-based coalitions that mobilize local resources to create friendly environments for children with asthma in home, school, and play settings. Asthma coalitions focus on identifying patients with asthma or those at risk for developing asthma, and include an educational component that promotes asthma awareness and self-management.

In 2001, the Robert Wood Johnson Foundation authorized $12.5 million to fund eight community-based coalitions for four years to implement comprehensive asthma management programs that include improved access to and quality of medical services, education, family and community support, and environmental and policy initiatives (Clark, Malveaux, and Friedman, 2006). CDC also funded thirty asthma partnership projects in 2001 under its National Asthma Control Program. In 2002, CDC funded Controlling Asthma in America's Cities, a five-year coalition-based project in eight U.S. cities that built on the experiences of the Allies Against Asthma project (University of Michigan, 2004). In 2002, the California Endowment launched its three-year initiative, Community Action to Fight Asthma (CAFA) that funded fifteen new asthma coalitions and linked them with thirteen other funded coalitions through four Regional Centers and a State Coordinating Office. The focus of CAFA is on reducing the prevalence of and exposure to indoor and outdoor environmental triggers for California's school-aged children. The established coalitions' focus on improving access to care and treatment for asthma was transformed to broader, collaborative goals of policy advocacy, media, and evaluation. Results from these combined asthma coalition initiatives, funded by national and private sources in over forty cities, are forthcoming.

Multiple Health Issue Coalitions: Turning Point Initiative

In 1997, the Robert Wood Johnson and W. K. Kellogg Foundations developed a program called Turning Point. Among other issues, the program issued a request for proposals that encouraged local and state applicants to rethink the delivery of public health, placing emphasis on state and local collaborative partnerships and eliciting ideas on intervention priorities from community partners. Individuals and organizations from different sectors in many communities and states came together to transform their public health systems to achieve the goals of preventing disease and injury, protecting the public from threats to health, and promoting healthy behaviors (Turning Point, 2005). The state grantees developed specific models for more effective and responsive public health systems. Through twenty-one state partnerships of state and local public health and community-based agencies and five national collaboratives, Turning Point (2005) accomplished the following objectives:

- Improved the accountability of public health efforts
- Developed a model law to update public health statutes
- Increased the effectiveness of public health information technology
- Motivated changes in behaviors to promote good health outcomes
- Promoted skills and competencies of public health practitioners and leaders

At the national level, Turning Point collaborated with other public health organizations to realize its goals. Specifically, state partnerships were focused on identifying the most important health needs of residents in their communities; creating effective and accountable structures to deliver public health services to their communities; developing population data that support decision making about public health priorities; generating strategies to improve the health status of individuals, families, and communities; targeting the best ways to eliminate health disparities among and within populations; and providing evidence of the effectiveness of their partnerships (Turning Point, 2005). These crosscutting partnerships developed many measurable outcomes that will be described in later chapters. The national office produced many effective training materials and modules on collaborative leadership, social marketing, performance management, and public health statutes that can be found online at http://www.turningpointprogram.org/.

Racial and Ethnic Approaches to Community Health (REACH) 2010

Launched in 1999, Racial and Ethnic Approaches to Community Health (REACH) 2010 is one of CDC's main efforts to eliminate racial and ethnic disparities in health, with appropriations of about $34 million per year to support forty projects, four of which serve the elderly. Other major funders and partners of this effort include the National Center on Minority Health and Health Disparities (NCMHHD) at the National Institutes of Health (NIH), Health Resources and Services Administration (HRSA), and the Administration on Aging.

REACH 2010 is designed to eliminate disparities among African Americans, Native Americans, Alaska Natives, Asian Americans, Hispanics, and Pacific Islanders in six priority areas: cardiovascular disease, immunizations, breast and cervical cancer screening and management, diabetes, HIV/AIDS, and infant mortality. REACH 2010 supports community coalitions to design, implement, and evaluate community-driven strategies to eliminate health disparities. Each coalition must have at least one community-based organization and three other organizations, one of which must be a local or state health department, or an academic or research organization. Coalition activities include continuing education for health care providers, health communication campaigns and health education, and promotion programs that utilize lay health workers to reach community members (Centers for Disease Control and Prevention, 2005).

Steps to a HealthierUS

Steps to a HealthierUS is a five-year cooperative agreement initiative from the U.S. Department of Health and Human Services that advances the goal of helping Americans live longer, better, and healthier lives. States, cities, and tribal entities receive funds to implement chronic disease prevention efforts that focus on reducing the burden of diabetes, overweight, obesity, and asthma, and address three risk factors—physical activity, poor nutrition, and tobacco use.

In 2003 and 2004, the Steps program allocated nearly $50 million to fund forty sites that represented seventeen large cities, three tribes, seven states, and twenty-five small cities and rural communities. Under the guidance of a coalition, each site must implement in school, health care, and workplace settings a community action plan that focuses on community interventions (for example, walking programs, media campaigns); environmental interventions (for example, smoking cessation, healthy food choices in schools); and educational interventions (for example, coordinated school health programs) (Centers for Disease Control and Prevention, 2004).

SUMMARY

The collaborative work involved in building coalitions to promote health and prevent disease has its roots firmly entrenched in the early history of America. From Benjamin Franklin's work in building associations to improve civic life and Alexis de Toqueville's observations of *Democracy in America*, succeeding generations of Americans continued to organize for social, economic, and political justice. *Community organizing* is a process by which ordinary people—most often with low to moderate incomes—are brought together to act in their common self-interest, while seeking the ideals of participatory democracy.

The community-organizing movements of the 1800s focused on improving Americans' health and quality of life through the work of feminists and abolitionists. In the twentieth century, three dominant types of community organizing emerged: social work approaches that resulted in settlement houses and trade unions; political activist approaches espoused by Saul Alinsky, such as those used in civil rights and student movements; and neighborhood maintenance–community development approaches to build and empower neighborhoods, used in postwar and antipoverty programs spearheaded by Kurt Lewin.

Community participation is broadly defined as the process of involving people in the institutions or decisions that affect their lives, and *citizen participation* is the mobilization of citizens for the purpose of undertaking activities to improve the conditions in the community. These activities defined the development of neighborhood block associations in the 1970s and 1980s, the precursors to modern coalitions. Finally, research in interorganizational relations focused on the formation of collaborative relationships in an effort to understand why organizations join collaborative alliances.

Modern coalitions for health promotion and disease prevention emerged in the late 1980s and early 1990s and continue to proliferate today. Multiyear funding for local, regional, state, and national coalitions is often substantial, and the expectations of success are high. Coalitions have been formed for single issues such as the promotion of immunizations and oral health; the prevention of alcohol, tobacco, and other drug abuse; teen pregnancy; and HIV/AIDS. Chronic disease prevention for cancer, cardiovascular disease, diabetes, and asthma are more recent issues around which coalitions mobilize. Finally, multi-issue coalitions for chronic disease prevention and for the elimination of racial and ethnic health disparities are the latest health improvement investments by federal and private funders.

QUESTIONS FOR REVIEW

1. What are the similarities and differences between coalitions and associations?
2. How do the community organizing approaches used by modern health coalitions differ from those used by coalitions developed to establish trade unions or promote civil rights?
3. Explain how each of these terms relates to the work of coalitions for health promotion and disease prevention: citizen and community participation, community empowerment, and social capital.

CHAPTER TWO

Principles of Collaboration
and Partnering:
Coalitions Defined

*We are caught in an inescapable network of mutuality, tied in a single
garment of destiny. Whatever affects one directly, affects all indirectly.*
—Martin Luther King, Jr. 1929–1968

The foundation of coalition building lies in the willingness and capacity of partners to collaborate to achieve common goals. Collaboration may take different forms and follow different pathways, but the intentionality and openness to envision accomplishments that are beyond the expectations of any single organization drives the need to collaborate. Definitions of the collaborative process and of coalitions in this chapter set the stage for dealing later in this book with how the actual work is accomplished and by whom.

DEFINING COLLABORATION

In general, we all know that collaboration occurs whenever people work together to achieve a common goal. However, for our purposes, we need to define more narrowly the concept of collaboration. Many formal definitions exist, but the most generally accepted is that collaboration is

> *a mutually beneficial and well-defined relationship entered into
> by two or more organizations to achieve common goals. The
> relationship includes a commitment to a definition of
> mutual relationships and goals; a jointly developed structure
> and shared responsibility; mutual authority and accountability
> for success; and sharing of resources and rewards.*
> —Mattesich, Murray-Close, and Monsey, 2005, p. 7

The expectation for organizations as regards collaboration is "to achieve results they are more likely to achieve together than alone" (Winer and Ray, 1994, p. 24). Others acknowledge that the commitment must be "formal and sustained" (National Assembly of National Voluntary Health and Social Welfare Organizations, 1991, p. 4). Finally, the strategic alliance should "enhance each other's ability to share risks and responsibilities" as well as resources and rewards (Himmelman, 1992, p. 3).

Gray (1989) describes the steps of collaboration as (1) recognition of stakeholder interdependence; (2) constructively dealing with differences; (3) development of joint ownership of decisions; (4) stakeholder assumption of responsibility for managing problems through formal and informal agreements; and (5) acceptance of the process as dynamic and continually emerging. Essential characteristics of collaboration (Rosenthal, 2000, p. 10) include these:

- Shared creation: joint action for mutual benefit
- Interdependence and reciprocity
- Mutual authority and accountability
- Shared responsibility, risks, resources, and rewards
- Inherent conflict and dynamic tensions

The Wilder Research Center conducted comprehensive research on collaborative relationships and developed a tool that describes twenty factors that influence successful collaborations (Mattesich, Murray-Close, and Monsey, 2001). Because these factors appear to be critical to coalition development as well, they are included as Exhibit 2.1. The factors are grouped into six categories related to the environment, membership characteristics, process and structure, communication, purpose, and resources. Besides the influencing factors, collaboration can be classified according to the levels of formality and intensity required and the roles that participants are expected to assume, as described in the following section.

INTENSITY AND LEVELS OF COLLABORATIVE WORK

Collaboration represents the highest level of working relationship that two or more organizations can enter into. Despite the rewards of collaboration, the effort must understand and respect each organization's self-interest (in other words, structure, agenda, values, and culture); its relationships and linkages; and how power is shared and distributed (Gray, 1996). Four types of working relationships have been identified: networking, cooperating, coordinating, and collaborating (Kagan, 1991; Himmelman, 1992). The levels and definitions follow (Habana-Hafner, Reed, and Associates, 1989; Himmelman, 1992; Kagan, 1991; National Network for Collaboration, 1996; Rosenthal, 2000):

Networking *("a net")* involves intermittent exchanging of information for mutual benefit through dialogue, common awareness, and understanding, and creating a base of support.

Cooperating *("to operate")* encompasses short and informal relationships without clearly defined missions or structure. The main purpose of cooperating is to get tasks done while limiting duplication of services. Each organization retains separate resources and authority, so no risk exists.

Coordinating *("to order")* includes exchanging information and altering activities for mutual benefit and to achieve a common purpose. These relationships are more formal, longer term, and focus on a specific goal, effort, or program. Coordination requires planning, division of roles and responsibilities, and communication. Resources and rewards are shared. Although each organization still retains separate resources and authority, risk increases.

Collaborating *("to labor")* signifies a more durable relationship. Separate organizations enter into a new structural arrangement with formal roles and full commitment to a common mission. Comprehensive planning and clear communication channels are needed at all levels. Consensus is used in shared decision making. Risk increases because each organization contributes resources as well as its reputation. Partners jointly secure or pool resources and share results and rewards. Trust levels and productivity are high. Power may not be equally shared.

Those involved in collaborative work are quick to point out that a continuum exists across collaborative relationships. As the work of relationships moves across the continuum, linkages become more intense and are influenced by common goals, tasks, decisions, rules, and committed resources. Purposes become more complex as information sharing gives way to joint problem solving, and agreements become more formal with the need for operating procedures and policies. Similarly, the relationships can take more time to develop and involve greater risks as well as greater opportunities or rewards. Figure 2.1 shows the continuum from networking relationships to collaborative ones.

Networking →	Cooperating →	Coordinating →	Collaborating
Intensity of Linkages	Less Intense	→	More Intense
Complexity of Purpose	Simple	→	Complex
Formality of Agreements	Informal	→	Formal
Amount of Risks and Rewards	Less	→	More

Figure 2.1 The Continuum for Building Relationships and Doing Work.

Source: Adapted from Kagan, 1991; National Network for Collaboration, 1996; Habana-Hafner and others, 1989.

Gray (1989) proposes a staged model of collaboration that moves from problem setting to direction setting, to implementation. Alter's and Hage's (1993) model of network development describes collaboration as evolving from *exchange* networks to *action* networks, to fully developed *systemic* networks. According to their model, action networks result when organizations can no longer meet a goal alone, due to environmental conditions. A network shifts from an exchange to an action network when members contribute private resources for access to collective output, depend on the collective output, and feel a normative obligation to comply with the coordinating mechanism.

An action network shifts to a *systemic* or collaborative network when its partners begin to produce together, with specialized roles. The different roles that organizations may assume in collaborations include convener, catalyst, conduit for funding, funder, advocate, community organizer, technical assistance provider, capacity builder, partner, and facilitator (Himmelman, 1994). These roles are not mutually exclusive; one role can lead to another or be integrated into another role.

In essence, collaboration changes the way organizations work together. Collaboration moves organizations from competing to building consensus; from working alone to including others from diverse cultures, fields, and settings; from thinking mostly about activities, services, and programs to looking for complex, integrated interventions; and from focusing on short-term accomplishments to broad systems changes (Winer and Ray, 1994, p. 24). Collaborative relationships for health promotion and disease prevention are most often called partnerships or coalitions, but a variety of other types of organizational entities have been developed that may on the surface appear to be similar. The next section describes the differences among them.

WHAT'S IN A NAME?

Joint efforts and strategic partnerships can be successful no matter how intense they are. The key elements for success are that organizations must agree on the level of intensity, and that the level must be appropriate for the kind of results expected. A partnership is a generic term that covers a wide range of across-organization relationships. Partnerships differ from single organizations in that organizations tend to have more regulations, more hierarchical leadership patterns, more established negotiation skills, clearer chains of command, more homogeneous organizational culture, and clear decision-making autonomy (Habana-Hafner, Reed, and Associates, 1989).

Although names are often used interchangeably, definitions do exist for each kind of partnering relationship, as shown here (Winer and Ray, 1994):

Network—a loose-knit, nonhierarchical group of individuals and organizations
    with flexible roles, and low-key leadership and decision making.
Advisory committee—a group that is formed at the request of an organization or
    person of authority (for example, mayor) to provide review, advice or services,
    ideas, and recommendations. The group exists for input into decision making,
    not decision making itself. Advisory committees can be made up of
    professionals or citizens who represent different community sectors.

Commission—a group that is appointed by an official body and is authorized to perform specific duties or steps or to take on certain powers.

Federation, consortium, alliance, or league—a union or connection of interests that have similar characters, structures, or outlooks; a semiofficial organization of organizations. Usually, a central body of communicators or facilitative leaders, or both, develops semiformal links and a joint budget and seeks new resources to coordinate tasks and limit duplication of services.

Executive board or committee—a formal group that holds delegated power in a particular arena and performs planning and governing functions for a larger collective body or organization. Participants are elected or appointed but represent specific organizations, sectors, or shareholders.

Task force—a self-contained group of "doers" that is not ongoing, but rather brought together due to a strong interest in an issue and for a specific purpose. Task forces are sometimes convened at the request of an overseeing body or committee.

Partnership—an association of two or more individuals or organizations who contribute money, property, or other resources to carry on joint business and share profits or losses. The partnership agrees to share resources, coordinate activities, address common issues, and merge their resource bases to create a new entity. A central, autonomous body of decision makers exists, with defined roles and formal links to outside organizations.

Coalition—a formal alliance of organizations that come together to work for a common goal. Unlike networks whose member organizations act independently, coalitions bring organizations together to act jointly. Coalitions may form to address a specific, time-limited issue or may establish a more sustained collaboration (Chavis and Florin, 1990, p. 20). They develop an internal decision-making and leadership structure that allows member organizations to speak with a united voice and engage in shared planning and implementation activities. Links to outside organizations and communication channels are formal. Member organizations are willing to pull resources from existing systems, as well as seek new resources to develop a joint budget. Agreements, benchmarks, roles, and assignments are often written.

MODELS OF COLLABORATION

Rosenthal (2000) presents four models of collaboration that are also useful for highlighting the differences in function among the previously defined entities: strategic partnerships, service integration efforts, comprehensive collaborations, and conflict resolution collaborations (pp. 11–18). She advises that the appropriate collaboration approach depends on the purpose, composition, timetable, and resources available for the collaboration.

Strategic partnerships include *joint ventures, partnerships,* and *public–private initiatives.* In this model, three to five organizations collaborate to develop a market, project, or product, each organization making a distinct contribution based upon its expertise or resources. Joining forces produces a strategic advantage and adds value to what each organization can do on its own. No governing body coordinates the work, and partners share responsibility, ownership of the results and products, and liability for any problems.

Service integration efforts include *networks, service linkages,* and *consortia.* Service integration involves collaboration between many organizations to streamline services, consolidate resources, save costs, increase service options, and broaden access. Partners provide similar or complementary services that are more efficient or cost-effective when united. Partners play a role in an integrated system, but each could be replaced if its functions or the scope of its services changed. These efforts can focus on populations, providers, programs, systems, organizations, or policies.

Conflict resolution collaborations include *negotiating team* or *mediation efforts.* These collaboratives involve organizations with previous relationships. Often they disagree about a shared condition or issue and seek common ground or a way to coexist while addressing their own self-interests. The goal of mediation is to understand and respect differences in order to find solutions that are acceptable to all partners.

Comprehensive collaborations involve *community-wide partnerships* and *coalitions.* These relationships can have a large number of diverse members who mobilize around an issue that affects all partners, but is larger than any one group can solve alone. These collaboratives intentionally include different perspectives and constituencies to achieve more power and reach. Although they rely on a central governance structure, they allow for organizational autonomy.

WHAT MAKES A COALITION A COALITION?

The word coalition comes from the Latin roots *coalescere,* to grow together, and *coalitio,* a union. Merriam-Webster's dictionary defines a coalition as "a temporary alliance of distinct parties, persons, or states for joint action" (Merriam-Webster, 2006). However, the term has gradually evolved to connote a collaboration that is durable and sustained over time (Butterfoss, Goodman, and Wandersman, 1993). Not surprisingly, the definitions for collaboration (a process) and coalition (an organization) are remarkably similar.

A *coalition* is classically defined as "an organization of diverse interest groups that combine their human and material resources to effect a specific change that members are unable to bring about independently" (Brown, 1984) or "a group of individuals representing diverse organizations, factions, or constituencies who agree to work together to achieve a common goal" (Feighery and Rogers, 1990). LaBonte (1993) elegantly describes coalitions as "groups of groups with a shared goal and some awareness that 'united we stand and divided we fall'" (p. 10). However, as we have seen before, unity and shared purpose are not distinguishing characteristics of coalitions.

Early work in defining coalitions agreed that coalitions are issue-oriented, structured, focused to act on specific goals external to the coalition, and committed to a diverse membership with unique talents and resources (Boissevain, 1974; Stevenson, Pearce, and Porter, 1985; Allensworth and Patton, 1990). Coalitions are "action sets," or groups of interested groups and individuals with a common purpose, whose joint actions are directed at achieving the coalition's goals. Another hallmark of coalitions is that members collaborate not only on behalf of the organization they represent but also on behalf of the coalition itself (Hord, 1986; Feighery and Rogers, 1990).

Coalitions are characterized as formal, multipurpose, and long-term alliances (Butterfoss and others, 1993). Bringing a variety of human and material resources to the table, coalition members work toward a specific change that they would not be able to bring about individually. These coalitions are multipurpose in order to accommodate more than one mission or set of goals (Black, 1983; Stevenson, Pearce, and Porter, 1985); exchange mutually beneficial resources (Hord, 1986; Allensworth and Patton, 1990); and direct such interventions as resource development and ecological change, at multiple levels (McLeroy, Bibeau, Steckler, and Glanz, 1988). Coalitions are also seen as durable and capable of being maintained long enough to accomplish health-promotion and disease-prevention goals (Sink and Stowers, 1989; Thompson and Kinney, 1999; Wandersman and Goodman, 1991).

TYPES OF COALITIONS

Coalitions may be categorized according to membership, patterns of formation, types of functions, and types of structures that accommodate these functions.

Based on *membership*, Feighery and Rogers (1990) describe three types of coalitions.

Grassroots coalitions are organized by volunteers in times of crisis to pressure policy makers to act on an issue. They can be controversial, but effective, in reaching their goals and often disband when the crisis ends, for example, when a neighborhood group pressures city council for more street lights to prevent crime.

Professional (agency-based) coalitions are formed by professional organizations either in time of crisis or as a long-term approach to increase their power and influence, such as when health professionals pressure their state licensing boards to establish more group homes for mental health patients. Although funding is provided to address community issues, the interventions usually come from professionals and institutions, and citizens are secondary players (Wolff, 2001b).

Community-based coalitions of professional and grassroots members are formed to influence more long-term health and welfare practices for their community, for example, the Smoke Free tobacco coalitions. Community ownership is higher in these groups, but external efforts are more likely to provide needed resources.

The size of coalition membership may vary from a few individuals or organizations to a few hundred (Boissevain, 1974). If a partnership is composed solely of individuals and not groups, then it is probably an organization or network and not a true coalition. Coalitions can also designate their membership according to degree of participation (Brown, 1984). Members can be *active* (or *core*) *members*, who assume central leadership positions, or *affiliates*, who desire a more networking type of relationship.

Coalitions may also be categorized according to patterns of formation, from those that form in response to a threat or adversary to those that are created as funding opportunities or for advocacy purposes (Butterfoss and others, 1993). For example, coalitions may be community-mandated or voluntary. Mandated coalitions are created through laws or regulations and are provided with resources to support their operations and, in some cases, to provide services (Rosenthal, 2000).

Often the agency or organization that mandated a coalition is perceived to hold greater ownership than the members of the community do. However, in some cases, the mandate is a positive action used to fund an existing coalition and move it toward action. The mandate may simply call for coalition formation but leave the details of coalition operation to the partners. However, sometimes mandates are specific and comprehensive, and can influence member recruitment and decision making.

Voluntary coalitions are initiated by service providers, grassroots community activists, and recognized community leaders as well as voluntary agencies or community-based organizations (CBOs) (Rosenthal, 2000). They may have an initial source of funding, rely on dues, or use a sponsorship-type funding ladder—in any case, the voluntary coalition makes the decision to address a worthy health issue while pursuing viable funding opportunities.

Coalitions may be classified by the *functions* they perform, although most coalitions function within one or more of the following categories: information and resource sharing, technical assistance and training, self-regulation, planning, and coordinating services (Croan and Lees, 1979). Similarly, Forsythe (1997) describes the difference between process coalitions, which accomplish networking, planning, and programming functions based on broad interests, and action coalitions that are more focused on specific goals, events, and results.

Finally, coalitions may be differentiated by *organizational structure* (Black, 1983). Roberts-DeGennero (1986) described three kinds of coalition structures.

Organization-set coalitions are groups of cooperative organizations that provide resources or services under an umbrella organization (for example, the United Way).

Network coalitions are subgroups of organizations loosely organized within an organizational system that provides services to a particular population or lobbies for a specific cause.

Action-set coalitions are issue-specific and can be more or less formal, depending on their purpose.

HOW COMMUNITY COALITIONS DIFFER FROM OTHER TYPES OF COALITIONS

All coalitions work toward reducing or preventing a problem by analyzing the problem, identifying and implementing solutions, and creating social change. Coalitions use data to identify populations in geographic areas with high risk and severity of disease or problems, develop and implement risk reduction strategies, and advocate for policies that reduce risk. However, the nature of these tasks changes when the geographical scope changes and coalitions become responsible for larger populations and issues. Although novice coalition builders assume that coalitions are the same regardless of scope, experience shows otherwise. Coalitions can be formed at the state, regional, national, or international levels.

Community Coalitions

Community coalitions are unique in that they represent defined communities and their memberships reflect the diversity and wisdom of those communities at both grassroots and "grasstops" (professional) levels (Feighery and Rogers, 1990; Butterfoss and others, 1993). The inherent wisdom and knowledge needed to solve the health or social problem at hand rests with these community stakeholders, who have direct experience with the issue. These community members should be actively engaged in decision making and problem solving in a collaborative, equitable way.

Clark and others (2006) define these important functions for a community coalition:

- Serves a defined community recognized by those within it as a community (a common location or experience) but also serves the broader community
- Is viewed by community residents as representing and serving them
- Reflects the community's diversity
- Addresses the problem(s) in a systematic, comprehensive, timely manner
- Builds community independence and capacity

State Coalitions

State coalitions have been developed through a number of funding sources as a way of facilitating communication and developing far-ranging strategies that cover a large geographic area. Although community coalitions by definition are "free-standing," in reality they are often short-lived and less effective if they do not have a relationship with statewide partners and organizations. Community coalitions usually partner and mobilize to form state coalitions when they realize the benefits of more widespread commitment and support for the issue. Likewise, a state coalition may form initially, then recognize the need for closer links to communities that can help disseminate information and interventions throughout the state. Both scenarios appear to work equally well—the key is to develop a thoughtful approach to linking local and state concerns and resources.

Stable management within a community coalition helps provide for regular interactions with the state program. In turn, the local coalition can help cover the gaps in the state's activities, for example, by more effectively educating legislators and others on the local level all year long. Community coalitions often work on integrating services at the local level; state coalitions, however, can address federal or state policies that affect eligibility for services or how resources are allocated. If policies at the state or federal level continue to create barriers to local action, then a broader coalition or umbrella group that includes other coalitions may be needed to address the policy barriers.

For example, a community coalition is more appropriate to help increase enrollment in state-sponsored child health insurance programs. However, the state insurance coalition is the more likely vehicle to change application forms, procedures, and waiting times that are sometimes barriers to enrollment in state social service and health agencies. Similarly, a local tobacco coalition can rally support to enact strict local clean indoor air ordinances, but with critical support from local legislators, a state tobacco coalition is the more appropriate group to pass initiatives to increase cigarette taxes. National-level tobacco coalitions, such as the National Coalition for Tobacco-Free Older Persons, use the experiences of their state counterparts to advocate for federal legislation that sets environmental clean air standards for smokestack emissions. Ideally, international coalitions, such as the International Non-Governmental Coalition Against Tobacco, will share their expertise with other nations who are beginning to address the issue of tobacco abuse.

However, if a state institution, such as the state health department, funds a coalition, the coalition is prohibited from lobbying against the state government's position and may be viewed as less self-sufficient and independent by other organizations. For example, a local coalition may rally the support of a local congressperson who sponsors a bill that requires immunization of children against influenza prior to school entry. However, the state health department may not have the funds to provide the vaccine for eligible children under its federal subsidy (Vaccines for Children), so it may not support the bill. In this case, the local coalition is restricted from advocating for the bill because it risks losing its funding from the state health department.

The most critical differences between local and state coalitions appear to be the kinds of partners who are recruited, the frequency of meetings, and the type of activities they undertake. Due to the need for developing strategic alliances with key officials, state coalitions should have more high-ranking professional members who are linked to organizations and individuals in positions of power and influence. Unlike community coalitions that ensure diversity by seeking a mix of professional and grassroots members, state coalitions must recruit a variety of organizations that serve residents of the state.

Coalition facilitators or coordinators should recognize that grassroots representation is a hallmark of community coalitions and is assured by linking closely with them. Realistically, local community representatives do not have the time, interest, or financial ability to attend state coalition meetings on a regular basis. Further, although interested volunteers often come to the community coalition table, state coalition members usually are appointed by their organizations.

State coalitions tend to meet less often than local coalitions; meetings are usually two to four times per year. The meetings last from two to four hours, with time built in for work groups or committees to convene. Many state groups provide for teleconferencing for the main meetings and for task or work groups that meet between times so that travel becomes less problematic for members. Often one of these quarterly coalition meetings will be convened as a larger conference or planning summit.

Finally, the types of activities that state coalitions engage in should be comprehensive but limited in their service orientation. Generally, these activities consist of one or more of the following: surveillance or needs-assessment activities; planning activities that result in a statewide plan; communications, media marketing, or large-scale educational campaigns; and legislative advocacy activities to change policies or enact new laws. Governors and secretaries of health have a strong voice in setting the agenda of these groups. Sometimes state coalitions pilot one or more strategies with community coalitions to determine effectiveness, acceptability, and cost of the strategy(ies) with local populations.

Regional or National Coalitions

Regional and national coalitions are convened to harness the success of, or connections with, statewide groups. These tend to be very visible organizations with strong educational and policy agendas. They may be convened by elected or appointed leaders (for example, surgeons general or cabinet members) or by television and movie personalities or well-known advocates. Membership is usually appointed or assumed by leaders of recruited organizations. As in state groups, the agendas of these groups are tied to national health policies and goals, often set by presidential decree. The Appalachia Leadership Initiative on Cancer (ALIC) is an example of a regional coalition, and the National Folic Acid Coalition is an example of a national coalition. International coalitions, such as Safe Kids International, are relatively rare but share many of the traits of national coalitions.

COMPETING COALITIONS

Conflict may emerge when a new coalition starts to deal with the same or related problem already addressed by a pre-existing coalition(s). Sometimes the new coalition may be unaware of the existing coalition, or sometimes the new coalition developed because the existing coalition was ineffective. It may even be possible that two coalitions developed simultaneously. In any case, the pre-existing coalition(s) may view the new coalition as trying to replace, duplicate, or preempt its efforts. Sofaer (2001) recommends the following options for coalitions that must deal with pre-existing coalitions (p. 10):

- Support and join the existing coalition instead of starting another one.
- Use the existing coalition as a foundation for building a stronger, broader, or more focused effort.
- Create a specialized coalition under the umbrella of the existing one.
- Start a new coalition anyway and coordinate efforts, if possible; the new coalition may have to deal with conflict, especially if the existing one is ineffective or destructive.

COALITION SPOTLIGHT: CHANGING WITH THE TIMES—THE CONSORTIUM FOR INFANT AND CHILD HEALTH (CINCH)

Coalitions are dynamic entities and must be responsive to their environments—by merging operations, relinquishing control, or setting up cooperative ventures. CINCH, a community child health coalition, has taken all of these options over its fifteen-year history. It was created and funded as a research project to increase immunizations for two-year-olds in one city in Virginia. The comparison city for the project, which was geographically separated by a major waterway, later initiated its own immunization coalition. Over a four-year period, CINCH expanded to become a regional coalition that covered seven cities and three counties, and continued to invite other groups under its umbrella. However, despite frequent invitations, the smaller immunization coalition did not join CINCH until its own base of support eroded nearly eight years later.

CINCH formed a perinatal work group to focus on reducing disparities in low-weight births and infant mortality. An existing coalition in the area had focused on the same issue for some time with little success. Expanding the diversity of the work group beyond health care providers and responding to pressure from local citizens to produce a resource guide and conduct an educational campaign on preterm labor led to improved birth outcomes. This success and coaching by CINCH encouraged the pre-existing coalition to develop new goals and a work plan. CINCH eventually dissolved its work group and developed a formal link with the existing perinatal coalition. In response to local pressure about the childhood obesity epidemic, CINCH also formed an obesity prevention work group, unaware that a similar coalition existed in another part of the geographic region. Both groups continue to thrive by sharing information and resources, and even coordinate annual Obesity Summits in the region.

Finally, CINCH was approached by an existing coalition for increasing enrollment in a state-sponsored child health insurance program (SCHIP). Aware of CINCH's reputation for producing results, the smaller coalition asked to come in under CINCH's umbrella as a new work group. CINCH agreed and the synergy led to years of success and significant foundation, state, and federal funding that increased enrollment in the SCHIP programs by over 300 percent.

SUMMARY

Four types of working relationships have been identified: networking, cooperating, coordinating, and collaborating. Collaboration is the most intense, formal, and complex of these relationships, and it implies specific characteristics: shared creation and joint action for mutual benefit; interdependence and reciprocity; mutual authority and accountability; shared responsibility, risks, resources, and rewards; and inherent conflict and dynamic tensions. Strategic partnerships, service integration efforts, comprehensive collaborations, and conflict resolution collaborations are four models of collaboration that are differentially used, depending on the collaboration's purpose, composition, timetable, and resources. Exhibits 2.1 and 2.2 (pages 39–44) present information influencing the success and risk factors of collaboration. Exhibits 2.3 and 2.4 (pages 45–48) offer checklists of strengths, challenges, and readiness for collaboration.

The majority of collaborative relationships for health promotion and disease prevention are called partnerships or coalitions. However, both these and other names (for example, alliances, task forces, boards) are used interchangeably, even though specific definitions exist for each. A coalition is a group of individuals representing diverse organizations, factions, or constituencies who agree to work together to achieve a common goal. Coalitions are characterized as formal, multipurpose, and long-term alliances. They may be categorized according to patterns of formation, types of functions, types of structures that accommodate these functions, or their membership.

Community coalitions represent defined communities, and their memberships reflect the diversity and wisdom of those communities at both grassroots and grasstops levels. The most critical differences between community and state coalitions appear to be the kinds of partners who are recruited, the frequency of meetings, and the types of activities they undertake.

QUESTIONS FOR REVIEW

1. What factors characterize collaborative relationships as they move across a continuum from networking to full collaboration?
2. How does collaboration change the way organizations work together?
3. What are the key characteristics of community coalitions?

Exhibit 2.1. Factors Influencing the Success of Collaboration.

These twenty factors were identified by the Wilder Foundation[1] as influential to the success of collaborations formed by nonprofit organizations, government agencies, and other organizations. These factors should be considered when forming coalitions and other partnerships for health promotion and disease prevention.

Factors Related to the ENVIRONMENT

1. **Existing history of collaboration or cooperation in the community**

   An existing history of collaboration or cooperation in the community offers the potential partners an understanding of the roles and expectations required in collaboration and enables them to trust the process.

2. **Collaborative group seen as a legitimate leader in the community**

   The collaborative group is perceived within the community as reliable and competent in relation to the goals and activities it intends to accomplish.

3. **Favorable political and social climate**

   Political leaders, opinion-makers, persons who control resources, and the general public support (or at least do not oppose) the mission of the collaborative group.

Factors Related to MEMBERSHIP CHARACTERISTICS

4. **Mutual respect, understanding, and trust**

   Members of the group share an understanding and respect for each other and their respective organizations—how they operate, their cultural norms and values, their limitations, and their expectations.

5. **Appropriate cross-section of members**

   To the extent that they are needed, the collaborative group includes representatives from each sector of the community that will be affected by its activities.

6. **Members seeing collaboration as in their self-interest**

   Partners believe that they will benefit from their involvement in the collaboration and that the advantages of membership will offset costs such as loss of autonomy and turf.

7. **Ability to compromise**

   Partners are able to compromise, because the many decisions within a collaborative effort cannot possibly fit the preferences of each member perfectly.

Factors Related to PROCESS AND STRUCTURE

8. **Members sharing a stake in both process and outcome**

   Members feel ownership of both the way the group works and the results and products of its work.

---

[1] Adapted from Mattesich, Murray-Close, and Monsey, 2001. From *Collaboration: What Makes it Work—A Review of the Research Literature on Factors Influencing Successful Collaboration*, 2nd ed., by P. Mattesich, M. Murray-Close & B. Monsey. Copyright © 2001 by Fieldstone Alliance. Reproduced with permission of Fieldstone Alliance via Copyright Clearance Center.

(continued)

Exhibit 2.1. Factors Influencing the Success of Collaboration. (*Continued*)

9. **Multiple layers of participation and decision making**

   Every level of management within each partner organization has at least some representation and ongoing involvement in the collaborative initiative.

10. **Flexibility**

    The group remains open to varied ways of organizing itself and accomplishing its work.

11. **Development of clear roles and policy guidelines**

    Partners clearly understand their roles, rights, and responsibilities, and they understand how to carry out those responsibilities.

12. **Adaptability**

    The group has the ability to sustain itself in the midst of major changes even if it needs to change some goals, strategies, or members to deal with changing conditions.

13. **Appropriate pace of development**

    At each point throughout the collaborative initiative, the structure, resources, and activities of the group change over time to meet the needs of the group without overwhelming its capacity.

Factors Related to COMMUNICATION

14. **Open and frequent communication**

    Group members interact often, update one another, discuss issues openly, and convey all necessary information to one another and to people outside the group.

15. **Established informal relationships and communication links**

    In addition to formal channels of communication, members establish personal connections, producing a better, more informed, and cohesive group working on a common project.

Factors Related to PURPOSE

16. **Concrete, attainable goals and objectives**

    Goals and objectives are clear to all partners and can realistically be attained.

17. **Shared vision**

    Members have the same vision, with clearly agreed-upon mission, objective(s), and strategy(ies). The shared vision may exist at the outset of collaboration, or the partners may develop a vision as they work together.

18. **Unique purpose**

    Either the mission and goals or the approach of the collaborative group differ, at least in part, from those of member organizations.

Factors Related to RESOURCES

19. **Sufficient funds, staff, materials, and time**

    The group has an adequate, consistent financial base, along with the staff and materials needed to support its operations. It allows sufficient time to achieve its goals and to nurture the collaboration.

20. **Skilled leadership**

    The individuals who provide leadership for the group have organizing and interpersonal skills and carry out the role with fairness. Because of these and other characteristics, the leaders are granted respect or legitimacy by the collaborative partners.

Exhibit 2.2. Risk Factors for Collaborative Participation.

Take this risk factor diagnosis to find out which parts of your partnership are at risk of discouraging active participation of members and could use a tune-up and which parts are in good shape. The results may surprise you! *Note*: This diagnosis may be more useful once your collaborative effort is up and running but can provide interesting insights at any stage of your initiative.

Rate the following parts of your partnership using the following scale:

Strong/Always				Weak/Never
5	4	3	2	1

1. Clarity of Your Vision and Goals

_____ A. Our vision takes into account what is happening in the community.

_____ B. The vision and goals are written down.

_____ C. Residents and institutions are all aware of the vision and goals of the collaboration.

_____ D. We periodically reevaluate and update our vision and goals.

_____ E. The activities of the effort are evaluated in relation to our vision and goals.

2. Effectiveness of Your Initiative's Structure

_____ A. Our effort has a regular meeting cycle that members can expect.

_____ B. There are active committees.

_____ C. All members have copies of the bylaws.

_____ D. There is frequent communication among staff, coordinating committee, and stakeholders.

_____ E. The coordinating committee meets regularly with good attendance.

3. Effectiveness of Your Outreach and Communication Tools and Methods

_____ A. The effort has a newsletter or another method of communication that keeps the community regularly updated and informed about its activities.

_____ B. We use surveys or other methods to collect information about members' interests, needs, and concerns.

_____ C. Survey results are always published and used to guide our projects.

_____ D. The survey is conducted every year or so because the community and residents change.

_____ E. The partnership goes where members are to do outreach, including where people live, shop, and work.

4. Effectiveness of Coalition Meetings

_____ A. Stakeholders feel free to speak at meetings without fear of being attacked.

_____ B. The initiative advertises its meetings with sufficient notice by sending out agendas or flyers in advance.

(continued)

Exhibit 2.2. Risk Factors for Collaborative Participation. (*Continued*)

_____ C. Child care and interpreters are provided at meetings when needed.

_____ D. The work of the meeting, as outlined in the agenda, gets accomplished. Meetings start and end on time.

_____ E. Meetings are held in central, convenient, and comfortable places and at convenient times for all members.

5. Opportunities for Member Responsibility and Growth

_____ A. The partnership makes a conscious effort to develop new leaders.

_____ B. Training and support are offered to new leaders as well as to more experienced leaders (by our own members or through outside agencies).

_____ C. A "buddy system" matches less experienced members with leaders to help them learn jobs and make contacts.

_____ D. Stakeholder committees are given serious work to do.

_____ E. Leadership responsibilities are shared (for example, chairing a meeting is a rotating job).

6. Effectiveness of Your Partnership's Planning and Doing

_____ A. At the beginning of each new year, the effort develops a plan that includes objectives and activities that it wants to accomplish during the year.

_____ B. Plans are based, at least in part, on information collected from surveys of stakeholders.

_____ C. After each activity or project, the leadership or the Coordinating Committee evaluates how things went in order to learn from the experience.

_____ D. We frequently organize visible projects that make a difference to members.

_____ E. When projects are undertaken, action plans that identify tasks, responsibilities, and target dates are developed.

7. Your Effort's Use of Research and External Resources

_____ A. The partnership works with other groups in the community on common issues and with citywide organizations that work on critical community concerns.

_____ B. The partnership uses resources and information of other organizations that can help the community (for example, training workshops on environmental organizing).

_____ C. We stay on top of issues affecting communities across the city and state.

_____ D. Outside speakers come to meetings to speak on topics of interest to stakeholders.

_____ E. Leaders know where to get necessary information (for example, statistics and forms).

Exhibit 2.2. *(Continued)*

8. Your Partnership's Sense of Community

_____ A. The initiative plans social time at meetings so that people can talk informally and build a sense of community.

_____ B. We plan fun social activities in addition to working meetings.

_____ C. We treat everyone in the group equally.

_____ D. We recognize all contributions, large and small.

_____ E. We make all residents feel welcome regardless of income, race, gender, or education level.

9. How Well Your Initiative Meets Needs and Provides Benefits

_____ A. We make resource lists and important contacts available to stakeholders.

_____ B. We hold workshops with experts who can provide concrete services to members.

_____ C. As much as possible, the effort helps out members with issues on individual needs.

_____ D. If a survey of the members indicated that personal issues (such as child care or landlord–tenant problems) were getting in the way of resident's involvement, the group would find a solution that enables the resident to participate in the organizing of the effort.

_____ E. We hold meetings and workshops where residents can meet elected officials and city service personnel to voice their opinions and learn about resources and programs in the community.

10. The Group's Relationship with the Elected Officials, Institutional Leaders, and Other "Power Players"

_____ A. Leaders know how to negotiate with "power players," such as elected officials and institutional leaders to successfully "win" on issues of concern to members.

_____ B. The group has regular representatives who attend important community meetings.

_____ C. All stakeholders understand the lines of authority, decision-making power, responsibilities, and other aspects of the power structure of the community.

_____ D. The leadership meets regularly with officials about the issues that concern members.

_____ E. The initiative participates in citywide activities and demonstrations that focus on community issues.

(continued)

Exhibit 2.2. Risk Factors for Collaborative Participation. (*Continued*)

Diagnosis Score Sheet

Add the scores from A through E together for each section of the Risk Factor Diagnosis. Fill out this score sheet using the total from each section as your total score. The next section will help you evaluate your score.

	Total Score
1. Vision and Sense of Purpose	_____
2. Effort's Structure	_____
3. Outreach and Communication	_____
4. Meetings	_____
5. Membership Responsibility and Growth	_____
6. Doing Projects	_____
7. Research and External Resources	_____
8. Sense of Community	_____
9. Needs and Benefits	_____
10. Relationship with Power Players	_____

For each section, follow the guidelines below. If you scored between

5–15 Checkup time! You may need an overhaul in this area. Take a look at the Suggestions and Strategies section in the workbook that follows!

15–20 Watch out! It's time for a "tune-up" to get everything in good working order. Look at the Suggestions and Strategies section in the workbook that follows for some ideas.

20–25 Congratulations! You're running smoothly and all systems are go! Keep up the good work! (You may want to read the workbook for some new ideas and inspiration.)

Do you need a complete overhaul of your meetings?
Are you looking for a "tune-up" of your organization or partnership's structure? Maybe you are running smoothly in the area of vision and goals but hoping for a few pointers?

Source: Rosenthal, 2000.

Exhibit 2.3. A Collaboration Checklist.

Each of the following factors influences the collaborative process. After reading a brief description for each of the areas, place an X in the box that best reflects your opinion of how your collaboration is functioning, using the following scale:

1 = Strongly Disagree, 2 = Disagree, 3 = Neither Agree nor Disagree, 4 = Agree, and 5 = Strongly Agree

Each of the factors is identified and defined:

1. **Communication.** The collaboration has open and clear communication. There is an established process for communication between meetings.

2. **Sustainability.** The collaboration has a plan for sustaining membership and resources. This involves membership guidelines relating to terms of office and replacement of members.

3. **Research and evaluation.** The collaboration has conducted a needs assessment or has obtained information to establish its goals, and the collaboration continues to collect data to measure goal achievement.

4. **Political climate.** The history and environment surrounding power and decision making is positive. Political climate may be within the community as a whole, systems within the community, or networks of people.

5. **Resources.** The collaboration has access to needed resources. Resources refer to four types of capital: environmental, in-kind, financial, and human.

6. **Catalysts.** The collaboration was started because of existing problem(s), or the reason(s) for collaboration to exist required a comprehensive approach.

7. **Policies, laws, and regulations.** The collaboration has changed policies, laws, or regulations to allow the collaboration to function effectively.

8. **History.** The community has a history of working cooperatively and solving problems.

9. **Connectedness.** Members of this collaboration are connected and have established informal and formal communication networks at all levels.

10. **Leadership.** The leadership facilitates and supports team building, and capitalizes upon diversity and individual, group, and organizational strengths.

11. **Community development.** This community was mobilized to address important issues. There is a communication system and formal information channels that permit the exploration of issues, goals, and objectives.

12. **Understanding community.** The collaboration understands the community, including its people, cultures, values, and habits.

(continued)

Exhibit 2.3. A Collaboration Checklist. (*Continued*)

	Strongly Agree 1	Somewhat Agree 2	Neither Agree nor Disagree 3	Somewhat Disagree 4	Strongly Disagree 5
A COLLABORATION PROGRESS CHECKLIST					
Factors					
Goals	____	____	____	____	____
Communication	____	____	____	____	____
Sustainability	____	____	____	____	____
Research and evaluation	____	____	____	____	____
Political climate	____	____	____	____	____
Resources	____	____	____	____	____
Catalysts	____	____	____	____	____
Policies, laws, and regulations	____	____	____	____	____
History	____	____	____	____	____
Connectedness	____	____	____	____	____
Leadership	____	____	____	____	____
Community development	____	____	____	____	____
Understanding community	____	____	____	____	____
Totals	____	____	____	____	____
Grand totals	____	____	____	____	____

Identifying the collaboration's strengths and challenges assists the collaboration in determining the best course of action to achieve its identified goals. For example, if the group scores from 0–30, it has many components that comprise a successful collaboration, such as goals, working members, and strong leadership. If the collaborative group scores 31–48, the group has some of these factors; however, there is a need to develop the interrelationships in the group's work to determine new ways of working together. However, if the group scores 49–65, the group may wish to refocus their goals and leadership. Establishing a group's strengths and challenges can serve as a springboard to building a more effective collaborative group.

Source: Borden and Perkins, 1999. From "Assessing your collaboration: A self evaluation tool," by L. M. Borden and D. F. Perkins in *Journal of Extension, 37*(2):1–3, 1999. Reprinted by permission of Journal of Extension.

Exhibit 2.4. Collaboration Readiness Checklist.

1. **Context or Conditions for the Collaboration**

   ☐ The problem, issue, or project we want to address requires a collaborative approach; it cannot be done effectively by one organization alone.

   ☐ We have sufficient resources or sponsorship to begin and implement the effort.

   ☐ We are aware of the qualities and resources needed for successful collaboration, and we believe we can obtain them.

2. **Organizational Self-Assessment for Collaboration**

   ☐ We have organizational protocols for collaboration and have prepared our representative.

   ☐ We have criteria for entering collaborations and selecting collaboration partners, and can use them to help us to commit to or decline collaboration opportunities.

   ☐ The goal of the collaboration is linked to our goals and priorities.

   ☐ We are aware of what might be a problem for our organization if we join the collaboration or if certain others participate, and we are prepared to address this.

   ☐ We are ready to meet the collaboration's expectations for participation and work.

   ☐ We are clear about the level of organization (for example, director, staff, board) we will involve in this collaboration.

   ☐ Our proposed role in this collaboration is appropriate, given our resources and priorities.

   ☐ Appropriate leadership endorses our participation in this collaboration.

3. **Things to Discern About Potential Collaboration Partners**

   ☐ What are their organizational mission and goals?

   ☐ What are their organization's philosophy, values, and cultures?

   ☐ What can they bring to the collaboration? Why is their involvement essential to the success of this effort?

   ☐ Why do they want to collaborate with you and others? What are their expectations of this collaboration's outcome?

   ☐ Where does this collaboration fit within organizational priorities?

4. **Things to Clarify About the Potential Collaboration**

   ☐ Is there a foundation of trust among the partners or members of this collaboration?

   ☐ What will collaboration success look like, and what will be the standards of practice?

(continued)

Exhibit 2.4. Collaboration Readiness Checklist. (*Continued*)

☐ How will we evaluate the effort and make mid-course adjustments? Are the partners open to developing shared evaluation criteria and conducting periodic evaluations to keep the project on course?

☐ What type and level of organizational representation is expected?

☐ How will the partners fulfill the different roles needed to make this collaboration function?

5. Individual Role and Readiness for Collaboration

Organizational Role:

Within my own organization I have influence and expertise in these areas:

_____

_____

My agency's expectations for me as a representative in this collaboration are

_____

_____

I have authority, on behalf of my organization, to

☐ Establish relationships.
☐ Generate ideas.
☐ Set policy.
☐ Plan activities.
☐ Implement activities.
☐ Spend money.
☐ Assign resources.
☐ Commit staff time.
☐ Sign position papers.
☐ Evaluate.
☐ Make recommendations.
☐ Make organizational or personal changes.

Source: Rosenthal, 2000. Copyright © 2006 Beth B. Rosenthal, M. S. Collaboration and Change, LLC. Reprinted with permission.

CHAPTER THREE

Why Coalitions?

A small, thoughtful group of people can change the world.
Indeed, it is the only thing that ever has.
—Margaret Meade, anthropologist, 1901–1978

I hesitated to include Meade's words in this text, wishing to avoid being trite and using phrases that have been repeated so often that they have become as well worn as an old carpet. But Meade speaks to the heart of the volunteer—the person who wonders, *Is it enough? Will it ever be finished?* And, of course, the answer is *no*. Still, her conviction lends strength to many, and so it is shared here.

The age-old riddle asks, *Which came first—the chicken or the egg?* We face a similar dilemma when we approach the notion of how coalitions began. Does the issue or concern drive coalition formation? Or does the collaborative power of a group of concerned citizens identify the issue that sustains their original partnership? In fact, both situations occur in real communities, and neither is preferable to the other. This chapter explores the many reasons for coalition formation, how coalitions relate (or do not) to community context, and the inherent benefits and challenges that arise in creating and sustaining coalitions.

WHY COALITIONS FORM

Coalitions are established for many different reasons and focus on a variety of issues (Butterfoss and others, 1993). In general, community coalitions often form in response to an opportunity such as new funding, exemplified by the tobacco settlement funds made available for coalition building around youth tobacco control and prevention. They may form because of a threat such as a national story about rising asthma prevalence or a local event, such as an outbreak of meningitis on a college campus. Local health organizations may voluntarily form or join coalitions to augment their limited resources of staff, time, talent, equipment, supplies, materials, contacts, and influence.

By sharing their resources, coalitions provide a multifocal approach to a community issue. Joining with other agencies and individuals can benefit an organization, giving it expanded access to printing and postage services, media coverage, marketing services, meeting space, community residents, influential people, personnel, community and professional networks, and expertise (Whitt, 1993). Additionally, coalitions may be mandatory or required by a funding source, such as the Robert Wood Johnson Allies Against Asthma initiative.

As related in Chapter One, the past twenty-five years have seen a dramatic rise in the number of coalitions formed to promote health and prevent disease. The reasons for the popularity of the coalition approach for dealing with health problems are, first, that most chronic health problems, such as asthma and heart disease, have multiple causes and consequences that require complex solutions; second, clusters of problems co-exist that require the action of multiple participants from many disciplines and organizations such as social services, mental health, housing, and education; and third, health professionals realize that they must work collaboratively with individuals, families, and communities who are affected by these health problems, if they are to solve them effectively (Sofaer, 2001a, pp. 6–7).

Wolff also suggests that coalitions form because prevention strategies require community-wide involvement, reinforcement, and dissemination; the federal government has cut back human services and shifted responsibility for programs to state and local levels; health and human services organizations are limited in addressing community needs due to duplication of efforts, fragmentation of services, multicultural insensitivity, and unequal access to resources; and coalitions are vehicles to counter the declining trend in civic engagement and to reengage residents in all sectors of the community to address local problems (2001a, pp. 169–171).

Finally, coalitions use multifaceted strategies aimed at environmental, behavioral, and social policy changes, not just changes in individuals. They employ an ecological approach to address multiple layers of influence on behavior and offer comprehensive methods for health promotion initiatives (McLeroy, Bibeau, Steckler, and Glanz, 1988). This approach has been used successfully for public health initiatives in worksite health promotion, food labeling requirements, and smoking and alcohol prevention (Green, Richard, and Potvin, 1996).

Ecological models take into account the physical environment and its relationship to people at intrapersonal, interpersonal, organizational, community, and public policy levels (McLeroy, Bibeau, Steckler, and Glanz, 1988). They engage the social processes and institutions that are major influences on individual behaviors and assume that behavior does not occur in a vacuum. Each coalition must determine for itself at which level(s) it expects to concentrate to have the most profound influence. As the levels are described below (McLeroy, Bibeau, Steckler, and Glanz, 1988), note that coalitions usually intervene at the organizational, community, and public policy levels to produce more far-reaching and sustained changes.

The intrapersonal level takes into account an individual's knowledge, attitudes, values, skills behavior, self-concept, and self-esteem. Strategies to intervene at this level include mass media campaigns, social marketing, and skills development.

The interpersonal level includes an individual's social networks, social supports, families, work groups, peers, and neighbors. Strategies at this level include enhancement of social supports and networks, changing group norms, and increasing access to services.

The organizational level includes norms, incentives, organizational culture, management styles, organizational structure, and communication networks. Interventions at this level include incentive programs, process consultation, coalition development, and agency linkage.

The community level includes community resources, neighborhood organizations, social and health services, organizational relationships, folk practices, governmental structures, and informal and formal leadership practices. Strategies at this level include community development, community coalitions, empowerment, conflict resolution, and mass media campaigns.

The public policy level includes legislation, policies, taxes, and regulatory agencies. Strategies include mass media campaigns, policy analysis, political change, and lobbying.

THE IMPORTANCE OF COMMUNITY CONTEXT

Coalitions are embedded in communities, and as a result, factors in the environment can have a significant impact on a coalition throughout all stages of its development (Butterfoss and others, 1993; McLeroy and others, 1994; Lasker, Weiss, and Miller, 2001). Contextual factors are described as conditions that either exist or are lacking within an environment and that can enhance or inhibit collaborations (National Network for Collaboration, 1996). A coalition's interaction with its environment is "dynamic and persistent during its life cycle" (Habana-Hafner, Reed, and Associates, 1989, p. 15). Reininger and colleagues (Reininger, Dinh-Zarr, Sinicrope, and Martin, 1999) discuss tension and mistrust between groups and how the lack of trust affected one coalition. Others have documented the impact of political and administrative contexts on coalitions (Dill, 1994; Clark, Baker, and Chawla, 1993; Nelson, 1994). Kegler and colleagues (1998b) noted the impact of tobacco-related politics on tobacco control coalitions in several stages of coalition development, from recruitment in the formation stage to types of activities conducted in the maintenance stage.

History of collaboration is cited as another contextual factor that can affect the formation of collaborative relationships, including coalitions (Gray, 1989; Matessich, Murray-Close, and Monsey, 2001), with positive norms for collaboration increasing the likelihood of future successful collaboration. Sofaer (2001) notes that "people's good and bad experiences will influence whether they come to a new one with optimism or serious skepticism, or whether they stay away all together!" (p. 11). The

National Network for Collaboration (1996) suggests six factors that contribute to the success of collaborative efforts within communities (p. 14):

- Connectedness, or the linkages between individuals, groups, and organizations
- History of working together in a cooperative or competitive way
- Political climate, or the history and environment surrounding power and decision making
- Policies, laws, and regulations which represent the concepts and activities used to resolve problems
- Environmental, in-kind, financial, and human resources
- Catalysts, or the existing problem(s), reason(s), or convener(s) that get the collaborative effort started

Mattesich and Monsey suggest eight similar community attributes that contribute to collaborative or community-building efforts, the last four of which were mentioned previously (2005, p. 14):

- Community awareness of an issue
- Motivation from within the community
- Small geographic area
- Flexibility and adaptability in problem solving and task accomplishment
- Pre-existing social cohesion (similar to connectedness)
- Ability to discuss, reach consensus, and cooperate
- Existing identifiable leadership
- Prior success with community building

Additional contextual factors that affect coalitions include social capital (including trust between segments of a community), geography, and community readiness (Wolff, 2001b). Mattesich and Monsey (2005) suggest that successful collaborations are more likely in communities with smaller geographic areas, where planning and implementing activities are more manageable. Geography and climatic conditions are especially important in deciding how, when, and where to hold coalition meetings (Sofaer, 2001). In a small town or state, or an island community, face-to-face meetings are desired and practical. However, in a large state, a city with traffic and parking barriers, or a mountain environment with hazardous weather conditions, conference-call meetings or teleconferencing with partners who live at a distance make sense.

The coalition must take into consideration the overall community attitude about the health issue as members begin working together. If teen pregnancy prevention is one of the coalition's goals, for example, care must be taken to work with parent groups and faith-based institutions to determine how to approach the sensitive issues of abstinence and birth-control education. Finally, the coalition must consider the cultural climate of the community and how people usually work together in the community (Sofaer, 2001). Coalition leaders must recognize and respond to racial and ethnic diversity and customs (for example, food served and times or days that meetings are held), as well the amount of formality in conducting meetings and making decisions (for instance, using Robert's Rules of Order versus informal meeting guidelines, and voting versus reaching consensus). Here are several contextual questions (adapted from Clark and others, 2006) that coalitions should consider as they begin their work in a given community:

- What are the agreed-upon boundaries for the community?
- What are the priority populations for coalition membership and coalition activities?
- How does geography affect the community and what is possible to do?
- What is the social, political, and economic history of the community?
- Is there a history and culture of collaboration in the community, or will the coalition be introducing the idea of cooperation and creating a new culture?
- What are the types and number of stakeholders or partners in the problem?
- What is the degree of trust among stakeholders?
- Are stakeholders in agreement about the problem and ways to resolve it? Are they ready to act?
- What potential resources can partners generate? Are competition and conflict likely?
- Is there a leader(s) who has the confidence and credibility to move the coalition idea forward?

BENEFITS OF A COALITION APPROACH

Ultimately, collaboration is possible when a perceived need exists and an organization anticipates deriving a benefit that is contingent on mutual action (Gray and Wood, 1991). Coalitions offer such benefits by serving as effective and efficient vehicles for the exchange of knowledge, ideas, and strategies. Advantages of working in partnership may be intermediate or long-term, direct or indirect. Through coalitions, individuals and organizations can become involved in new, broader issues without assuming sole responsibility. Coalitions can also demonstrate and develop community support or concern for issues; maximize the power of individuals and groups through collective action; improve trust and communication among community agencies and sectors; mobilize diverse talents, resources, and strategies; build strength and cohesiveness by connecting individual activists and organizations; build a constituency for a given issue; reduce the social acceptability of health risk behaviors; and change community norms and standards (Whitt, 1993).

The synergy that is created from working collaboratively results in greater accomplishments (with less fragmentation of efforts and resources) than each group working on its own could ever achieve (Lasker, Weiss, and Miller, 2001). Lasker's and colleagues' (2001) study of sixty-three partnerships (815 members) indicated that those with a high level of synergy have leaders that promote productive interactions among diverse participants as well as the ability to make good use of their participants' in-kind and financial resources and time (partnership efficiency). High levels of synergy were also related to more collaborative administration and management capacities and to the ability of partnerships to obtain sufficient nonfinancial resources from their participants (such as skills, information, connections to people and groups, endorsements, convening power).

When real community involvement exists, coalitions can address community health concerns while empowering or developing capacity in those communities. Coalition membership can lead to increased community participation and leadership, skills, resources, social and inter-organizational networks, sense of community, community power, and successful community problem solving (Goodman and others, 1998; Kegler, Steckler, McLeroy, and Malek, 1998b).

Learning why members participate in voluntary organizations helps us understand people's motivations and provides an opportunity to intervene on factors that improve coalition functioning (Chinman and others, 1996). Studies of member benefits and costs suggest that participants and organizations decide to invest their energy in collaborative relationships only if the expected benefits outweigh the costs that are entailed (Gray, 1989; Norton and others, 1993; Prestby and others, 1990; Roberts-DeGennaro, 1986; Rich, 1980; Whetten, 1981). Potential benefits of collaboration include increased networking, information sharing, and access to ideas, materials, and resources (Hord, 1986; Kaplan, 1986); being involved in an important cause and attaining desired outcomes from the coalition's efforts (Rich, 1980; Zapka and others, 1992); enjoying the coalition's work (Benard, 1989); receiving personal recognition (Bailey, 1996; Benard 1989; Wandersman and Alderman, 1993); and enhancing one's skills (Rich, 1980; Roberts-DeGennaro, 1986; Wandersman and Alderman, 1993).

Improved communication between agencies and organizations will result in the delivery of more consistent and reliable information to the client or priority population. Shared information across agencies may increase public support, use of programs and services, and partners' awareness of policy and legislative issues that affect community members. Finally, improved communication among partners may provide better evaluation of the total impact of programs (Jackson and Maddy, 2001).

Clark and Wilson (1961) described a typology with three general types of benefits from participation: *material* (tangible rewards such as improved skills, money, and increased property value), *solidary* (interpersonal relationships and status, group identification, and increased cooperation), and *purposive* (personal organizational goals such as improving the community, doing one's duty, and feeling a sense of responsibility). Prestby and others (1990) reduced this model to two main sources of motivation: *personal gain benefits*, such as learning new skills and gaining personal recognition, and *social–communal benefits*, such as improving the neighborhood and helping others. Wandersman and colleagues (1987) found that members and nonmembers agreed that the greatest benefits were making a contribution and helping others rather than satisfying self-interest or a need for personal gain. Participants who are more active further reported receiving significantly more social–communal and personal benefits than less active participants and reported higher benefit-to-cost ratios (Prestby and others 1990). Similarly, in studying coalition committees, Chinman and others (1996) found that those members in committees with high attendance rates experienced more benefits and less costs than those in committees with low attendance rates. Finally, a recent study found that increased involvement was initially associated with decreased costs and increased satisfaction up to a point, beyond which costs increased and satisfaction decreased despite increasing benefits (Ansari's paradox). The favorable cost-to-benefit ratio occurred when benefits were at least 60 percent more than costs (Ansari and Phillips, 2004).

Additional benefits of participating in coalitions include the potential to minimize duplication and use resources efficiently; the opportunity to reduce uncertainty in the environment and achieve legitimacy; the ability to negotiate potential conflict through power distribution within coalitions; and the sharing of costs and associated risks (Alter and Hage, 1993; Bazzoli and others, 1997; Butterfoss, Goodman, and Wandersman, 1993; Gray, 1989; Gulati, 1995; Penner, 1995; Whetten, 1981; Wandersman and Alderman, 1993; Zapka and others, 1992).

CHALLENGES OF A COALITION APPROACH

Unfortunately, not every coalition has been successful, and not every coalition has achieved its results without having its members pay a high price for its success (Dowling, O'Donnell, and Wellington Consulting Group, 2000; Wolff, 2001a). Although coalitions are usually built from unselfish motives to improve communities, they still may experience difficulties that are common to many types of organizations as well as some that are unique to collaborative efforts. Specific costs involved in participation include *personal costs* (for example, time, effort, the things people give up in other parts of their lives in order to participate) and *social–organizational costs* (for example, interpersonal conflict and lack of organizational progress) (Wandersman, Florin, Friedmann, and Meier, 1987). Furthermore, the least active coalition members often report more social–organizational costs than do more active members (Prestby and others, 1990). Such costs may act as a barrier to participation that is more active.

With the initiation of a coalition, frustrations often arise. Despite common concerns, each organization may have its own take on the problem, with its own set of assumptions and preferred solutions (Boydell, 2003). Due to limited budgets, promised resources may not be made available, and some organizations that would be valued partners may be unable to participate in coalition activities. Member organizations may also face budget cuts, changes in administration, or other short-term changes that affect their commitment. In these cases, devoting resources to a collaborative effort may detract from their other priority projects.

Conflicting interests may prevent a coalition from having its desired effect in the community. If a coalition takes a position that is inconsistent with the policy of one of its partners, the partner may become uncooperative or ineffective, or may eventually withdraw from the coalition. Withdrawal of support by a key member, or outside pressures from individuals or groups who disagree with or do not understand the coalition's purpose, may strain the coalition or cause a crisis. Sometimes turf protection and mistrust arise in coalition work. If coalition members do not trust their partners, they will not be open to new ideas. During a conflict with a partner or the coalition, members may not be willing to cooperate or share resources and burdens.

Other costs associated with coalition membership may include loss of autonomy and the ability to unilaterally control outcomes, conflict over goals and methods, expenditure of scarce resources (time, money, information, status), risk of losing competitive position, possible delays in solving problems, inequality of power, too many compromises, and overcoming any unfavorable image held by other partners (Alter and Hage, 1993; Bailey 1996; Rich 1980; Schermerhorn, 1975; United Nations Association of the United States of America, 2005).

Reaching consensus may take time, and many partners may not be able to move forward without approval by a higher authority or more study. Depending on how well the group communicates or how often it meets, decision by consensus could make acting on a problem slow and ineffective (Jackson and Maddy, 2001).

Member organizations may also perceive a lack of direction from coalition leadership or staff, lack of recognition or appreciation, burnout, lack of necessary skills, or pressure for additional commitment (Wandersman and Alderman, 1993). Community coalitions that survive over time must provide ongoing benefits that outweigh the costs of membership.

"Breaking Barriers to Success in Your Coalition" (Kaye and Wolfe, 1995) is an activity adapted for group use to identify and suggest solutions to the barriers that a coalition might face. This activity is done in a coalition setting with several groups of five to eight persons, or in a training activity with several groups of coalitions. First, the facilitator introduces a list of the thirteen barriers to success in a coalition:

- Lack of direction or focus
- Turf battles and competition
- History
- Failure to plan, act, or both
- Dominance by professionals
- Poor links to the community
- Minimal organizational capacity
- Funding—too much or too little
- Failure to develop, maintain, or rotate leadership
- Unequal sharing of responsibility and decision making
- Time and loyalty conflicts
- Lack of ongoing staff and member training
- Burnout or unrealistic demands on members and staff

Then the facilitator asks if the group can think of any other barriers, which are duly noted on a flip chart. Within groups, each participant selects up to three barriers from the list, flip chart, or both, and writes them on a worksheet. One person selected as the group recorder asks the others to each name barriers in round-robin fashion. Once all have participated, the group uses a consensus method to decide which barrier was stated most often or is most important to the group. Then the group brainstorms a list of potential strategies that might be used to overcome that barrier. If time permits, the group can go on to prioritize Barrier Two. After thirty minutes, the groups are asked to name their top barriers and the strategies to overcome them. After each group presents, the facilitator asks other groups whether they chose the same barrier and inquires about their strategies. The process continues until all groups have reported.

APPLYING DEMOCRATIC PRINCIPLES TO COALITION BUILDING

One key reason why coalitions and partnerships are so attractive to so many is that they mirror the very principles of democracy that permit and encourage their formation. Pickeral (2005) outlines these principles as follows:

Civic participation. In building and sustaining a coalition, members have a right and responsibility to participate, which includes being informed, attending meetings, contributing to discussions, and making critical decisions for the public or the coalition's good.

Equality. Partners should be treated equally and without discrimination and given equal opportunities to contribute to, learn from, and represent the coalition.

Tolerance. Coalitions should ensure the rights of minority opinions; in other words, all members should be allowed to express their opinions and help move the coalition's agenda forward.

Human rights. Coalitions should establish agreed-upon rights and freedoms, and protect the rights of individuals and organizations.

Rule of law. Coalitions must ensure that no individual or organization is above the law, including its leadership. Everyone should adhere to accepted processes and protocols that are equally, fairly, and consistently enforced.

Accountability. Coalitions should be accountable to members for their actions such as how decisions are made and carried out.

Transparency. Coalitions should be open to partners and the public about their actions and should seek input before decisions are made.

Discussion, deliberation, and decision making. Coalitions should guarantee fair and regular opportunities for members to engage in discussions and deliberations to meet short- and long-term goals.

Controlling abuse of power. A coalition should operate in the best interest of its mission and not allow individual members or organizations to abuse shared power.

WHEN COALITIONS ARE NOT THE SOLUTION

Coalitions are not a panacea. Even the most successful coalition cannot provide easy answers for dealing with the numerous issues that impact a community from the outside. Because coalition building involves a long-term investment of time and resources, a coalition should not be established if a simpler, less complex structure will get the job done or if the community does not embrace this approach. First, coalitions are not automatic links to the grassroots or the "real people" of a community. Often coalitions are composed mostly of agency and institutional members and must make special efforts through extensive outreach if they are serious about reaching agencies that have deep community roots, or the grass roots themselves.

Second, coalitions should not be established primarily as human service organizations, but work best as catalysts to action. The more they deliver direct services, the harder it is to focus on their role as catalysts for community change. They *can* serve to coordinate and integrate services policies and activities or to develop and deliver model programs and services, as long as those roles are seen as rather temporary (Clark, Friedman, and Lachance, 2006).

Third, no data yet exist to prove that coalition building is efficient for either time or resources. Although desirable, building consensus and trust within a community both take time. Even though the intent of collaboration is to bring together human service providers to reduce overhead and avoid duplication of services, saving money has not yet been a proven outcome.

Finally, a coalition should not be established if the potential organizational partners have a history of noncooperation or competitiveness; if needed coalition resources are unlikely to be available in the near future; or if one or two resourceful partners already have the time, money, and people to solve the problem alone (Dowling, O'Donnell, and Wellington Consulting Group, 2000). Because these conditions rarely occur in public health, a coalition approach is often warranted.

Here are some questions that organizations and individuals should consider before committing to forming a coalition:

- Does the problem affect a broad range of people?
- Is the problem complex, requiring information and expertise from various sectors of the community, state, region, or country?
- Is broad public awareness or education needed?
- Does a gap in services or programs exist, such that no existing organization is clearly mandated to take on this work?
- Do other organizations see this problem as a priority?
- Are other organizations willing to work together to address this problem?
- Is this problem best addressed through the joint ownership and responsibility of a number of organizations?

- Are potential coalition members willing to relinquish individual control over coalition activities and outcomes and actively engage in a collaborative process?
- Are potential coalition members willing to commit to and abide by democratic decision-making procedures?
- Do organizational goals and policies of potential members align with of the coalition?
- Are there resources that can be shared or obtained to assist with the work?
- Is there a true commitment to work together and produce results, regardless of funder commitments for collaboration?

If the answer to any of the above items is *no,* careful thought should be given as to whether a coalition is the best organizational structure for a group.

The alternative to working within a coalition structure is to continue networking to build and maintain new individual and organizational relationships. If no one else is ready to work on the issue, an organization should get started anyway and keep others informed about its work. It should also consider collaborating with other organizations in less intense ways, such as working on a single event or a short-term project. The trust and respect that are built under these conditions may lead to productive and collaborative future work.

TO BE OR NOT TO BE?
SHOULD COALITIONS EVER DISBAND?

In a well-known refrain from a Kenny Rogers song, the gambler advises us to "know when to hold 'em and know when to fold 'em." This is good advice for coalition builders. Knowing when to close a coalition and its work is as critical as knowing when and how to establish one. Most people acknowledge that health coalitions are not meant to be permanent bodies. However, the same people feel conflicted when forced to acknowledge that their group is, in fact, temporary. Nothing is more demoralizing than trying to breathe life into a coalition that has outlived its usefulness or whose members are no longer committed.

The lifespan of a coalition should be tied to the accomplishment of its goals and objectives. When goals are measurable, then an end date tied to accomplishing those goals is implied. If goals are broad or indefinite, the task of deciding when to terminate the group becomes more difficult. Even if goals are indefinite, the group should agree to revisit long-term goals at least every three to five years to determine whether to disband or whether more time or expanded goals are needed. In the case of the Virginia Coalition for a Healthy Future, its goal was to increase the tax on cigarettes and tobacco products. In 2004, after five years of effort, the tax was passed by the legislature. This would have been a logical end for the coalition, but after reassessment and celebration, the coalition decided to build on their success and expand their goals to include clean indoor air and clean smokestack advocacy efforts.

SUMMARY

Coalitions are established for many different reasons, such as a response to an opportunity, a threat, or a local event. Local health organizations may voluntarily form or join coalitions to augment their limited resources, or coalitions may be mandated or required by a funding source or governmental entity. Coalitions are popular vehicles for disease prevention and health promotion because health problems are complex and often have multiple causes and effects. These issues require collaboration among diverse organizations and wide dissemination of strategies among populations that will be served by the coalition effort. The recent downsizing of federal initiatives and reliance on local agencies and community-based organizations makes coalition building essential to avoid duplication of efforts and resources. Contextual factors in the environment can have a significant impact on coalitions. These factors include the history of collaboration, tension and mistrust among groups, politics, economics, geography, climate, ethnic and racial diversity, community readiness, attitudes about the health issue(s), and working styles.

Coalitions provide many benefits such as allowing individuals and organizations to become involved in new, broader issues without assuming sole responsibility; demonstrating and developing community support or concern for issues; maximizing the power of individuals and groups through collective action; improving trust, cohesiveness, and communication among groups; mobilizing diverse talents, resources, and strategies; minimizing duplication and using resources efficiently; negotiating potential conflict through power distribution within coalitions; and sharing responsibilities, risks, and rewards. Coalition members may also experience difficulties such as expending time, effort, and resources without appropriate recognition or appreciation; experiencing interpersonal conflict and lack of organizational progress; losing autonomy and control; and feeling burned out or pressured for additional commitment. Coalitions that survive over time must provide ongoing benefits that outweigh the costs of membership. Ideally, a coalition should not be established if a simpler, less complex structure will get the job done or if the community does not embrace this approach.

QUESTIONS FOR REVIEW

1. Why are coalitions a popular approach to solving health problems?
2. What motivates members to join and remain involved in coalitions and partnerships? What disincentives are incurred by coalition membership?

CHAPTER FOUR

The Community Coalition
Action Theory (CCAT)

Action will remove the doubts that theory cannot solve.
—Tehyi Hsieh, Chinese educator

Communities, organizations, businesses, and even nations are forming alliances, joint ventures, and public–private partnerships more than ever before. Indeed, over the past three decades, community coalitions have served as excellent vehicles for consensus building and active involvement of diverse organizations and constituencies in addressing community problem(s). The advantages of partnership approaches are widely accepted by government agencies and foundations, and as a result, the majority of prevention initiatives over the past fifteen years required the formation of community coalitions. Public health professionals have most eagerly embraced the practice of coalition building. They have looked for an effective, inclusive approach to complex health issues, and coalitions have seemed most appropriate. Previous research has concluded that although clear and definite theoretical underpinnings exist for community coalitions, the practice of coalition building has outpaced the development of coalition theory (Butterfoss and Kegler, 2002). This chapter will serve to elucidate the various models and frameworks that have served as critical precursors to the comprehensive theory that I co-developed with Michelle Kegler, the Community Coalition Action Theory (CCAT) (Butterfoss and Kegler, 2002). Because its constructs and propositions are fundamental to the chapters that follow, this theory will be explained fully here.

61

THE COMMUNITY COALITION ACTION THEORY (CCAT): ORIGIN AND ROOTS

In the first chapter of this book, we learned that the underlying theoretical basis for the development and maintenance of community coalitions was borrowed from many arenas, including community development, citizen participation, community empowerment, political science, interorganizational relations, and group process.

Chapters Two and Three explained that community approaches—including those that build coalitions—attempt to alleviate community problems by organizing the community to bring about modifications in systems, rules, social norms, or laws, eventually changing the social acceptability of certain behaviors. We also learned that these community-wide approaches recognize that behaviors are inextricably tied to the environment (Milio, 1989; Thompson and Kinney, 1990; Stokols, 1992; Tesh, 1988).

Community coalitions have the potential to involve multiple sectors of the community, pool resources, mobilize talents and diverse approaches, and conduct multiple interventions that focus on both individuals and their environments (McLeroy and others, 1994). Building on the social movements of the 1960s and 1970s, coalitions must ultimately involve community members to help ensure that interventions meet the needs of the community and are culturally sensitive. Community participation through coalitions facilitates ownership, which in turn is thought to increase the chances of successful institutionalization into the community (Bracht, 1990).

Finally, we have learned that community coalition building is a promising strategy for building among member organizations the capacity and competence to address future critical health issues in the communities they serve (Chavis, 2001; Goodman and others, 1998; Kegler, Steckler, McLeroy, and Malek, 1998b).

COALITION FRAMEWORKS AND MODELS

No theory should be developed in a vacuum but rather should be built upon previous knowledge and wisdom. In developing CCAT, Michelle Kegler and I stood on the shoulders of many innovators whose work stimulated our thinking and helped us crystallize our ideas into a cohesive theory. Their creative models and frameworks are summarized in the following sections. We expect that CCAT will evolve as promising students, experienced researchers, and practitioners use it in their work.

Community Organization and Development Model

An early planning model for partnership building is the Community Organization and Development Model (COD) (Braithwaite, Murphy, Lythcott, and Blumenthal, 1989), which is based on the belief that health-promotion efforts are likely to be more successful among minority and poor populations when the communities at risk are empowered to identify their own problems. Community residents participate in developing interventions and form coalition boards to make policy decisions and manage resources. The seven-step model that follows borrows from the empowerment education approach of Paulo Friere (1973) and still provides relevant guidance for health educators and community organizers.

1. *Learning the community layout.* Entry to the community should be preceded by a study of the community, that is, its geography and health-status measures, among others.
2. *Learning the community ecology.* This includes identifying places where people congregate, as well as meeting community leaders and gatekeepers and learning their relationships to one another.
3. *Community entry process.* The process must be negotiated with gatekeepers, and the community organizer must be "validated" by the formal and informal community networks.
4. *Building credibility.* Offering tangible resources is helpful at this step.
5. *Development of a community coalition board.* The board described in this step is consumer-dominated (at least 60 percent) but also includes academic, agency, and organizational representatives as well as elected officials.
6. *Conducting a community needs assessment.* This involves a survey or similar method to identify those health issues felt by community residents to be most important.
7. *Planning the intervention.* The planning step is followed by providing feedback to the community on the results of the intervention.

In later adaptations of the model, Braithwaite and colleagues proposed the formation and effective functioning of a community coalition that incorporates community-organizing and community-building practices in a culturally competent context (Braithwaite, 1994; Braithwaite, Taylor, and Austin, 2000).

Framework for Partnerships for Community Development

During the same period that the COD Model was developed, Habana-Hafner, Reed, and Associates (1989) from the Center for Organizational and Community Development (University of Massachusetts, Amherst) developed the Framework for Partnerships for Community Development. The Framework, shown in Figure 4.1, has two abstract concepts at its core: (1) *identity*—the membership, its shared sense of meaning and goals, values and culture, interpersonal relations, shared resources, history, and synergy; and (2) *productive work*—leadership, decision making, communication, policies and rules, roles, evaluation, organizational structure, and group dynamics.

The partnership must interact with a dynamic and persistent external *environment* with influences such as geography, history, politics, economics, power structure, and ethnic and cultural diversity. Three stages of development occur as organizations work together in the partnership. Prior to Stage 1 is *Preparation: Knowing the Environment*, which involves clarifying broad concerns, exploring environmental influences, and defining the membership. Stage 1 is *Negotiation and Problem Clarification*; Stage 2 is *Direction Setting, Trust Building, and Empowerment*; and Stage 3 is *Developing Structure and Operation*. Following Stage 3 is *Assessment:*

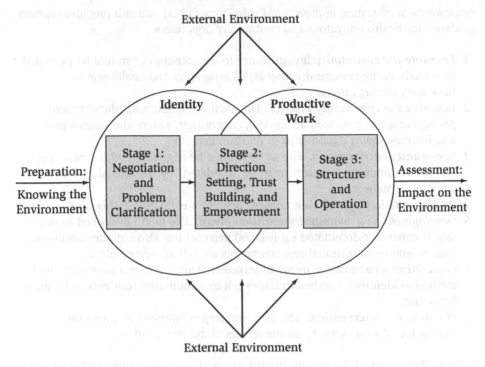

Figure 4.1 Framework for Partnerships for Community Development.

Source: Habana-Hafner, Reed and Associates, 1989, p. 22. From Habana-Hafner, Reed and Associates, *Partnerships for Community Development: Resources for Practitioners and Trainers.* Amherst, MA: University of Massachusetts Center for Organizational and Community Development. Reprinted by permission, www.umass.edu/cie.

Impact on the Environment, in which the partnership evaluates its outcomes. At this point, the partnership may disband, look at other ways of addressing the problem, or focus on another problem.

Framework of Organizational Viability

In 1978, Katz and Kahn developed an open-systems perspective on how organizations function and maintain momentum as they interact with the surrounding environment. They proposed that organizations could be seen as mechanisms for processing resources obtained from the environment into products that affect that environment.

Prestby and Wandersman (1985) developed a Framework of Organizational Viability, based on Katz's and Kahn's work, that suggests four components of organizational functioning: (1) resource acquisition, (2) maintenance subsystem (organizational structure), (3) production subsystem (actions or activities), and (4) external goal attainment (accomplishments). This model indicates that any organization that fails to obtain adequate and appropriate resources, develop an organizational structure for obtaining resources and conducting work, mobilize resources efficiently

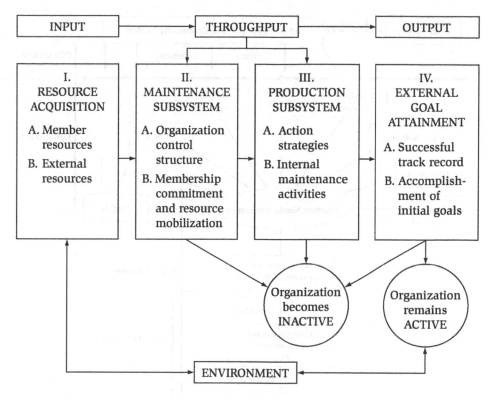

Figure 4.2 An Open-Systems Framework of Organizational Characteristics Related to Coalition Funding.

Source: Prestby & Wandersman, 1985; Minkler 2003, p. 296. From "An empirical exploration of a framework of organizational viability: Maintaining block organizations," by J. Prestby and A. Wandersman in *The Journal of Applied Behavioral Science, 21*(3), 287–305 (fig. on p. 296). Copyright © 1985 by Sage Publications, Inc. Reproduced with permission of Sage Publications Inc. via Copyright Clearance Center.

and effectively, turn out appropriate "products" (such as action or benefits to members), or accomplish something will eventually cease to operate. The elements of the open-systems framework are diagrammed in Figure 4.2.

Community Coalition Model

Butterfoss, Goodman, and Wandersman (1993) further developed a Community Coalition Model that described the development of community coalitions, while evaluating community coalitions for alcohol, tobacco, and other drug abuse (ATOD) prevention for the Centers for Substance Abuse Prevention (CASP). In Figure 4.3, these authors show how a coalition forms and develops in four specific stages:

Formation stage occurs as a lead agency is granted funding to convene an ad hoc committee of local leaders. This committee nominates influential citizens to serve on committees representing different sectors of the community and provides training on prevention goals, issues, and tasks.

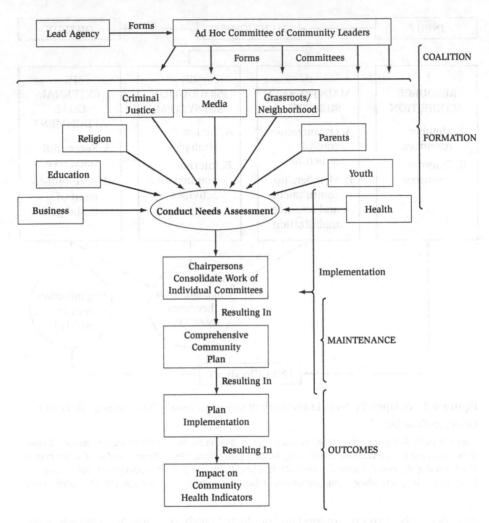

Figure 4.3 Overview of the Development of a Community Coalition.

Source: Butterfoss, Goodman, and Wandersman 1993, p. 320. Fig. 1 from "Community Coalitions for Prevention and Health Promotion," by F. Butterfoss, R. Goodman and A. Wandersman in *Health Education Research, 8*(3), p. 320. Copyright © 1993 by Oxford University Press. Reproduced with permission of Oxford University Press via Copyright Clearance Center.

Implementation stage occurs as each committee conducts a needs assessment to determine the extent and nature of its constituents' concerns and resources around ATOD abuse and develops a community-wide intervention plan.

Maintenance stage consists of the monitoring and upkeep of the committees and the planned activities.

Outcome stage consists of impacts that result from the deployment of community-wide strategies.

At each stage, different sets of factors may be important in enhancing coalition function.

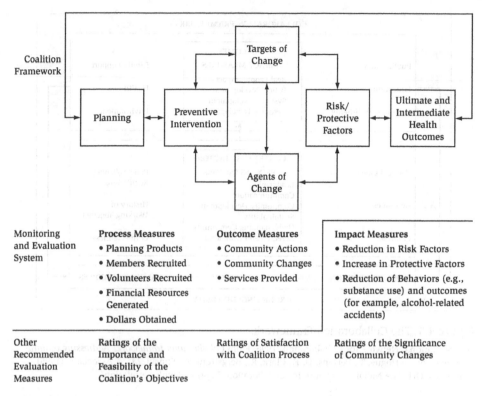

Figure 4.4 A Framework for Community Health Coalitions and Their Evaluation.

Source: Fawcett et al., 1993, p. 405. Fig. 1, p. 405 from "A Methodology for Monitoring and Evaluation Community Health Coalitions," by V. T. Francisco, A. L. Paine & S. B. Fawcett in *Health Education Research, 8*(3), pp. 403–416. 1993. Copyright © 1993 by Oxford University Press. Reproduced with permission of Oxford University Press via Copyright Clearance Center.

Work Group on Health Promotion and Community Development Model

In 1993, the Work Group on Health Promotion and Community Development developed a framework to guide both the process of coalition development and the design of the evaluation for their CSAP coalitions (Francisco, Paine, and Fawcett, 1993). The framework shown in Figure 4.4 is based on an adaptation of the Predisposing, Reinforcing, and Enabling Constructs in Educational/Ecological Diagnosis and Evaluation (PRECEDE) model (Green and Kreuter, 1991). According to this framework, community coalitions plan for and launch preventive interventions for targets of change (for example, youth and elected officials) and agents of change (for instance, peers and elders). These interventions are designed to have an impact on risk and protective factors and, eventually, on intermediate and ultimate health outcomes (such as substance use and its consequences). The framework also depicts the monitoring system whereby coalition members and the evaluation team develop process, outcome, and impact measures.

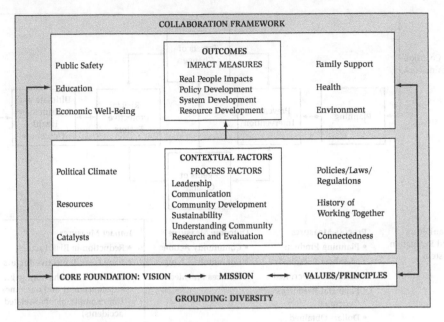

Figure 4.5 The Collaboration Framework.

Source: National Network for Collaboration, 1996. From *Collaboration framework: Addressing community capacity,* by Hogue, T., Perkins, D. F., Clark, R., Bergstrom, A., Slinski, M., & Associates (1995). Columbus, OH: The National Network for Collaboration. Reprinted with permission.

The Collaboration Framework

Another model, known as the Collaboration Framework, was developed through the joint efforts of eleven land-grant universities and the Cooperative States Research Education and Extension Service as a comprehensive guide to form new collaborative efforts, enhance existing efforts, and evaluate the progress of developing collaborations. Although not specifically focused on coalitions, it is included here because it serves as an invaluable tool for communicating, setting direction and focus, defining results, leveraging new resources, and diagnosing problems in coalitions. The Collaboration Framework, shown in Figure 4.5, depicts the common elements of collaboration as follows:

Grounding, the foundation of collaboration, is the diversity of gifts and talents that individuals, groups, organizations, and communities bring to the collaborative effort.

Core foundation is the shared vision, mission, values, and principles of the collaboration.

Contextual factors are characteristics of the ecology or environment that are related to the effectiveness of the collaboration (connectedness; history of working together; political climate; policies, laws, and regulations; resources; and catalysts).

Process factors deal with specific skills and components that are needed to build effective working relationships (for example, understanding the community, community development, leadership, communication, sustainability, research, and evaluation).

Outcomes are the specific conditions to be achieved in areas such as public safety, education, economic well-being, family support, health, and environment.

Impacts are specific measures that are related to these outcomes, such as real people impacts (behavior changes) and policy, systems, and resource developments.

Typology of Community Organization and Community Building

Minkler's and Wallerstein's (2005) Typology of Community Organization and Community Building has already been described in Chapter One (p. 11) as having great relevance for coalition work because it incorporates the classic need-based models (*community development* and *social action*) with the newer asset-based models (*community and capacity building* and *social action*) (p. 33).

The Conceptual Framework for Coalition Assessment

Sofaer developed The Conceptual Framework for Coalition Assessment in 1993 for the National Cancer Institute, to help evaluate coalitions that were associated with the ASSIST tobacco control program, and refined it in 2000. The model, as shown in Figure 4.6, shows that environmental characteristics, such as history of collaboration, community response, and geographic and cultural diversity, directly affect the structural and functional characteristics of the coalition as well as its programs and interventions. These interventions lead to, and are affected by, intermediate outcomes such as member commitment, involvement, perceptions of success, and expectations of effectiveness. Finally, the intermediate measures lead to longer-term outcomes of programs and policies, and institutionalization of the coalition itself.

Model of Community Health Governance

Finally, the Model of Community Health Governance (Lasker and Weiss, 2003) is a road map that lays out the pathways by which participatory processes lead to more effective community problem solving and to improvements in community health. According to Figure 4.7, the model proposes that communities need collaborative processes that achieve three intermediate outcomes: individual empowerment, bridging social ties, and synergy. All three of these intermediate outcomes are needed to strengthen community problem solving that directly improves health. These intermediate outcomes also improve health indirectly by enhancing the collaborative process to solve problems, which leads to improvements in community health.

The model also hypothesized that a collaborative process must have special kinds of leadership and management that lead to certain characteristics needed to achieve these intermediate outcomes. Leadership and management involve a variety of people, in both formal and informal capacities, who have different skills than those

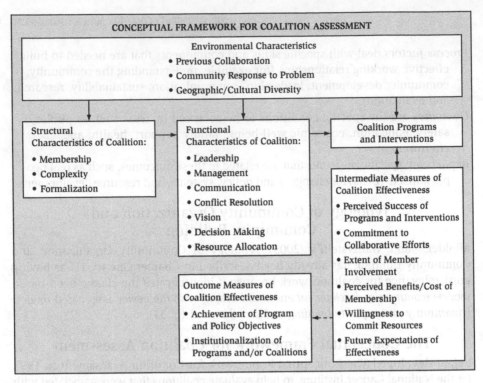

Figure 4.6 Conceptual Framework for Coalition Assessment.

Source: NCI, Sofaer, A Manual to Support Effective Community Health Coalitions, 2000, p. 2. NCI, S. Sofaer, *Working Together, Moving Ahead: A Manual to Support Effective Community Health Coalitions*, 2000, p. 2. Reprinted by permission of Shoshanna Sofaer.

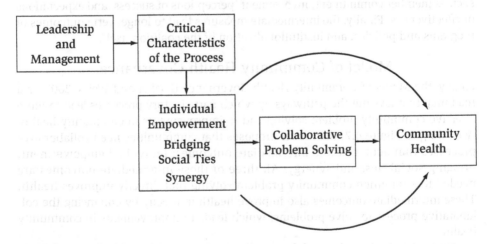

Figure 4.7 Model of Healthy Governance.

Source: Lasker & Weiss, 2003. From "Broadening Participation in Community Problem Solving: A Multi-disciplinary Model to Support Collaborative Practice and Research," by R. D. Lasker & E. S. Weiss in *Journal of Urban Health: Bulletin of the New York Academy of Medicine,* 80(1): 14–34, 2003. Reprinted with permission.

required to coordinate a program or its services. These leaders are collaborative—that is, they understand and appreciate different perspectives, bridge diverse cultures, and are comfortable in sharing ideas, resources, and power.

The other critical characteristics of the process are that a broad group of people and organizations must be involved, including people directly affected by the issues; all phases of problem solving should be designed and run by a diverse group of participants who are engaged as part of a learning community; and the process should focus on multiple issues and problems—including agenda setting, planning, and action—and should be iterative and ongoing. According to this model, social ties must be created among people and organizations from a broad range of backgrounds, disciplines, and sectors, including ties between community residents directly affected by problems and people with various kinds of professional expertise both from and beyond the local community. Further, the model proposes that the number, strength, and reciprocity of social relationships may actually increase the physical health, stress-coping mechanisms, sense of belonging, and social identity among people.

All of the aforementioned models and frameworks helped us to develop the Community Coalition Action Theory (CCAT). From these models and the practice literature, a wealth of practice-proven propositions have arisen. These propositions provide the basis for the development of a grounded theory about the development and maintenance of coalitions, as well as how they result in successful actions and health outcomes. CCAT is an attempt to provide a comprehensive theory that will lead to an increased understanding of how community coalitions work in practice. The next section describes the theory, constructs, and assumptions developed to further our understanding of these community-building entities.

COMMUNITY COALITION ACTION THEORY: ASSUMPTIONS AND CONSTRUCTS

It should be emphasized that the Community Coalition Action Theory applies primarily to community coalitions. A community coalition is different from other types of community entities in that a structured arrangement for collaboration among organizations exists in which all members work together toward a common purpose. If a group is composed solely of individuals and not organizations, then it is not a coalition in its truest form.

As an action-oriented partnership, a coalition usually focuses on preventing or ameliorating a community problem by analyzing the problem; gathering data and assessing need; developing an action plan with identified solutions; implementing those solutions; reaching community-level outcomes, such as health behavior changes; and creating social change (Whitt, 1993). This theory does not apply to short-term grassroots coalitions that form for a specific purpose, such as opposing a landfill, and then disband when the goal is achieved.

In addition, community coalitions are characterized as formal, multipurpose, and long-term alliances (Butterfoss, Goodman, and Wandersman, 1993). The scope of community coalition work tends to be local or regional, and coalitions usually have some paid staff whose time is dedicated to coalition efforts. The size of its membership varies, as does the diversity of professional and grassroots organizations and the individuals who represent these organizations. The degree of formalization of working relationships and role expectations ranges from very formal, with strict adherence to bylaws and contractual relationships, to rather informal.

The constructs behind the Community Coalition Action Theory are provided in a series of figures that dissect the model to explain it more clearly (Figures 4.8–4.12).

Outline of the CCAT Theory

In the complete CCAT Model, shown in Figure 4.8, coalitions progress through stages from formation to institutionalization, with frequent loops back to earlier stages as new issues arise or as planning cycles are repeated (Propositions 1 and 2). The theory also acknowledges contextual factors of the community, such as the sociopolitical climate, geography, history, and norms surrounding collaborative efforts that will impact each stage of coalition development from formation to institutionalization (Proposition 3). Figure 4.9 shows the details of how Propositions 1–3 relate to the model.

In the formation stages, depicted in Figure 4.10, a convener or lead agency with given strengths and linkages to the community brings together core organizations, which recruit an initial group of community partners to initiate a coalition effort focusing on a health or social issue of concern (Propositions 4–8).

Figure 4.11 illustrates how the coalition identifies key leaders and staff, who then develop structures (for example, committees and rules) and operating procedures (processes) that promote coalition effectiveness (Propositions 9–16). Structural

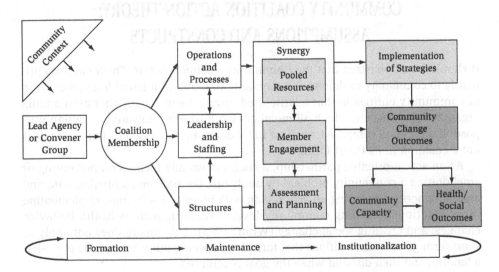

Figure 4.8 Community Coalition Action Theory.

Source: Butterfoss & Kegler, 2002.

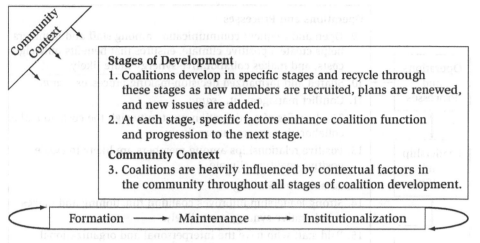

Figure 4.9 Community Coalition Action Theory: Propositions 1–3.

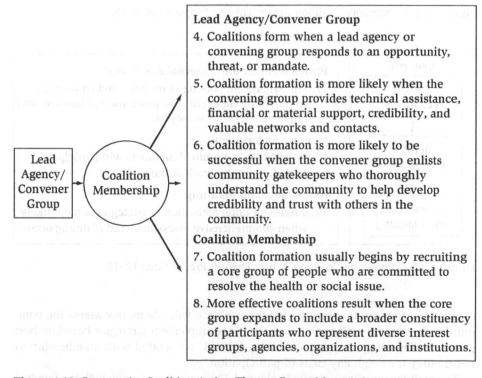

Figure 4.10 Community Coalition Action Theory: Propositions 4–8.

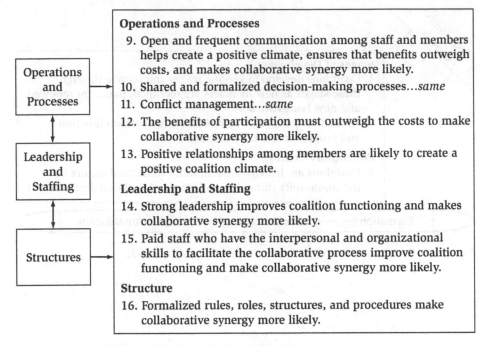

Operations and Processes

9. Open and frequent communication among staff and members helps create a positive climate, ensures that benefits outweigh costs, and makes collaborative synergy more likely.
10. Shared and formalized decision-making processes...*same*
11. Conflict management...*same*
12. The benefits of participation must outweigh the costs to make collaborative synergy more likely.
13. Positive relationships among members are likely to create a positive coalition climate.

Leadership and Staffing

14. Strong leadership improves coalition functioning and makes collaborative synergy more likely.
15. Paid staff who have the interpersonal and organizational skills to facilitate the collaborative process improve coalition functioning and make collaborative synergy more likely.

Structure

16. Formalized rules, roles, structures, and procedures make collaborative synergy more likely.

Figure 4.11 Community Coalition Action Theory: Propositions 9–16.

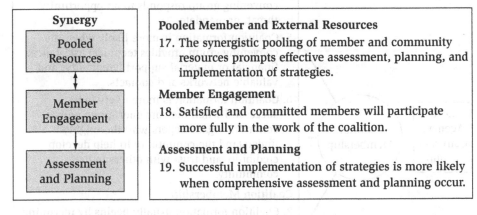

Pooled Member and External Resources

17. The synergistic pooling of member and community resources prompts effective assessment, planning, and implementation of strategies.

Member Engagement

18. Satisfied and committed members will participate more fully in the work of the coalition.

Assessment and Planning

19. Successful implementation of strategies is more likely when comprehensive assessment and planning occur.

Figure 4.12 Community Coalition Action Theory: Propositions 17–19.

elements in the coalition ensure that the coalition will adequately assess the community, develop an action plan, and select and implement strategies based on best practices. This stage requires balancing benefits associated with membership to ensure they outweigh any costs of participation.

The maintenance stage, shown in Figure 4.12, involves sustaining member involvement and taking concrete action steps to achieve the goals of the coalition. In public

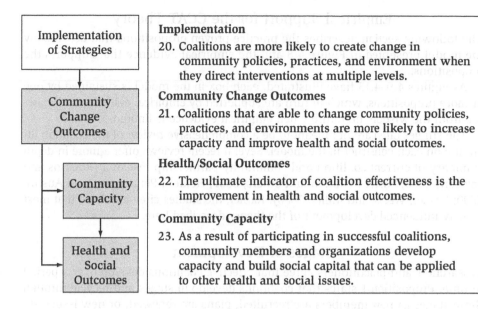

Implementation
20. Coalitions are more likely to create change in community policies, practices, and environment when they direct interventions at multiple levels.

Community Change Outcomes
21. Coalitions that are able to change community policies, practices, and environments are more likely to increase capacity and improve health and social outcomes.

Health/Social Outcomes
22. The ultimate indicator of coalition effectiveness is the improvement in health and social outcomes.

Community Capacity
23. As a result of participating in successful coalitions, community members and organizations develop capacity and build social capital that can be applied to other health and social issues.

Figure 4.13 Community Coalition Action Theory: Propositions 20–23.

health, these steps usually involve assessing, planning, selecting, and implementing strategies (Propositions 19 and 20). Success in this stage also depends on the mobilization and pooling of member and external resources (Proposition 17). The coalition relies on resources from members and external sources to design and then implement the planned strategies. Acquisition of resources, combined with a competent planning and implementation process, are precursors to successful transition to the institutionalization stage. With adequate resources, members become engaged in assessing, planning, and implementing strategies, and experience increased levels of commitment, participation, and satisfaction (Proposition 18).

In Figure 4.13, we see that by implementing strategies of sufficient duration and intensity according to the action plan, shorter-term outcomes such as changes in individual knowledge, beliefs, self-efficacy, and behavior, as well as changes in community systems, policies, practices, and environment, should occur (Propositions 20 and 21). These intermediate changes should lead to long-term outcomes, such as reductions in morbidity and mortality, or substantive progress toward other social goals (Proposition 22).

In the institutionalization stage, successful strategies result in outcomes. If resources have been adequately mobilized and strategies effectively address an ongoing need, coalition strategies may become institutionalized in a community as part of a long-term coalition or be adopted by organizations in the community. The coalition itself may or may not be institutionalized in a community. Both maintenance and institutionalization stages have the potential to increase community capacity to solve problems. Progress in ameliorating one community problem can potentially increase the capacity of local organizations to apply these skills and resources to address additional issues that resonate with the community (Proposition 23).

Empirical Support for the CCAT Theory

The following section describes the practice-proven propositions that accompany the model presented in Figure 4.8 and the empirical evidence that supports the propositions.

As Figures 4.9–4.13 have illustrated, each box in the model is sustained by one or more propositions, which in turn are supported by empirical evidence and material from the wisdom literature when empirical evidence is limited.

The studies cited are not meant to be a comprehensive review of the coalition literature on each construct in the model. Several recent reviews offer a more in-depth summary of current coalition and community-partnership research (Roussos and Fawcett, 2000; Foster-Fishman and others, 2001; Holden, Pendergast, and Austin, 2000; Lasker, Weiss, and Miller, 2000). Rather, the studies cited are those that most heavily influenced development of the theory described here.

Stages of Development

Researchers and practitioners agree that effective coalitions develop over a period of time. Proposition 1 states that coalitions develop in stages and recycle through these stages as new members are recruited, plans are renewed, or new issues are added. Thus, the process of building and maintaining coalitions is not linear, but rather cyclical, with coalitions returning to earlier stages as community situations dictate (McLeroy and others, 1994). The naming of those stages and the specific tasks that should be accomplished at each stage, however, differ. Several different series of stages have been proposed, including formation, implementation, maintenance, and outcomes (Butterfoss, Goodman, and Wandersman, 1993); planning, intervention, and outcomes (Fawcett, Paine, Francisco, and Vliet, 1993); and mobilizing, establishing structure and function, building capacity for action, planning for action, implementation, refinement, and institutionalization (Florin, Mitchell, and Stevenson, 1993).

Researchers and practitioners agree that the following tasks must occur at some stage to assure coalition effectiveness: recruiting and mobilizing coalition members, establishing organizational structure, building capacity and planning for action, selecting and implementing strategies, evaluating outcomes, refining strategies and approaches, and institutionalizing those strategies or the coalition itself (McLeroy and others, 1994). The same authors agree that at each stage, certain factors enhance coalition function and progression to the next stage (Proposition 2). In a recent study of coalition development, seven community coalitions established to address childhood asthma management took an average of twelve months to form, and five of seven coalitions progressed to the institutionalization stage by their fourth year (Butterfoss and others, 2006). Important factors in how well they progressed thorough the stages were community context, their maturity as coalitions, and whether they had experience in working collaboratively.

The detailed tasks that are likely to occur at each stage have also been described (Mizrahi and Rosenthal, 2001). In the asthma study by Butterfoss and colleagues (2006), staff self-rated their coalitions as having completed 98 percent of formation tasks, 95 percent of implementation tasks, 86 percent of maintenance tasks, and

62 percent of institutionalization tasks. The percentage of accomplished tasks decreased as tasks later in the life cycle became more difficult. Finally, those who study or work in coalition settings agree that to accomplish their objectives, attention must be paid to maintaining coalitions and constantly recruiting new organizations in order to increase the coalition's impact (Kreuter, Lezin, and Young, 2000; Kaye and Wolff, 1995; Dowling, O'Donnell, and Wellington Consulting Group, 2000; Butterfoss and others, 1998). Most of the research to date focuses on the early stages of coalition development; consequently, less is known about the factors related to coalition success in the later stages of development.

Community Context

Coalitions are embedded in communities, and as a result, factors in the environment can have a significant impact on a coalition (Butterfoss and others, 1993; McLeroy and others, 1994; Lasker and others, 2000). Proposition 3 asserts that coalitions are heavily influenced by contextual factors throughout all stages of development. Several studies support this proposition. For example, Reininger and colleagues (1999) discuss tension and mistrust between groups and how the lack of trust affected a coalition. Others have documented the impact of political and administrative contexts on coalitions (Dill, 1994; Clark and others, 1993; Nelson, 1994). Kegler, Steckler, Malek, and McLeroy (1998a) noted the impact of tobacco-related politics on tobacco control coalitions in several stages of coalition development, from recruitment in the formation stage to types of activities conducted in the maintenance stage. History of collaboration is widely cited in the wisdom and theoretical literature as another contextual factor that can affect the formation of collaborative relationships, including coalitions (Gray, 1989), with positive norms for collaboration increasing the likelihood of future successful collaboration. Additional contextual factors that affect coalitions include social capital (including trust between segments of a community), geography, and community readiness (Wolff, 2001a).

Lead Agency or Convener Group

Proposition 4 states that coalitions usually form when a lead agency or convener group responds to an opportunity, threat, or mandate. Propositions 5 and 6 state that a lead agency begins coalition formation by recruiting a core group of community leaders and providing initial support for the coalition. The lead agency or convener is the organization that has the vision or mandate to initially mobilize community members to form a coalition focused on a specific issue of concern. This organization may or may not have written a grant or otherwise procured funds for coalition operation. The convener does, however, accept responsibility to host an initial meeting and recruit prospective partners. The lead agency may also provide physical space for coalition operation and a part- or full-time staff person to manage the initiative.

Although the practice literature acknowledges that the convening agency must have sufficient organizational capacity, commitment, leadership, and vision to build an effective coalition, research on these and other factors that lead agencies should possess is sorely lacking (Butterfoss and others, 1993). In one of the few studies comparing coalitions with differing reasons for initiation, Mansergh and colleagues

(1996) found that researcher- and community-initiated coalitions were similar in terms of perceived coalition efficiency, outcome efficacy, benefits of involvement, and interagency collaboration. The only difference between the two was that action committee effectiveness ranked higher in the researcher-initiated coalition. The researchers concluded that factors other than the impetus for initiation may be more critical for coalition effectiveness. A related area with little research is whether coalitions develop anew or simply evolve from other pre-existing coalitions and networks in a community (Herman, Wolfson, and Forster, 1993; Nezlek and Galano, 1993).

Coalition Membership

Again, limited research has focused on the defining characteristics of the founding members of community coalitions. Common wisdom holds that previous experience with the health issue or with coalitions increases the commitment of these core members. Research shows that members participate in coalitions with varying levels of intensity, what Brager, Sprecht, and Torczner (1987) describe as "active, occasional, and supporting participants." Flexible participation is essential when working with volunteers.

Composition of the core group may affect its ability to engage a broad spectrum of the community. Propositions 6, 7, and 8 state that the core group must recruit community gatekeepers, those committed to the issue, and a broad constituency of diverse groups and organizations. This pooling of diverse views, perspectives, and resources is one of the hallmarks of coalitions and gives them the potential to solve problems that individual agencies could not address alone. As such, effective coalitions make concerted efforts to recruit diverse memberships, in terms of expertise, constituencies, sectors, perspectives, and backgrounds. Additionally, funders are often concerned about increasing the diversity of coalition members, as evidenced by the recent focus on reducing health disparities in such efforts as CDC's REACH initiative.

Coalition Operations and Processes

Coalitions must fulfill certain basic functions such as making decisions, communicating, and managing conflict (Propositions 9–11). Indeed, much of the research on coalitions has focused on internal processes and operations, with the assumption that effective internal functioning is necessary for progress in achieving goals. The quality of interactions among member networks is demonstrated by the frequency and intensity of contacts as well as the benefits that members receive from them, such as emotional or tangible support and access to social contacts (Israel, 1982). Research demonstrates that the extent of regular contacts among community members can foster cooperation (Putnam, 1993). Similarly, members can be empowered by building networks and experiencing positive social relationships (Kumpher, Turner, Hopkins, and Librett, 1993). Research has also shown that frequent and productive communication and networking among members increases satisfaction, commitment, and implementation of strategies (Rogers and others, 1993; Kegler and others, 1998). Similarly, staff is most satisfied and committed when good communication exists between members and themselves (Rogers and others, 1993).

Members who report an increase in the number and type of linkages with outside organizations participate more in the coalition (Butterfoss and others, 1996; Mayer and others, 1998). Coalition studies have also examined decision making and shown that the influence that participants have in making decisions is vital to a partnership. Influence in decision making is related to increased satisfaction, participation, and reporting of more positive benefits (Butterfoss and others, 1996; Mayer and others, 1998).

Another internal process that must be initiated to ensure smooth internal functioning is conflict management. Mizrahi and Rosenthal (1993) argue that conflict is an inherent characteristic of partnerships. Conflict may arise between the partnership and its priorities for social change or among partners concerning issues such as loyalty, leadership, goals, benefits, contributions, and representation. Conflict has been shown to lead to staff turnover, avoidance of certain activities, and difficulty in recruiting members (Kegler, Steckler, Malek, and McLeroy, 1998a). Conflict transformation is the process whereby resolution of conflict strengthens the coalition and builds capacity. Research shows that it results from effective coalition planning and contributes to coalition goal attainment (Mayer and others, 1998).

Proposition 12 posits that benefits must outweigh costs to ensure ongoing participation in assessment, planning, and resource development. The literature points out several examples where member costs and benefits were related to the process of engagement. In general, providing incentives and reducing costs increased member participation in voluntary associations (Wandersman, Florin, Friedmann, and Meier, 1987; Prestby and others, 1990) and in coalition committees, especially during the formation and early maintenance stages (Butterfoss and others, 1996; Butterfoss and others, 1998; Chinman and others, 1996; Mayer and others, 1998). The wisdom literature is consistent in encouraging coalition leaders to provide incentives for continued participation (Kaye and Wolff, 1995).

Another factor related to member engagement is the organizational climate of the coalition. Proposition 13 states that positive relationships among members are likely to create a productive coalition environment or climate. Organizational climate refers to members' perceptions of the "personality" of an organization and is typically measured by ten factors: cohesion, leader support, expression, independence, task orientation, self-discovery, anger and aggression, order and organization, leader control, and innovation (Moos, 1986). Organizational climate characteristics (for example, leader support and leader control) are related to satisfaction with the work, participation in the partnership, and costs and benefits (Butterfoss and others, 1996) as well as implementation of action plans (Kegler, Steckler, McLeroy, and Malek, 1998b). Researchers have also found that task focus is related to satisfaction (Kegler, Steckler, McLeroy, and Malek, 1998b) and psychological and organizational empowerment (McMillan, 1995). Similarly, the wisdom literature points out the value of promoting positive group climate and relationships among members (Kaye and Wolff, 1995; Dowling, O'Donnell, and Wellington Consulting Group, 2000).

Leadership and Staffing

Propositions 14 and 15 emphasize the importance of leadership and staffing in coalitions. Without these, coalitions are unlikely to move beyond the initial steps in the formation stage of development. Coalition leaders and staff organize the structure through which coalitions accomplish their work and are responsible for coalition processes such as communication and decision making, which keep members satisfied and committed to coalition efforts. Effective coalition leadership requires a collection of qualities and skills that are typically not found in one individual, but rather in a team of committed leaders. A common approach to leadership in coalitions is the formation of steering committees composed of leaders from action-focused work groups. Empirical research on coalitions shows a consistent relationship between leader competence and satisfaction.

Leadership is complex and researchers have examined many facets in addition to member perceptions of leader competence (Glidewell, Kelly, Bagby, and Dickerson, 1998). For example, Kumpher and colleagues (1993) studied leadership style and found that an empowering style was related to action-plan quality. Butterfoss and colleagues (1996) found that leader support and control were related to several member-related outcomes, but not to plan quality. Reininger and colleagues (1999) explored whether leaders being indigenous affected coalitions. In a study of ten rural coalitions formed to prevent drug abuse, Braithwaite, Taylor, and Austin (2000) noted that the most successful coalitions had strong leadership and a commitment to a common goal. Others have found that the ability of a coalition to develop a clear and shared vision, a likely result of good leadership, is associated with success (Kegler, Steckler, McLeroy, and Malek, 1998b; Center for Substance Abuse Prevention, 1998).

In many coalitions, leadership and staffing are intertwined, with paid staff fulfilling many leadership functions, such as setting agendas and facilitating meetings. Staff often support the coalition, encourage membership involvement, and build community capacity (Sanchez, 2000). Some research suggests that coalitions with staff who play a supportive role for the coalition, rather than a visible leadership role, have higher levels of implementation (Kegler, Steckler, Malek, and McLeroy, 1998a).

Several studies of coalitions have examined how staffing is related to intermediate indicators of effectiveness, including member-related outcomes, plan quality, resource mobilization, and implementation of planned activities. Two of these studies demonstrate relationships between staff competence and member satisfaction (Rogers and others, 1993; Kegler, Steckler, Malek, and McLeroy, 1998a). Butterfoss and colleagues (1996) found an association between staff competence and member benefits. Kegler and colleagues (1998a) also found a relationship between staff time devoted to coalition efforts and the amount of resources mobilized and the level of implementation of planned activities, thereby lending support to the need for paid staff with sufficient time to devote to the coalition. Minimal or nondisruptive staff turnover has also been linked to positive outcomes (Center for Substance Abuse Prevention, 1998; Kegler, Steckler, Malek, and McLeroy, 1998a).

Coalition Structures

Proposition 16 asserts that coalitions are more likely to engage members, pool resources, and assess and plan well when they formalize rules, roles, structures, and procedures by precisely defining them. Examples of formal structures include committees; written memoranda of understanding; bylaws; policy and procedures manuals; clearly defined roles; mission statements, goals, and objectives; and regular reorientation to the purposes, goals, roles, and procedures of collaboration (Butterfoss and others, 1993; Goodman and Steckler, 1989). Formal structures often result in the routinization or persistent implementation of the partnership's operations. The more routinized operations become, the more likely they will be sustained (Goodman and Steckler, 1989). Research shows that the existence of formal structural elements such as bylaws, agendas, and minutes are related to organizational commitment (Rogers and others, 1993). Additionally, structuring a coalition to focus on action, for example, by creating task forces or action teams, is associated with increased resource mobilization and implementation of strategies (Kegler, Steckler, Malek, and McLeroy, 1998a).

Pooled Member and External Resources

A major premise underlying the widespread adoption of coalitions to address community problems is that working together creates a synergy that enables individuals and organizations to accomplish more than they could achieve independently (McLeroy and others, 1994). Proposition 17 asserts that this pooling of resources ensures more effective assessment, planning, and implementation of strategies. Resource sharing also gives coalitions unique advantages over less collaborative problem-solving approaches. Lasker, Weiss, and Miller (2001) correctly point out that much of the research on coalitions focuses on internal functioning but does not explicate the pathways through which collaboration increases the likelihood of achieving outcomes over traditional single agency interventions. They propose that synergy is the mechanism through which partnerships gain advantage over more traditional, less collaborative approaches. Further, they hypothesize that synergy is the proximal outcome that links partnership functioning to achievement of outcomes.

Resources, defined broadly, are one of the major determinants of synergy as conceptualized by Lasker and colleagues. Coalition members are the greatest asset in a coalition-based initiative. They bring energy, knowledge, skills, expertise, perspectives, connections, and tangible resources to the table. The pooling of these diverse resources enables coalition members to achieve together what they could not accomplish alone. Research has shown that staffing and structure of coalitions are related to resource mobilization, which in turn is related to effective implementation of coalition strategies (Kegler, Steckler, Malek, and McLeroy, 1998a). Successful resource mobilization allows for more solutions that are creative and more practical, comprehensive approaches (Lasker and others, 2000).

Resources from outside the membership, and even outside the community, are also helpful, as they often fund staff and pay costs associated with implementing planned activities. Such resources relieve some of the burden faced by communities with limited financial resources. External resources may also provide additional expertise, meeting facilities, mailing lists, referrals, additional personnel for special projects, grant funding, loans or donations, equipment, supplies, and co-sponsorship of events (Chavis, Florin, Rich, and Wandersman, 1987; Prestby and Wandersman, 1985; Braithwaite, Taylor, and Austin, 2000).

Member Engagement

Member engagement is best defined as the process by which members are empowered and develop a sense of belonging to the coalition. Positive engagement is evidenced by commitment to the mission and goals of the coalition, high levels of participation both in and outside of coalition meetings and activities, and satisfaction with the work of the coalition. Two factors enhance engagement, namely, that the benefits of membership outweigh the costs and that members experience a positive coalition environment (Propositions 12 and 13) (Butterfoss and others, 1996).

As previously stated, members who experience more benefits than costs participate more fully and are more satisfied with the work of the coalition. Proposition 18 asserts that satisfied and committed members will have higher levels of participation than less satisfied members.

Research supports this assertion and consistently demonstrates that satisfied and committed members will also participate more in the work of the coalition (Butterfoss and others, 1996; Kumpher, Turner, Hopkins, and Librett, 1993; Roberts-DeGennaro, 1986; Rogers and others, 1993; Mayer and others, 1998). Although satisfied and highly participating members are valued, the same studies did not demonstrate that these factors lead to desired intermediate outcomes (for example, producing high-quality action plans) or long-term outcomes (reducing ATOD use). However, case examples of coalitions exist where practitioners attribute their intermediate and long-range successes to the commitment and satisfaction of their members (Butterfoss and others, 1998).

Assessment and Planning

Achieving a coalition's goals involves assessing the situation and deciding on what action to take. A coalition-based initiative—such as one that is a part of a state or national program—usually engages in an extensive assessment and planning process. This process, lasting as long as two years in some initiatives, is typically followed by a three- to five-year implementation phase. Several coalition studies have examined the quality of the action plans produced by these types of coalition efforts. Analyses of activities selected by coalitions have shown a tendency toward activities that promote changes in awareness (Florin, Mitchell, and Stevenson, 1993). Kreuter, Lezin, and Young (2000) note that despite a strong emphasis on needs assessment, written objectives, and logic models that depict cause-effect relationships between interventions and outcomes, many collaborative efforts fail to produce rigorous plans. Quality plans, associated in several studies with competent staffing, leadership, and resource mobilization, contribute to successful implementation (Butterfoss, 1996; Kumpher, Turner, Hopkins, and Librett, 1993; Kegler, Steckler, Malek, and McLeroy 1998a). Proposition 19 states that successful implementation of strategies is more likely when comprehensive planning and assessment occur.

Implementation of Strategies

Successful implementation depends on numerous factors such as sufficient resources, completion of tasks on schedule, fidelity to the planned intervention strategies, and a supportive (or non-turbulent) organizational and community environment. Assuming the interventions link logically to planned outcomes, the likelihood of achieving these outcomes depends on the extent to which the strategies are implemented and reach the priority populations. Adaptations of interventions that have been previously evaluated (evidence-based) or are commonly accepted as best practices increase the likelihood that interventions will result in community change and, ultimately, desired health and social outcomes. Using best practices or evidence-based interventions should minimize the tendency of coalitions to focus so heavily on building community awareness. This tendency to focus on quick wins may help to maintain member interest but is unlikely to lead to more valued outcomes; and it may help explain why some coalition-based efforts are not able to achieve systems or health outcomes change (Kreuter, Lezin, and Young, 2000).

Most researchers and practitioners agree that effective health-promotion efforts require change at multiple levels, including environmental and policy change (McLeroy, Bibeau, Steckler, and Glanz, 1988). Goodman and colleagues (1996) further suggest that as coalition interventions become more complex and focus less on individual behavior change, the assessments of such coalitions should focus across multiple levels and take into account community readiness. Proposition 20 emphasizes the importance of implementing interventions at multiple levels to create change in community policies, practices, and environments.

Community Change Outcomes

By implementing interventions at multiple levels, coalitions are able to create change in communities that can reduce risk factors and increase protective factors. Fawcett and colleagues (1997) categorize these into changes in programs, changes in policies, and changes in practices of community agencies, businesses, and government entities. Coalitions can also create change in communities by enhancing the skills of individuals, increasing the sense of community, and providing new perspectives on community-problem solving for residents. At other levels, coalitions can create change in opportunities for civic participation, linkages between organizations, and the physical and social environment of a community (Kegler, Twiss, and Look, 2000). The Community Coalition Action Theory posits that coalitions that are able to create these types of community change are more likely to increase community capacity to address other issues of concern and to realize their long-term goals (Proposition 21).

Health and Social Outcomes

Proposition 22 states that the ultimate indicator of coalition effectiveness is improvement in health, social outcomes, or both. Several recent reviews have been published documenting only modest evidence of effective collaborative partnerships. Roussos and Fawcett (2000) reviewed 34 studies that represented 252 collaborative partnerships. The authors categorized the studies into those that provided evidence for more distant population-level outcomes, community-wide behavior change, or environmental change. The review stated that research is insufficient to make strong conclusions about the impact of partnerships on population-level outcomes, largely due to design issues (most of the research consists of case studies). With respect to community-wide behavior change, Roussos and Fawcett concluded that partnerships can make modest contributions. Strongest evidence existed for the contribution of partnership to environmental change, broadly defined to include changes in programs, services, and practices.

Similarly, Kreuter, Lezin, and Young (2000) reviewed sixty-eight published descriptions of coalitions and consortia with evaluation protocols in place and found only six examples of documented health status or systems change. Numerous reasons have been discussed in the literature as possible explanations for the disappointing findings associated with collaborative initiatives (Roussos and Fawcett, 2000; Mittelmark, 1999; Kreuter, Lezin, and Young, 2000; Berkowitz, 2001). In addition to design issues and secular trends that make detecting community-level change challenging, some note that coalitions tend to focus on "quick wins" and awareness activities. These strategies alone will not lead to significant changes in systems or health status. Proposition 22 states that the ultimate indicator of coalition effectiveness is the improvement in health and social outcomes.

Community Capacity

In addition to coalition outcomes associated with health or social issues, another set of outcomes is associated with increases in a community's capacity to solve problems. Proposition 23 asserts that coalitions can enhance community capacity. Community capacity has been discussed both as a possible prerequisite to community problem solving and as an outcome of community health-promotion efforts (Goodman and others, 1998; Norton and others, 2002). It includes dimensions that coalitions can theoretically impact (either positively or negatively) such as participation and leadership, networks of individuals and organizations, skills and resources, and sense of community. Crisp, Swerissen, and Duckett (2000) identify the development of partnerships as one of four distinct approaches to building capacity, arguing that two-way communication between groups not previously working together can result in more resources for planning and implementation. Little coalition research has focused on outcomes associated with community capacity, although current evaluation research is examining these issues (Norton and others, 2002).

APPLICATION OF CCAT: CONSORTIUM FOR THE IMMUNIZATION OF NORFOLK'S CHILDREN (CINCH)

To ground the CCAT theory, a community coalition known as the Consortium for the Immunization of Norfolk's Children, or CINCH, will be used to illustrate how the theory works in practice. In 1992, the CDC National Immunization Program established Norfolk, Virginia, as a site to demonstrate how a community coalition could improve immunization rates for children under two years of age. Norfolk was selected due to its low immunization rates (49 percent of two-year-olds in 1993); ethnic diversity; and public, private, and military health care systems. By helping citizens develop and implement comprehensive, effective strategies, CINCH worked to increase childhood immunization rates by 17 percent. The following section shows how CINCH followed the community coalition model that was presented in Figure 4.8.

Stages of Development

CINCH was in the formation stage for approximately six months. During this time, under-immunization was defined as a community problem; coalition members were recruited; mission, rules, and roles were specified; and members were trained. During the next stage—maintenance—coalition membership was sustained and actual work began. Coalition members assessed needs, collected and analyzed data, developed a plan, initiated and monitored strategies, and supported and evaluated their group process. After three years, the coalition expanded geographically to include the Hampton Roads region, and was renamed the Consortium for Infant and Child Health (same acronym). CINCH subsequently recycled through formation and maintenance stages as it engaged in new recruitment and a needs-assessment process.

Community Context

In February 1997, CINCH released the Report on the Health of Children in Hampton Roads. After engaging in a priority-setting process, the coalition decided to focus on immunization and add perinatal issues (such as low birth weight, teen pregnancy, infant mortality) to its mission. CINCH collaborated with and re-energized an existing perinatal council, and eventually relinquished responsibility for this health issue (institutionalization stage).

In March 2000, the Second Report on the Health of Children in Hampton Roads identified childhood asthma as the number one diagnosis for regional hospital admission as well as emergency room and physician visits. CINCH then launched an asthma work group, and applied for and received funding from Robert Wood Johnson in 2001. The coalition recruited new members with asthma expertise and concern, and conducted an asthma-related needs assessment. Finally, in March 2005, a third report identified childhood obesity as a priority, and once again new partners were recruited and a new work group (Obesity Prevention) was formed. CINCH recycled through the developmental stages at least three times during eight years as new issues arose, strategies were revised, or new members were recruited.

Lead Agency or Convener Group

The Center for Pediatric Research, a joint program of a children's hospital and a medical school, convened CINCH and serves as its lead agency. Although the Center was new, the region valued collaborative efforts and embraced the concept of coalition building as proposed by the Center staff, who were experienced with this strategy. The staff recruited a core group of organizations, which then recruited fifty-five more organizations, including service agencies; academic, civic, and faith-based institutions; health care providers; and parents.

Coalition Membership

Members from various grassroots and professional organizations provided diversity in age, occupation, race, and ethnicity. They willingly put aside differences in order to share responsibility for all of the community's children. Relying on new knowledge and core values, the coalition developed its mission to improve immunization rates for children less than two years of age. This common mission and commitment to community improvement helped members overcome barriers that often stall new coalitions, such as lack of direction and turf battles (Kaye and Wolff, 1995; Butterfoss, Goodman, and Wandersman, 1996).

Coalition Operations and Processes

Members reported that they had either a great degree of influence (74 percent) or some influence (26 percent) in determining policies and actions of the consortium. When conflict arose, 82 percent reported that they were able to resolve it effectively. Content analysis of meetings showed that activities were balanced among tasks of orienting members, assessing needs, planning and revising coalition structure and functions, sharing information, and developing and evaluating products or services. Members evaluated meetings to identify successful elements (Goodman and Wandersman, 1994) and rated work group and general meetings as 88 percent and 92 percent effective, respectively. Leaders and staff debriefed about barriers to effective meetings and recommended improving agendas, attendance, timeliness, participation, leadership, and grassroots representation.

Leadership and Staffing

From the onset, CINCH had a full-time staff coordinator and part-time administrative assistant. The leaders of the coalition were community members who were elected by the membership. The steering committee, which consisted of coalition and work group chairs and vice-chairs, as well as staff and other non-voting honorary members, prepared the job description, advertised, interviewed, and hired the coalition coordinator. The coordinator had previously served as a coalition member but now worked for the coalition.

Leaders were sensitive to member needs by allowing varying levels of participation during each coalition stage. They reduced burnout and maximized resources by recognizing that some members are better *planners*, whereas others are better *doers*. Staff supported members by preparing draft documents, minutes, rosters, meeting reminders, and mailings. They helped leaders set agendas, run effective meetings, and plan strategies to promote member retention. To engage members, lead agency staff provided training on a variety of issues related to immunization.

Membership and commitment may waiver when a coalition realizes that it takes time to accomplish its goals. To keep members involved, CINCH participated in health fairs, marches, and other community health efforts. Leaders worked to maximize member participation. Meetings provided opportunities to cultivate and renew relationships and to celebrate incremental achievements. Members received written reminders and phone calls about meetings, and follow-up when they were absent. Member surveys measured satisfaction and participation, and defined areas for improvement.

Coalition Structures

Members developed written rules of operation, criteria for membership, and roles for members, leaders, and staff. CINCH also developed work groups focused on specific tasks and populations that complemented each other. Chairs and vice-chairs were elected for work groups and the coalition at large.

Pooled Member and External Resources

Each member brought individual skills to the coalition, but also represented an organization that brought resources to the table. Member organizations contributed financially or in-kind to implement strategies, because grant funds were earmarked only for research. When personal agendas are put aside, resources may be effectively pooled. Work group members invited health department and hospital directors, as well as professional and voluntary agencies from neighboring cities, to join them at the table. As previously competitive organizations learned the value of collaborating to accomplish tasks, the level of trust improved.

Funding restrictions prompted CINCH to develop community support for its activities and increased the likelihood of it sustaining its efforts beyond the grant period. Private foundation funding enabled the coalition to hire an outreach coordinator, conduct a media campaign, and implement key strategies. In-kind contributions from CINCH members included printing posters, flyers, and brochures; arranging satellite teleconferences; and contributing parent incentives. In this way, the resources from the federal grant, local foundation, and member organizations complemented each other and created synergy.

Member Engagement

Training, clearly defined roles, and ongoing contact with participating institutions were essential for member retention. Member involvement was bolstered by achievement of objectives and positive results. An explicit vision of leadership and commitment to a quality process kept members interested. CINCH also made good use of each member's linkage with others. Members constantly recruited others who provided resources or represented the priority population. New recruits stimulated creativity and renewed effort among founding members. Member surveys showed that 86 percent were satisfied with the work of the coalition (Butterfoss and others, 1998). Average attendance over 130 CINCH meetings was 59 percent, considered acceptable by coalition research (Prestby and Wandersman, 1985).

Assessment and Planning

Following formation, CINCH's major tasks focused on needs assessment, data collection, analysis, feedback, and plan development. First, work group members participated in a needs assessment to diagnose local causes of under-immunization. Parent focus groups, patient exit interviews, household and health care provider surveys were planned and conducted (Houseman, Butterfoss, Morrow, and Rosenthal, 1997; Butterfoss and others, 1998).

Staff conducted workshops to train work group members to develop quality action plans. Once trained, each work group used data to identify a prioritized set of needs related to their priority group (for example, parents, health care providers). Goals, objectives, and strategies were developed to address each identified community need. The groups considered the strengths of their community and the resources they could draw on to implement various strategies. Linkages among community agencies were identified, and evaluation of strategies was planned. Work group leaders combined the individual plans into one overall two-year strategic immunization plan. The plan focused on parent and provider education and support for at-risk families, thereby increasing access to immunizations and improving immunization delivery. The intrinsic negotiation involved in this process cemented relationships among group leaders and strengthened internal support for the plan. The planning process led to the creation of a steering committee that still meets regularly to share successes and challenges. Members also learned that planning is a continuous process, and later they developed timelines, management plans, and budgets.

Implementation of Strategies

During this time, new strategies were initiated and others were maintained and monitored. Work groups collaborated on strategies and responsibilities and even merged to streamline operations. Some activities were initiated and finished quickly, while others were not achieved until after funding ended. CINCH had an impact on the Norfolk community by effectively implementing sixty-one of seventy-nine planned strategies (77 percent). An evaluation component for each strategy helped members to decide whether it was based on need and had been implemented as planned, and whether it could be improved. Action plans were revised annually.

Community Change and Health Outcomes

CINCH accomplished some of its more difficult objectives such as WIC linkage, physician practice assessment and feedback, hospital birth reminder systems, and legislative action. Members not only directed the course of community events but also wielded power to influence larger institutions, such as hospitals and the state legislature. Although change in immunization levels for two-year-olds could not be attributed to CINCH alone, rates rose from 48 percent in 1993 to 66 percent in 1996 (Morrow and others, 1998). Higher rates were reported among hospital and military clinics.

Community Capacity

Through training and practice in leadership, meeting facilitation, needs assessment, and planning, coalition members developed skills that improved their participation and could be generalized to other civic areas. Members and staff also provide technical assistance to other local partnerships that deal with tobacco use, child safety, and school health. Additionally, CINCH collaborates with projects focused on case management, community policing, and neighborhood improvement. Moreover, CINCH fostered new state contracts and federal grants that promote environmental change. A contract between CINCH's lead agency and the state health department was forged to develop and manage a state immunization coalition, Project Immunize Virginia (PIV). PIV used the CINCH model to help other localities develop community partnerships to advocate for immunizing children across the state. Under an Association of Teachers of Preventive Medicine grant, the Coalition

Training Institute was established in Norfolk in 1995. The Institute trains key health agency staff who coordinate immunization coalitions in eighty-eight urban, state, and territorial sites (Butterfoss, Webster, Morrow, and Rosenthal, 1998).

STRENGTHS AND LIMITATIONS OF THE THEORY, OR MODEL

Any new theory is bound to have strengths and limitations and must be open to constructive criticism from practitioners and researchers who have a stake in the related work. Although the Community Coalition Action Theory is long overdue, the benefit of the delay is that it is based on almost two decades of practice and research. Perhaps one reason that this theory has not been developed before is that the complexity of community coalitions and the multifaceted nature of their work overwhelms researchers and practitioners alike. The model that describes our theory is likewise complex and takes into account the diverse factors that influence the formation, implementation, and maintenance of coalitions.

Although community coalitions are found in a variety of settings that range from urban to rural, the empirical research and subsequent findings have focused mostly in the area of alcohol, tobacco, and other drug abuse prevention. This is not surprising, when one considers that the highest level of foundation and governmental agency funding for coalition work has centered on this health issue. Though coalitions exist for many other health issues, including cardiovascular disease, HIV/AIDS, unintentional injury prevention, and immunization, large-scale evaluative research findings on the coalitions themselves have not yet been reported for these issues. Similarly, much of the research that forms the basis of the Community Coalition Action Theory is from studies conducted in the early 1990s and tends to focus on coalition functioning and intermediate indicators of effectiveness, such as satisfaction, participation, action plan quality, and implementation. Because of the widely acknowledged difficulty in attributing health outcome change to community collaborative efforts, much of the more recent research uses case study methodology. Although very informative, case study findings are difficult to generalize from, and they focus less often on associations among constructs.

The constructs that are used in the theory are informed by research, yet we speculated on how they interrelate with one another. We used a set of propositions to help order the constructs in a logical sequence and develop reciprocal or directional linkages among them. But the research evidence does not totally assure that these assumptions are correct. In addition, we have not weighted each variable in our model—how important are coalition processes, for example, compared to coalition structures? The model does not quantify the resources needed to implement successful strategies, nor the level of member engagement that leads to effective assessment and planning. Further research should help clarify the constructs, their importance to the whole, linkage patterns, and directionality.

The model is further complicated by the complexity of each of the constructs. For example, the operation and processes construct includes communication, decision making, and conflict management. All of these are likely related to organizational climate, but which are more important and in what situations and stages? Similarly, we identify several dimensions of community context and assert that context affects each construct in the model and each stage in coalition development. Yet much research remains to be done to understand how distribution of power in a community, for example, affects what organization serves as the lead agency, who makes up the core group, and whose needs are assessed.

Numerous types of collaborative relationships exist. We focused on community coalitions and defined them as long-term community structures that enable organizations and individuals to work collaboratively to address community problems. We also were careful not to cite research done with other types of collaborative initiatives, because in the past, careful distinctions have not been made when summarizing "coalition" findings. Different types of collaborative partnerships (state-level, grassroots, mandated, voluntary, and so on) may function differently and be influenced by different factors in each stage of coalition development. It may also be necessary to conceptualize stages of coalition development variously for diverse types of partnerships. For example, a grassroots coalition formed to keep a landfill out of a neighborhood may not need to institutionalize anything, once the landfill is sited elsewhere.

FUTURE DIRECTIONS

With the advent of evidence-based medicine and outcome-based interventions, coalitions have recently been criticized for not meeting expectations for success (Green, 2000). Given the tremendous infusion of resources, both monetary and in donated volunteer time, some feel this criticism is well deserved. In truth, the overall evidence for positive coalition outcomes is lacking. Traditional scientific methodology may not be adequate to capture the outcomes of these complex collaborative organizations (Berkowitz, 2000). We cannot underestimate the amount of time that it takes to create and sustain viable coalitions, the difficulty in identifying and implementing "best practices," the reluctance to accept qualitative methods of evaluation, the identification of realistic intermediate and long-term outcomes, and finally, the understanding of long-term benefits and unintended positive outcomes for communities. However, we should be careful lest we "throw the baby out with the bathwater" by criticizing coalitions for not achieving measurable outcomes.

Some are beginning to argue for more research focusing on what coalitions contribute to community-based interventions, beyond more traditional approaches (Lasker, Weiss, and Miller, 2001; Berkowitz, 2001; Butterfoss, Cashman, Foster-Fishman, and Kegler, 2001). For example, do coalition approaches develop more innovative strategies due to the pooling of expertise and resources? Do they reach previously untapped community assets? Are they better able to implement certain types of interventions than traditional public health and social service agencies, such as policy or media advocacy efforts? A logical future direction for research on coalitions, and this theory in particular, would be to document what Lasker and colleagues term partnership synergy.

Unfortunately, community coalitions are in the same situation as almost all community-level initiatives in facing the challenges associated with documenting long-term outcomes and attributing resulting changes to the initiative. Michelle Kegler and I contend that by strengthening the theoretical base and developing a model of action for community coalitions, we will advance this area of scientific inquiry. We encourage theoreticians to test the logic of this model. We challenge researchers to use the model, at both the case-study and large-scale levels, to field test our assumptions and advance the understanding of which coalition characteristics and interactions are most likely to fuel goal attainment. Finally, we ask practitioners, the front-line coalition pioneers, to determine whether this model is useful to increase local support and capacity for further coalition development. This theoretical model is a starting point—we welcome all contributions that improve its validity, reliability, and utility.

SUMMARY

Several different frameworks and models were presented in this chapter: the Community Organization and Development Model, the Framework for Partnerships for Community Development, the Framework of Organizational Viability, the Community Coalition Model, the Work Group on Health Promotion and Community Development Model, the Collaboration Framework, the Typology of Community Organization and Community Building, and the Model of Community Health Governance. Butterfoss and Kegler's Community Coalition Action Theory (CCAT) consists of fourteen constructs and twenty-three testable propositions and is based on many of these models, as well as on research and practice with community coalitions. A local community coalition is used to illustrate how the theory works in practice.

QUESTIONS FOR REVIEW

1. In what way was the development of CCAT a way to "put the horse before the cart"?

2. How does CCAT build on earlier frameworks and models? How were CCAT's theoretical constructs and propositions derived?

3. How can this theory be tested further?

PART TWO

BUILDING EFFECTIVE COALITIONS AND PARTNERSHIPS

CHAPTER FIVE

Lead Agency, Coalition Staff, and Leadership

Leadership is not wielding authority—it is empowering people.
—Becky Brodin

At the core of any successful organization is effective leadership. It takes leadership from all fronts to create and sustain a viable organization. Coalitions and partnerships demand a delicate balance of leadership that is neither bureaucratic nor autocratic. It starts with a founding organization that has compassion for its community and values collaboration and diversity. This organization creates the conditions that make principled leadership possible and foster the emergence of capable, visionary leaders. Those leaders, whether paid or voluntary, have members' interests at heart and are able to effectively share their vision for a better community.

The sustainability of a coalition or partnership depends not only on the leadership capacity within the local community but also on long-term training and technical assistance that contributes to capacity (Butterfoss, Goodman, and Wandersman, 1993, 1996, and 2001; Fawcett and others, 1997; Florin, Mitchell, and Stevenson, 1993; Goodman and others, 1996; Goodman, Wheeler, and Lee, 1995; Kegler, Steckler, McLeroy, and Malek, 1998b; Rowitz, 1999; Steckler, Goodman, and Alciati, 1997). Coalitions must develop the capacity to perform competent assessment, planning, implementation, and evaluation (Kreuter, Lezin, and Young, 2000; Wandersman and others, 1996). This chapter will show how specific structural elements, along with adequate training and technical assistance, can help coalitions flourish.

WHO IS THE LEAD AGENCY?

Coalitions usually form when a lead agency or convener group responds to an opportunity, threat, or mandate by recruiting a core group of community leaders and providing initial support for the coalition. This is usually a practical matter, because someone has to receive and manage funds on behalf of the group. What appears to be quite variable is how the lead agency is identified. In some cases, the lead agency or convener is the organization that has the vision or mandate to initially mobilize community members to form a coalition focused on a specific issue of concern. In other cases, a funding source specifies who the lead agency must be; and in yet others, the lead agency may have written a grant or otherwise procured funds for coalition operation. Finally, in some cases, a convened group makes a decision as a whole body as to which is the most appropriate agency among them to take the lead.

Sometimes competition arises over who should be the lead agency, especially if the position promises recognition, prestige, or financial gain. Choosing a visible, well-regarded, powerful, or wealthy organization to take the lead is a good idea because action and resources may follow, but care must be taken so that the less powerful organizations in the coalition do not feel left out of influencing the coalition's agenda, structure, and activities. Finding the most neutral group with adequate resources is a good strategy. Sofaer (2001, p. 23) offers two critical questions regarding lead agencies: Who is in the best position to carry out the administrative and financial function of a lead agency, and who is most likely to be respected and trusted by other coalition members and by the community and constituencies the coalition needs to reach?

Types of Lead Agencies

A lead agency does not have to be a specific type of organization. Commitment and a sense that the organization is the right fit for the coalition are key ingredients. Some coalitions adopt a structure where more than one agency shares lead agency responsibilities, or they develop a rotation of administration over time. Coalitions should be aware that these adaptations might be problematic if these agencies develop turf issues about the coalition or compete over other issues that are entirely unrelated to the coalition. The coalition may end up the loser here, especially if disagreements arise over coalition stances that are unpopular or contrary to the lead agency position(s). Looking at coalitions for health promotion and disease prevention across the country, lead agencies may be any of these:

- *Governmental institutions,* such as health departments or social service agencies
- *Voluntary agencies,* such as the American Heart Association, American Lung Association, or American Cancer Society
- *Statewide organizations or professional societies*
- *Academic or health institutions*

- *Community-based organizations,* such as the Young Men's Christian Association (YMCA) or Young Women's Christian Association (YWCA), Boys and Girls Clubs, ethnic organizations, and other neighborhood organizations

The Role of Lead Agencies

Lead agencies can often help the coalition and its staff by taking many of the more mundane and time-consuming, although necessary, business activities off their hands. The agreed-upon convener accepts responsibility to host initial meetings and recruit prospective partners, and may also provide physical space for coalition operation and a part- or full-time staff person to manage the initiative. The lead agency may also agree to be the fiscal agent and provide basic communication and administrative services (e-mail, phone, mail). These agencies can manage payroll, benefits, facility and space, and some professional development.

The lead agency usually is seen as having significant, and sometimes undue, influence about the direction of the coalition's policies, programs, and resources. This may be problematic, but it can be managed as long as members understand that as well as having greater influence, the lead agency agrees to assume more risks and responsibilities. Ellis and Lenczner (2000) report that the time that coalition staff from six Community Anti-Drug Coalitions of America (CADCA) spent dealing with the logistical details of running an organization took away from the time they spent on affecting change in their communities. They maintain that even though the potential exists for coalitions to feel constrained by their lead agencies, these issues can be avoided by competent staff and clear, frequent communication. Danger only arises when the lead agency exerts influence that is not aligned with the will of the coalition and its members (Sofaer, 2001).

What Makes a Good Lead Agency?

Although the coalition literature generally acknowledges that the convening agency must have sufficient organizational capacity, commitment, leadership, and vision to build an effective coalition, research on these and other factors that lead agencies should possess is lacking (Butterfoss, Goodman, and Wandersman, 1993).

Listed here are some of the characteristics a good lead agency should possess:

- Strong links to and respect for the local community
- The respect of community organizations and key leaders, or at least the perception that the agency is a neutral entity
- A deep understanding of community health issues, priority populations, and local politics
- Belief in collaboration and the patience and confidence to "trust the process" of community engagement and shared decision making
- Adoption within its own walls of positive health practices that support the activities of the coalition (for example, adopting clean indoor air policies, immunization services, wellness activities, and nondiscriminatory health benefits)

- Ability to serve as an umbrella organization to provide private, not-for-profit status (501(c)(3)) for the coalition
- "Deep pockets" or at least a reserve of resources to support the basic administrative needs of the coalition, in other words, office space, telecommunication and mail services, computer connections and services, printing, and funds to sustain the coalition between times of outside funding
- Staff support through its employment and benefits structure
- Development, media, and advocacy capabilities to positively promote the coalition and its work

COALITION STAFF

Some coalitions survive for quite some time with part-time administrative support staff who can schedule and arrange meeting logistics, contact members, and copy materials. However, more complex tasks, such as developing agendas and assessment activities as well as identifying potential organizations to recruit, will require professional staff or technical assistance from committed coalition members. Without competent leadership and staffing, coalitions are unlikely to move beyond the initial steps in the formation stage of development (Butterfoss, Goodman, and Wandersman, 1996; Edwards and Stern, 1998; Feighery and Rogers, 1990; Lee and Jackson, 1997; Mulroy, 1997).

Staff persons are not hired only to help coalitions survive, however; they should be hired to make coalitions strong and productive. Although many coalitions function without designated staff, field experience shows that these coalitions have difficulty taking on multiple issues, keeping members engaged, completing essential tasks, and producing results, compared to staffed coalitions (Wolff, 2001b).

Coalition staff must be committed to working with coalition leaders to organize the structures through which the coalition accomplishes its work, and they are responsible for coalition processes such as communication and decision making, which keep members satisfied and committed to coalition efforts. Staff can be most helpful when they possess an appreciation of the voluntary nature of coalitions, have the organizational and interpersonal skills to facilitate the collaborative process, and are skilled in diplomacy and negotiation (Croan and Lees, 1979; Wandersman and Alderman, 1993).

Coalition research has examined how staffing is related to intermediate indicators of effectiveness, including member-related outcomes, plan quality, resource mobilization, and implementation of planned activities. Butterfoss and colleagues (1996) found an association between members' positive relationships with staff and member benefits. Two studies demonstrate relationships between staff competence and member satisfaction (Rogers and others, 1993; Kegler, Steckler, Malek, and McLeroy, 1998a). For example, coalitions with staff who lack community organization skills (for example, lack of follow-up on recruitment or maintenance of rosters, no follow-through on coalition member suggestions, or unwillingness to share leadership roles with members) have been identified as those with lower levels of implementation and vice versa (Kegler, Steckler, Malek, and McLeroy, 1998b).

Kegler, Steckler, Malek, and McLeroy (1998a) also found that lack of staff time for planning, combined with inflexible deadlines for deliverables (action plans and reports), led to a trend among coordinators to complete these activities with little input from coalition members. Thus a strong relationship can be seen between staff skills and staff time devoted to coalition efforts and the amount of resources mobilized and level of implementation of planned activities, lending support to the need for paid staff with sufficient time to devote to the coalition.

The barriers of staff availability, conflicting priorities, and turnover can potentially cause tension among organizations, staff burnout, weaknesses in program delivery, and a lack of continual representation (Gottlieb, Brink, and Gingiss, 1993). Minimal or nondisruptive staff turnover, therefore, also has been linked to positive outcomes (Center for Substance Abuse Prevention, 1998; Kegler, Steckler, Malek, and McLeroy, 1998a). Finally, staff must manage their time between obtaining funds and resources and developing coalition infrastructure. They must also coordinate a multitude of programs among many organizations and deal with volunteers who have different skill sets and levels of commitment (Dowling, O'Donnell, and Wellington Consulting Group, 2000).

Rogers and colleagues (1993) found that staff were most satisfied when organizational bylaws and procedures were in place; they had sufficient control over the process; and communication with members was good. In large initiatives, where local coalitions are supported by state-level or national-program office staff, the activities that are supported by these staff (for example, through technical assistance, training, and translating research to practice) are more likely to be implemented (Kegler, Steckler, Malek, and McLeroy, 1998a; Clark and others, 2006). Several studies have documented an increased change in community programs, practices, and policies when staff and community organizers were hired (Roussos and Fawcett, 2000).

STAFF ROLES

In many coalitions, leadership and staffing are intertwined, with paid staff fulfilling many leadership functions, such as setting agendas and facilitating meetings. Staff usually support the coalition, encourage membership involvement, and build community capacity (Sanchez, 2000). The difficulties in finding the right staff person(s) are many (Sofaer, 2001). First, staff should maintain a neutral position that presents an unbiased view of the issues, facilitates decision making, and supports members' priorities—not necessarily their own. Exerting undue influence in decisions is unethical and contrary to true collaboration. Second, staff members should facilitate linkages with the community through its members by connecting members to influential leaders, policy makers, and the media, instead of taking the limelight themselves. Third, members and staff must clarify the staff's job description so that coalition tasks are shared among staff, members, and coalition leaders. Often staff members complain that they are left to do all or most of the work, because members easily abdicate their responsibilities.

Finally, the question of accountability arises. To whom is the staff accountable—the members or the agency that pays their salary (if it is not the coalition itself)? The coalition leaders should function in a supervisory role for the coalition coordinator or at least ensure that they have significant input in performance reviews that are part of the lead agency's operating structure. The coordinator, in turn, should supervise administrative staff.

Another strategy is to hire a consultant or outside firm to manage the coalition. The advantage of flexibility with respect to supervisory responsibilities, however, may be outweighed by the disadvantages of other clients who compete for the consultant's time, the potential for conflicts of interest, and the higher cost related to such a strategy (Sofaer, 2001). On the other hand, consultants are invaluable for short-term or specific tasks, such as facilitating meetings; planning sessions or retreats; writing grant proposals and reports; managing websites and media campaigns; or designing logos, brochures, and educational materials.

Staff issues and roles should be clarified early in the life of the coalition so that staff can educate members on coalition issues and help shape members' roles and responsibilities in carrying out the coalition's work (Feighery and Rogers, 1990; Reininger, Dinh-Zarr, Sinicrope, and Martin, 1999). Examples of job descriptions that clearly outline the role of the coalition coordinator and administrative staff are included in Exhibits 5.1–5.5. Lack of clarity, role delineation, and loose coalition structure may

(Text resumes on page 104.)

Exhibit 5.1. Job Description: Coalition Coordinator.

Coalition Coordinator will be responsible for planning, implementing, and evaluating activities associated with the coalition to include providing general oversight for coalition activities and associated projects; grant development, submission, and management; state and national reporting; and technical assistance to local and regional coalitions and partnerships that focus on [topic]. The Coordinator will work to develop and implement strategies that will lead to long-term involvement of medical practices, institutions, insurers, and community partners in health promotion, assessment, and evaluation activities.

Job Duties and Responsibilities

- Reports to lead agency and coalition leadership
- Works as team member with lead agency staff and administrators to meet program goals
- Continually broadens expertise in the area of [topic specific] and serves as resource person
- Conducts literature and resource reviews to identify best practices to apply to coalition activities and associated projects
- Represents coalition through professional associations locally, statewide, and nationally

Exhibit 5.1. (Continued)

- Recruits and maintains a diverse coalition membership with state and national partners
- Serves as Coordinator or Health Planner for the coalition by coordinating all activities such as these:
  - Directs needs-assessment activities
  - Develops evaluation instruments and protocols for testing the effectiveness of strategies developed by the coalition
  - Conducts community health-planning activities
  - Collects, manages, and analyzes community health-indicators data
  - Directs coalition in developing health policies related to [topic]
  - Collaborates with other local, state, and national organizations focusing on [topic]
- Assists coalition members in conducting annual strategic planning and guides coalition to develop a comprehensive action plan based on needs assessment and strategic planning
- Develops and implements data collection methods, tools, and evaluation measures for coalition activities and associated projects in conjunction with coalition members
- Coordinates and facilitates coalition meetings and communicates effectively with members to promote collaboration, negotiation, and problem solving
- Plans, coordinates, and conducts educational and training activities for immunization providers statewide. Develops training, reference materials, and workshops for coalition and community members, coalition activities, and associated projects
- Continually maintains and develops content for the coalition website
- Collaborates and works closely with the health department administrators, legislators, heads of health plans, hospitals, physicians' health organizations, related businesses, academic institutions, and community-based organizations to promote the mission, goals, and strategies of the coalition
- Develops marketing and media materials, campaigns, and opportunities in conjunction with the external affairs staff and statewide media consultants and network
- Directs and assists coalition to develop legislative action that promotes the coalition mission by developing position statements, reviewing and recommending endorsements of policies regarding immunizations, and advocating for policies and legislation at state and federal levels
- Advocates and expands the use of Continuous Quality Improvement processes in service delivery

(continued)

Exhibit 5.1. Job Description: Coalition Coordinator. (*Continued*)

- Serves as a consultant in the area of developing community partnerships for [issue]. Works with local and regional groups throughout the state in the following areas:
  - Coalition development and maintenance
  - Community health planning and needs assessments
  - Health outcomes evaluation
  - Improving immunization delivery
  - Developing effective health plans and policies
- Conducts annual site visits to other local and state coalitions and provides consultation
- Continuously evaluates coalition effectiveness and coalition strategic plan
- Documents findings and progress of programs and activities in written quarterly reports to lead agency, other funding agencies, and coalition members
- Manages and oversees expenditures of coalition budget (or contract). Seeks and writes grant proposals to obtain additional funding
- Reports and presents coalition progress and program findings through publications and presentations at national meetings and conferences
- Directs the work and activities of coalition administrative support staff; supervises, mentors, and directs the work activities of students and assigned temporary staff

Qualifications

- Master's degree or relevant experience in public health or related field such as health education, administration, policy and planning, or in community or organizational psychology; or bachelor's degree and five years of appropriate experience in managing or coordinating a community-based public health or voluntary health-related agency could be substituted for advanced degree.
- At least two years of experience with health-education programs in community setting
- Proven ability to work independently
- Public relations or marketing skills
- Excellent organizational skills
- Excellent interpersonal and communication skills
- Knowledge of the research process
- High proficiency with Microsoft Office® and general computer skills

Exhibit 5.2. Job Description: Coalition Administrative Assistant.

Administrative Assistant will be responsible for supporting all activities associated with the coalition. The Administrative Assistant will report to the Coalition Coordinator and will provide administrative support to the coalition and all of its work groups to include meeting scheduling and support, event planning, coalition project and program support, and other administrative duties as assigned.

Job Duties and Responsibilities

- Supports coalition, steering committee, and work group meetings
  - Schedules rooms or arranges for outside venue
  - Makes contact with host site to confirm room, audio-visual needs, chair setup and other specific details for meeting, if applicable
  - Arranges for refreshments for meetings, if applicable
  - Attends all meetings to take minutes and transcribe them in timely manner for Coordinator's review prior to distribution to members
  - E-mails and makes phone call reminders to all members a week prior to the meeting
  - Compiles meeting agendas for Coalition Coordinator's and Work Group Chair's review prior to emailing
  - Prepares handouts for distribution at meetings
- Plans events
  - Assists Coordinator in finding location for conference or event
  - Sends out mailing to all past attendees of conference or event, notifying them of date, directions, parking, and so on
  - Creates Microsoft Excel® file with names of all attendees, addresses, titles, and organizations in order to prepare labels, letters, and name tags
  - Accepts registration forms
  - Helps design and arranges for printing of conference materials (brochure, forms, signs, name tags, handouts, compendium of resources and educational materials and syllabus)
  - Arranges for coalition volunteers to assist with preparing packets needed for conference
  - Contacts vendors to place orders for program materials and conference incentive items
  - Prepares signs to assist with registration at conference
  - Confirms menu selection with catering department at event site
  - Confirms meeting room selections with representative at event site
  - Visits site to confirm all arrangements are in place prior to conference date
  - Remains on-site during event to oversee details and supervise volunteers

(continued)

Exhibit 5.2. Job Description: Coalition Administrative Assistant. (*Continued*)

- Supports coalition project or program
  - Conducts basic searches using PubMed® and other bibliographic databases to support projects
  - Manages databases for research projects utilizing Microsoft Excel, Microsoft Access®, and Statistical Package for Social Sciences (SPSS®)—data sorting and routine frequency analyses
  - Assists in preparing budget worksheets as per federal guidelines and acquiring required grant materials, letters of support, appendices
  - Creates presentations in Microsoft PowerPoint® and diagrams and flowchart graphics for oral presentations, manuscripts, poster presentations, and grant proposals
  - Prepares posters to be presented at national meetings, including oversight of data layout
  - Assists with completing required forms and obtains appropriate signatures
  - Maintains program hardware, for example, digital camera, cell phones, and pagers
- Provides general help
  - Orders supplies and materials, recruits volunteers, places printing orders
  - Enters data for surveys, evaluations, and so forth
  - Creates newsletters reminding members of submission dates
  - Assists with formatting of surveys and questionnaires
  - Processes checks and purchase program incentives
  - Acquires and archives publicity generated by programs
  - Maintains annual records of program activities
  - Designs and writes text for coalition or program brochures and flyers

Qualifications

- Proven ability to work independently
- Excellent organizational skills
- Excellent interpersonal and communication skills
- Highly proficient with Microsoft Office (Word®, PowerPoint, Excel, Access, Publisher®, Outlook®), basic SPSS, and general computer skills

---

contribute to the members' perceived lack of commitment to the organization. Some research suggests that coalitions with staff who play a supportive role for the coalition, rather than a visible leadership role, have higher levels of implementation (Kegler, Steckler, Malek, and McLeroy, 1998a). Coalition staff and member relationships are more harmonious when roles are clarified and staff have the latitude to carry out simple daily tasks (Brown, 1984).

(*Text resumes on page 107.*)

Exhibit 5.3. Job Descriptions: Coalition Chair and Vice-Chair.

Coalition Chair is responsible to the coalition.

Job Duties and Responsibilities

- Maintains and or expands current work group membership with assistance from Coalition Coordinator
- Serves as liaison for work group to steering committee and coalition
- Develops work group agenda with staff assistance
- Serves as moderator of work group meeting (stays fifteen minutes after meeting to network and evaluate meeting)
- Designates a recorder for each work group meeting
- Contacts members and coordinates work group responsibilities with them
- Represents coalition in the community (with staff assistance)
- Consults with Coalition Coordinator as needed
- Deals with members and staff fairly, sensitively, and confidentially
- Promotes collaboration, conflict resolution, and decision making
- Is open to diverse opinions and points of view

Time Commitment

- Approximately three hours per month
- Attends two work group meetings per year, steering committee and coalition meetings, and major coalition activities
- One-year availability

Qualifications

- Ascribes to coalition mission, goals, and bylaws
- Possesses strong leadership and organizational skills
- Is familiar with or willing to learn principles of parliamentary procedure

Coalition Vice-Chair is responsible to the Chair and the coalition

Job Description

- Presides over work group meetings in the absence of the work group Chair
- Assumes the role of Chair in the event of the Chair's inability to complete a responsibility or term
- Consults with work group Chair as needed
- Performs other duties as directed by the Chair

Time Commitment

- Approximately one to two hours per month
- Attends two work group meetings per year, steering committee and coalition meetings, and major coalition activities
- One-year availability

Qualifications

- Ascribes to coalition mission, goals, and bylaws
- Possesses strong leadership and organizational skills
- Is familiar with or willing to learn principles of parliamentary procedure

---

Exhibit 5.4. Job Description: Coalition Secretary-Treasurer.

Coalition Secretary-Treasurer

The Coalition Secretary-Treasurer is responsible to the Coalition Chair

Job Description

- Serves as secretary to coalition and steering committee
- Assists with coalition and steering committee meeting agenda layout and distribution
- Notifies all coalition and steering committee members of upcoming meetings two weeks in advance
- Locates and secures facilities and arranges lunch for meetings
- Takes minutes at coalition and steering committee meetings and distributes them electronically to all members within two weeks of meeting
- Maintains current roster
- Serves as custodian for all records and reports
- Prepares annual budget and works with auditor for routine audits
- Collects dues (if any) and maintains financial records

Time Commitment

- Approximately two to four hours per month
- Attends quarterly coalition and steering committee meetings
- One-year availability

Qualifications

- Ascribes to coalition mission, goals, and bylaws
- Possesses strong mathematical and accounting skills

Exhibit 5.5. Job Description: Work Group Chair and Vice-Chair.

Work Group Chair is responsible to the Coalition Chair.

Job Description

- Maintains and or expands current work group membership with assistance from Coalition Coordinator
- Serves as liaison for work group to steering committee and coalition
- Develops work group agenda with staff assistance
- Serves as moderator of work group meeting (stays fifteen minutes after meeting to network and evaluate meeting)
- Designates a recorder for each meeting of the work group
- Contacts members and coordinates work group responsibilities with them
- Represents coalition in the community (with staff assistance)
- Consults with coalition coordinator as needed

Exhibit 5.5. (*Continued*)

- Deals with members and staff fairly, sensitively, and confidentially
- Promotes collaboration, conflict resolution and decision making
- Is open to diverse opinions and points of view

Time Commitment

- Approximately two hours per month
- Attends work group, steering committee, and coalition meetings and major work group activities
- One-year availability

Qualifications

- Ascribes to coalition mission, goals, and bylaws
- Possesses strong leadership and organizational skills
- Is familiar with or willing to learn principles of parliamentary procedure

Work Group Vice-Chair is responsible to Work Group Chair

Job Description

- Presides over work group meetings in the absence of the Work Group Chair
- Assumes the role of Chair in the event of the Chair's inability to complete a responsibility or term
- Consults with Work Group Chair as needed
- Performs other duties as directed by the Chair

Time Commitment

- Approximately one to two hours per month
- Attends work group, steering committee, and coalition meetings and major work group activities
- One-year availability

Qualifications

- Ascribes to coalition mission, goals, and bylaws
- Possesses strong leadership and organizational skills
- Is familiar with or willing to learn principles of parliamentary procedure

Based on qualitative reports of staff from local tobacco coalitions, Kegler and colleagues (1998a, p. 232) describe five roles that staff often are asked to play, namely Coach, Director, Linking Agent, Doer, and Coordinator. Staff may play each of these roles at some point in the life of the coalition or, more often, play several simultaneously. Kegler and colleagues also found that the way staff perceived their roles influenced the level of coalition implementation. For example, the coalitions where the coordinator perceived herself as primarily responsible for carrying out the coalition's activities (Doer) had the lowest levels of implementation. Descriptions of these different leadership roles follow.

Coach provides training and technical assistance to increase the community's capacity for public health work.

Director takes an authoritative stance to direct coalition members to accomplish needed tasks.

Linking agent serves as a liaison between the state and locality to provide information needed for action.

Doer primarily acts as jack-of-all-trades to assist coalition members in tasks; sometimes acts single-handedly to accomplish tasks like reporting and fundraising.

Coordinator prepares, organizes, attends meetings, and reports work of coalition work groups.

COALITION LEADERSHIP

Leadership, even if it is informal, is essential to coalition survival. Staff members can hold a coalition together for the short term, but if leadership is not forthcoming from members, the coalition will eventually succumb. Leadership is the most often reported internal, or organizational, factor that helps a coalition create effective community and systems change (Roussos and Fawcett, 2000). Mizrahi's and Rosenthal's (2001) focus group study of seventy past and current organizers and leaders also identified leadership as the factor most often linked to coalition success. A community's readiness for collaborative work is dependent on the quality of its leaders because "they bring hope, energy, and vision to the launching of coalitions" (Wolff, 2001b, p. 176). By using democratic and consensus-based decision making, leaders may increase members' satisfaction, broaden community participation, and improve overall coalition effectiveness (Roussos and Fawcett, 2000). Key leaders' involvement in building community capacity may also lead to greater program effectiveness (Griffin and others, 2005).

Coalition leadership is complex, and researchers have examined its many facets. In her early work on coalitions, Brown (1984) noted that coalitions were more cohesive, maintained operations, and reached out to peripheral members when leaders were attentive to and supportive of individual member concerns, and competent in negotiating, garnering resources, solving problems, and resolving conflict. Empirical research on coalitions shows a consistent relationship between *leader competence* and *satisfaction* (Glidewell, Kelly, Bagby, and Dickerson, 1998b). Butterfoss, Goodman, and Wandersman (1996) found that *leader support and control* were related to several positive member-related outcomes, but not to plan quality. Reininger and colleagues (1999) reported that indigenous leaders were overall more effective than outside leaders. In a study of ten rural coalitions formed to prevent drug abuse, Braithwaite, Taylor, and Austin (2000) noted that the most successful coalitions had strong leaders who were *committed to a common goal*. Others have found that the ability of a coalition to develop a *clear and shared vision*, a likely result of good leadership, is associated with success (Kegler,

Steckler, Malek, and McLeroy, 1998b; Center for Substance Abuse Prevention, 1998).

Foster-Fishman and colleagues found that the ability to engage coalition members in productive work (organizational capacity) was most related to coalition leaders who have the "skills (for example, communication, conflict resolution, resource development, and administration), internal and external relationships, and vision to transform individual interests into a dynamic collective force that achieves targeted outcomes" (2001, p. 253). The authors maintain that because leaders are so critical and their tenure is relatively short, coalitions must "continually foster and build a cadre of emerging leaders" (2001, p. 254). Planning for succession is critical so that a sense of continuity and momentum exists. A succession plan also allows more leadership opportunities for other members and opens up the coalition to new ideas. When coalitions use term limits for leadership and vice or co-chair positions, this grooms new leaders by giving them an opportunity to manage smaller tasks and numbers of volunteers in preparation for larger leadership roles.

Coalitions should decide in advance whether to set terms of office (for example, one or two years), whether leaders can serve more than one term, and whether a succession from vice-chair to chair should be planned. Experience with community- and state-level coalitions has taught that one-year renewable terms of office are ideal, because coalitions often meet infrequently and it takes a while to orient new leaders. This scheme also prevents long terms of office if the leader does not work out as expected.

Coalitions must also be committed to identifying skilled indigenous or local community leadership if capacity is to be built (Reininger and others, 1999). According to Lasker, Weiss, and Miller (2001), the effectiveness of leadership is the most powerful determinant of partnership synergy. Such leadership facilitates productive interactions among partners by bridging diverse cultures, spanning boundaries, and challenging assumptions that limit creative thinking and action. Successful leaders create an internal work environment that is efficient and task oriented (Butterfoss, Goodman, and Wandersman, 1996), is empowering, fosters member satisfaction and commitment, and is effective (Butterfoss, Goodman, and Wandersman, 1993; Butterfoss, Goodman, and Wandersman, 1996; Kegler, Steckler, Malek, and McLeroy, 1998a; Kumpher, Turner, Hopkins and Librett, 1993; Rogers and others, 1993; Roussos and Fawcett, 2000).

Leadership is a skill that can be fostered throughout the life of the coalition. Different leadership skills may be more useful during various stages of coalition development. Whereas earlier stages may require greater facilitation and listening skills to recruit and engage diverse members, negotiation and advocacy skills may be needed to bring about more complex environmental changes during subsequent stages of development (Roussos and Fawcett, 2000). Exhibit 5.6, adapted from DeLizia's (2002) work with professional associations, provides five steps to developing quality volunteer leaders.

Collaborative or Transformational Leaders

Effective coalition leadership requires a collection of personal qualities and skills that are typically not found in one individual, but rather in a group of committed leaders who have grassroots community support (Roussos and Fawcett, 2000).

Exhibit 5.6. Developing Quality Volunteer Leaders.

Looking to harvest a bumper crop of volunteer leaders? Consider the following five steps first.

Step 1: Be clear about what you want.

What do you require of leaders? Do you expect them to testify on key professional issues? Serve as media contacts? Plan and run productive meetings? A member who has valuable contacts with elected officials may make an effective legislative chair but may not have what it takes to be a coalition chairperson. Be clear—and be proactive—in identifying requirements for coalition leadership positions. Developing a clear set of leader job descriptions is better than the hit-or-miss strategy of seeing who steps forward for the position. The person who has the time and desire to lead may not necessarily be the best candidate for the job.

Sample strategy: Identify leadership skills, qualities, and experience necessary for each position, and use this information as a guide for the nomination and appointment processes.

Step 2: Make cultivation everyone's job.

Whose job is it to develop future leaders? The steering committee's? The staff's? The committee chairs'? The answer is yes. Every leader and staff member has the opportunity to get to know a variety of members and observe them in a number of situations. What contributions do members make? How do they interact with others? What questions do they ask? These observations provide clues to potential volunteer or leadership opportunities.

Sample strategy: Ask each new member to complete a profile to capture valuable information on professional, personal, and volunteer experience and interests. Add personal observations from your colleagues and contacts to this information base to build a volunteer resource bank.

Step 3: Position the job right . . . right from the start.

Properly matched with interests and skills, most jobs in the coalition can further a member's personal and professional goals, as well as provide the coalition with valuable expertise and support. The perception that most people have is that volunteerism is a one-way street: give, give, give. Participating, volunteering, and assuming leadership roles can be a member benefit that is as valuable as educational seminars, advocacy efforts, or member discount programs.

Sample strategy: Focus the new-member orientation on helping members get the most value from their membership. Explain how personal and professional goals can be matched up with the right coalition benefits and services.

Exhibit 5.6. (*Continued*)

Step 4: Create an environment that will grow leaders.

Seeds sprout stronger roots in prepared soil. What messages do members receive about the value of volunteerism in the coalition's print and electronic communication? What support is available to ensure success if a member steps forward to volunteer? Do members see past leaders still involved and getting value? Don't underestimate intangible rewards as a powerful strategy to stimulate interest in volunteerism and leadership. At the very least, ensure that no conflicting messages come from the coalition about volunteerism.

Sample strategy: Ask a small group of members or trusted outsiders to critique the coalition environment for volunteerism. Ask one person to review the last few newsletters, get another to scan the coalition website, and let another attend one or two membership meetings. All should attempt to view the organization through a new member's eyes to understand your message about the value of involvement.

Step 5: Take the long view.

Although some members will come into the coalition ready to take on leadership roles, most will not. Some have not yet developed the right skills, whereas others have not realized the value of taking on volunteer roles. Waiting to find leaders until you need them is risky. Identifying and building leaders is a system of cultivation that takes place from the recruitment process to encouragement from past leaders to stay involved.

Sample strategy: Examine each of the crucial stages in a member's involvement in the coalition, identify any barriers to increased involvement, and develop strategies to address those barriers: *new member* to *participating member, participating member* to *volunteer, volunteer* to *leader,* and *leader* to *past leader.*

Adapted from "A Bumper Crop," by James S. DeLiza in *Volunteer Leader,* October 2002. Reprinted with permission.

Collaborative leadership involves having leaders broadly share power to set priorities, allocate resources, and evaluate coalition performance (Weiner, Alexander, and Shortell, 2002). Having multiple leaders supports the ideals of diversity and a nonhierarchical structure; promotes principles of shared responsibilities and decision making; allows for flexibility, thereby helping to prevent burnout; and creates a broad base of former leaders who represent the history of the coalition and can mentor its future leaders. Collaborative leadership is an encompassing approach that describes a wide range of leadership, from narrow one-on-one approaches to broad approaches that influence whole organizations and cultures. For example, in public health and business, a team or community-centered view of leadership is favored over a single-leader approach (Avolio, 1999). At the same time, the complex situations that abound in these fields call for "skills and abilities that are as complex as the situations in which they are found" (Turning Point, 2001a, p. 14).

Laissez-faire ⟶ Transactional ⟶ Transformational

Figure 5.1 Leadership Continuum.

One type of collaborative leadership is called *transformational* (also called servant, or facilitative, leadership). Although first coined by Downton (1973), the classic work *Leadership* by Burns (1978) describes how certain leaders are able to inspire followers to accomplish great things and how leaders and members are inextricably linked in the transformation process. Transformational leaders are change agents who are good role models, create and articulate a clear vision for an organization, empower followers to achieve at higher standards, lead as peer problem solvers, build broad-based involvement and participation, act in ways that make others want to trust them, and give meaning to organizational life (Chrislip and Larson, 1994; Northouse, 2001, p. 158). Mohandas Gandhi is a good example of a transformational leader, because he raised the hopes and demands of millions of his people and in the process was changed himself. Likewise, Ryan White raised awareness about AIDS and in the process became a spokesperson for increasing government support of AIDS research. Bass (1985) describes a leadership continuum from laissez-faire, to transactional (exchange process between leaders and followers), to transformational leadership as illustrated in Figure 5.1. These four factors define transformational leadership:

Charisma, or idealized influence, is a quality of leaders who are strong role models with very high standards of moral and ethical conduct. Followers want very much to conform to their vision and emulate them. Nelson Mandela characterizes the charisma factor, because his standards and vision resulted in monumental changes in governance that transformed the entire nation of South Africa.

Inspirational motivation is provided by leaders who communicate high expectations to followers, inspiring or motivating them to become committed to and part of the organization's shared vision.

Intellectual stimulation is imparted by leaders who stimulate followers to be innovative and to challenge their own beliefs and values, as well as those of the leader and the organization, in order to solve problems.

Individualized consideration is shown by leaders who provide a supportive climate in which they carefully listen to the individual needs of followers and act as coaches to help individuals become fully actualized or empowered (Bass, 1985).

Figure 5.2 shows how transformational leadership leads to greater effects than transactional leadership.

Researchers have proposed a distinction between *transformational* leadership and *transforming* leadership. *Transformational* leadership works to accomplish systems changes within an organization to improve its efficiency and effectiveness—in other words, for organizational purposes directly—and those enacted for social and political

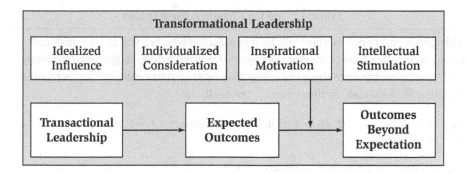

Figure 5.2 Transformational Leadership.

purposes only indirectly, if at all. *Transforming* leadership works to accomplish social and political changes within and through organizations. In this way, a higher moral plane is expected in *transforming leadership,* which shares the same characteristics as *social capital* (Burns, 1978). The moral resources and public goods of social capital are the distinguishing characteristics of transforming leadership, or "significant change," according to Burns (Couto, 1997). For example, Franklin D. Roosevelt's New Deal brought forth new public goods and moral resources to address the basic needs of many Americans in a way that was unprecedented for the federal government. Franklin expressed a higher value for a group of people and a bond of mutuality between that group and the rest of society that previously had been disregarded or denied. When leaders work to create new and increased forms of social capital, they attempt to move their communities up the scale of human values and development.

This distinction being acknowledged, *transformational leadership* will be used to describe the collaborative type of leadership that is desirable for coalitions and partnerships. Transformational leadership is useful for a coalition approach in that it has been widely researched, has intuitive appeal, treats leadership as a process that occurs between leaders and followers, and provides an expanded picture that includes not only the exchange of rewards but also leaders' attention to the needs and growth of followers (Northouse, 2001, p. 146). Exhibit 5.7 provides a self-assessment for determining if one is a transformational leader. Exhibit 5.8 describes the traits of transformational leaders.

Coalitions may broaden their leadership by supporting community champions who work for change within their sectors or for a specific objective. A coalition that disperses leadership across the organization may be more efficient and less likely to disband than one that depends on one or two leaders (Roussos and Fawcett, 2000). A common approach that builds collaborative leadership in a coalition is the formation of a steering committee composed of officers of the coalition, chairs of its working groups, and other influential members. The role of the steering committee will be discussed in more detail in Chapter Eight on governance.

(Text resumes on page 117.)

Exhibit 5.7. Are You a Transformational Leader?

This paper-and-pencil exercise will help you decide whether you use a transformational style of leadership. Twelve statements are listed below. Judge how frequently each statement fits you. The word *others* may refer to your coalition members, other coalition leaders, staff, or those outside the coalition.

Key 0 = Never 1 = Once in a while 2 = Sometimes 3 = Fairly often
4 = Frequently or always

1. I make others feel good to be around me.	0	1	2	3	4
2. I express with a few simple words what we could do.	0	1	2	3	4
3. I help others to think about old problems in new ways.	0	1	2	3	4
4. I help others develop themselves.	0	1	2	3	4
5. Others have complete faith in me.	0	1	2	3	4
6. I provide appealing images of what we can do.	0	1	2	3	4
7. I provide others with new ways to look at things.	0	1	2	3	4
8. I let others know how I think they are doing.	0	1	2	3	4
9. Others are proud to be associated with me.	0	1	2	3	4
10. I help others find meaning in their work.	0	1	2	3	4
11. I get others to rethink ideas not questioned before.	0	1	2	3	4
12. I pay personal attention to others who seem dejected.	0	1	2	3	4

Scales   **Totals**

Idealized influence (Items 1, 5, and 9)   _____ Factor 1

Inspirational motivation (Items 2, 6, and 10)   _____ Factor 2

Intellectual stimulation (Items 3, 7, and 11)   _____ Factor 3

Individualized consideration (Items 4, 8, and 12)   _____ Factor 4

Score Range   High = 9–12   Moderate = 5–8   Low = 0–4

Score Interpretation

Factor 1.   *Idealized influence* indicates whether you hold others' trust, maintain their faith and respect, show dedication to them, appeal to their hopes and dreams, and act as their role model.

Factor 2.   *Inspirational motivation* measures the degree to which you provide a vision, help others focus on their work, and try to make others feel their work is significant.

Exhibit 5.7. (*Continued*)

Factor 3	*Intellectual stimulation* shows the degree to which you encourage others to be creative in looking at old problems in new ways, create an environment that tolerates opposition, and nurture people to question their own values and beliefs and those of the organization.
Factor 4	*Individualized consideration* indicates the degree to which you show interest in others' well being, assign projects individually, and pay attention to those who seem less involved in the group.

Source: Adapted from the Multifactor Leadership Questionnaire (MLQ-6S) by B. M. Bass and B. J. Avolio, 1992 (in Northouse, P. G., *Leadership,* 2nd ed. Thousand Oaks, Calif.: Sage, 2001, pp. 156–157). Complete scale can be obtained from Mind Garden, Inc., 1690 Woodside Road, Suite 202, Redwood City, Calif., 94061, or by calling (650) 261-3500.

Exhibit 5.8. Ten Traits of Transformational Leaders.

Transformational Leaders . . .

1. **Let go of things others can do.**
   - Let go of tasks and responsibilities that will help others develop.
   - Let go of authority to make decisions about the work.
   - Know what others in the group can do and want to do.
   - Build people's skills to take over by involving them in the work.

2. **Encourage initiative, ideas, and risk taking.**
   - Actively seek ideas and suggestions from the work group.
   - Allow people to run with an idea, even if it might involve some risk.
   - Recognize ideas and initiative through compliments, formal recognition, and tangible rewards.
   - Are careful not to put down or discount ideas.

3. **Ensure that people have goals and know how they're doing.**
   - Encourage work group to take lead role in setting goals and assessing *the leader's* performance.
   - Ensure that goals are clear and understandable.
   - Let people know how they're doing in meeting goals and provide needed guidance and support.

4. **Delegate to challenge, develop, and empower.**
   - Delegate to challenge and develop people.
   - Delegate authority to make decisions about the work.
   - Provide clear understanding of responsibility, authority, expectations, and constraints.
   - Support delegation within and outside the work group.
   - Set up controls that keep themselves apprised of progress but aren't seen as restrictive.

(continued)

Exhibit 5.8. Ten Traits of Transformational Leaders. (*Continued*)

5. **Coach to ensure success.**
   - Coach *before* person begins task or assumes responsibility *and along the way*.
   - Use coaching to guide and instruct people while maintaining and enhancing their self-esteem.

6. **Reinforce good work and good attempts.**
   - Use verbal *praise frequently*.
   - Know kind of reinforcement that works best for each person.
   - Provide tangible reinforcement when possible (for example, recognition letters, awards, or gifts).
   - Remember to reinforce what someone does well even when his or her work has a few flaws.

7. **Share information, knowledge, and skills.**
   - Meet with group regularly to share and update information.
   - Make sure people have or know how to get information they need to succeed in the task or responsibility.
   - Share their insights, knowledge, expertise, and skills.

8. **Value, trust, and respect each individual.**
   - Show trust and respect by encouraging people to take control of their jobs and give them authority to take action.
   - Take opportunities to compliment people for good work, creative ideas, and contributions to group.
   - Listen to people and empathize with their problems and concerns.
   - Never put people down or minimize their contributions.

9. **Provide support without taking over.**
   - Understand that support is essential and know when it's needed.
   - Know how to support others, for example, by coaching, reinforcing, preparing for resistance, gaining others' commitment.
   - Resist temptation to take over when things go wrong.

10. **Practice what they preach.**
    - *Support* people through rough spots of new task instead of punishing them for errors or taking over.
    - Ask for ideas and empower people to *implement* them—especially those that involve risk.
    - Tell people that they are important and *show* them through actions.

Leadership Recruitment

Although the benefits of developing and rotating leaders are clear, coalitions often struggle with the reality of finding able leaders and sustaining their involvement. We will explore the basics of recruiting and sustaining member involvement in Chapter Seven, but the issues surrounding leadership identification and recruitment deserve special attention.

Coalitions should recruit leaders in three categories: formal, voluntary, and informal leaders.

Formal leaders are the obvious recruits in any community, in other words, those who already hold visible leadership positions in mainstream organizations. Chief executive officers (CEOs) of businesses, government, and private institutions (for example, hospitals and health departments), and not-for-profit agencies (for example, the American Heart Association and March of Dimes)— these leaders are seen as tried-and-true and bring assets ranging from management skills to business savvy. However, coalitions should be aware that these leaders are more experienced in leading an executive board and may be untested in collaborative decision-making environments. Additionally, even though they are respected and inspire confidence, they may be too busy to give the coalition the attention it needs.

Voluntary leaders are those who hold leadership positions in voluntary organizations, for example, other coalitions and community-based organizations. These people are also natural choices for leadership because they bring respect and tested leadership skills to the coalition. Voluntary leaders are more accustomed to working in a democratic, decision-making environment, but they may also work under a board-type leadership and management.

Informal leaders have not usually held previous elected or appointed leadership positions. They represent the natural leadership or authentic voices of the community. The concept of natural leaders is inspired by Eng's and Parker's (2002) work with *natural helpers,* who serve as lay health advisors in their communities, to improve access to and use of screening exams (for example, for hypertension and breast cancer) . These natural helpers are "particular individuals to whom others naturally turn for advice, emotional support, and tangible aid" (Eng and Parker, 2002, p. 126). By engaging natural leaders, coalition credibility is enhanced, and community members who may have been hesitant to join coalition efforts may be more likely to step forward and volunteer to help these leaders.

Informal leaders are also invaluable sources of information in a community. Even if they do not agree to hold formal office or regularly attend coalition meetings, they are in tune with the community's pulse, know other key community stakeholders, and may recommend and mentor others to join, and eventually lead, coalitions.

How can coalitions encourage people to serve in leadership positions? Like members, leaders must perceive that the benefits of leadership outweigh the costs. When the potential leader is recruited, he or she already knows that certain costs will be incurred. Extra time will have to be spent in preparing for, traveling to, and facilitating or attending meetings, and extra responsibilities will be added to the leader's regular workload. To compensate for these burdens, staff and volunteer recruiters must make potential leaders aware of the benefits that come with leadership. Building on the adage "leadership has its privileges," recruiters should emphasize what these privileges entail. Experience with coalitions for all health issues shows that leaders value some or all of the following benefits:

- Expanding opportunities to network with other leaders, movers, and shakers
- Developing leadership skills, such as public speaking, facilitation, problem solving, and decision making, that can be transferred to other leadership settings
- Increasing connection to community and coalition members
- Opportunities to represent the coalition via print, radio, and televised media outlets and in other community forums; and opportunity for travel to national issue meetings or grantee meetings to represent the coalition leader
- Increased visibility and prominence for the leaders' organization
- Opportunity to add leadership experience to resumes that require or value volunteer or community service
- Ability to obtain letters of reference or recommendation from coalition staff that attest to leader's involvement and impact in the coalition
- Satisfaction from making a concerted contribution to a worthwhile effort

Leadership Styles

No two people lead in exactly the same way. Every leader has a natural style that is a function of many things, including his or her personality, experience, and training. Leaders must also learn to adapt to different situations and adjust their leadership styles accordingly. Kumpher, Turner, Hopkins, and Librett (1993) found that the *leadership style* most associated with an effective team and a quality action plan was one that empowered team members by building networks, providing planning, and supporting team members. Similarly, in SmokeLess States coalitions, Sofaer (2001) found that leaders needed to balance both process and outcome. Leaders who were reported to be more controlling were more likely to take advantage of limited opportunities to get things done (for example, pass a cigarette excise tax increase). However, leaders who were reported to have a more inclusive and less directive style were associated with members who were more satisfied and committed to the coalition and who reported that the benefits outweighed the costs of participation.

In the leadership literature, a distinction has been made between leaders and managers, especially in the business or corporate sector. Grace Murray Hopper, a retired U.S. Navy admiral, once said, "You manage things; you lead people."

However, a coalition leader needs to be skilled in managing things *and* in leading people. The skills of leader and manager are complementary and essential and can be cultivated over time. (See Exhibit 5.8, Heim and Chapman's Management and Leadership Assessment Scale, to appreciate the duality of these skills.)

Dowling and colleagues provide a summary of five different styles of leadership, noting that leaders that are more skilled have many or all of these approaches in their skill sets (Dowling, O'Donnell, and Wellington Consulting Group, 2000, p. 62):

Strategic approach. Leader has a vision for the future and develops a plan to move the organization forward.
Human assets approach. Leader analyzes available people and other resources and focuses on them to manage for success.
Expertise approach. Leader's professional expertise, shared by no others or only a few, is the power behind his or her leadership (often seen in health-focused coalitions where the leader is a physician or health director).
Box approach. Leader uses a highly developed systematic set of principles, rules, and procedures to lead others.
Change approach. Leader sees the future as filled with change and leads by creating an organization that is dynamic and responsive to change.

Himmelman describes collaborative leadership as one that facilitates mutual enhancement among those working together for a common purpose. His ten collaborative leadership characteristics are presented here (Rosenthal, 2000, p. 67):

1. A commitment to improve common circumstances based on values, beliefs, and a vision for change that is communicated both by talking it and walking it

2. An ability to persuade people to conduct themselves within ground rules that provide the basis for mutual trust, respect, and accountability

3. An ability to respectfully educate others about the relationship of processes to products and outcomes, and of organizational structure to effective action

4. An ability to draw out ideas and information in ways that contribute to effective problem solving rather than ineffective restatements of problems

5. A willingness to actively encourage partners to share risks, responsibilities, resources, and rewards, and to offer acknowledgments of those making contributions

6. An ability to balance the need for discussion, information sharing, and storytelling with timely problem solving and staying focused on responding to action-oriented expectations of those engaged in common efforts

7. An understanding of the role of community organizing as the basis for developing and expanding collaborative power

8. A commitment to and active engagement in leadership development activities, both informal and formal, that can take the collaborative process to higher levels of inclusiveness and effectiveness

9. An ability to communicate in ways that invite comments and suggestions that address problems without attacking people and, when appropriate, to draw upon conflict resolution and win-win negotiating to resolve differences

10. A very good sense of humor, especially whenever collaborative processes get ugly, boring, or both

To see how collaborative or transformative leaders differ from traditional, transactional leaders, a summary of the differences between the styles of both are compared in Table 5.1.

Lolly (1996) conceptualizes leadership style according to five levels that start with a very hierarchical, top-down model and proceed to a horizontal, flat model, while moving from an unempowered environment to one that is highly empowered.

In Level One (Chain of Command), the leader is positioned *above and separate* from the work group and has sole authority for decision making.

In Level Two (Leader Is Central), the leader moves from above to the center of the work group, but a clear distinction still exists between what the leader does and what other work group members do. The leader is central to most of the communication within the group, directs everyone's activities, and channels the communication from upper management to the group.

In Level Three (Transition), the leader begins to shift decision-making authority for basic tasks to the work group. Some members may begin to take on responsibilities

Table 5.1. Comparison of Collaborative Versus Traditional Leaders.

Collaborative Leaders	Traditional Leaders
Share power	Impose hierarchy
Holistic views of organization or community	Fragmented view
Focus on facilitation and process	Focus on decision making
Flexible	Controlling
Decentralized	Centralized
Inclusive	Exclusive
Proactive	Reactive
Focus on process and product	Focus on product

Source: Wolff and Kaye, 1998, p. 3.

belonging traditionally to the leader. The leader also encourages communication, cooperation, and teamwork among group members whenever possible. The leader is still central to the group, especially as the initiator of transition to empowerment.

In Level Four (Partnership), the leader's role becomes increasingly supportive. No longer central to decision making, the leader becomes a partner within the work group. Links between group members might become even stronger; they might depend on each other as much as on the leader for information, help on decisions, and support. Group members are empowered to make decisions about how they do their jobs, as well as to assume many responsibilities and decisions once held by the leader.

In Level Five (Highly Empowered), the group members are self-directed. The leader's primary role is to coach, counsel, and support them. Group members take responsibility for and make decisions about tasks and jobs, including most that were formerly the leader's responsibility. The leader still provides direction and acts as a resource, often tackling issues outside of the group (Lolly, 1996).

Leadership Traits, Skills, and Roles

Research on leadership in every kind of organization has failed to come up with a definitive set of leadership traits that define the ideal leader. However, in *Principle-Centered Leadership,* Covey (1990) identifies seven behavioral traits common to effective leaders:

Proactiveness. Leader instills in people the belief that quality begins with the leader and that the leader should be a stakeholder and responsible for the performance of the organization.

Imagination and conscience. Leader shares vision, hopes, and purpose, as well as social responsibility, for people and their families.

Willpower. Leader maintains a disciplined personal and professional life with high moral values, and focuses on important activities while minimizing crisis management.

A win-win mindset. Leader shares recognition and power by tapping the capabilities of all people and routinely provides constructive feedback and praise; he or she recognizes that strength lies in diversity, creates an environment of trust, and attempts to reduce friction.

Courage balanced with consideration. Leader actively listens to others to clearly understand their ideas, fosters mutual respect, and builds teams where each individual strength is made productive and each weakness is made irrelevant.

Synergy. Leader solves problems by promoting open communication between respectful individuals and achieves creativity, improvement, and innovation beyond individual capacities.

Continuous improvement or self-renewal. Leader avoids being closed to new ideas and pursues innovation and refinement in himself or herself and in others. He or she expands cooperation, communication, trust, and synergy within the organization.

In *The Tao of Leadership*, John Heider (1985) espouses only three essential leadership traits: compassion, material simplicity or frugality, and a sense of equality or modesty. A compassionate leader "acts in behalf of everyone's right to life"; material simplicity "gives one an abundance to share," and a sense of equality "is, paradoxically, one's true greatness" (p. 133).

In coalition leadership research, the personal traits and skills that have been cited as important include self-efficacy, membership in other community organizations, and level of education (Prestby and Wandersman, 1985); a high degree of political knowledge, commitment, and competence (Rich, 1980; Prestby and Wandersman, 1985); trustworthiness, patience, energy, and hope (W. K. Kellogg Foundation, 1994); proven administrative skills for setting agendas and running efficient meetings, garnering resources and delegating responsibilities (Feighery and Rogers, 1990); skill in communication and interpersonal relations (Brown, 1984; Andrews, 1990); the ability to promote equal status and encourage overall collaboration (Croan and Lees, 1979; Hord, 1986; Lindsay and Edwards, 1988); flexibility (Cohen, 1989); and easy access to the media and decision makers in the community (National Assembly of National Voluntary Health and Social Welfare Organizations, 1991). Leaders must recognize conflict as an inherent and positive aspect of collaboration and must be, at the same time, assertive and responsive. Good leadership is good "follower-ship," as leaders must follow the lead of the other stakeholder groups and find new paths to manage these complex systems (Bailey and Koney, 1996). Mizrahi and Rosenthal (2001) identified specific values such as trustworthiness, commitment, persistence, persuasiveness, and credibility, as well as skills in facilitation, negotiation, looking for commonalities among coalition members, strategy development, and politics.

Roussos and Fawcett (2000) argue that different stages of coalition development require different leadership skills. Although coalitions in formation may need greater listening and facilitation skills to recruit and engage members, coalitions that are heavily involved in implementing and maintaining programs may need negotiation and advocacy skills to bring about environmental changes. Exhibit 5.9 offers a leadership assessment scale, and Exhibit 5.10 outlines a composite description of the traits of an ideal coalition leader (Sofaer, 2001, p. 36; Dowling, O'Donnell, and Wellington Consulting Group, 2000, p. 65).

As discussed earlier with reference to staff, leadership is a team effort. In a study of leaders within twenty-one diverse organizations that collaborated to build capacity for heart health promotion in Nova Scotia, Canada, researchers found that leaders served three main roles: as *innovators* of new processes and interventions, as *linkers* that fostered individual and organizational collaboration, and as *enablers* that created environments that facilitated capacity building among their members (Joffres and others, 2004). Dowling and colleagues further define the roles that should be carried out by different leaders within the coalition (Dowling, O'Donnell, and Wellington Consulting Group, 2000, p. 63). Key leaders, namely the coalition coordinator and chair, must assure that these roles are competently filled.

Public leader presents coalition vision and key messages to the community and gives the coalition a public face.

(*Text resumes on page 125.*)

Exhibit 5.9. Management and Leader Assessment Scale.

This survey describes twenty practices that are commonly demonstrated by excellent managers and twenty more commonly demonstrated by effective leaders. Read all statements carefully and decide on the score that you would assign yourself for each practice or characteristic as demonstrated in your work life.

Indicate your decision by circling the appropriate number for each practice.

1 = Seldom   2 = Sometimes   3 = Frequently   4 = Very Frequently   5 = Always

1. Gets tough when needed	1	2	3	4	5
2. Speaks well to groups	1	2	3	4	5
3. Establishes consistent, clear discipline line	1	2	3	4	5
4. Motivates others with a clear message	1	2	3	4	5
5. Provides environment conducive to a feeling of cohesiveness	1	2	3	4	5
6. Communicates sense of being in charge	1	2	3	4	5
7. Has full backing from those reporting to him or her	1	2	3	4	5
8. Converts employees into followers	1	2	3	4	5
9. Strives to win by allowing employees to also win	1	2	3	4	5
10. Attracts others to join his or her group	1	2	3	4	5
11. Provides important rewards to staff	1	2	3	4	5
12. Utilizes sources of power in a sensitive, consistent manner	1	2	3	4	5
13. Shows compassion	1	2	3	4	5
14. Strong track record for making solid and decisive decisions	1	2	3	4	5
15. Good listener	1	2	3	4	5
16. Formalizes and "stages" communication announcements	1	2	3	4	5
17. Expresses thoughts clearly	1	2	3	4	5
18. Prudent risk taker	1	2	3	4	5
19. Keeps employees fully informed	1	2	3	4	5
20. Articulates an inspiring mission	1	2	3	4	5
21. Highly ethical	1	2	3	4	5
22. Generates a feeling of pride in followers	1	2	3	4	5
23. Delegates effectively	1	2	3	4	5
24. Ties short-term work goals to mission	1	2	3	4	5
25. Shares large and small victories with staff	1	2	3	4	5
26. Gets others caught up in his or her positive force	1	2	3	4	5
27. Makes work enjoyable	1	2	3	4	5
28. Creates active tempo	1	2	3	4	5
29. Maintains positive, upbeat attitude	1	2	3	4	5
30. Highly energetic, not "desk-bound"	1	2	3	4	5
31. Admits to mistakes	1	2	3	4	5
32. Good negotiator; knows when to compromise	1	2	3	4	5
33. Follows logical steps in making decisions	1	2	3	4	5

(continued)

Exhibit 5.9. Management and Leader Assessment Scale. (*Continued*)

34. If he or she resigned, others would consider following	1	2	3	4	5
35. Consults with others in making decisions	1	2	3	4	5
36. Builds commitment to his or her cause	1	2	3	4	5
37. Uses management role with sensitivity	1	2	3	4	5
38. Stands firm on principle	1	2	3	4	5
39. Respected by employees when authority is used	1	2	3	4	5
40. Communicates a power image	1	2	3	4	5

Management and Leadership Assessment Scale Results

All of the practices that are found in effective *managers* have odd numbers. Those practices not always found in managers but usually found in *leaders* have even numbers.

To calculate your response scores:

- Add all the responses to the odd numbered questions. The total of your responses to the twenty Management Practices Statements is _____ out of 100 possible.
- Add all the responses to the even numbered questions. The total of your responses to the twenty Leadership Practices Statements is _____ out of 100 possible.

Look at the twenty management statements. Do any of these surprise you?

Now, look at the twenty leadership statements. Do any of these surprise you?

Will you do your work in a new way so as to challenge these management and leadership styles? Explain your answer.

Source: Heim, P. and Chapman, E. N. (1990). *Learning to lead: An action plan for success.* Los Altos, CA: Crisp Publications, Inc.

Exhibit 5.10. Characteristics of an Ideal Coalition Leader.

- Has a clear vision and is goal- and task-oriented; keeps the coalition focused
- Is unafraid to challenge the status quo
- Is inclusive—appreciates and respects diverse perspectives and contributions
- Respects each coalition member and, in turn, is respected by him or her
- Trusts members and is trustworthy (keeps promises)
- Is fair, equitable, and ethical, both within and outside of the coalition
- Gives and receives feedback in a constructive manner
- Often takes the blame and sees mistakes as learning opportunities
- Acts as a coach, appealing to the best in people and moving them to action
- Achieves closure on decisions without cutting off input and participation prematurely
- Is accessible to members
- Thinks of ways to make people and processes more productive and efficient
- Simplifies—makes the job look easy
- Works collaboratively—creates balance of responsibility among members and between members and staff
- Is a good listener and elicits input, especially from quiet or new members who feel like outsiders
- Is skilled at framing issues, distilling complex ideas into simple messages, and managing and resolving conflict

Consensus builder brings coalition members together, summarizes decisions, and helps resolve differences.

Organizer coordinates the various parts of the coalition in an efficient and effective way.

Cheerleader brings energy and enthusiasm to coalition tasks, stirs other people up with that same enthusiasm, and prevents the work of the coalition from being dull and lifeless.

Coach provides guidance and direction to coalition members and ensures that all opinions are heard.

In their classic research work with public and private business organizations, Kouzes and Posner (1987) outline the practices and commitment of successful leaders, as shown in Table 5.2. Although not created specifically for coalition leadership, they are relevant to our discussion.

Similarly, the Turning Point Leadership Development National Excellence Collaborative (2001b) identified six practices of collaborative leaders based on an extensive literature review, interviews, focus groups, and expert panel debates. These practices, or competencies, are especially useful for coalition

Table 5.2. Ten Commitments of Leadership

Practices	Commitments
Challenge the process	1. *Search out* challenging opportunities to change, grow, innovate, and improve.
	2. *Experiment,* take risks, and learn from the accompanying mistakes.
Inspire a shared vision	3. *Envision* an uplifting and ennobling future.
	4. *Enlist* others in a common vision by appealing to their values, interests, hopes, and dreams.
Enable other to act	5. *Foster* collaboration by promoting cooperative goals and building trust.
	6. *Strengthen* people by giving power away, providing choice, developing competence, assigning critical tasks, and offering visible support.
Model the way	7. *Set* the example by behaving in ways that are consistent with shared values.
	8. *Achieve* small wins that promote consistent progress and build commitment.
Encourage the heart	9. *Recognize* individual contributions to the success of every project.
	10. *Celebrate* team accomplishments regularly.

Source: Adapted from Kouzes and Posner, 1987.

leaders and follow the themes that lead to collaboration described in Chapter Two (p. 33):

- *Assessing the environment,* or understanding the context for change before one acts
- *Creating clarity,* or defining shared values and engaging people in positive action
- *Building trust,* or creating safe places for developing shared purpose and action
- *Sharing power and influence,* or developing synergy of people, organizations, and communities to accomplish a shared vision
- *Developing people,* or committing to people as a key asset through coaching and mentoring
- *Self-reflection,* or understanding one's own values, attitudes, and behaviors as they relate to one's leadership style and its impact on others

TEAM LEADERSHIP

As the coalition develops, more work will be done by work groups that function as teams. Teamwork can be used to build the base of leaders and to give members a sense of belonging and control that does not occur when the coalition is convened as a large group. Team leadership follows many of the principles proposed in this chapter, but some unique issues involved in leading small groups will be covered in Chapter Eight.

TRAINING, TECHNICAL ASSISTANCE, AND ORIENTATION

Practitioners increasingly find themselves in the role of coordinating community coalitions to promote health and prevent disease. However, they often do not possess the skill set needed to build and maintain partnerships that deal with complex issues such as consensus building, conflict resolution, and advocacy. To fulfill their duties, members and leaders obtain training in coalition building from professional conferences, workshops, self-help manuals, peers in similar positions, or by hiring consultants to offer on-site training. In this section, we will focus on the training that leaders, as well as members, need to be competent.

Borrowing from the literature on learning organizations, coalitions must develop individuals' levels of personal mastery, their skills with mental models, and their willingness to interrelate, to build team learning approaches and shared vision (Senge, 1990). Similarly, Kotter (1995) uses a business paradigm that can be applied to public health, namely, that the capacity to compete in a changing world is a function of an organization's commitment to develop competitive new skills and abilities, and engage in lifelong learning. Thus, coalitions that survive must be learning organizations that are committed to adapting, changing, and learning new skills through training and technical assistance.

Training

Training should be based on a review of relevant training literature and the external policies that may affect a coalition's operation, because members have different theoretical backgrounds, levels of experience, and opinions about how tasks should be accomplished (Andrews, 1990; Cohen, Baer, and Satterwhite, 2002). With the demand for more sophisticated competencies at the local coalition level, training strategies must also be created to meet the needs of leaders from many backgrounds who face multiple issues (Doble and Johnson, 1991; Matthews, 1994; Stevens and Lodl, 1999).

Overall, coalitions have found that training works. In a study of thirteen community coalitions in Nebraska, youth members completed an advocacy training program and as a result became more comfortable about taking public policy action for their coalitions. With training and encouragement from the group, coalition members moved from beginning level actions (talking to others about public opinions, considering various alternatives to local issues, exploring the consequences to alternatives) to more complex actions (contacting policy makers, becoming involved in policy) (Stevens and Lodl, 1999). In Robert Wood Johnson's Faith in Action program, early training of coalition volunteers resulted in a competent pool of members in faith-based coalitions who were able to recruit more participants to take part in their programs (Pepper, Herrera, and Leviton, 2003).

Florin, Mitchell, and Stevenson (1993) discovered that over 75 percent of the task forces they studied that were exposed to training and written resource materials found them helpful in promoting their coalitions' efforts. Less is known about which knowledge areas for coalitions can be easily and efficiently acquired with written materials; which require the skill-building practice found in face-to-face training sessions; and which call for the intensity of on-site consultation (Florin, Mitchell, and Stevenson, 1993).

The authors describe several levels of technical-assistance and training needs based on the coalition's stage of development; that is, coalitions need training for initial mobilization, establishing a sound organization, capacity building, and planning for action. Within the coalition stages, they offer several recommendations regarding technical assistance and training:

- Avoid moving too quickly into action before engaging all the relevant community constituencies and sectors. Special attention should be paid to developing appropriate recruitment strategies to increase cultural and age diversity and underrepresented community sectors. Coalitions should develop special mechanisms to maintain contact with community sectors that are unrepresented in the coalition, such as businesses and religious organizations.
- Provide clear options for organizational structuring and specific guidelines for operating procedures. Train coalitions on leadership techniques, such as managing meetings, delegating responsibilities, and assigning reporting duties to keep the coalition focused.

- Help communities analyze problem conditions and connect identified problems to goals and effective actions. Most coalitions focus on providing information and raising awareness. Instead, they should be oriented to the full range of intervention strategies and innovative programs that can be adopted, perhaps by conducting regional meetings for information sharing. Information on research that has practical implications for the strategies, programs, and populations of interest would also be helpful for coalitions.

- Build evaluation capacity into the coalitions, or find a supporting organization to take on a consultative role to carry out this function.

Technical Assistance

Technical assistance involves the transfer of knowledge and practice skills to groups, which helps them to develop or improve organizations, programs, products, services, delivery systems, and internal operations (Suarez and Montgomery, 1989). As an intervention, technical assistance introduces external people, practices, or products into an existing organization (Suarez and Montgomery, 1989). However, the ability to foster real change through new practices requires that the coalition or organization be provided with opportunities and assistance to put the new ideas and information into practice (Senge, 1990). Technical assistance can take many forms such as consultation, training, dissemination, network building, and materials development.

Bruner (1993) describes several reasons for seeking technical assistance and support, for example: the desire to know what others in similar situations have done and to learn from their experience; the need for time- and resource-limited assistance, which can be provided by an expert; and the need for an independent perspective from a legitimate, impartial party. Another reason may be that the expertise does not exist, is not available, or is not available within the required timeframe.

As a supportive and helping process, technical assistance embodies principles of counseling and consultation, such as establishing credibility and a trusting relationship, maintaining confidentiality, and matching compatible providers with recipients (Suarez and Montgomery, 1989). The authors acknowledge that certain influential contextual and historical factors are critical, such as leadership support, local commitment, political influences, organizational setting, and the policy environment.

The technical-assistance provider must pay close attention to the recipient's expectations of the provider and the reasons this organization has for seeking assistance. In addition, both parties must have a clear understanding of the specific roles and responsibilities of technical-assistance providers and recipients (Russell, 2002).

The development of capacity for systemic change requires that technical-assistance providers and recipients consider the following questions regarding the nature of their relationship (Mojkowski, 1995; Trohanis, 1998):

- Who are the recipients and what are their needs?
- What contextual issues must be addressed before planning and implementing the intervention?
- Do the philosophies of the provider and the recipient align?

- How should technical-assistance services be provided to this particular recipient?
- Can the provider and recipient meet each other's needs? (In other words, what amount of technical assistance is needed in terms of scope, intensity, and cost? How will recipients support the assistance? What impact can realistically be achieved by providing technical assistance to this recipient?)
- How and by whom will the technical-assistance services be evaluated?

Trainers' and Technical-Assistance Consultants' Roles, Responsibilities, and Characteristics

Effective technical assistance is based on a strong interpersonal relationship in which the provider is perceived as being warm, open, and nonjudgmental, and as providing the support that builds trust in recipients and encourages them to openly specify needs and share contextual aspects (Suarez and Montgomery, 1989). In other words, trainers and technical-assistance providers should be more than just experts. They must demonstrate that they are primarily helpers to the people who perform the actual work, and they must listen to and work with the coalition to develop appropriate solutions to their most significant problems (Buckley and Mank, 1994).

Providers must help the coalition understand, reflect upon, and develop the capacity necessary to manage change. Effective providers are proactive and responsive to recipients' needs (Yin and White, 1984). Key provider attributes are expertise, consulting skills, interpersonal skills, and quality performance (Suarez and Montgomery, 1989). The provider must possess extensive content and process knowledge that comes from experience. Consulting skills enable the provider to diagnose recipient needs, set goals and formulate plans, take action and provide feedback, and extend or terminate the relationship as the recipient's capacity expands (Block, 1981).

Coalition Roles, Responsibilities, and Characteristics

Coalitions must recognize the need for help, be clear about the type of assistance needed, and prepare the organization for the infusion of new knowledge in order for change to occur (Russell, 2002). Prior to any change initiative, leaders at every level have to ensure that their organizations and staff are *adept to change* (Kanter, 1999). Change-adept organizations share three key attributes, each associated with a particular role for leaders: (1) the imagination to innovate, (2) professionalism and competence to perform, and (3) the openness to collaborate (Kanter, 1999). Other desirable characteristics of coalition recipients include incentive for reform, continuity of staff and resources, ownership over the technical-assistance process, and some capacity, skills, or training in the subject (Yin and White, 1984).

Building and Sustaining Technical-Assistance Consultant–Coalition Relationships

Open communication between partners is the vehicle by which trust is established and good partner relationships are sustained (Justice, 1993). Timely introductions of key participants, thorough and continuous needs assessments, mutually agreed-upon evaluation systems, and ongoing communication will engender trust and respect between the provider and the coalition (Bruner, 1993). Additional efforts that sustain a trusting relationship include sharing decisions, recognition, and credit; recognizing and appreciating differences in values; working toward a common vision; building shared ownership; getting to know each other on a personal level; acknowledging that all contributions are important; and using a win–win approach (Miller, Rossing, and Steel, 1992).

Skills training leads to increased reporting of issues by members, improvements in the chairpersons' ability to conduct action-oriented meetings, and overall improved effectiveness within an advocacy coalition (Balcazar, Seekins, Fawcett, and Hopkins, 1990). How well leadership and participation are applied and transferred is crucial for community change (Goodman and others, 1998).

Training and Technical-Assistance Venues

An array of coalition-training options have been offered throughout the United States. Many issue-specific area conferences sponsored by federal agencies, such as the Centers for Disease Control and Prevention (CDC), Health Care and Finance Administration (HCFA), Health Resources and Services Administration (HRSA), and the Center for Substance Abuse Prevention (CSAP), have focused on coalition training. Academic institutions have conducted intensive training institutes to develop coalition-building skills (for example, the Annual Tobacco Control Conference by the University of North Carolina School of Public Health, the Coalition Training Institute by the Center for Pediatric Research, the HIV/AIDS Leadership Institute by the University of South Carolina School of Public Health).

However, despite the breadth and quality of such training opportunities, researchers question whether a transfer of training actually occurs after these workshops (Ottoson, 1997; Cividin and Ottoson, 1997). Regardless, other than these short intensive training sessions, community coalitions have had to rely on presentations or workshops to augment or individualize their coalition training. Evidence from focus groups with coalitions after intensive training suggests that coalitions need ongoing technical assistance and support over a formative period to accomplish tasks related to coalition building and maintenance (Butterfoss, Webster, Morrow, and Rosenthal, 1998; Butterfoss, Morrow, Webster, and Crews, 2003).

To address this need, the Coalition Technical Assistance and Training (CTAT) Framework is a six-step process that may be initiated by a consultant or by a coalition itself (see Exhibits 5.11–5.13). The framework uses an empowerment approach that helps coalition staff and members to be more effective and efficient by diagnosing coalition strengths and challenges themselves, and coming up with a prescription for action. Re-evaluation after a specified time helps determine whether a coalition adopted recommended changes in coalition participants, structures, and processes, and progressed through stages of development. This process should take six months to one year to accomplish, depending on the level of coalition development and the number of suggested recommendations. This framework can be used for coalitions that are local or distant to the consultant, because few site visits are required.

Building on years of work with health-promotion coalitions, the framework was formally piloted with seven perinatal councils in Virginia that focused on preventing low-weight births and infant mortality. By using the framework, the coalitions adopted 75 percent of the recommended actions within one year. Results from a pre-and post-coalition assessment after three years showed significant progress in the coalitions' ability to develop effective participants, structures, and procedures (Butterfoss, 2004). The six steps are assessment, site visit, written recommendations, telephone consultation, training, and evaluation as described in Exhibit 5.11. And Exhibit 5.12 provides a sample follow-up report, Exhibit 5.13 is a needs assessment tool, and other tools used in this process are included in Chapter Thirteen on evaluation.

Chavis, Florin, and Felix (1992) advocate setting up an intermediary organization that can provide training and technical assistance to multiple coalitions with minimal staff, and is affordable, easily accessible, culturally sensitive, and manageable over a long period of time. In addition to offering technical assistance, such an "enabling system" creates linkages, supplies resources, and removes barriers common to all the coalitions it serves (Chavis, Florin, and Felix, 1992). The enabling system would include training programs for skills development; telephone and on-site consultation; information and referral services; mechanisms for creating

Exhibit 5.11. Coalition Technical Assistance and Training Framework.

STEP 1:   **ASSESSMENT**

- Complete written self-assessments (coalition staff and/or leaders):
  - Initial Coalition Needs Assessment (CNA)
  - Coalition Effectiveness Inventory (CEI)

STEP 2:   **SITE VISIT**

- Consult with staff.
- Review CNA, CEI, and historical documents.
- Attend and evaluate meetings.
- Take a Meeting Effectiveness Inventory (MEI).
- Out-process with staff.

STEP 3:   **WRITTEN RECOMMENDATIONS**

Send site report with recommendations for action to staff.

STEP 4:   **TELEPHONE CONSULTATION**

Consult by telephone with staff to explain or clarify recommendations.

STEP 5:   **COALITION TRAINING**

Provide training on issues related to building or sustaining coalition.

STEP 6:   **EVALUATION**

- Evaluate success of actions taken (staff and consultant).
- Identify new recommendations for action (repeat Steps 4–6).

Source: From "Building Effective Coalitions with Consultation and Technical Assistance: Virginia's Healthy Start Initiative," by F. D. Butterfoss in *Health Promotion Practice,* 5(2), 118–126. Copyright © 2004 Sage Publications, Inc. Reproduced with permission of Sage Publications, Inc. via Copyright Clearance Center.

Exhibit 5.12. Sample Follow-Up Report to Coalition (Step 3).

SITE VISIT to Coalition X (date)

Activities

- Met with coordinator and outreach educator (time).
- Discussed progress of coalition to date and issues with grant as implemented.
- Reviewed needs assessment and CEI.
- Attended and evaluated membership meeting (time).
- Shared findings at debriefing (date and time).

Overall Impression

- Strong, professionally driven coalition.
- Coordinators open to re-evaluating coalition and its direction.

Recommendations

- Create committee structure either by issue areas or geographic locations (for example, four health districts). Geographic focus would eliminate travel barriers and develop local support for perinatal initiatives.
- Meetings should occur quarterly or, if subcommittees are established, could alternate with quarterly general membership meetings.
- Elect chair and vice-chair positions for coalition and for each subcommittee.
- Recruit more diverse membership to include social service, voluntary agencies, grassroots community groups and consumer representatives.
- Review and update original bylaws.
- Create organizational chart for coalition and job descriptions for staff, members, and leaders.
- Develop recruitment and new member orientation mechanism and packet.
- This year, encourage each committee to develop one goal that is realistic and measurable; then entire coalition should develop one overall focus (goal).
- Convene task force to react to above recommendations and plan coalition-building training session for members.

Source: From "Building Effective Coalitions with Consultation and Technical Assistance: Virginia's Healthy Start Initiative," by F. D. Butterfoss in *Health Promotion Practice,* 5(2), 118–126. Copyright © 2004 Sage Publications, Inc. Reproduced with permission of Sage Publications, Inc. via Copyright Clearance Center.

linkages among coalitions; methods of recognizing group achievement; and publications and other public education materials (Chavis, Florin, and Felix, 1992). One such model program is available through the Community Anti-Drug Coalitions of America (CADCA). They offer programs that answer the training and technical-assistance needs of most coalitions:

Satellite broadcasts. CADCA, the National Guard Bureau (NGB), and the Multijurisdictional Counterdrug Task Force Training Program (MCTFT) co-sponsored live satellite broadcasts on varied topics related to substance abuse prevention, intervention, and treatment. Visit the institute's website for the current schedule.

Exhibit 5.13. Coalition Initial Needs Assessment.

1. If your coalition has a written mission statement, please write it below.

2. If your coalition has written goals or objectives, please write them below. If you have an action plan, please include a copy.

3. In general, what are the main functions of your coalition? (Check as many as apply.)

   ☐ Information and resource sharing

   ☐ Planning and coordination

   ☐ Technical assistance and training

   ☐ Advocacy and community change

4. How many organizations are represented in your coalition? _____

5. List your coalition's most active member organizations (or attach member roster).

6. How often does your coalition meet?

7. If your coalition has working committees, please list them below.

8. If your coalition has elected leadership, please list the offices held.

9. What are your coalition's most significant successes; in other words, what accomplishments would your members be most proud of? (Name at least three.)

10. What are your coalition's most significant challenges (for example, lack of resources, commitment, time, and organization)?

11. If your coalition could develop further to implement real change, what could you imagine being achieved?

    Within the next few months . . .

    Within the next year . . .

    Within the next five years . . .

Source: Butterfoss F. D., "Building Effective Coalitions with Consultation and Technical Assistance: Virginia's Healthy Start Initiative," *Health Promotion Practice,* 5(2), 2004, pp. 118–126.

Audio teleconferences. CADCA's National Coalition Institute offers regular no-cost audio teleconferences on substance abuse topics of interest to coalitions. Visit the institute's website for the current schedule and archived events.

On-site training workshops. Arrangements can be made for trainers from the National Coalition Institute to come to your location to train your coalition on a variety of topics, including strategic planning, evaluation, and cultural competency.

Training at national, regional, and state conferences. CADCA and the National Coalition Institute plan, sponsor, and participate in a number of national, regional, and state coalition-focused conferences throughout the year.

Specifically, two other programs offered by CADCA are on the cutting edge of coalition training, namely the National Coalition Academy and the Leader Mentor Program. The National Coalition Academy combines classroom instruction with video teleconferencing, mentoring, and a comprehensive online support system to help participants learn to become more effective coalition leaders. The training equips coalition leaders with vital skills and techniques necessary to make real change happen in a community. The National Coalition Academy is offered to coalitions free of charge through support from CADCA's Institute and the National Guard Bureau. Participants receive instruction on core competencies essential for a highly effective coalition; these range from developing strategic action plans and building partnerships to enhancing cultural competency and writing grant applications. In addition to classroom sessions, trainees participate in six video-teleconferencing community broadcasts, where they communicate with their classmates and work together to implement essential coalition strategies. The year-long training also includes an interactive website that allows participants to obtain additional resources and communicate with their instructors and classmates.

CADCA's National Coalition Institute's Coalition Leader Mentor Program is a formal, structured relationship between two coalitions. Novice coalitions are guided through a process to achieve skills and gain knowledge that will help them reach their goals to create and sustain their community antidrug coalitions and generate outcomes. Program objectives include developing an environment of mutual learning between new coalitions and experienced coalitions with documented success in their communities, and expanding the amount of technical assistance available to forming coalitions. Coalitions are matched based the following criteria: geographic proximity, culture or language, geographic similarity (rural, urban, and so forth), size of coalition, size of area served (local, county, state, and so on), and socioeconomic similarities. Leader mentors also advise the Institute, as well as the National Coalition Academy participants, and work cooperatively on a national project to benefit the field.

SUMMARY

The lead agency is an organization that acts as the convener of the coalition and has the vision, mandate, credibility, funds, and other resources to mobilize community members to form a coalition focused on a specific issue of concern. Lead agencies may be governmental institutions or social service agencies, voluntary agencies, professional societies, academic or health institutions, or community-based organizations. The lead agency may provide any or all of the following functions: host meetings, recruit prospective partners, provide physical space for coalition operation, provide or manage staff, serve as the fiscal agent, and provide basic communication and administrative services (e-mail, phone, mail).

Although coalitions may survive without support staff, they are unlikely to move beyond the initial steps of formation to become strong and productive without staff. Research shows a strong relationship between staff and volunteer leader competence and coalition member satisfaction as well as coalition survival. When leaders support member concerns and are skilled in negotiating, garnering resources, solving problems, and resolving conflict, coalitions are more cohesive and sustainable. Transformational leadership is a collaborative type of leadership that is desirable for coalitions and partnerships. Transformational leaders are change agents who are good role models and trustworthy, create and articulate a clear vision for the organization, encourage participation, empower members to achieve at higher standards, and lead as peer problem solvers.

Coalition leaders must learn to adapt to different situations and adjust their leadership styles. Personal traits that have been cited as important for partnership leaders include self-efficacy; membership in other community organizations; level of education; a high degree of political knowledge, commitment, and competence; trustworthiness; patience; energy; and hope. The leader also needs skills in collaboration, setting agendas and running efficient meetings, garnering resources, delegating responsibilities, communication and interpersonal relations, and advocacy.

High-quality training and technical assistance necessitates that both trainers and trainees be cognizant of their roles, strengths, and limitations. Sound planning requires that partners openly discuss and agree upon goals, work toward mutual agreements and understandings, be flexible, and adhere to established objectives. This means that both trainers and trainees should agree on the definition of success; establish not only clarity of mission but also mutual understanding of the other's characteristics and roles; understand not only the values, goals, and constraints of the relationship itself but also the values, goals, and constraints of each other; and translate broad goals into accomplishable interim targets and timeframes (Russell, 2002). By examining and paying attention to each other's responsibilities as well as characteristics such as trust, communication, and collaboration, an effective technical-assistance provider-recipient relationship can develop. When done well, high-quality technical assistance will provide the support needed for improvement.

QUESTIONS FOR REVIEW

1. What are the roles that a lead agency may be asked to play in a coalition setting? What are the roles for a coalition coordinator or a voluntary leader?

2. How will the choice of lead agency, staff, and leadership affect the operations and outcomes of the coalition? How can balance in leadership be achieved?

3. How does transformational and collaborative leadership differ from transactional leadership?

4. Refer to the statement, "Good leaders are born, not made." Do you think this is true? What are the implications for coalitions?

RESOURCES

Center for Creative Leadership (CCL) is the leading nonprofit institution dedicated exclusively to leadership. CCL integrates cutting-edge research with innovative training, coaching, assessment, and publishing to create proven impact for leaders and organizations around the world. CCL offers print resources, training, coaching, and a list serve for leaders. Address: Center for Creative Leadership, Attn.: Client Services, P.O. Box 26300, Greensboro, N.C. 27438-6300.Tel: (336) 545-2810; fax: (336) 282-3284; e-mail: info@leaders.ccl.org;www. ccl.org

Community Change is an organization that helps low-income people, especially people of color, build powerful, effective organizations through which they can change their communities and public policies for the better. The site offers resources and tools for administration, funding, applying for nonprofit status and evaluation. Headquarters: 1536 U Street, N.W., Washington, D.C. 20009. Tel: (202) 339-9300 or (877) 777-1536; e-mail: info@communitychange.org. Field Office: 8201 Fourth St., Suite G, Downey, Calif., 90241. Tel: (562) 862-2070; e-mail: LAOffice@communitychange.org;www.communitychange.org

Robert F. Greenleaf Center for Servant Leadership is an international, not-for-profit institution headquartered in Indianapolis, Indiana. Their goal is to help people understand the principles and practices of servant-leadership; to nurture colleagues and institutions by providing a focal point and opportunities to share thoughts and ideas on servant-leadership; to produce and publish new resources by others on servant-leadership; and to connect servant-leaders in a network of learning. The site provides an extensive reading list, articles, and links to other servant leader resources. Address: 770 Pawtucket Drive, Westfield, Ind. 46074. Tel: (317) 669-8050; fax: (317) 669-8055; e-mail: webmaster@greenleaf.org; www.greenleaf.org

International Leadership Association (ILA) is the global network for all those who practice, study, and teach leadership. The ILA promotes a deeper understanding of leadership knowledge and practices for the greater good of individuals and communities worldwide. This membership organization provides annual conferences and publications to its members and general information to the public. Address: Academy of Leadership, University of Maryland, College Park, Md. 20742-7715. Tel: (301) 405-6100; fax: (301) 405-6402; e-mail: learning@academy.umd.edu; www.academy.umd.edu

Just Associates (JASS) is a global advocacy learning network dedicated to building movements for human rights, equality, and justice by strengthening the leaders, strategies, and organizations that share their vision. The JASS network is comprised of activists, popular educators, and researchers in fourteen countries on a range of rights and justice issues, such as education, gender and racial equality, jobs, corruption, and land. JASS offers training and a number of publications. Address: 2040 S Street, N.W., Suite 203, Washington, D.C. 20009. Tel: (202) 232-1211; fax: (202) 234-0981; e-mail: info@ justassociates.org; www.justassociates.org

W. K. Kellogg Foundation Leadership Program is an online resource for the seasoned and developing leader with an interactive learning center, list serve, publications, and grant opportunities. Address: One Michigan Ave. East, Battle Creek, Mich. 49017-4012. Tel: (269) 968-1611; fax: (269) 968-0413; e-mail: ali.webb@wkkf.org; www.leadershiponlinewkkf.org

Leadership Learning Community (LLC) has the goal of strengthening the work of those dedicated to developing leadership that can address a range of significant social issues. LLC connects a diverse group of leadership development practitioners, grant writers, and thought leaders who identify successful practices, conduct research, evaluate current leadership efforts, and exchange information and tools. Through its website and regional and national meetings, LLC generates and disseminates publicly accessible knowledge to promote effective leadership support and development. Address: 1203 Preservation Parkway, Suite 200, Oakland, Calif. 94612. Tel: (510) 238-9080; fax: (510) 238-9084; e-mail: bella@leadershiplearning.org; www.leadershiplearning.org

CHAPTER SIX

Coalition Membership and Teamwork

Every single person has capabilities, abilities, and gifts. Living a good life
depends on whether those capabilities can be used, abilities expressed, and gifts
given. If they are, the person will be valued, [and] feel powerful and well
connected to the people around him or her. And the community around
the person will be more powerful because of the contribution
that person is making.
—John P. Kretzmann and John L. McKnight, 1993, p. 13

Members are the *lifeblood* of a coalition—without them, there is no organization at all. I have repeated this phrase often, but it is no less true or clear to me now than in 1989, when I began my research and work with coalitions for health promotion. Members determine the vision, the course, and the outcomes of effective coalitions. Capable coalition members are sought after, recruited, trained, and valued. They represent or actually are the *authentic voices* of the community.

Membership structure in coalitions is dynamic and may often be ambiguous, given the different linkages among stakeholders inside and outside of the partnership. Membership may not always be clear, because the same person may represent different organizations in different arenas, and the role a person represents often changes (Huxham, 2003). Members may not be certain about who is responsible for a given activity—the coalition itself, one of its members, or even an individual acting independently from the coalition. This chapter will explore how to develop and sustain members' interest in collaboration and partnering in order to accomplish coalition goals.

MEMBER ORGANIZATIONS VERSUS INDIVIDUAL MEMBERS

In most coalitions, the majority of members represent organizations, because coalitions desire the rich resources, commitment, and accountability that an entire organization can bring to the coalition table. However, some feel that organizational members pose barriers because the organizations' agendas may compete with those of the coalition. Most coalitions do have some individual members who self-select into the group or are recruited because their particular expertise, experience, skills, or connections are valued. An individual member may be a committed citizen concerned about the issue, a professional, retiree, student, or homemaker. An individual member may also belong to an organization without his or her affiliation with that organization being related to the role this person has in the coalition. A mix of both types of members keeps the coalition vital.

CATEGORIES OF MEMBERSHIP

Some coalitions maintain different categories of membership. Members rarely stay active throughout the life of the coalition and may experience burnout if they do. Having different categories of members provides flexibility so that members can move in and out of activity over time if competing loyalties or demands from home or work become excessive. To streamline operations and communication, coalitions should review their rosters at least annually and ask for annual letters or indications of the level of commitment their members desire. Experience shows that members participate in coalitions with varying levels of intensity that can be described as active, occasional, and supporting (Brager, Sprecht, and Torczyner, 1987). Himmelman (2005) distinguishes between *convening members* who provide ongoing coordination, communication, and decision making and *participating members* who actively work on activities specific to their interests. Here is a description of a typology of participation that fits many community coalitions:

Active members are actively involved in the work of the coalition, attend most coalition meetings and activities, serve on work groups, assume leadership roles, recruit members, and help fund-raise.

Less active members may be essential to the coalition because they lend their names and credibility to its efforts (and the letterhead), publicly promote its work in the community, and provide valuable connections to key organizations or populations, even if they only attend occasional coalition meetings or functions. These members may include community leaders, administrators, school officials, politicians, or religious leaders. Sofaer (2001) refers to these members as *symbolic,* and Dowling, O'Donnell, and Wellington Consulting Group (2000) describe them as *cooperating members*.

Inactive members are *networkers,* or those who want to stay informed, remain on the roster, and receive mailings, but who may never come to meetings. It is worthwhile to keep a secondary roster of inactive members because circumstances may change, and a former networker may begin to see active membership as valuable.

Shared members are sometimes appointed by organizations that wish two individuals to share a membership, with one or both members attending meetings and divvying up responsibilities. This works well for smaller organizations and when members do a good job of keeping each other informed about coalition activities. However, having organizations designate a different member to attend each meeting can be problematic, because valuable time is lost in catching members up with what is going on, and these members are often unprepared to make decisions. Continuous membership, especially in work groups, leads to progress in reaching goals.

Dukes, Piscolish, and Stephens (2000) describe another way to categorize members:

Full, or voting, members are directly involved in making decisions as part of the coalition.

Resource members regularly provide expertise but do not vote or participate in consensus decisions.

Conveners bring together the participants and may be responsible for implementing any decision. Conveners may also serve as voting members or resource members.

Alternate members take part in decisions when a regular member is absent and may attend meetings regularly as well.

Facilitators advocate for a fair and effective process but take no stand on any major decisions. The facilitator may also serve as a recorder.

Observers represent a constituency that either has decided not to participate or was not invited to do so, but wants to monitor the process.

MEMBER CHARACTERISTICS, CAPACITIES, AND SKILLS

Little has been published on the traits or characteristics that good coalition partners should possess. Dowling and colleagues suggest that effective members are able to follow a plan, make and fulfill all commitments, act in an egalitarian manner with all members, support all members of the coalition, communicate well, and provide and respond to leadership (Dowling, O'Donnell, and Wellington Consulting Group, 2000, p. 48). Individual and organizational members bring different sets of skills and resources to the coalition. Examples of resources include providing space, transportation, or refreshments for meetings; assisting with staff duties, recruitment, or fund-raising; and providing access to and influence with relevant policy makers (Butterfoss, Goodman, and Wandersman, 1993). The pooling of assets is critical when participation is voluntary and the coalition has few material resources (Butterfoss, Goodman, and Wandersman, 1993; Prestby and Wandersman, 1985). For a partnership to be effective and perceived as legitimate, coalition members must also have the skills or capacity to participate (Gray, 1989). Member competence and performance were positively related to coordination among organizations and negatively related to conflict in a coalition that worked with problem youth (Hall and others, 1977).

The essential competencies that members need to be effective include skills and knowledge to collaborate with others, such as how to

- Cooperate with and respect others, resolve conflict, communicate effectively, and deal with diversity.

- Build effective programs, such as program planning, implementation, and evaluation skills.
- Understand the priority population, the community, and change processes.
- Build an effective coalition infrastructure (Foster-Fishman and others, 2001, pp. 243–248).

Collaboration and participation are also fostered when members are committed to the collaborative process and have positive attitudes toward the need for, value, and benefits of collaboration; the proposed project or the priority issue; themselves and their own competencies; and the other stakeholders (in other words, they see these other members as capable, experienced, and legitimate) (Foster-Fishman and others, 2001, pp. 248–249). In fact, the relationships among members, or organizational climate of the coalition, is related to how well members participate and engage in coalition work. Attention to group dynamics is essential, because coalition members may share a history of conflict and misunderstandings or have little experience working in partnership with others (Bartunek, Foster-Fishman, and Keyes, 1996; Wischnowski and McCollum, 1995).

Organizational climate refers to members' perceptions of the "personality" of an organization and is typically measured by ten factors: cohesion, leader support, expression, independence, task orientation, self-discovery, anger and aggression, order and organization, leader control, and innovation (Moos, 1986). The value of promoting positive group climate and relationships among members is well supported (Dowling, O'Donnell, and Wellington Consulting Group, 2000; Kaye and Wolff, 1995; Kegler and Butterfoss, 2002). Organizational climate characteristics (for example, leader support and leader control) are related to satisfaction with the work, participation in the partnership, costs and benefits, and implementation of action plans (Butterfoss, Goodman, and Wandersman, 1996; Kegler, Steckler, McLeroy, and Malek, 1998b). Specifically, task focus is related to satisfaction and psychological and organizational empowerment (Kegler, Steckler, McLeroy, and Malek, 1998b; McMillan and others, 1995).

Positive internal relationships can be fostered by creating a climate that is cohesive, trusting, and capable of resolving conflict; identifying and uniting around shared vision; and creating an inclusive culture where decision making is shared and diversity (especially related to status or priorities) is openly addressed and accounted for in the coalition's plans (Foster-Fishman and others, 2001).

In Chapter Three, we learned that members who perceive more benefits of participation are more likely to collaborate and engage in voluntary associations and coalitions than those who perceive membership as more costly (Butterfoss and Kegler, 2002; Butterfoss and others, 1998; Chinman and others, 1996; Kaye and Wolff, 1995; Mayer and others, 1998; Prestby and others, 1990; Wandersman, Florin, Friedmann, and Meier, 1987). Likewise, members who report more benefits than costs also report higher levels of satisfaction and commitment (Butterfoss, Goodman, and Wandersman, 1996; Kegler, Steckler, McLeroy, and Malek, 1998b; Knoke and Wright-Isak, 1982). Member satisfaction has also been linked to more organized, task-focused, cohesive, and durable coalitions (Giamartino and Wandersman, 1983; Kegler, Steckler, McLeroy, and Malek, 1998b; Prestby and Wandersman, 1985).

MEMBER RESPONSIBILITIES

Members provide the links between their organizations and the coalition. Every member representing an organization should understand as a condition of membership that serving as a liaison between that organization and the coalition is a primary duty. Members should regularly update the coalition about events, issues, and policy changes that occur in their organizations so the coalition can keep its member organizations in mind when deliberating about issues and making decisions. Similarly, members should ensure that their organizations are alerted to key decisions that the coalition makes. For example, if the coalition decides to advocate a clean indoor air policy, the organizational member should be aware of this stance and help promote it within his or her organization, if possible. Minutes, reports, flyers, and e-mail alerts should regularly be distributed to member organizations (as well as to their coalition representatives). If a major decision that has particular policy implications for an organization is made by the coalition, it behooves a staff member to confer directly with the executive staff of that organization to be certain the critical information is communicated. Presented here is a complete list of member roles and responsibilities (University of Florida Extension, 2002):

- Participate in determining direction of the coalition.
- Serve as liaison to the represented organization; report progress of discussions to that organization and ensure that other members do the same for their organizations. Share concerns and ideas of the represented organization with the coalition.
- Invest in developing ground rules for group behavior.
- Candidly share interests and concerns, and assure that others are invited to do the same.
- Listen and fully understand views of others.
- Participate in the completion of a comprehensive community needs assessment.
- Assist in drafting a strategic plan and in prioritizing goals and objectives into an action plan.
- Assist in implementing activities, including those that directly involve or relate to the represented organization.
- Serve as a resource for the development of program activities.
- Help to represent the coalition at key meetings and events.
- Serve as ambassador for the work of the coalition and promote its mission when and wherever possible.
- Gather and relay appropriate information to the coalition to serve as a basis for decisions.
- Prepare for and attend meetings on a regular basis.
- Help to develop and implement a plan to develop resources to sustain the coalition.

Sometimes individual representatives of organizations are more committed to coalition goals and activities than to those of their organizations. Coalition staff should not assume that an organization is willing to commit resources or outward support based on the coalition representative's word. Some coalitions use annual *commitment letters* to clarify members' roles, organizational intentions, and levels of support. An example of such a letter is included as Exhibit 6.1.

Exhibit 6.1. Model Commitment Letter: Coalition Organizations.

Our organization, [NAME], is committed to be an active member of the [NAME] Coalition. We are committed to the vision, goals, objectives, and strategies that have been and/or will be decided by the Coalition. We are committed to the planning and collaboration that such coalitions undertake and understand that it will take time. We acknowledge the contributions and expectations of the other members of the Coalition. Benefits of membership include newsletters, access to Coalition website and its resources, educational events, connection to other members and priority populations, and _____ [SPECIFY ANY OTHERS THAT APPLY].

As general evidence of our commitment, we agree to do the following:

☐ Appoint a representative(s) to attend coalition meetings and activities.

☐ Authorize that representative to make decisions on our behalf, except for decisions regarding _____ [SPECIFY EXCEPTIONS, IF APPROPRIATE].

☐ Read minutes, reports, and newsletters to keep abreast of coalition decisions and activities.

☐ Disseminate relevant information to organizational members or employees through list serves, websites, and newsletters.

☐ Keep coalition informed of our organization's related activities.

Specifically, our organization will commit the following resources to the coalition:

☐ Access to our volunteers for coalition tasks

☐ A financial commitment for $ _____ [OR DUES, IF APPROPRIATE]

☐ In-kind contributions of staff time, material resources, meeting space, refreshments, and incentive items _____ [SPECIFY]

☐ Connections to other key organizations or individuals _____
[PLEASE SPECIFY]

MEMBER ROLES

Himmelman (2001) describes common roles played by partners in collaborative processes. These roles are not mutually exclusive, and one can lead to or be integrated into another.

Convener encourages discussion on a significant community issue that may or may not lead to further action.

Catalyst uses organization's influence and resources to encourage other partners to get on board with the coalition and its issue(s). This partner makes an early, deep commitment to participate in long-term community problem solving.

Conduit serves as a channel for funding, a role similar to that of the lead agency or founding partner.

Funder provides funds for the collaborative effort.

Advocate supports or actively promotes individuals or groups that are the priority of the coalition's activities, or supports and promotes policy and systems changes that emerge from the coalition's work.

Community organizer conducts ongoing recruitment, welcoming, and sustaining participation of community, neighborhood, and constituency-based organizations and individuals.

Technical-assistance provider provides training and technical-assistance resources on data collection and assists in preparing funding applications, lobbying, planning, and obtaining legal opinions and other specific expertise on a wide variety of subjects.

Capacity builder helps community-based organizations and individuals prioritize issues and secure resources to address their issues. Work might involve mapping community assets, acknowledging and valuing individual contributions, providing skill development opportunities, setting realistic goals and time frames, and facilitating access to resources.

Partner shares risks, responsibilities, and rewards. Good partners establish respectful and trusting relationships, take time to understand each other's motivations and expectations, and define and address challenges in ways that provide opportunities for others to share in their solutions.

Facilitator helps community problem-solving initiatives work more effectively. When effective, facilitation is valued as a fair, affirming resource to all partners.

MEMBER RECRUITMENT

Coalitions face the difficult task of recruiting potential members to the coalition, an issue similar to that of identifying the priority population within communities (Chapter Five). In *Good to Great*, business entrepreneur and researcher Jim Collins (2001) speaks to the issue of making sure the right people are recruited and retained in a business venture or company. The same central issues hold true for not-for-profit organizations and coalitions. Collins uses a bus on a long distance trip as a metaphor of the organization. He advises that there is a need to make sure that the right people are *on the bus* (recruited) and that they are sitting *in the right seats* (assuming the roles for which they are well-suited or trained, or both). Moreover, he admonishes organizations to take responsibility to get the wrong people off the bus as quickly as possible because their attitudes can undermine the efforts of others.

Coalitions might recruit for convenience, necessity, or experience (Dowling, O'Donnell, and Wellington Consulting Group, 2000). However, they should begin by asking these questions:

- Which groups, organizations, or agencies have missions, goals, and objectives compatible with the issue?
- What are the values and cultures of the identified groups, organizations, and agencies?
- What are the relationships among the identified groups, organizations, and agencies?
- What are the experiences and work records of the identified groups, organizations, and agencies?
- What do the identified groups, organizations, and agencies bring to the collaboration?
- What are their public records and positions about the issue(s) of concern? Who has supported the issue or the coalition in the past? Who has not and why?
- Are these groups, organizations, and agencies willing to develop mutual trust with current or potential partners?

The next question coalitions need to consider in recruitment is, *Why do people volunteer?* David McClelland (1998) identified three types of needs that motivate members to join and lead organizations: the need for (1) achievement, (2) authority or power, or (3) affiliation. The volunteer who is motivated by the need for achievement seeks attainment of realistic but challenging goals and advancement in the organization. These types of members thrive on accomplishment and need feedback on achievement and progress. The volunteer who is motivated by a need for authority and power desires to be influential and effective and to make an impact. These individuals have strong needs to lead, for their ideas to prevail, and to increase their personal status and prestige. Finally, the volunteer who is affiliation-motivated has a need for friendly relationships and is galvanized toward interacting with other people. These people are team players who desire to be liked and held in popular regard.

According to McClelland (1998), most people possess and exhibit a combination of these characteristics. Coalitions and partnerships can appeal to all three of these member needs. By definition, coalitions focus on goal achievement and empower volunteers to lead and develop their human potential and build camaraderie and a sense of belonging. By interviewing perspective members, recruiters can get a sense of what might motivate them to participate in coalitions and then appeal to their most pressing needs.

Cohen and Gould describe specifically some of the less obvious reasons why people would volunteer to join a coalition (2003, p. 4). First, because they believe in the particular mission for which the coalition has formed, they might hope that their organization's work could be part of something bigger; in other words, they want to participate in creating a broader vision. Second, a community organization may join a coalition because it experiences a threat to its power and fears that the coalition might reframe the public debate and undermine the organization's position, credibility, or funding streams. Third, the organization and its representatives may simply want to remain up-to-date on a particular issue and be part of the movement that the coalition represents. Finally, organizations and individuals are often mandated to join a coalition by their funders.

Ballenger (1981) describes four general member recruitment strategies: self-interest, transactional, altruistic, and social needs. Each type of strategy can be effective under specific circumstances, and using more than one strategy to recruit an individual or organization is advised. Coalition image often depends on the right mix of members. The reputation of members can either bring power and legitimacy to the coalition or discourage others from joining. Understanding the issue(s) and image that the coalition wishes to project is critical when deciding whom to recruit.

Self-interest approach. Appealing to individuals and organizations based on self-interest can be quite effective, especially if the interests and general mission of the organization whose members are being recruited matches that of the coalition. For example, in developing an injury-prevention coalition, recruiting members from a regional day-care cooperative would be based on appealing to their interest in child safety. However, the recruiter should make it clear that the coalition cannot serve the self-interest of any *one* organization. Similarly, the recruiter should communicate that a recruited organization's self-interest could be served as the coalition addresses a particular issue, but should take care not to raise expectations beyond the coalition's ability to deliver (Reinheimer and Jenkins, 1994).

Transactional approach. This approach is a direct sales appeal based on some transaction between the coalition and the organization or individual being recruited. The coalition is sold to the recruit based on offering a commodity (for example, monthly newsletters, listing the organization on the coalition letterhead, educational opportunities). This can send a message that involvement only encompasses that exchange. The recruiter must use the potential rewards as a starting point upon which to build a relationship so that members join the coalition for solid reasons and not only for a product which may or may not be satisfactory.

Altruistic approach. This approach is most often used in public health and relies on the concept of the public good. Even though organizations and individuals care about the issue and contribute their time, they may not contribute as much as the coalition hoped for in terms of talents or resources. Altruism may quickly build membership, but not the deep participation and investment that are needed to sustain the coalition. Members who are recruited on the basis of altruism should be engaged early on to participate fully in the work of the coalition.

Social-needs approach. This strategy appeals to potential members' need to belong, associate with others, and conform to what others are doing, or to alleviate a sense of guilt or shame. This type of recruitment is effective, for example, when individuals join a cancer prevention coalition because they or close acquaintances have experience with the disease.

Coalitions should also build on pre-existing relationships. Individuals and organizations that are already well connected and trusted in the community provide legitimacy and help attract others to the coalition. Often these potential members have important qualities for effective participation, for example, a strong commitment to the issue, a collaborative approach to problem solving, an ability to influence their peers, a willingness to be constructive, or some combination of these traits.

Kaye (2001) describes several ways to reach out and recruit coalition members and recommends hiring a community organizer to do outreach and recruitment, develop and engage leaders, facilitate meetings, and organize strategies. The following outreach methods have been used by coalitions (Kaye, 2001, pp. 270–272; Dowling, O'Donnell, and the Wellington Consulting Group, 2000, pp. 47–48):

Personal contact or face-to-face meetings with community leaders to build trust and learn about community perspectives and issues. These leaders can be invaluable in promoting one's coalition and identifying other leaders and community members who should be involved. For example, in recruiting partners to teen pregnancy prevention coalitions, talking face-to-face helped coalition leaders learn about potential members' values and priorities. With an issue as controversial as this, potential partners were more likely to say "yes" if given the opportunity to voice their concerns and express their views (National Campaign to Prevent Teen Pregnancy, 2003).

Town meetings can be used to publicize the work of the coalition, acknowledge the critical role of the community and its leaders, and obtain opinions from community members about community assets and potential solutions to community problems.

Less formal meetings in homes, a local business, or community centers can accomplish similar purposes, and the more intimate nature of these meetings may be more comfortable and trust building for some people.

Conferences or trainings on coalition-specific issues can also be used to recruit members.

Door-to-door visits are especially helpful for recruiting members and publicizing events. These visits can build credibility and visibility, and help obtain first-hand perspectives from community members. Residents can be asked to complete opinion surveys during these visits.

Street outreach can be used to build support and recruit members, and can occur wherever people congregate—on the street corner, at a shopping area, or at a recreational event. This type of outreach works best when a community leader initiates it or helps a coalition staff person do so.

Attending community meetings as an observer or presenter is an effective way to spread the word about the coalition and shows that the coalition cares about other community activities.

Community assessments that mobilize coalition and community members to collect data about the community are an excellent way to engage the community.

The Internet or flyers can be used to build a coalition's visibility and recruit new members.

Investing in Recruitment

Often coalitions hurry the recruitment phase of coalition building due to pressures imposed by the coalition itself as well as from grantors or the community. However, member recruitment should be carefully orchestrated. Recruiting and engaging individuals as community representatives begins with a commitment to acknowledging the presence of power differentials among representatives of professional organizations and individual community members. These differentials affect who attends meetings, who participates, whose opinions are considered valid, and who influences decisions (Israel, Schulz, Parker, and Becker, 1998).

Additionally, coalitions should realize that recruitment is never finished. A coalition that does not grow or refine its membership is surely entering a phase of decline. New members can revitalize a group that has grown stagnant or is no longer able to see issues clearly. The best course of action is to adopt an open-door membership policy that builds on diversity and new ideas, while approaching new organizations and individuals with full awareness of their capabilities and resources. When recruiting new members, the recruiter should describe how the potential organization can contribute and why their participation is needed. Members who are initially involved in specific activities that fit their talents and interests may eventually be willing to be more involved as their comfort and trust levels with other members and the coalition grow. Certain groups or individuals should be recruited early in the life of the coalition because they are good organizers or planners. Similarly, some organizations (especially businesses and parents) are better recruited later, when actual visible tasks and activities must be accomplished.

Coalitions should acknowledge that their recruitment efforts will not always be successful. Often, coalitions have trouble in recruiting representatives from certain segments of the community, for example, parents, grassroots members, business owners, and physicians. Several strategies to solve this conundrum include gathering and sharing data that are meaningful to the group being recruited, appealing to those who are affected directly by the health issue, illustrating how a coalition approach and involvement have been successful in the past, and emphasizing the tangible benefits of participation (Kelly and others, 2006, p. 74S).

When a potential member declines the invitation to join the coalition, it is helpful to ask why, if enough trust has been established. Sometimes people are not comfortable joining a group that is newly established and unproven or one that has already made many key decisions. The potential recruit might be put on a mailing list and asked again later, or solicited to provide suggestions for other recruits (also known as the snowball method of recruiting).

Although coalitions tend to recruit individuals and organizations that they know already, know about, or whose resources they know they have access to, Winer and Ray (1994) describe other issues that should be explored during member recruitment. These include the number of members required to accomplish coalition goals; unusual or difficult partners or those from other disciplines who may move a coalition to action; special relationships that exist outside of the group (for example, friendships, marriages, business partners) that may be helpful or detrimental; persons or organizations with similar purposes, expertise, community ties, and clients; organizations with a history of positive working relationships; the power of members' connections, expertise, resources, position, persuasion, charisma, visibility, and integrity; and achieving a mix of persons who are planners or process-oriented, as well as those who are doers and implementers.

Coalitions can develop a potential member matrix that lists potential partner organizations or individuals to recruit; their reputations, related activities, and achievements; their possible contributions (power, time, talent, resources); their self-interests (organizational and personal gains); and potential conflicts. By conducting this research and reviewing the matrix, coalitions can decide whether to recruit organizations, which ones have what the coalition needs to succeed, and what incentives will attract or deter partners. Exhibits 6.2 and 6.3 help identify potential collaboration partners, and how to engage such partners at your initial collaboration meeting. When considering recruitment, member diversity becomes a key issue, and it will be discussed next.

Building Member Diversity

According to traditional melting pot theory, immigrants who settled in America would shed the ways of their own countries and blend into one people, ignoring the significance of their own cultures. However, gradually the notion of *one* American

(*Text resumes on page 153.*)

Exhibit 6.2. Identifying Potential Collaboration Partners.

Worksheet #1: Targeting Necessary Participants

The first thing most coalitions do is to identify potential partners. Partnership selection is a strategic process. Initially, cultivate those organizations or individuals that possess whatever the collaboration needs to succeed—resources, technology, constituencies, skills, reputation, and power. Pay attention to what incentives will attract or deter partners. Later in a collaboration's life, focus shifts to retaining, cultivating, and replenishing partners who bring important contributions to the effort. These worksheets can help you to identify diverse organizations to consider as potential partners in your collaboration and guide you in doing field research on organizations that you are considering. For each type of organization, find out specific details: names, relevant activities or experiences, reputation, potential contributions, incentives, and conflicts.

(continued)

Exhibit 6.2. Identifying Potential Collaboration Partners. (*Continued*)

Types of Organizations to Consider as Partners

	Organizations and Groups	Details
1.	Advocacy and lobbying organizations	
2.	Businesses—local	
3.	Cancer control organizations	
4.	Civic and community organizations	
5.	Civil rights organizations	
6.	Consultants, technical assistants, planners	
7.	Consumer and patient groups	
8.	Corporations	
9.	Cultural institutions	
10.	Educational institutions	
11.	Elected officials and legislators	
12.	Environmental organizations	
13.	Financial institutions	
14.	Governmental agencies	
15.	Health care providers and hospitals	
16.	Housing organizations	
17.	Labor unions	
18.	Media	
19.	National health and medical organizations	
20.	Nutrition experts and organizations	
21.	Parents' organizations	
22.	Personal identity or constituency groups	
23.	Policy and research organizations	
24.	Private foundations and philanthropic organizations	
25.	Professional organizations	
26.	Religious institutions and organizations	
27.	Senior citizen organizations	
28.	Social service organizations	
29.	Support groups	
30.	Survivor organizations	
31.	Women's or men's organizations	
32.	Youth groups	
33.	Others	

Exhibit 6.2. Identifying Potential Collaboration Partners. (*Continued*)

Worksheet #2: Researching Prospects

Collaboration name: _____

Collaboration goal: _____

Step 1: For each category of organization that would be helpful to include in your coalition, do research on specific groups you are considering.

Step 2: Once you have identified potential partners, you can use another form, the *Collaboration Readiness Checklist*, to explore more details.

Name of Potential Collaboration Partner	Current Relevant Activities or Achievements	Resources and Talents: What will the partner contribute?	Buy-In: What will the partner gain?	Conflicts: What issues are related to the partner's involvement?

Source: Rosenthal, 2000. Copyright © 2000 Beth B. Rosenthal, M.S. Collaboration and Change, LLC. Reprinted with permission.

Exhibit 6.3. Engaging Potential Partners Worksheet.

Tasks for Your Initial Collaboration Meeting

1. Review the background information about the collaboration to make sure that everyone is aware of the context and initial purpose.

2. Group should introduce themselves to one another.

3. Collectively explore whether to begin this collaboration by answering the following questions:

   - What can each partner bring or contribute to the effort?

   - What are the necessary requirements or constraints that should be addressed for each partner?

   - What are the issues for negotiated agreement?

Partner Name	Contribution	Requirements and Constraints	Issues to Negotiate
1.			
2.			
3.			
4.			
5.			
6.			

Source: Rosenthal, 2000. Copyright © 2000 Beth B. Rosenthal, M.S. Collaboration and Change, LLC. Reprinted with permission.

culture has been replaced by one of a pluralistic society that evolves by integrating many cultures. Our country and world are becoming increasingly diverse, and problems and solutions are interconnected. Community-based organizations, such as coalitions, have begun to realize that multiple perspectives benefit their approach to opportunities and problem solving (Cox, 1991; Loden and Rosener, 1991).

Cultural differences can either enrich or deter coalition function. Working closely with diverse partners challenges members to deal with differences and use them to strengthen the coalition to accomplish far-reaching goals. By combining the perspectives and experiences of people from multiple cultures, coalition members are exposed to different and creative approaches to problem solving. Diversity is not only about uniting diverse groups around common goals. Coalitions must become *multicultural* and embrace diversity in every aspect of their work. In a multicultural coalition, "diverse groups interact to shape the coalition, make decisions, create a unique organizational culture, and guide all actions. [The coalition] defines and redefines itself as a result of the interaction of people with diverse values, perspectives, and experiences, and celebrates the contributions of each culture" (Rosenthal, 1995, p. 52).

A diverse coalition membership is one that has a range of stakeholders invested in or affected by the coalition's issue(s), and is representative of the local community (Foster-Fishman and others, 2001, p. 249). Thus members must be recruited that represent the various sectors (for example, health care, faith-based institutions, business, human services, government, consumers) and demographics of the community. Demographic dimensions of diversity include age, educational background, ethnicity, family status, gender, income, military experience, geographical area of origin, ownership of property and assets, physical and mental ability, race, sexual orientation, social class, spiritual practice, and work experience (Ohio State University, 2005). Finally, the coalition members should reflect the special needs and issues relevant to their mission. For example, a coalition focusing on chronic disease issues would recruit members who represent the range of diseases (such as cancer, diabetes, cardiovascular disease) within the community. In essence, the coalition should be held up as a mirror that reflects the rich differences of the community it serves.

According to Mizrahi and Rosenthal (1993), unity and diversity push in opposite directions. Too much unity among members weakens the ability of the coalition to create synergy, whereas too much diversity slows down progress toward goals, because building trust, familiarity, and common vision take time. Mizrahi and Rosenthal (1993) consider the following potential sources of diversity among coalition members: differences in goals, ideology, expected outcomes, power, levels of commitment, and demographic composition, or social identity (class, gender, sex, race). Diversity within the coalition membership accounts for its strength, and awareness of its relevance is critical to moving from tolerating to valuing the diversity that each organization brings. However, diversity in characteristics, strengths, goals, and interests may generate tensions and difficulties when members are trying to collaborate and reach common ground.

But representing diversity is not enough. Wolff argues that coalitions must make diversity and social justice part of their "agenda for change" (2001c, p. 265). Discussions must cross racial, ethnic, class, and gender lines, and actions must address issues such as racism, sexism, homophobia, and discrimination against new immigrants in order to "celebrate the wholeness of the community" (Wolff, 2001c, p. 265). Kaye speaks of "community-committed" coalitions that challenge assumptions about how organizations should operate and create climates where diverse members can share power, knowledge, and access to the coalition (Wolff, 2001c, p. 275). Such coalitions schedule meetings at times and places that are convenient for all members; provide transportation, child care, and translation services, if needed; do not use professional jargon or acronyms; hold regular member orientations; and build in time for socializing and expressing care and concern for each other.

The first phase of building diversity is to make a serious effort to become aware of and acknowledge the dimensions of cultural diversity that exist within an organization. Appreciating and understanding cultural diversity means not only tolerating differences among individuals or groups but supporting and nurturing them (Ohio State University, 2005). First, providing a supportive and nurturing environment enhances other coalition goals by exposing members to new issues, ideas, and information. In the second phase, people talk about their cultural differences. Appreciating and accepting both commonalities and differences is essential to effective working relationships. Diversity builds character by teaching tolerance and respect for people and by encouraging concern for equity. More people will choose to participate in an organization which values and nurtures members from all backgrounds. However, as diversity grows, so does the complexity of communication and the need to spend more effort improving communication skills within the coalition.

Overall, coalition members should represent the organization and its best interests. Tokenism promotes only symbolic commitment to a population group or interest. To avoid creating token positions, coalitions must start with a firm commitment to diversity, then declare it and put it in writing. Creating a sense of ownership is difficult if recruitment of new coalition members is based purely on representation of a specific group in the constituency. No member wants to fill a quota, and no member can represent an entire subsection of the population. Coalition members contribute according to their skills and knowledge. Therefore, the primary emphasis should be on the coalition as a diverse mixture, not on individual representation. Second, each person should be treated equally and be expected to fulfill his or her responsibilities as a member. Every new member should be involved immediately in the work of the coalition, with tasks assigned independently of cultural or ethnic background. Ideally, several members should be recruited at the same time from the same group (BoardSource, 2003).

Several steps must be embraced to build effective multicultural coalitions (Loden and Rosener, 1991; Rosenthal, 1995, p. 55):

- Articulating a pluralistic, shared vision and values
- Conducting strategic outreach and membership development
- Setting ground rules that maintain a safe, nurturing atmosphere
- Establishing structure and procedures that reinforce equity and eliminate discrimination in all its forms inside the coalition and in the coalition's relationships to other people, groups, and organizations
- Encouraging and supporting discussion about the meaning of diversity and how it can be incorporated into existing programs

- Valuing ongoing personal learning and change; soliciting views and opinions of diverse people; inviting feedback about behavior; and being open to modifying beliefs and actions based on feedback

- Practicing new modes of communication by using inclusive and valuing language, quoting diverse sources, adapting to differences in communication styles of diverse people, and displaying respect for differences and comfort in dealing with them

- Creating leadership opportunities for everyone by mentoring and empowering diverse individuals, and encouraging others to do so as well.

- Engaging in activities that celebrate differences in food, customs, and culture.

Exhibit 6.4 may be used as a tool for developing multicultural coalitions (Rosenthal 1995, pp. 69–70). Exhibit 6.5 offers concrete suggestions for how to begin to recruit more organizations with diversity to the coalition table.

(*Text resumes on page 158.*)

Exhibit 6.4. Inclusivity Checklist.

Use this tool to measure how prepared your coalition is for multicultural work and to identify areas for improvement. Place a check in the box next to each statement that applies to your coalition. If you cannot put a check in the box, this may indicate an area for change.

☐ The leadership of our coalition is multiracial and multicultural.

☐ We work hard to recruit members who represent the diversity of our community.

☐ We make special efforts to cultivate new leaders, particularly people of color.

☐ Our mission, operations, and products reflect contributions of diverse cultural or social groups.

☐ Members of diverse cultural or social groups are full participants in all aspects of our coalition's work.

☐ Meetings are not dominated by speakers from any one group.

☐ All segments of our community are represented in decision making.

☐ We are sensitive and aware of different religious and cultural holidays, customs, and food preferences.

☐ We communicate clearly and people of different cultures feel comfortable sharing their opinions and participating in meetings.

☐ We prohibit the use of ethnic, racial, and sexual stereotypes and prejudicial comments, slurs, or jokes.

Source: Adapted from Rosenthal, 1995, p. 69. From "Multicultural issues in coalitions," by Beth B. Rosenthal in" *From the Group Up: A Workbook on Coalition Building and Community Development,* G. Kaye and T. Wolff, eds., Amherst, MA: Community Partners, 1995. Reprinted with permission.

Exhibit 6.5. Building More Diverse Coalitions: Groups to Contact.

LABOR AND EMPLOYMENT

☐ Workers and their unions (for example, hotel workers, automobile workers, and so on)

☐ American Federation of Labor–Congress of Industrial Organizations (AFL–CIO) and its chapters

☐ American Federation of State, County and Municipal Employees (AFSCME) and its chapters

☐ Service Employees International Union (SEIU) and its chapters

☐ Businesses (especially local and community businesses)

RELIGIOUS/FAITH-BASED

☐ Local places of worship (for example, churches, synagogues, mosques) and groups based in places of worship

☐ National religious organizations

☐ Other faith-based organizations (for example, religious student groups, and so forth)

LOCAL COMMUNITY

☐ Community action and consumer advocacy groups

☐ Community health centers and their staff

☐ Clients of community health centers

☐ Local housing and homeless coalitions

☐ Recognized community and neighborhood leaders

FAMILY/CHILDREN

☐ Organizations focusing on children and families

☐ National and local chapters of March of Dimes

☐ Parents of children with special needs

SENIOR/ELDERLY

☐ Senior advocacy groups

☐ National and local chapters of American Association of Retired Persons (AARP) or the Gray Panthers

☐ Others: United Seniors

Exhibit 6.5. *(Continued)*

ETHNIC

☐ Organizations protecting health needs/rights of people of color

☐ National and local chapters of National Association for the Advancement of Colored People (NAACP)

☐ National Council of Negro Women

☐ National Council of La Raza

☐ North American Indian Legal Services, National Congress of American Indians

WOMEN

☐ Organizations protecting health needs and rights of women

☐ National Organization for Women

☐ League of Women Voters

☐ National Women's Health Network/National Women's Health Organization

☐ Others: Young Women's Christian Association (YWCA), Big Sister Association, Mothers Against Drunk Driving (MADD)

GAY AND LESBIAN

☐ Organizations protecting health needs/rights of gays and lesbians

☐ Gay Men's Health Crisis, AIDS Action

☐ Others: Parents, Families and Friends of Lesbians and Gays (PFLAG), Act Up

HEALTH ADVOCACY/MEDICAL ISSUES

☐ University-based health law and health care justice advocates

☐ Representatives and employees of local health clinics/hospitals

☐ Disability rights organizations (for example, National Alliance for the Mentally Ill)

☐ Medicaid and Medicare beneficiaries and their advocates

☐ Health services and health reform advocates

☐ Others: American Cancer Society, American Lung Association

(continued)

Exhibit 6.5. Building More Diverse Coalitions: Groups to Contact. (*Continued*)

PROFESSIONAL/TRADE ASSOCIATIONS

☐ Primary care associations

☐ Hospital associations (for example, National Association of Children's Hospitals)

☐ Medical societies, American College of Physicians

☐ Nurses, nurse-midwives, and physician assistants associations

☐ Small business associations

MULTIPLE INTEREST GROUPS

☐ Lesbian and Gay Law Association, Gay and Lesbian Medical Association

☐ National Latina Health Organization, National Hispanic Employee Association

☐ National Black Women's Health Project

☐ National Asian Women's Health Organization

☐ Catholic Health Association, Catholic Charities, National Council of Jewish Women

OTHER POSSIBILITIES

☐ Student groups [for example, fraternities, sororities, alumni associations, Students Against Drunk Driving (SADD)]

☐ Immigrant interests: migrant worker rights groups

☐ Regional: National Rural Health Association

☐ Local affiliates of national organizations (for example, AARP, NAACP, YMCA)

☐ Political groups

Source: Community Catalyst, 2003, pp. 19–20.

MEMBER RETENTION

Once the coalition has devised a solid recruitment plan based in diversity, the question often arises, *Why do members choose to remain in coalitions?* As mentioned before, members mentally calculate whether the benefits outweigh the costs of participation. Organizations are likely to retain their membership in coalitions when coalition mission and values match theirs; positive social interactions occur; they have access to information, visibility, credit, decision-making influence, and resources; and the coalition is efficient and effective (Sofaer, 2001). Membership is more likely to be maintained in coalitions that pay attention to orientation and training of members, provide varied and fulfilling opportunities for participation, link new members to experienced members, and recognize the need for different levels of involvement over time. Butterfoss (1997) devised the following "Buddy System" steps for recruitment and retention:

1. Each time a new strategy is introduced, the Work Group Chair asks members to consider this question: Who is not at the table that might help us enact this strategy or idea? For each identified organization, a work group member who has the best connection to that organization is asked to begin the recruitment process and volunteer to be a "buddy."

2. The buddy contacts the prospective member and asks him or her to join the coalition effort. The buddy encourages the recruit and answers any immediate questions about participation or the coalition. Successful contact information is forwarded to the Work Group Chair and Coordinator.

3. The Coordinator follows up with a phone call and sends an orientation packet to the new member. The packet contains the coalition brochure, member roster, bylaws, minutes of the last full coalition and work group meetings, a map, a calendar of meetings, recent program materials, and press coverage.

4. As soon as the buddy receives notice of the next work group meeting, he or she phones the recruit, makes sure that the notice was received, and encourages the new member to attend. Babysitting or transportation needs are attended to as well.

5. At the meeting, the buddy introduces himself to the new member, helps acclimate the member to the surroundings and meeting protocol, and introduces the new member to others. The new member is given an opportunity to introduce him- or herself to the group. A personal welcome and offer of assistance by the chair occurs at some point during the meeting.

Following are seven tips for retaining coalition members adapted from the University of Nevada Cooperative Extension's Community Leader Guide (2005):

1. Provide members with meaningful tasks that are suited to their interests and abilities.

2. Conduct regular member orientations to the coalition and its activities. These should cover mission statement, goals, action plans, roles, and expectations of coalition members.

3. On a regular basis, conduct formal and informal training that give members the knowledge and skills needed to be effective partners.

4. Recognize and accommodate members' personal needs as much as possible.

5. Evaluate members' performance regularly and provide feedback and encouragement to ensure that tasks are accomplished and that their potential for growth is maximized.

6. Recognize members in ways that can range from simply thanking them to offering tangible rewards and incentives for continued participation. Some members may want public recognition, whereas others prefer personalized, one-on-one forms of recognition.

7. Seek feedback from members as goals and action plans are updated and to make sure that they make sense to those who will execute them.

Kaye has developed the "The Six 'R's' of Participation" to describe how coalitions can increase member involvement (2001, p. 273). Members will continue to participate in coalitions when they are *recognized* for their service, *respected* for themselves and their values by others, have a valued *role* in the coalition, have opportunities to network and develop *relationships* with others, are *rewarded* for their participation through coalition benefits and material incentives, and see visible *results* for their efforts (see Exhibit 6.6).

(*Text resumes on page 162.*)

Exhibit 6.6. The Six "R's" of Participation: Involving and Mobilizing Grassroots Residents in Coalitions.

By understanding why community members participate in a coalition, you take the first step toward developing strategies to ensure their inclusion. Prospective grassroots residents expect to have certain roles and kinds of power. Why would someone want to be involved in your coalition? How does it benefit him or her? Your coalition can be successful when it meets the needs of your membership, as outlined in the following "Six 'R's' of Participation."

1. Recognition. People want to be recognized for their leadership. We all want to be known, initially by the members of our own group and then by others, for our contributions to a better quality of life.

Tip: You can recognize contributions through awards and dinners, and by highlighting and praising members at public events.

2. Respect. Everyone wants respect. By joining in community activities, we seek the respect of our peers. People often find that their values, culture, or traditions are not respected in the workplace or community, so they seek recognition and respect for themselves and their values by joining community organizations and coalitions.

Tips: Do not schedule all of your planning meetings during regular working hours, but meet in the evenings and provide dinner and child care. Translate materials into languages for non-English-speaking members and provide translators.

3. Role. We all like to feel needed; we want to belong to a group in which our unique contribution is appreciated. Groups must find a role for everyone if they expect to maintain a membership.

Exhibit 6.6. (*Continued*)

Tip: Grassroots leaders and members may have experienced being "tokens" on coalitions. Create roles with real power and substance.

4. Relationship. Organizations are networks of relationships; often a personal invitation convinces someone to join. People may sign up for private reasons (say, to make new friends) and for public reasons as well (to broaden a base of support or influence, for example). People may also join to get connected to a "power player" in your coalition. Organizations draw us into a wider context of community relationships that encourage accountability, mutual support, and responsibility.

Tip: Provide real opportunities for networking with other institutions and leaders.

5. Reward. Organizations and coalitions keep members and attract new ones when the rewards of membership outweigh the costs. Not everyone is looking for the same kind of rewards. To sustain members' role in your coalition, try to identify their interests and find out what public and private rewards suit them.

Tip: Schedule social time and interaction into the agenda of the coalition so families can participate. Make sure there is an ongoing way to share resources and information, including funding opportunities and access to people in power.

6. Results. Nothing works like results! An organization that cannot deliver the goods will not continue to attract people and resources. If your coalition is formed in response to negative forces in the community (for example, rising crime rates), safer streets will obviously be welcome and will enhance your coalition's credibility. Build in visible, short-term successes to your work.

Tip: To many grassroots leaders and residents, visible projects and activities that directly affect conditions and issues in their communities are the results they want in return for their participation.

1. RECOGNITION

What do we do now?	What could we do?

2. RESPECT

What do we do now?	What could we do?

(*continued*)

Exhibit 6.6. The Six "R's" of Participation: Involving and Mobilizing
Grassroots Residents in Coalitions. (*Continued*)

3. ROLE

What do we do now?	What could we do?

4. RELATIONSHIP

What do we do now?	What could we do?

5. REWARD

What do we do now?	What could we do?

6. RESULTS

What do we do now?	What could we do?

Source: Adapted from Kaye and Wolfe, 1995.

DOES SIZE MATTER?

People often ask whether they should approach a specific number of organizations about joining the coalition. Consensus is lacking about the effective number of organizations required for successful collaboration in a coalition. In gaming theory, participants create coalitions that are as large as they believe they need to ensure that they will win, and no larger—the *minimum winning coalition* (Riker, 1962). Similarly, Kanter (1994) suggests that as many people as possible should be involved in order to bridge interpersonal and interorganizational differences in structures, processes, and skills. In contrast, some researchers conclude that complexity must be kept low and membership numbers limited, and that strong, trusting relations may only be maintained with a limited number of members (Huxham and Vangen, 2000; Klijn and Teisman, 2000). Optimal coalition size may vary according to its stage of development, its mission, what it needs to accomplish, and whether it represents an urban, rural, or county level population. As productive communication is affected by the size of a gathering, group dynamics may become a criterion for structuring the coalition (Andringa and Engstrom, 2001).

Obviously, pros and cons can be identified for having large versus small memberships. Large size provides enough people to more easily manage the workload and divide responsibilities, as well as diverse perspectives on issues. However, larger coalitions have drawbacks as well, namely: meetings are difficult to schedule; every member may not be engaged in a meaningful activity, which can result in apathy and loss of interest; cliques and core groups are more likely to form, which hinders overall cohesion; individual accountability is threatened; and interactive discussions are difficult to sustain (Andringa and Engstrom, 2001).

On the other hand, in small coalitions, communication and interaction are easier and members get to know each other as individuals. Personal satisfaction from service can be greater for members, due to constant and meaningful involvement. However, small memberships require heavier workloads that may create burnout. Key points of view also might not be represented when the coalition is small (Andringa and Engstrom, 2001).

In practical terms, coalitions usually start with a smaller group and expand as is appropriate to accomplish their objectives. The magical number of twelve to eighteen people has been espoused as the ideal number of group members for efficiency and effectiveness. However, even though a larger group may require more resources and take longer to gel—in other words, to develop a common mission and cohesion—the number of members should not be decided ad hoc. The size of a coalition is not critical; rather, how the coalition is organized and managed matters. If the group is large, then to be efficient, the work should be divided among committees or work groups of approximately ten to fifteen members. Work groups can be further subdivided into task groups that meet individually and then convene occasionally as a whole work group. Team building is essential to the success of work groups and will now be covered in depth.

BUILDING EFFECTIVE TEAMS AND WORK GROUPS

Structuring a coalition to focus on action, such as creating task forces or action teams, is associated with increased resource mobilization and implementation of strategies (Kegler, Steckler, Malek, and McLeroy, 1998a). Team building within coalitions sets the stage for developing effective work groups and task groups. To build quality teams, we must understand the traits that uniquely define teams and distinguish them from small groups.

Teams are more than collections of individuals, and teamwork is more than an aggregate of their individual behaviors (Paris, Salas, and Cannon-Bowers, 2000). When labeling a group as a team, one should not automatically expect that it will perform as a team (Bass, 1980). A team is "a distinguishable set of two or more people who interact dynamically, independently, and adaptively toward a common and valued goal, objective, or mission and who have each been assigned specific roles or functions to perform" (Salas, Dickinson, Converse, and Tannenbaum, 1992, p. 4).

If a team is a group of people working toward a common goal, then team building is the process of enabling that group of people to reach their goal. Peter Grazier, founder and president of Teambuilding, Inc., argues that "teams are a formal way of actualizing collaboration" (Shinn and Williams, 2005, p. 2). Teamwork helps a group to leverage its time, talent, and resources for the benefit of the organization. However, Glazier also notes that we tend to think of teams in relation to sports and play, not as a tool for real work (Shinn and Williams, 2005).

Stages of Team Development

Teams are not instantly functional and effective. The well-known descriptive stages of team development are "Forming, Storming, Norming, Performing, and Re-forming" (Tuckman and Jenson, 1977). Team development is a continuously changing and recursive process. Often, no sooner has a team begun to function efficiently in stage four than something will happen requiring it to *reform*, even if only in part. Sometimes teams pass easily from one stage to another, but more often teams fail to progress and do not maximize their potential. The stages of team development are aptly named and can easily be used to recount the development of work teams and groups described here (The Teal Trust, 2002; University of Nevada Cooperative Extension, 2005a).

Forming. This honeymoon stage is where team members are becoming acquainted. Basically, they are concerned with the question, *What are we here for?* People will tend to look for a strong leader to get things moving in a new unstructured environment. Discussion focuses on different perceptions of the reason the group has come together and what types of information may be needed. Conflicts may emerge, individual differences are expressed, and the leader's role may be challenged. The value and feasibility of the task(s) may also be challenged. People are checking one another out to decide whether they want to be a part of the group. Normally, little work is accomplished at this stage because anxiety exists about the new situation, and members may be confused about how to proceed. However, two important things must be achieved at this stage: members must feel welcome and included and have a sense that their opinions will be respected; and they need to develop consensus, or group agreement, about the basic mission or goal they are seeking to work toward. The first is a "maintenance" concern (maintaining good group relations), and the second is a "task" concern (getting the work done). During this stage, the team needs to provide orientation, create structure, and define goals, direction, and roles as well as tasks and skills.

Storming. During this stage, more conflicts emerge as team members negotiate work assignments; they may also disagree on the course of action that should be taken. Even though members have "bought in" to the team and its goals, power plays may occur regarding who is in charge and what actions will be taken to reach a goal. The leadership established during formation may be challenged by other team members, and individuals with special interests may try to assert themselves. Frustration about how to proceed may trigger intense feelings of instability and polarization. Some groups may move through the storm phase in one meeting, whereas other groups remain in this phase for a while. Group facilitators can help to bring conflict out in the open, encourage good communication skills, and confirm that disagreement is healthy and can be resolved. Team tasks are to develop skills; redefine goals, roles, and tasks; and learn to work together.

Norming. After the storm comes the calm of norming. After discussion and negotiation, the team reaches a stage where ground rules are established, members learn to work together productively, and team pride develops. Team tasks are to deepen skills and understanding, increase productivity, share opinions and skills, and evaluate critically and constructively. By exploring their differences, the group should reach general agreement on their roles in relationship to one another and on the ground rules for getting their work done. These ground rules, or "norms," will address how people treat one another, how meetings are conducted, who will do what work, and how that work will be accomplished. The leader or facilitator can be less directive because members feel comfortable with each other and cohesive.

Performing. During the final and shortest phase, the group becomes a functional team. The team must focus on task achievement, deal with group issues, continue to deepen knowledge and skills, and make efficient use of time. Now that the team has established its norms, it is capable of diagnosing, solving problems, and making decisions. This is the stage where a great deal of work can occur, and the team may become quite creative. As new tasks emerge, members confidently tackle them. The whole team works together or may delegate work to task groups and individuals. Initiative in leadership may come from any group member, and most members share responsibility.

Mourning or re-forming. Some groups may choose to disband at this time, and a period of celebrating achievements or mourning the loss of the group may ensue. For continuing groups, most return to the forming stage, either because their original purpose has been achieved and they need to refocus on new goals, or because of membership or leadership turnover. Once a group has progressed through these stages of team development, subsequent team building should progress at a faster rate.

Each stage of team development has its own characteristics, with distinct forms of team leader and member behavior, emotional climate, and task outcomes. These characteristics are summarized in Table 6.1, adapted from the classic work of theorists in group and team development (Bennis and Sheppard, 1956; Tuckman and Jenson, 1977; Drinka, 1991).

Traits of Teams and Work Groups

Teams are different from small groups in that they have multiple sources of information, task interdependence, coordination among members, task-relevant knowledge,

Table 6.1. Integration of Team and Group Development Theories.

Stage of Development	Leader Behavior	Member Behavior	Emotional Climate	Task Outcome
Forming	Directs	Dependence	Uncertain	Committing
Storming	Persuades	Resistance	Conflict	Clarifying
Norming	Participates	Cohesion	Support	Developing rules
Performing	Delegates Negotiates	Interdependence	Pride	Achieving
Reforming	Evaluates Reviews	Maintaining	Satisfied	Consolidating Renewing

intensive communication, and adaptive strategies to help respond to change (Paris, Salas, and Cannon–Bowers, 2000). Teams tend to be more successful than individuals in implementing complex plans and developing creative solutions to difficult problems.

People may resist working in teams if they are convinced that teams are not worth the effort or are risky, or if they feel uncomfortable (Katzenbach and Smith, 1993). Coalitions can facilitate member empowerment in teams (for example, work groups) by keeping the focus on the mission and the structured task(s) at hand, delegating responsibility, stretching the ability of others, creating a climate for risk taking, providing appropriate resources and training, and assuring clear and open communication (Waterman, 1987). To be effective, teams must develop and build upon several critical competencies (Linder and Ledlow, 2005):

- *Cohesiveness*, or valuing of group membership. *Social cohesiveness* is the interpersonal attraction that links members, whereas *task cohesiveness* is the way that skills and abilities of members mesh to allow optimal performance.

- *Roles and norms*, or the rules that govern group behavior. Personal agendas should be left at the door.

- *Effective interpersonal communication*, such as listening and responding to others in an objective and productive way and being open about one's values, ideas, and concerns.

- *Commitment to specific and clear goals.*

- *Interdependence*, or an understanding that each member's success is determined at least in part by the success of the other members. Members should take on different roles in the team—in other words, follow as well as lead.

Working on teams can be rewarding, but members often face difficulties such as the increased time needed to make group decisions, pressure to conform to the group's wishes, and the potential for real conflict over decisions (Katzenbach and Smith, 1993). Team building is enhanced when all members work jointly on a task of mutual importance. Each member can then provide his or her technical knowledge and skills to help solve the problem, complete the project, or develop new programs. Although members of highly functional teams report a strong feeling of control within the team, they also must be patient and willing to allow change to occur in order to accomplish desired results (Adams, 1988). In addition, team members should be willing to manage conflict, evaluate group performance, and provide feedback and support that encourages commitment to the team and, ultimately, to the partnership.

Specific exercises can be used to build on member competencies, such as designing a team logo, producing a mission or goals statement, discovering characteristics that team members have in common, assessing team strengths and weaknesses, creating ground rules for communication, identifying and assigning roles to team members, practicing active listening or giving and receiving feedback, and team ranking of priorities (Solomon, Davidson, and Solomon, 1993).

Team and work group leadership. The team leader is the liaison between the team or work group and the entire coalition. The team leader should take risks and encourage team member growth by having team members provide leadership for specific tasks. The leader should be recognized as one who can make final judgments and give support and direction to the team as needed. Team leadership differs from traditional leadership in the following ways (Yukl, 2005):

- Group effectiveness and maintenance is not only the leader's responsibility but is shared by the group.
- Final decisions are not controlled by the leader but left to the group. The leader's power and position are de-emphasized.
- The leader sees the group as an interactive team, not as a group of individuals.
- Tasks are shared by the entire group.
- Leaders encourage members to express needs and feelings and deal openly with them in meetings.

What makes a good team leader? The Teal Trust (2002) identifies five essential traits of good team leaders. (1) They are committed to people and spend time building the team, not only initially but also whenever a new member joins the team or committee. Good team leaders understand that team members are concerned about relationships and being valued, as well as about the task at hand. (2) Team leaders have a desire to become servant leaders, that is, to support members in the coalition's work, as well as serve as their leaders. (3) Leaders must have the enthusiasm and energy to inspire and motivate team members, as well as the expertise to lead the team in the right direction. (4) The leader must be willing to shoulder the responsibility of ensuring that the team meets the challenges to goal attainment and is strengthened in the process. (5) The team leader understands that more is accomplished when a team works well together. He or she must be willing to share the leadership role within the team; understand the roles, strengths, and talents of the team; establish mutual accountability within the team; and create an open, healthy, and productive team environment.

Leadership styles are critical in building work groups and teams that are effective in reaching their goals. Although the general leadership styles described in Chapter Five apply to small groups as well as the entire community coalition, different factors emerge when specific task accomplishment is warranted. Hersey and Blanchard's model of *situational leadership* enables leaders to knowingly adjust their leadership styles, depending on different situations (Hersey, 1984). According to the model, leaders should adapt their styles to team development (or "maturity"), based on how ready and willing team members are to perform required tasks (in other words, their competence and motivation). Team leaders can choose from four styles of behavior that range from highly directive to highly laissez-faire, and match them to the development of their team members, depending on the situation:

Director has a directive or telling style.
Coach uses a persuasive or selling style.
Supporter is characterized by a participative or consultative style.
Delegator has a style of mandating or appointing.

The model also illustrates the ideal development of a team from immaturity (stage 1) through maturity (stage 4), during which the leadership style progressively develops from relatively detached task directing (1), through the more involved stages of explanation and persuasion (2), to participation (3), to the final stage of relatively detached delegation (4), at which time ideally the team is largely self-directing. Each of these styles is based on the team leader's diagnosis of whether the group is willing and able to take on and complete a particular task. For example, a group may be able to easily accomplish a task; therefore, the leader may delegate the task and take no further part in it. The same group, on another task, may be either immature, unwilling, or unable to complete the task. Here, the leader may have to take a directive role to determine what should be done and tell people what to do and how to do it (Hersey, Blanchard, and Johnson, 2005). Exhibit 6.7 outlines the various behaviors of team leaders and members in more detail and Exhibit 6.8 provides tips for effective team leadership.

Team membership. The Teal Trust (2002) outlines five characteristics of good team members. A good team member can aid the team process as much as a good team leader. First, members must be committed to the team above themselves. Second, they must make positive contributions to improving the

Exhibit 6.7. Situational Leadership: Team Member and Leader Styles.

Telling or Directing

Team Member: Low competence, low commitment; unable and unwilling

Team Leader: High task focus, low relationship focus

Team members cannot do the job and are not motivated. The leader must take a highly directive role, telling them what to do without a great deal of concern for the relationship.

Selling or Coaching

Team Member: Some competence, low commitment; unable and willing

Team Leader: High task focus, high relationship focus

Team members want to do the job but lack the skills or knowledge. The leader must act in a friendlier manner as he or she persuades and helps the members to complete the task.

Participating or Supporting

Team Member: High competence, variable commitment; able and unwilling

Team Leader: Low task focus, high relationship focus

Team members can do the job but refuse to do it. The leader must find out why the members are resistant and persuade them to cooperate.

Delegating

Team Member: High competence, high commitment; able and willing

Team Leader: Low task focus, low relationship focus

Team members can do the task and are motivated. The leader must trust them and leave them to it.

team's process of working together and delivering team goals. Third, team members should learn to use their individual expertise and talents to inspire and motivate each other to contribute. Fourth, team members should be willing to take responsibility for some elements of the team's work such as tasks or aspects of team development. Finally, team members must deliver on commitments. This means that if a member agrees to carry out certain action steps at a meeting, then the team expects that these will be carried out unless that expectation is changed. Exhibits 6.9–6.11 provide short tools that coalitions can use to diagnose the perceived effectiveness of their teams and work groups.

(*Text resumes on page 174.*)

Exhibit 6.8. Tips for Effective Team Leadership.

- *Coach, do not demonstrate.* When under a deadline, it is easier to demonstrate a task than to provide supportive directions, but this can undermine the team's skill development and make members overly dependent on the leader.

- *Provide constructive criticism.* When providing feedback, communicate the good, the bad, and clear suggestions on how team members can improve. Instead of providing all the solutions, guide the group by sharing knowledge and experience.

- *Back off.* After assigning a team project, provide some initial guidance and be available for additional questions that may arise. Instead of getting overly involved, demonstrate to the team that you believe in their abilities and talents by providing them opportunities to perform without interference.

- *Be positive.* If the leader is excited about the group's project, members are likely to follow suit. Team members look to the leader for direction; if the group's motivation and output are low, discuss what needs to be changed and listen to what the team suggests.

- *Value your team's ideas.* Do not devalue the team's ideas with phrases such as, "I know, but . . ." or "We have already tried that." An idea that failed before may have resulted from poor execution or timing. Consider all ideas that the team generates and encourage them to communicate their insights regularly.

- *Communicate.* If you have a problem with a group member, talk to him or her about it. Letting feelings out avoids isolating you from the group and is better for the team.

- *Do not blame others.* Group members understand heavy workloads and the inability to meet deadlines. Apologizing in earnest will earn more respect than making it seem like it is everyone else's fault that the leader missed a deadline.

- *Do not brag.* Rejoicing in successes with the group is fine, but bragging will make others regret the leader's personal successes and may create tension within the team. Have faith that people will recognize when good work is being done and will let the leader know how well he or she is doing.

- *Listen actively.* Look at the person who is speaking, nod, ask probing questions, and acknowledge what is said. If uncertain, ask for more information to clear up any confusion before moving on. Effective communication and listening are vital parts of any team.

- *Get involved.* Share suggestions, ideas, solutions, and proposals with team members, and take the time to help them. If the leader routinely helps members, teammates will willingly lend a helping hand later.

Exhibit 6.9. Building Effective Work Teams: Team Effectiveness Questionnaire.

This activity is designed to improve work group or team effectiveness by resolving conflict, establishing norms, and improving problem-solving capacities. It is designed to help a team discover and agree upon factors that affect their effectiveness. It clarifies the factors that help and hinder team effectiveness, and establishes areas to work on to make needed changes. Follow these steps to promote team development:

Step 1: The Team Effectiveness Questionnaire (see below) is introduced and explained at a meeting of the entire work group. Each team member reviews the questionnaire without scoring it. Any questions are clarified.

Step 2: Each team member now completes the questionnaire (which takes just a few minutes), reflecting on the group as a whole.

Step 3: The facilitator then writes the scale and each category on newsprint. Categories are dealt with one at a time, and team members sequentially give their scores. This is done for all eight categories.

Step 4: The team members discuss each category in turn. Time is devoted to discussing major discrepancies between team member scores in any category, and the team focuses discussion on areas of work group functioning that clearly need improvement.

Step 5: The team decides which areas to work on. It sets goals for change, discusses ways to strengthen positives, and plans activities and follow-up interventions.

A. Goals

Poor					Good
Confused, diverse; conflicting; indifferent; little interest.					Clear to and shared by all; all care about goals, feel involved.
	1	2	3	4	5

B. Participation

Poor					Good
A few dominate, are passive or ignored; many talk at once or interrupt.					All members involved and are listened to.
	1	2	3	4	5

C. Feelings

Poor					Good
Feelings are ignored or criticized.					Feelings are freely expressed.
	1	2	3	4	5

D. Diagnosis of Group Problems

Poor					Good
Jump directly to remedial proposals; treat symptoms rather than basic causes.					When problems arise, they are fully diagnosed before solutions that attack basic causes are proposed.
	1	2	3	4	5

(continued)

Exhibit 6.9. Building Effective Work Teams: Team Effectiveness Questionnaire. (*Continued*)

E. Leadership

Poor						Good
Group needs for leadership not met; group depends too much on one or two persons.	1	2	3	4	5	As needs for leadership arise, various members volunteer.

F. Decisions

Poor						Good
Needed decisions do not get made; decisions made by part of group; others uncommitted.	1	2	3	4	5	Consensus sought and diversity appreciated—used to improve decisions that are fully supported.

G. Trust

Poor						Good
Members distrust one another; are polite and guarded; outwardly listen but reject what others say; afraid to criticize or be criticized.	1	2	3	4	5	Members trust one another and share with group; respect and use group solutions; express negative reactions without fear of reprisal.

H. Creativity and Growth

Poor						Good
Members and group in a rut; operate routinely; persons stereotyped and rigid in their roles; no progress.	1	2	3	4	5	Group is flexible, seeks new and better ways; creative; individuals changing and growing; individually supported.

Source: Schein, 1969, pp. 42–43. From *Process Consultation: Its Role in Organizational Development* by E. Schein. Copyright © 1969, pp. 42–43. Reprinted by permission of Pearson Education, Inc., Upper Saddle River, NJ.

Exhibit 6.10. Team Effectiveness Checklist.

	Yes	No
1. We strongly believe in mutual purpose and interdependence.	☐	☐
2. The values we preach are the values we practice.	☐	☐
3. Our mission statement has been discussed and jointly agreed upon.	☐	☐
4. Our team has clearly defined objectives.	☐	☐
5. Expectations of how we are going to operate have been collectively decided.	☐	☐

Exhibit 6.10. *(Continued)*

6. Effective mechanisms exist to deal with interpersonal or intercultural conflict. ☐ ☐

7. Each person on the team is clear about each person's job. ☐ ☐

8. Group trust builds because people carry out their commitments. ☐ ☐

9. Group members help each other out when needed. ☐ ☐

10. Team members can easily talk about their joys and frustrations. ☐ ☐

11. Members of our team do not compete with each other. ☐ ☐

12. Effective processes exist for solving systemic and interpersonal problems. ☐ ☐

13. Cultural differences (for example, promptness) are acknowledged and dealt with. ☐ ☐

14. Official communication is more reliable than the grapevine. ☐ ☐

15. *Nonjudgmental* accurately describes this team's attitude toward diversity. ☐ ☐

Source: Adapted from the Centraide Canada Board Basics Kit Manual, United Way of Canada at http://www.boarddevelopment.org/display_document.cfm?document_id=110. Accessed October 24, 2005.

Exhibit 6.11. Team Effectiveness Critique.

Directions: Circle the number on each scale that best describes your team. Use this tool for the most recent team meeting or for how the team generally functions. Scores should be summarized, reported to the group, and discussed.

1. Goals and Objectives Commonly understood goals and objectives are lacking.	Team members understand and agree on goals and objectives.
1 2 3 4 5 6 7	

2. Utilization of Resources Member resources are not fully recognized and/or used.	Members' resources are fully recognized and used.
1 2 3 4 5 6 7	

3. Trust and Conflict Little trust exists among members; conflict is evident.	A high degree of trust exists among members; conflict is not evident.
1 2 3 4 5 6 7	

(continued)

Exhibit 6.11. Team Effectiveness Critique. *(Continued)*

4. Leadership						
One person dominates; leadership roles are not carried or shared.				Full participation in leadership occurs; leadership roles are shared by members.		
1	2	3	4	5	6	7

5. Control and Procedures						
Little control occurs; procedures to guide team functioning are lacking.				Effective procedures guide team functioning; team members support these procedures and regulate themselves.		
1	2	3	4	5	6	7

6. Interpersonal Communications						
Communications between members are closed and guarded.				Communications between members are open and participative.		
1	2	3	4	5	6	7

7. Problem Solving						
Team has no agreed-upon approaches to problem solving and decision making.				Team has well-established and agreed-upon approaches to problem solving and decision making.		
1	2	3	4	5	6	7

8. Experimentation and Creativity						
Team is rigid, does not experiment with how things are done.				Team experiments with different ways of doing things and is creative in its approach.		
1	2	3	4	5	6	7

9. Task Completion						
Team does not get much done.				Team carries out its goals.		
1	2	3	4	5	6	7

Team and Work Group Roles

Teams function better if roles are defined. Movement between roles should be allowed and even encouraged. The various functional roles that members should assume were outlined earlier in this chapter; however, members may also play different "meeting roles," as described here. (The last two roles may be assumed by the facilitator or leader.)

Initiator puts ideas on the table.
Facilitator or leader helps define the problem and set the agenda.

Recorder or secretary records all ideas.

Timekeeper keeps meeting on track.

Devil's advocate, or skeptic, reviews ideas for potential problems.

Optimist keeps a positive frame of mind and facilitates the search
  for solutions.

Reflector does not participate in meeting activities but observes process and
  gives feedback to the group.

Summarizer, or clarifier, summarizes and clarifies results.

Liaison, or spokesperson, maintains contact with the rest of the coalition.

BUILDING COMMUNITY OWNERSHIP
OF THE COALITION

To involve community members in coalition work, the following factors appear to
be critical: a shared commitment to outcomes, trust in the process, feasible and comfortable participation, community-identified needs, and leadership development
opportunities (Peterson and others, 2006). To develop ownership of the coalition by
volunteers and community members, certain principles must be followed. First, as
discussed in Chapter Five, members must be involved in defining the issues that
the coalition addresses. In this bottom-up approach, members will see their
contributions not only as helpful but also as necessary. Coalition leaders, especially
those who represent the professional health and human services community, will
begin to realize that success lies in having community members and coalition volunteers identify their assets as well as their problems. Second, they must develop
workable, acceptable solutions. Finally, they must be integrally involved in actually
implementing those solutions with guidance from public health professionals. Guidance must come not only in the form of wisdom and knowledge but also in providing material resources, such as training, funds, and tools.

Partners that represent mainstream or majority groups often experience difficulty in involving minority, grassroots, or end-user groups. Initiators need to
attract these groups by making personal contact, building relationships, making
sure that participation is beneficial, and developing clear roles and feasible activities for members to accomplish (Winer and Ray, 1994). Although this approach
makes sense, it usually involves major shifts in attitudes, focus, and the balance
of power. Building credibility with the community takes patience and perseverance. To engender real involvement by the grassroots community, the coalition
must recognize the community's historical perspective and communicate that it
cares about building an equal partnership *with* community members. Gillian Kaye
expresses this concern:

> The history of many coalitions is here today, gone tomorrow. Programs and
> resources appeared in communities and disappeared overnight. Promises were
> made to community residents and never kept, resources promised and never

delivered, and, as is often the case, residents were never involved in the ownership process and, instead, were delivered services and programs in which the community had no investment or say [2001, p. 273].

Coalition members also need to build relationships *outside* of the coalition to increase access to resources and support for coalition programs (Butterfoss, Goodman, and Wandersman, 1993, 1996; Coe, 1988; Foster-Fishman and others, 2001; O'Donnell and others, 1998; Lin, 1999; Roussos and Fawcett, 2000). First, coalitions should reach out to stakeholders from community sectors that are not represented in the coalition (for example, faith-based organizations and businesses) to promote access to resources and adoption and implementation of coalition programs. Second, coalitions should involve community residents in order to build community support and ensure that programs are relevant and culturally sensitive. Third, coalitions must build relationships with key opinion leaders and lawmakers to ensure that coalition policies will change existing institutions and systems. Last, coalitions need to interact with other related community coalitions to keep apprised of new, promising practices.

SUMMARY

Members are the *lifeblood* of a coalition. Although individuals may belong to coalitions, the majority of members represent organizations that commit their resources and are accountable to the coalition. Members participate in coalitions with varying levels of intensity that can be described from very active to inactive, but supportive. Individual and organizational members bring varied resources to the coalition, such as providing space or refreshments for meetings, funds for incentives, or assisting with staff duties. Pooling of assets is critical when participation is voluntary and the coalition has few material resources. Members must also have needed skills and capacity to participate, such as skills in recruitment or fund-raising, or access to and influence with policy makers. Collaboration and participation are fostered when members are committed to and have positive attitudes about collaboration, the coalition's issues, themselves, and other stakeholders. Members who report more benefits than costs of participation are likely to participate more and report higher levels of satisfaction and commitment than those who perceive membership as more costly. Members provide the links between their organizations and the coalition. Every member representing an organization should understand that he or she serves as a liaison between that organization and the coalition and should keep their organization informed about key decisions that the coalition makes.

Member recruitment should be carefully planned and ongoing. A coalition may recruit members out of convenience, necessity, or experience. However, understanding the issue(s) and image that it wishes to project is critical when deciding whom to recruit. Methods of recruitment include personal contact or face-to-face meetings with community leaders, conducting or attending public meetings or trainings, door-to-door visits, street outreach, conducting community assessments, and distributing recruitment notices via print or Internet. Membership is likely to be maintained in coalitions that pay attention to members' needs and desire for meaningful involvement.

Teams tend to be more successful in implementing complex plans and developing more creative solutions to difficult problems than individuals. Team building within coalitions sets the stage for developing effective work groups and task groups. The stages of team development are Forming, Storming, Norming, Performing, and Re-forming. Team development is a continuously changing and recursive process. Sometimes teams pass easily from one stage to another, but more often, teams fail to progress and do not maximize their potential. To be effective, teams must build upon several critical competencies, such as cohesiveness, or valuing of group membership; roles and norms, or the rules that govern group behavior; effective interpersonal communication; commitment to specific and clear goals; and interdependence.

Diversity is essential in coalitions. Members should include a broad range of stakeholders who are invested in or affected by the coalition's issue(s) and represent the sectors, demographics, and special needs of the community. Furthermore, coalitions should operate in ways that allow diverse members to share power and knowledge and to access decision-making. To develop community ownership of the coalition, members must help define the issues that the coalition will address, develop workable solutions, and implement them.

QUESTIONS FOR REVIEW

1. Why is it desirable for coalitions to have different categories of membership?
2. What issues should coalitions consider when recruiting new members?
3. What are the keys to sustaining member involvement and participation?
4. How is diversity an asset to a coalition? How can diversity make collaboration more difficult?

RESOURCES

Organizations

BoardSource: Building Effective Nonprofit Boards. Many print resources that apply mostly to nonprofit boards but can be applied to coalitions as well. Address: 1828 L Street, N.W., Suite 900, Washington, D.C. 20036-5114. Tel: (202) 452-6262; fax: (202) 452-6299; www.boardsource.org

Center for Community Change. The Center is a progressive social justice organization whose central project is to support the emergence of one or more movements for social and economic justice in the United States. It strives to transform the national debate and national politics as well as the institutions, economic systems, and policies that affect low-income and working-class people, especially people of color. It helps grassroots leaders build strong organizations, develop the skills and resources they need to improve their communities, and change the policies and institutions that adversely affect their lives. This site offers print resources and information on classes and technical assistance. Address: 1536 U Street, N.W., Washington, D.C. 20009. Tel: (202) 339-9300 or (877) 777-1536; e-mail: info@communitychange.org

Collaboration and Change, LLC provides programs in leadership and organizational, collaborative, and community development. Their goal is to strengthen leaders, institutions and communities to be inventive, compassionate, adaptable, and sustainable; to create collaborations that maximize the power of diverse skills and perspectives; and to produce inclusive solutions to collective challenges. They specialize in: (1) collaborations, coalitions, and partnerships; (2) advocacy, community organizing, and planning; (3) organizational change and capacity building; (4) leadership and board development; and (5) applied research for policy, community, and program development. Services include consultation, training, facilitation, coaching and organizing, research, writing, and project management for nonprofit organizations, coalitions, networks, government agencies, and foundations focusing on a broad spectrum of social and environmental issues. Workshops are offered on Organizing, Advocacy, and Community Development; Collaborations and Coalitions; and Leadership Development and Organizational Capacity Building. They offer an assortment of checklists, worksheets, exercises and outlines, and workbooks and study guides such as the Strategic Partnerships Workbook. Address: Collaboration and Change, 267 E. 7th Street, Suite 5, New York, N.Y. 10009. Tel: (212) 673-9118 or (212) 452-7112; fax: (212) 420-6026; e-mail: info@collaborationandchange.com; http://www.collaborationandchange.com/index.htm

Community Catalyst, Inc. This national nonprofit advocacy organization builds consumer and community participation in the shaping of the U.S. health system to ensure quality, affordable health care for all. It uses a capacity-building approach to establish institutional and policy-maker engagement with communities for expanding access to health care. Its multidisciplinary staff provide technical assistance to community-based, statewide, and national organizations on a wide range of policy and organizational capacity-building issues. This assistance constitutes a blend of policy analysis, legal intervention, organizational development, and public education through the media. Address: 30 Winter Street, 10th floor, Boston, Mass. 02108. Tel: (617) 338-6035; fax: (617) 451-5838; www.communitycatalyst.org

National Network for Collaboration. A self-directed team of twenty-one land-grant universities that facilitates collaboration among professionals at the local, state, and national levels (across program areas, among university departments, among universities, and among Extension and its partners, including collaborations with nontraditional partners) to build their capacity to solve their own problems. The network publishes reports on the results of a nationwide survey of successful community coalitions across a variety of disciplines. For information about network services and resources, contact Jeff Miller, 4-H Youth Development, North Dakota State University Extension Service, 219 FLC, P.O. Box 5016, Fargo, N.D. 58105-5016. Tel: (701) 231-7253 or 701-231-7259, fax: (701) 231-8568; e-mail: jpmiller@ndsuext.nodak.edu; http://crs.uvm.edu/nnco/

Partnership Self-Assessment Tool. http://www.partnershiptool.net

Teambuilding, Inc. Offers training, resources, and publications on team building, mostly with a corporate focus, but can be easily applied to coalitions. Address: One Pine Lane, Chadds Ford, Penn. 19317. Tel: (877) 358-1961 or (610) 358-1961; e-mail: inquire@teambuildinginc.com; http://www.teambuildinginc.com/about.htm

TeamBonding. Offers training, resources, and publications on team building and the power of play. Has a corporate focus but can be applied to coalitions. Address: 18 Washington Street, 200, Canton, Mass. 02021. Tel: (888) 398-8326, ext. 203 or (781) 793-9706; fax: (781) 784-4887; e-mail: inquire@teambuildinginc.com; http://www.teambonding.com/contact.html

Publications

American Cancer Society National Advisory Group on Collaboration with Organizations. *1 + 1 = 3: A Collaboration Guidebook,* 2nd ed. Code No. 5033. American Cancer Society National Distribution Center, 2000.

Couto, R., Simpson, N., and Harris, G. *Sowing Seeds in the Mountains: Community-Based Coalitions for Cancer Prevention and Control* (NIH Monograph No. 94-3779). Bethesda, Md.: National Institutes of Health, National Cancer Institute, 1994.

Dowling, J., O'Donnell, H., and Wellington Consulting Group. *A Development Manual for Asthma Coalitions.* Northbrook, Ill.: The CHEST Foundation and the American College of Chest Physicians, 2000.

Feighery E., and Rogers, T. *Building and Maintaining Effective Coalitions.* Published as Guide No. 12 in the series *How-to Guides on Community Health Promotion.* Palo Alto, Calif.: Stanford Health Promotion Resource Center, 1989.

Habana-Hafner, S., Reed, H., and Associates. *Partnerships for Community Development: Resources for Practitioners and Trainers.* Amherst, Mass.: University of Mass., Center for Organizational and Community Development, 1989.

Harvey, T. B., and Drolet, B. *Building Teams, Building People: Expanding the Fifth Resource,* 2nd ed. Lanham, Md.: Rowman and Littlefield Publishers, Inc., 2004.

Kaye, G., and Wolff, T. (eds.). *From the Ground Up: A Workbook on Coalition Building and Community Development.* Amherst, Mass.: University of Massachusetts, Area Health Education Center/Community Partners, 1995.

Kretzmann, J., and McKnight, J. *Building Communities from the Inside Out: A Path Toward Finding and Mobilizing a Community's Assets.* Evanston, Ill.: Northwestern University, Center for Urban Affairs and Policy Research, 1993.

National Assembly of National Voluntary and Social Welfare Organizations. *The Community Collaboration Manual.* Washington, D.C.: Author, 1993.

Pertschuk, M., and Erickson, A. *Smoke Fighting.* Washington, D.C.: American Cancer Society, 1987.

Sofaer, S. *Working Together, Moving Ahead: A Manual to Support Effective Community Health Coalitions.* New York: Baruch College, Robert Wood Johnson Foundation, 2001.

Winer, M., and Ray, K. *Collaboration Handbook: Creating, Sustaining and Enjoying the Journey.* Saint Paul, Minn.: Amherst H. Wilder Foundation, 1994.

CHAPTER SEVEN

Essential Coalition Processes

No great thing is created suddenly.
—Epictetus, c. 55–135 C.E.

C oalitions face two types of work: *Inward* work includes the activities needed to build, nurture, and maintain the coalition. *Outward* work focuses on task-oriented behaviors to achieve the coalition's goals, independently or through its members (Shortell and others, 2002). Developing its vision and goals, setting up its structure, and attracting, recruiting, and keeping its members (in other words, building community) are inward tasks that all coalitions must accomplish (Agranoff and McGuire, 2001; Vangen and Huxham, 2004; Kickert, Klijn, and Koopenjan, 1997; Shortell and others, 2002). Identifying and proposing issues for common work and setting up structures and processes for interaction promote collaboration and honor diversity. Members and leaders should be oriented and trained to develop the self-efficacy and skills needed to function effectively. Promoting participation and respect helps members to feel valued and to experience a balanced distribution of power and ownership (Huxham, 2003). When members engage in satisfying personal relationships, they learn to value their differences, find common ground, and support each other in the process.

In contrast to tasks that involve building community, tasks associated with outward work focus on what needs to be done to influence an external target. Outward-oriented work encompasses at least three different tasks. First, it includes work with the coalition members, so they can engage outside organizations and allies. Second, some of the outward work is oriented toward developing alliances and partnerships with individuals, organizations, and coalitions who will enhance the coalition's ability to leverage power. Finally, coalition members must spend considerable energy engaging members of the population and institutions that the coalition intends to influence.

Moving the coalition's agenda forward depends on the resources coalition members either pool together or provide separately as well as on the members' willingness and capacity to engage in the actual outward-oriented work. Outward-work effectiveness will depend on the quality of the internal coordination of the coalition and on the level of trust developed via inward work with coalition members. Chapters Eight through Ten focus on this inward work so critical to a coalition's ultimate success.

Once a coalition has developed the structural elements needed to govern and maintain its operation, it is ready to deal with the more difficult process issues. How will it communicate effectively, solve problems, make decisions, and resolve conflicts? How well a coalition handles these tasks will determine its effectiveness and longevity.

COMMUNICATION

Effective internal communication among the membership and staff may be the most essential ingredient for keeping staff and members informed and enhancing the positive climate of the coalition (Andrews, 1990; Cohen and others, 2002). Communication is defined as an exchange of words and meanings, or a two-way process of sending and receiving messages between one person and another person or among a group of people. Effective communication occurs when there is shared meaning; in other words, the message that is sent is the same one that is received and understood. According to Beckham and King (2005), effective communication happens in coalitions when members

- Use language that is appropriate to others' levels of understanding.
- Make sure that others receive the intended information or knowledge.
- Develop networks and relationships with other members.
- Talk with others in ways that facilitate openness, honesty, and cooperation.
- Provide feedback.

Face-to-face communication includes both verbal and nonverbal interaction. However, in a coalition setting, communication often occurs via written or telephonic means. Open communication helps the group focus on a common mission, increases trust and sharing of resources, provides information about one another's programs, and allows members to express and resolve misgivings about planned activities (Butterfoss, Goodman, and Wandersman, 1993).

The quality of communication has been positively related to coordination and negatively related to conflict (Hall and others, 1977). The quality of interactions among member networks is demonstrated by the frequency and intensity of contacts and the benefits that members receive from them, such as emotional or tangible support and access to social contacts (Israel, 1982). Social network analysis has been used to study connections among individuals and organizations (Scott, 2000).

Research demonstrates that the extent of regular contacts and positive relationships among community members can foster cooperation (Putnam, 1993) and empowerment (Kumpher, Turner, Hopkins, and Librett, 1993). Members who report an increase in the number and type of linkages with *outside* organizations tend to participate more in the coalition (Butterfoss, Goodman, and Wandersman, 1996; Mayer and others, 1998). Frequent and productive communication and networking among members increases satisfaction, commitment, and implementation of strategies (Rogers and others, 1993; Kegler, Steckler, McLeroy, and Malek, 1998b; Valente, 1995). Similarly, staff is most satisfied and committed when good communication exists between members and themselves (Rogers and others, 1993). However, the centralization of power that helps mobilize members within a strong network may sometimes result in diminished levels of shared decision making, accountability, and commitment (Valente, 1995; Jasuja and others, 2005).

Positive relationships among members are likely to create a productive coalition environment or climate (Kaye and Wolff, 1995; Dowling, O'Donnell, and Wellington Consulting Group, 2000). As we learned in Chapter Six, organizational climate characteristics are related to satisfaction with the work, participation, psychological and organizational empowerment, costs and benefits, and implementation of action plans (Butterfoss and others, 1996; Kegler, Steckler, McLeroy, and Malek, 1998b; McMillan and others, 1995).

Of all the group climate characteristics, group cohesion is one that must be developed over time to develop a "we" versus "I" atmosphere in the coalition. Holli and Calabrese (1998) identify several factors that can increase group cohesiveness:

- All members complete worthwhile tasks and feel appreciated by the group.
- Members clearly understand the group goals and deem them realistic.
- Members feel that the group's issues are important.
- Members perceive the group as an entity in its own right, calling it "the group" or "our group."
- The group has prestige.
- Members have knowledge or material resources needed by the group.
- Personal interactions are based on equality, and no member exercises authority over another.
- Members do not openly compete with one another.

The Communication Process

Effective communication involves a simultaneous two-way sending and receiving process. The elements of the communication process are these:

Sender initiates the communication.
Receiver is the person or persons for whom the message is intended. Receivers usually interpret and transmit messages simultaneously. They listen to what is

being said, think about what they are going to say, and may react in nonverbal ways depending on how they interpret the message.

Message is the information that the sender wants the receiver to know, which includes both the verbal message (content) and nonverbal messages inferred from the sender and the environment.

Feedback is the response that ideally will lead to mutual understanding about the message.

People communicate in at least three important ways: symbolic, verbal, and nonverbal communication (McNeese, 1991):

Symbolic communication. Symbols can be defined as things or objects that represent something abstract. Often the basis for people's reactions to others, they may include where people live and work, their job titles, clothes, or other personal characteristics, such as age, gender, educational level, ethnic background, and cultural heritage. People often make assumptions and misjudge others based on this symbolic information. Thus the way people behave toward others is often based solely on observations not backed by real knowledge.

Verbal communication. Verbal communication includes the actual words used to send messages and the way in which they are arranged into thoughts. Because words are the primary symbols used in this type of communication, it includes both oral and written messages.

Nonverbal communication. For interpersonal communication to be effective, people must send verbal and nonverbal messages that are in accord. If the verbal and nonverbal messages being sent are not in agreement, receivers generally will believe what they "hear" nonverbally. Nonverbal communication falls into four major categories:

- *Eye contact.* Effective eye contact includes spontaneous glances and looking at another person in a way that communicates interest and support. Appropriate eye contact lets people know that others are interested in them and respect them enough to openly communicate with them. Ineffective eye contact (for example, staring, glaring, not looking at another person) tells people that others do not respect them and are not interested in what they have to say.

- *Body orientation.* Appropriate posture, body movements, facial expressions, and limb placement enhance communication. Having a relaxed face, and leaning toward and directly facing the sender of a message communicate interest and attention. Communication is hindered if the person is physically distant from or does not face the sender, slouches or has a rigid posture, does not use gestures, or has no facial expression.

- *Verbal quality.* To be effective, the tone of voice must match the message; in other words, it must be an audible tone of voice that communicates confidence and directness. If the tone is inappropriate, the speaker appears to be passive or demanding. If he or she often pauses, is repetitive, or uses incomplete sentences, the listener will stop paying attention.

- *Energy level.* Energy level is contagious in groups. A person's positive energy level communicates interest and enthusiasm about a coalition project, whereas a negative energy level may lead to breakdowns in the communication process.

Miscommunication

While senders talk, they receive nonverbal reactions from receivers. Senders make inferences based on the receivers' reactions and adjust their tone or language to help make a message better understood. However, sometimes the message sent is not the message received, resulting in miscommunication that may cause time loss, feelings of resentment, rumors, and poor relationships.

Beckham and King (2005) identify several barriers that can lead to breakdowns in communication, especially in groups like coalitions, where one or more of these factors are likely to be present. These barriers include environmental factors, such as room size, shape, lighting, color, temperature, and furniture arrangement; personal attributes of the sender and receiver, for example, appearance, educational backgrounds, and the physiological state of each communicator; culture and psychological interference due to origin or birth, upbringing, ethnicity, race, religion, or socioeconomic identity; the tendency to perceive information selectively—in other words, people hearing what they want to hear, especially if it reaffirms established beliefs and values or supports personal decisions; and unconscious substitution, addition, or simplification of the received message before it is sent to others.

Communication Channels

Many modes of group communication currently exist, including face-to-face conversations; meetings; telephones and cell phones; memos, letters, and telegraphs; electronic mail, text messaging, and fax messages; and media methods, such as newspapers, magazines, radio, and television. When choosing the best method to communicate, considerations include the importance of the message, the effectiveness of the chosen method, and the kind of feedback needed in return. If the message is important, it should be written, especially if it must be sent to several people or if sharing it must be documented. If the message is sensitive or intended for only one or two people, a phone call or note may be more appropriate; getting verbal feedback is easier than getting written feedback. The message can be discussed immediately and questioned for clarification, and misunderstandings can be resolved.

Some methods are more effective in certain situations than others. For example, when sharing information with group members is time sensitive, the message can be sent via electronic mail or fax. Sometimes multiple communication methods may be used to deliver the same critical message, for example, by both providing handouts and writing on a flip chart during a meeting discussion.

Electronic communication via the Internet and e-mail poses a challenge for coalition staff. The efficiency of one-on-one communication by e-mailing copies of agenda, minutes, and reports is vastly improved over previous phone, meeting, and mail systems. However, the Internet compresses time and hurries the pace of decision making in coalitions. It demands "sharper organizational reflexes, compelling staff to digest information without delay, change their websites with the regularity of a daily newspaper, and respond instantaneously to events provoked by their constituent's e-mail" (Social Marketing Institute, 2000a, p. 3). Eventually, these technologies will shift power within organizations and favor those who are technologically savvy for leadership positions, leaving behind all reluctant learners (Social Marketing Institute, 2000a).

Features of Effective Group Communication

Communication in healthy, effective groups has several key features: openness, trust, honesty, and full participation (University of Nevada Cooperative Extension, 2005a).

Openness involves sharing information that is needed for effectively accomplishing work and developing group-centered orientation, attitudes, and behaviors.

Trust and honesty occur when members take risks during open communication. Often the first crisis that coalition members face is the ability to trust each other enough to risk self-disclosure. When members are able to express feelings of anger or frustration, as well as satisfaction and pleasure, without fear of ridicule or group reprisal, group cohesion usually results. Actions that generate trust include making only those promises that can be kept (for example, providing certain kinds of information or offering a certain level of participation), and then keeping those promises; demonstrating through active listening an interest in meeting others' needs and concerns; asserting values and goals consistently and openly; raising the question of trust and explaining its meaning and importance; being willing to admit wrongdoing; focusing on doable issues (for example, reviewing existing information about key issues or developing a plan for a noncontroversial policy); contributing to the coalition, for instance, by offering information, meeting space, or refreshments; and developing and living by realistic and principled ground rules (Dukes, Piscolish, and Stephens, 2000).

Full participation happens when members' contributions, feelings, and ideas are valued by the group. Because members are critical resources for accomplishing tasks and goals, the group must strive to involve everyone in discussions and deliberations.

Communication among group members is inhibited by *binding* responses and facilitated by *freeing* responses (University of Nevada Cooperative Extension, 2005a). *Binding responses* include changing or diverting the subject without explanation; attributing motives to others; advising and persuading; judging and criticizing others; naming or labeling; commanding or ordering; and moralizing or expressing approval or disapproval of others based upon certain standards. Exhibit 7.1 provides a guide for dealing with communication roadblocks such as these. *Freeing responses* include paraphrasing to check whether what was heard was actually said; perception checking to see whether impressions of others' feelings are accurate; describing influencing behaviors; and describing feelings about others' communication ("I" messages).

Exhibit 7.1. Guide to Getting Past Communication Roadblocks.

JUDGING OR CRITICIZING

What it is:	Even if intention is to be supportive, by judging and criticizing, blame is placed on speaker who is already struggling with his or her problems.
What it sounds like:	"You're wrong," "I disagree," or "You're not thinking clearly."
Alternative:	Step back from your own situation and try to see the problem from the speaker's point of view.

NAMING OR LABELING

What it is:	By attaching a stigma to the speaker, his or her problem, or behavior, the person is made to feel foolish. The person is *seen* as this label, and it prevents others from getting to know him or her.
What it sounds like:	"That's a silly idea," "You're being shy," or "Why are you so irresponsible?"
Alternative:	Try to see through immediate response and truly listen to the speaker.

COMMANDING OR ORDERING

What it is:	Responding with command or order about what speaker should do implies that his or her judgment is poor; no collaboration on solution occurs.
What it sounds like:	"You must" or "You have to" statement are used.
Alternative:	Try to work together to develop a solution.

MORALIZING

What it is:	The listener tells the speaker what he or she should do and backs up the solution with moral or theological authority. Moralizing is demoralizing; it implies that the speaker lacks moral compass to come up with a responsible solution by himself or herself.

(continued)

Exhibit 7.1. Guide to Getting Past Communication Roadblocks. (*Continued*)

What it sounds like:	"It's the right thing to do" or "You know what you're doing is wrong."
Alternative:	Recognize that everyone has a personal choice and set of values and that the speaker does not necessarily share yours.

DIVERTING

What it is:	Attempting to throw aside a speaker's problems by switching to a more comfortable topic. In so doing, the listener loses the opportunity to understand the speaker's concern and to strengthen the relationship.
What it sounds like:	"Just forget about it," "Yeah, something similar happened to me; let me tell you about it," or "Not at the dinner table."
Alternative:	Try to put speaker's issues ahead of your own. Before you move on, ask if speaker has had his or her full say.

ADVISING

What it is:	Prematurely telling the other person how to solve his or her problem. We tend to see our solution as the only way to solve the problem and imply that speaker is not able to solve the problem himself or herself.
What it sounds like:	"What I think you should do is" or "Why don't you" statements are used.
Alternative:	Let the speaker talk through the problem. Often, he or she will come to his or her own solution with just a few nods or words of encouragement.

Adapted from Zook, L., *November Newsletter,* Carlsbad, Cal.: Buffini and Co., 2005.

Other key features of effective communication include the following:

Paraphrasing is crucial in bridging the interpersonal gap because it increases the accuracy of communication and the degree of mutual or shared understanding. The act of paraphrasing implies a desire to improve a relationship by being interested in the other person and concerned to see how he or she views things.

Perception checking describes the others' feelings without expressing disapproval or approval, and conveys a genuine concern for accurately understanding the other person's feelings.

Behavior description is the reporting of specific, observable actions of others without valuing them as right, wrong, bad, or good, and without making accusations or generalizations about others' motives, attitudes, or personality traits.

"I" messages are used when a person identifies his or her own specific feeling to be a result of a specific behavior or event. "I" messages have two parts: (1) feelings—"I felt angry and disappointed, . . ." and (2) behavior or event—". . . when I arrived at the meeting on time and no one else did." "I" messages are effective because they place responsibility with the sender of the message, reduce the receiver's defensiveness and resistance to further communications, and provide information about the receiver's behavior without evaluating it. A combination of "I" messages and active listening achieves effective communication by providing clarity, empathy, and understanding, and keeping communication channels open.

Active listening requires mental effort. In *active listening,* the listener focuses or looks at the person who is speaking and keeps his or her mind on the speaker's words and body language; respects the speaker by not interrupting even if he or she thinks the speaker has nothing important to say; shows interest while the speaker is talking by nodding or asking questions if the meaning is unclear; lets those with different opinions have their point of view; is quiet and does not give advice unless asked; and asks questions or paraphrases to clarify the speaker's words.

Groups within a coalition may either be productive or unproductive in their methods and styles of communication, as shown in Table 7.1 (University of Nevada Cooperative Extension, 2005a).

The Advocacy Institute (2005) suggests several practices that coalitions may engage in to develop effective communication. These practices will help members address conflicts and tensions as they emerge, voice concerns and frustration, and identify creative solutions that come from multiple perspectives.

First, the coalition must set the example that all voices should be heard. Coalitions must develop and observe ground rules that prevent some members from dominating discussions and encourage participation from quieter members or members from groups with less traditional power (for example, minorities or smaller organizations). Second, coalitions must create safe and comfortable environments where members feel heard when they voice concerns. One-on-one conversations, anonymous feedback, caucuses, or full-group discussions can be effectively used as the situations warrant.

Third, members must learn to listen well, get to the heart of issues, and draw out possible solutions. Blocks to effective listening include talking without allowing others to speak; forming an opinion before a person finishes speaking or others have been heard from; mentally rehearsing responses while a person is still speaking; agreeing with a speaker to avoid conflict; trying to win an argument rather than focusing on solutions; and being afraid to be wrong or assuming you are right. Fourth, coalition members should be open to discussing the underlying tensions or conflicts that usually are not discussed for fear of causing offense. Finally, coalitions must set aside time to solve problems and resolve conflicts.

Table 7.1. Communication in Productive Groups and Communication in Less Productive Groups.

Productive Groups	Less Productive Groups
Members discuss the subject at hand.	The discussion jumps from one idea to another.
All ideas and suggestions are welcomed.	Some members' ideas do not count; some members do not act as if they belong to the group.
All members have a chance to state their views.	One or two members do all the talking.
The group uses its agenda as a discussion guide.	The agenda is unclear or unwritten.
One or two members summarize the discussion after everyone has a chance to speak.	No one checks to see whether everyone who wants to speak has done so. Discussions continue until people get tired.
Members know and use problem-solving steps.	No order is followed for identifying or solving problems.
Members are clear about decisions and committed to group.	Decision making is unclear; members are not committed to the group's plans.

Source: Adapted from *Community Leader's Guide* developed cooperatively by: Community Colleges of Spokane, Institute of Extended Learning and Washington State University Cooperative Extension. Reprinted with permission.

PROBLEM SOLVING

Every coalition has to solve problems at one time or another. Not all problems are equal, and coalitions should keep their relative significance in perspective. To be effective, work groups should have an agreed-upon procedure for problem solving. Although many problem-solving models exist, they usually contain the following steps (McNeese, 1991; Rebori, 1997, 1998a, Tagliere, 1993).

1. *Define the problem.* One of the causes of coalition ineffectiveness is jumping to solutions before properly defining the problem. A good problem definition states the current situation and the desired situation. The statement of the problem should be clear and concise, contain the facts, and not imply any solutions or causes. The desired situation, or what the coalition wants to happen, should be defined as a concrete and realistic objective.
2. *Identify and define the root causes.* To permanently solve problems, the coalition must identify and define root causes (in other words, reasons for the problem) rather than symptoms, which merely indicate the presence of a problem.

Four techniques to use when structuring discussion about root causes are brainstorming, creating a brain pool, nominal group technique, and constructing a fishbone diagram.

- *Brainstorming* is a widely used tool to stimulate creative thinking developed in 1939 by Alex Osborn, an advertising executive who believed that anyone could learn to generate creative solutions for a wide variety of problems. Members are asked first to generate a list of the positive and negative aspects of a topic. These comments are recorded on an easel, and similar items are sorted and grouped according to simple categories, such as cost, effectiveness, desirability, and potential barriers. The purpose of brainstorming is to quickly gather the extent of opinions on the issue and make sure that everyone is heard. After grouping or categorizing, a discussion should be held to clarify the ideas, add missing points, and decide how to move to next steps. A step-by-step brainstorming method is found in Exhibit 7.2 (page 193).

- *The brain pool method* combines elements of brainstorming and the Delphi Technique (Rebori, 1998a). To begin, each member writes the problem in the form of a question on the top of a sheet of paper (for example, *How can we generate 50 percent more financial resources for the coalition?*). During the next five minutes, each member individually develops two or three ideas and writes them under the question. During this time, no discussion is allowed. Members place their papers in the middle of the table and exchange them for someone else's. Then each examines his or her new sheet and records any new ideas or modifications. The exchange continues in silence until the agreed-upon time limit is reached (for example, twenty to thirty minutes). Members process the ideas by listing those on the papers in front of them and then begin discussing alternative solutions; or the ideas can be summarized and discussed at a subsequent meeting.

- *The Nominal Group Technique (NGT)* is a time-tested technique often used for generating ideas, identifying issues and potential solutions, and promoting consensus (Moore, 1990). NGT focuses group discussion around one question; therefore, a specific question presented to a group usually results in more useful responses. The technique is a combination of brainstorming, the dot method (described later on), and the brain pool. NGT can be used when a coalition is uncertain about an agreed-upon solution to a complex community or organizational problem, or when disagreement about an issue exists among members. NGT works best with small groups of five to ten participants; however, larger groups can also employ this technique. Exhibit 7.3 (page 194) lists the steps for this method.

- *The fishbone diagram* (or cause and effect diagram) consists of a horizontal line (the spine) with a box at one end (the head), where the problem is stated. Several angled lines come off the horizontal line, forming the ribs of the fish, and at the end of each rib is listed a probable cause of the problem. Contributors to the cause are usually small branches off the ribs. If the group has defined the problem statement satisfactorily, the fishbone diagram builds naturally by repeating the question, *What is a potential cause of. . . ?*

The best use of a fishbone is when the group knows that a specific area needs to be analyzed but is not sure which part of it is creating the problem. When all root causes are identified and organized on the fishbone, the group should discuss the potential causes to verify their relevancy and impact to the problem. Some groups may choose to verify potential causes by gathering data or using some form of analysis besides group discussion.

3. *Generate alternative solutions.* Once the group has identified and defined root causes, it brainstorms alternative solutions. The focus of this step is to generate, *not* evaluate. When groups generate and evaluate at the same time (in other words, when one member suggests a solution, and other members offer reasons why it will not work), the number of potentially viable solutions often is reduced (Rebori, 1997). After the group has provided all their solutions, similar aspects of the solutions may be combined. The solution(s) that integrate the best aspects of various ideas are more likely to lead to group consensus.

4. *Evaluate the alternatives.* Before evaluating alternatives, the coalition must consider the possible consequences and results of each. Questions should be asked such as, *Who is affected?* or *Who pays?* Coalitions should establish criteria for judging solutions that are objective and measurable.

For a structured approach, a matrix can be created with criteria listed on one axis and solutions on the other. Criteria can be weighted if some are more important than others. For each solution, members assign a score (for example, on a scale of one to ten) based on the extent to which that solution meets the criterion. The ratings for each solution are multiplied by the weight given to each criterion. The products for each solution are added and written in a total score column, and the solution with the highest total score is the group's choice. Less formal approaches include multi-voting and a zero to ten rating, which will be described later in this chapter. These techniques should not be thought of as formulas that will produce correct answers, nor should they substitute for valuable group discussion or collective judgment about the selected solution or idea.

5. *Select the best solution.* Agreeing on the best solution requires that the group have some ground rules for making decisions, such as consensus or majority vote. If reaching consensus is difficult, members or a facilitator should work to clarify specific areas of disagreement and then identify ways to integrate similar interests into the solution. Disagreement may sometimes result in the group identifying new solutions supported by group consensus.

6. *Implement the solution.* A solution that involves coalition members and builds their commitment is likely to be implemented effectively and on time. During the action-planning phase, the questions to be answered include these (Conone, Brown, and Willis, 2005):

(*Text resumes on page 195.*)

Exhibit 7.2. A Guide to Effective Brainstorming.

1. Before starting, briefly explain the issue and its history to help participants prepare mentally for the session and focus on the particular issue.

2. It may be appropriate to invite to the meeting guests with different expertise or backgrounds. A new outlook may come from someone who is not considered an expert or close to the problem.

3. Limit brainstorming sessions to thirty or forty minutes. If a satisfactory idea has not emerged, move on to the next agenda item or adjourn the meeting. Encourage participants to think about the problem, because great ideas can come anytime and anywhere.

4. Review the rules of brainstorming before beginning:
   - Criticism of ideas isn't allowed.
   - All ideas, no matter how wild, are encouraged.
   - The more ideas, the better.
   - Every participant should try to build on or combine the ideas of others.

5. Provide red and green cards for each participant. When flow of ideas is positive, participants hold up green cards. If someone uses a "Killer Phrase" (a negative phrase that inhibits participation), participants hold up red cards. This helps the group identify "killer" behaviors and lets participants know when they should be more supportive of others' input.

6. If more than ten members participate, break into teams of five to six people and have each team brainstorm the issue. Smaller groups are less formal and make people more at ease to share ideas.

7. Write brainstorming objective where everyone can see it. Put it in question form, starting with either "How can we . . . ?" or "What can be done to . . . ?" Here are examples: "How can we better understand what our community needs?" and "What can be done to improve the quality of care?"

8. Capture group's ideas on a flip chart, eraser board, or interactive whiteboard (ideal for brainstorming because ideas can be easily edited and saved to a computer file). Whichever tool you use to record ideas, be sure they're saved for future reference.

9. If flow of ideas begins to fizzle, use the following strategies: (1) Re-read every third idea to generate new ideas. (2) Ask a participant to select an idea and give reasons why he or she likes it so that others can build on it. (3) Save an idea or two to share to initiate more discussion.

10. After all ideas are exhausted, have group members sort the brainstorming notes and arrange the ideas in related groups. Ask each member to select the five ideas he or she thinks are best and explain why these ideas are most promising and how they could be implemented. Although less ideal, if time is short, the notes can be mailed to members. Members then sort and prioritize the ideas as above and return them to the facilitator, who summarizes the information and presents it to the group via mail or at the next meeting.

Adapted from Hawkins, 1998.

Exhibit 7.3. Nominal Group Technique.

1. Select a neutral facilitator (member or non-group member).

2. The facilitator introduces a list of suggested ground rules. Following a discussion of them, participants are asked to honor the rules. Two key rules include: (a) All ideas count and (b) arguments are not allowed.

3. Distribute small sticky notes or index cards to participants (five to ten cards each). The facilitator states the issue or problem as one question and writes it on a flip chart.

4. Participants write their responses on cards (one per card), working silently and independently. Allow four to six minutes maximum for this task.

5. Collect and randomly redistribute participants' written responses. If a participant receives his or her own card back, the participant should not share this information with the group. Rather, the assumption is that no one knows who the actual author of the idea is.

6. Participants take turns reading one card at a time. Ideas are recorded on a flip chart. Participants are reminded that this is not the time to evaluate ideas and responses. If an idea is not understood, the facilitator asks volunteers from the group to speculate what the author meant, protecting author anonymity.

7. The facilitator continues recording ideas until all cards have been discussed.

8. The facilitator asks the group to identify ideas that are similar to one another and asks for permission to eliminate duplicates. The facilitator assigns each idea a letter of the alphabet.

9. The facilitator now asks participants to identify their top five preferences. For example, five dots of the same color or five sticky notes of the same color are given to each participant, who then affixes them to the ideas voted on. The scores are recorded, tabulated, posted, and discussed by the group.

10. From the results of the prioritization exercise, the facilitator might ask the group what next steps they would like to take regarding the results. Here are some issues the facilitator could raise to help the group discuss next steps:

    • *Do the ideas add clarity to the issue, creating a better understanding of members' opinions?*

    • *Do the top five ideas lend themselves to a plan of action or strategies for the group?*

    • *What would the group like to do with this information?*

Source: Adapted from *Community Leader's Guide* developed cooperatively by: Community Colleges of Spokane, Institute of Extended Learning and Washington State University Cooperative Extension. Reprinted with permission.

- What should be done? (goal)
- How should each step be accomplished? (strategy)
- When will it be done? (time frame)
- Who is responsible for each step?
- What is the expected outcome?

Solutions should be implemented according to the action plan. Sometimes, however, unintended consequences occur that require changing the plan midstream. The coalition can adapt quickly by adding project updates to each meeting's agenda.

7. *Evaluate the solution.* Evaluation is probably the step most groups underemphasize when problem solving, due to constraints such as time, cost, political climate, uneasiness in evaluation, and fear of being challenged in their agreed-upon solution (Rebori, 2005b). The purpose of evaluation is to determine how well the solution is working or why it may not be working. The evaluation should be based on the complexity of the problem and the agreed-upon solution, and can be as simple as interviews with key individuals or as complex as surveys and in-depth content analysis.

Objectives and approaches for problem solving will depend on the severity of the problem and the quality of solution desired. For minor problems, the coalition may focus on quickly reaching a solution. Coalitions concerned with finding a quality solution as the main objective will need more time for the problem-solving process. To be effective, coalitions must agree on a solution that gets the job done, uses available resources efficiently, promotes cooperation, and fosters competence among its members (Rebori, 1997).

EFFECTIVE DECISION MAKING

Napoleon Bonaparte once said, "Nothing is more difficult, and therefore more precious, than to be able to decide." And he should have known. When he made the decision to invade Russia, he committed his army to a thousand-mile trek in cold weather, with no food and inadequate clothing, and surrounded by hostile locals.

The word "decide" comes from the Latin *decidere* meaning "to cut off." Making a decision takes courage because it forces people to close the door on other opportunities and brings with it a degree of uncertainty. Because most of us hate, and will do almost anything to avoid, uncertainty, we continually defer decisions or make snap decisions with little forethought.

Fortune magazine's Jerry Useem says that making decisions means "inviting uncertainty into your home, offering it a drink, and asking it to stay for dinner" (2005, p. 56). He advises that the first step to good decision making is to overcome anxiety about it, and the second step is to let go of the idealistic notion that any decision is ever perfect. Useem acknowledges the difference between making a *wrong* decision, which is an *outcome* that you cannot control, and making a *bad* decision, a *process* that you can control. Wrong decisions are inevitable, but bad decisions are avoidable.

Business guru Jim Collins, author of *Built to Last* and *Good to Great*, echoes this sentiment. His research into companies that are committed to excellence convinced him of two things. First, decisions are not as much about *what* as about *who*—in other words, they are people decisions. Second, great outcomes are the result of a stream of decisions, made over time, that are brilliantly executed (Collins, 2005). He further asserts that the worst error you can make is *not* to decide; most mistakes can be overcome; debate and conflict are healthy; and major decisions are usually not reached by unanimous agreement.

We can also learn about decision making from others' mistakes. The National Aeronautics and Space Administration's (NASA) *Challenger* space shuttle explosion in 1986 and the fire disaster on Colorado's Storm King Mountain in 1994 are examples of tragedies where a series of small, poorly executed decisions led to disasters. In the wake of these tragedies, both NASA and the U.S. Forest Service revamped their training procedures and leadership models. These valuable, real-world lessons apply to coalitions as well. We cannot always tell our partners *what* to decide, but they can help us select competent leaders and train them *how* to decide.

Coalition studies have shown that the influence that participants have in making decisions is vital to a partnership. Influence in decision making is related to increased satisfaction and participation and increased reporting of positive benefits (Butterfoss, Goodman, and Wandersman, 1996; Mayer and others, 1998). Exhibit 7.4 presents a diagnostic tool for assessing a coalition's participant involvement.

Coalitions often encounter problems that interfere with effective decision making, such as vague or inconsistent goals and procedures, long meetings, unequal group involvement and commitment, group conflicts, low communication and literacy skills, different communication styles, extreme power differences, and poor memory of the group's past (Gastil, 1997). When discussion is open, free-flowing and idea-based, everything is fairly loose and agreeable. However, when the partnership moves to a decision phase, members' views of reality may change. Suddenly, members may be unsure of when, how, and whether a decision should be made.

Decision Making Styles

To maximize work group effectiveness, members should decide which of the following decision-making styles should be used, depending on the situation.

No decision. Some groups may unconsciously or consciously avoid making decisions and thus make the decision *not to decide*. This style may be exhibited by shifting to another topic before a decision is reached or by giving no response when a member initiates an idea or decision.

Self-appointed decision maker. In this scenario, a member initiates a decision under the assumption that other members consented. The member states a decision, which no one else agrees or disagrees with, and so he or she makes a decision for the entire group that does not necessarily reflect its collective opinion. The chair or facilitator often takes this role.

Minority rule. A minority of members makes a decision while other members remain silent. A vote is not usually taken, but based on the discussion, a few

(*Text resumes on page 198.*)

Exhibit 7.4. What's Your Coalition's Participant Involvement Score?

Key

1 = Always/Definitely/Strongly Agree
2 = Usually/Probably Agree
3 = Generally/Maybe/Neutral
4 = Sometimes/Rarely Disagree
5 = Almost Never/We have a big problem/Strongly Disagree

How do (or would) members and other participants respond to these statements?

1. All members have a fair say in decisions about the coalition's actions that affect their interests.

    1   2   3   4   5

2. Coalition's leadership is committed to having participants' contributions influence the decision.

    1   2   3   4   5

3. Coalition's leadership seeks out and facilitates the involvement of participants and others who are potentially affected.

    1   2   3   4   5

4. Coalition's governing process involves members in defining how they participate.

    1   2   3   4   5

5. Coalition leadership communicates to participants how their input was, or was not, utilized.

    1   2   3   4   5

6. Coalition leadership provides participants with information needed to participate in meaningful ways.

    1   2   3   4   5

7. Coalition leadership gives consideration to the various ways of engaging participants and uses processes that are suited to the issues and participant interests.

    1   2   3   4   5

TOTAL SCORE: _____

Evaluating the Participant Involvement Scorecard: How Did Your Coalition Do?

7–12   CONGRATULATIONS! Your coalition is on the cutting edge of effective shared decision making. You have probably made your way to this level through some hard-earned lessons. You may want to offer assistance to other coalitions.

13–18   You are doing a lot right! Give yourself some well-deserved credit, and realize the only way you can improve is through awareness and continued work. To keep improving, consider finding a consultant who can help you work through your coalition issues.

(continued)

Exhibit 7.4. What's Your Coalition's Participant Involvement Score? (*Continued*)

19–23	You are on the right track but may need help. It may be that the will is there, but the know-how is weak. Or it may be that the knowledge is fine, but the will is weak. Depending on which you think is holding you back, you may want to seek a consultant or you may wish to seek special training for your coalition.
24–28	Your coalition has a shaky grasp of participant involvement and leadership and needs a major transformation in its approach.
Above 28	Major culture or attitude issues need to be addressed before any coalition work is attempted.

From E. Franklin Dukes & Madeleine Solomon, 2000. *Reaching Higher Ground: A Guide for Preventing, Preparing for and Transforming Conflict for Tobacco Control Coalitions*. pp. K1–K2. San Francisco: Tobacco Technical Assistance Consortium. Reprinted with permission.

people make a decision for the entire group. This style does not consider other, quieter members' values or their opinions about the decision reached, and can be frustrating for those who feel that their views do not matter.

Majority rule. This style requires agreement of at least 51 percent of members to reach a decision. Groups often reach majority rule through holding a brief discussion, after which a final vote is taken, usually by a show of hands. When used for complex or high-stake decisions, majority rule may produce competitive, win-or-lose solutions. Although majority rule moves decisions quickly, it can result in divisiveness and frustration on the part of those whose opinions were not in the majority.

Consensus. Members make a decision based on all members supporting the decision. Consensus is not unanimity; it is reached when members mutually agree to a decision and feel as though their concerns regarding the issue have been addressed. Such a decision is not a compromise, because members work to seek mutual agreement. Although time-consuming, consensus fosters empowerment, group cohesion, accountability, and improved relationships, especially when decisions are complex or critical. Consensus is favored by many coalitions because everyone can live with the final decisions without compromising issues of fundamental importance. Even though some decision points reached by consensus may be less than ideal, the overall package is worthy of support; most individuals will work to support the full decision and not just the parts they like the best (Dukes, Piscolish, and Stephens, 2000).

Most coalitions make decisions through majority rule (voting) or consensus. Both methods have their strengths and limitations: Voting is efficient, but a simple majority may not lead to effective implementation. Consensus may take longer to achieve but can lead to higher levels of support for implementation and fosters group cohesion by incorporating everyone's opinions. Obviously, the no decision, self-appointed decision maker, and minority support styles are not recommended for decision making, but they are often used just the same. When deciding whether to use majority support (voting) or consensus, Rebori (2000) suggests considering these factors:

- *Timeliness*. How much time has been given to making the decision? If time is short, then the most efficient method should be used—in other words, majority rule.

- *Appropriateness*. How complex is the decision? If the decision is simple, consensus is not needed. If the decision is complex (for example, budgets, action plans), then all concerns must be heard.

- *Relationship*. How will the decision affect the group members' relationships? If the decision-making style could jeopardize one or more relationships within the group, then a more collective, consensus-building approach is required.

Techniques for Building Majority-Rule Decisions. A variety of techniques can be used to reduce frustration among members and prevent the divisiveness that often accompanies majority-rule decisions, especially when the vote is close (University of Wisconsin, 2001).

70/30 vote. This technique requires at least 70 percent of the members to agree with the decision and usually calls for more discussion. The discussion builds a deeper understanding of why members feel a certain way about a decision. The U.S. Marine Corps espouses a similar "70 percent solution": If you have 70 percent of the information, have done 70 percent of the analysis, and feel 70 percent confident, then decide. A less than ideal decision, quickly executed, stands a chance of success, whereas taking no action stands no chance.

Blind vote. This technique is recommended with high-stake or complex decisions and can be as simple as a secret ballot that gives anonymity to the voting and reduces divisiveness.

Dots. Dots can be used as a visual way to demonstrate majority support among a variety of possible decisions. See a full discussion of this method under "Prioritizing" later in this chapter.

Devil's advocate. In this technique, one member plays the devil's advocate to the potential decision by stating all the opposite possibilities. By having someone do this, members are encouraged to discuss the merits of the potential decision without worrying about blocking the group's momentum or slipping into "groupthink" (when members suppress their dissenting view because they think it is unpopular).

Techniques for Building Consensus. Rather than approaching consensus from an "I can live with it" standpoint, several methods may be used to make this technique easier and more likely to succeed.

Levels of consensus. Susskind (1994) offers an alternative framework for arriving at consensus, based on a series of levels of support. Coalitions can decide whether to use these or adopt their own levels.

- *Level One:* I can easily support the decision or action.
- *Level Two:* I can support the decision or action, but it may not be my preference.
- *Level Three:* I can support the decision or action with minor changes.
- *Level Four:* I support the will of the group, but I do not necessarily agree with the decision or action.
- *Level Five:* I *cannot* support the decision or action.

In the case of a decision where agreement does not seem imminent, the facilitator would call for a preliminary vote to gauge the level of consensus by asking members to hold up one, two, three, four, or five fingers. For Levels Four and Five, direct questions should then be asked to bring forth member concerns. If the issue is particularly contentious, the facilitator may call for a secret straw vote by having members close their eyes and raise their hands to indicate their level of support. This can reduce the pressure on the single member or small number of members who may feel coerced into consenting. Coalition members should decide at the outset what constitutes consensus. Should consensus mean that everyone has to have a One, Two, or Three level of support? When time is a consideration, coalitions may want to adopt a 70/30 rule, where 70 percent of members must have a Level Four or above to reach consensus.

Consensus log. Keeping a running list of actions or decisions where consensus was reached creates a clear record of what decisions have already been reached on complex issues, such as approving a strategic plan.

Distilling concerns. As members' concerns arise, they should be recorded on a flip chart. Once all concerns have been raised, the group can cluster similar ones to give members a sense of those that must be resolved.

Straw man. Draft a proposal or solution (the straw man) and encourage members to criticize and pull it apart. Providing a straw man gives the group a starting point for members' opinions and values about the potential proposal and builds ownership in a non-threatening way.

Prioritizing

In Robert's Rules of Order, the chief decision-making tool is a vote by the committee or group members. For some committees, the majority-rule approach is adequate. Other groups may wish to use a prioritizing process either before or in place of voting. Prioritizing tools share a common focus on the feasibility of the ideas or options, regardless of who first presented them, and help keep the purpose of the decision in the forefront. All three prioritizing techniques presented here assume that the choices from which the committee must select are written out for all to see on a board or chart. This visual record of choices is essential for decision making because most people can only hold five items in short-term memory (plus or minus two). That means that if you have more than three alternatives, some people in the room cannot remember all of them without a visual listing. Thus a visual list is essential if all the choices are to be equally considered. Two common and easy-to-use prioritizing tools include *multi-voting* and *zero to ten rating* (University of Wisconsin, 2001).

Multi-Voting. This is a very simple and quick method for committees or groups to use in setting priorities when there are many options. *Which are most important? What must be done this year? Which project should be started first? What core values are most important?* It is a variation of the Nominal Group Technique but is used here to reach a decision rather than to generate ideas. Multi-voting is a fun, participative activity that yields clearly visible priorities and limits lengthy discussions. Typically, for a group of ten, this would take twenty to thirty minutes to complete. The steps are presented here:

1. Brainstorm possibilities. Suppose you have a group that has generated a list of things they believe the coalition should address this year but know they cannot do them all. This method would provide a sense of which items are most important and should be addressed first. Therefore, begin by brainstorming all options, listing them on a flip chart in any order and leaving enough space between items for the self-stick dots.

2. Give each person in the group ten self-stick dots. (For this exercise, color is irrelevant.) Instruct them that in choosing their priorities, they are to use all ten dots but no more than four on any one item. Therefore, four dots would indicate a person's top priority, whereas some items might get no dots. Participants walk up to the flip charts and place their dots next to their items of choice.

3. When everyone has placed his or her dots, count the dots for each item and make a priority listing on a new flip-chart page. Usually a few clear winners emerge. Discuss with the group whether they agree these should be top priorities for coalition work. This does not necessarily mean that the other items on the list are eliminated.

4. If the list is still too long, give each person in the group two or three self-stick dots and ask everyone to vote for their top priorities from the existing priority list (one vote per item).

Zero to Ten Rating. Zero to ten rating is a technique to use when a coalition must decide something about its own operations. For example, the coalition is developing

its action plan for the coming year, and a number of possible options have been suggested (the multi-voting method may have been used to narrow down the possibilities). However, more ideas exist than are feasible to complete. The value of the zero
to ten rating is that it prevents people from forcing their views onto the group and
can be a reality check for those who say, "The whole coalition thinks this," or "I am
sure we all agree. . . ." The steps to the zero to ten rating follow:

1. Draw a scale with numbers from zero to ten below each item on the flip
   chart. At the left end, label zero "Can Wait." At the right end, label ten
   "Essential to Do Now." (You will have as many scales as you have items
   from which to choose.)

2. Each person goes up to the flip chart and places a self-stick dot or sticker
   on each item's scale, according to his or her opinion of the importance
   of the item. (Note that if extreme trust or confidentiality issues exist
   within the group, the chart can be turned around and each person can go
   up to the chart individually. The facilitator or leader may even place the
   first dots.)

3. After all self-stick dots have been placed, the group will have a clear
   visual representation of clusters of agreement. The facilitator may say, for
   example, "We will not spend time on items that received only one to five
   dots but will instead focus on the items that collected six or more." This
   exercise may show the group that they are "all over the board" in terms of
   what they believe is most important. Data will probably be needed at this
   point to help clarify priorities.

Ethical Decision Making. In coalitions, issues arise that may force members to make
difficult decisions. Often these ethical issues involve conflicting personal and organizational values. Ethics involves the ability to distinguish right from wrong and the
commitment to do what is right. Ethics, therefore, is concerned with how a person
should behave, in contrast to values, which concern the beliefs and attitudes that
determine how a person actually behaves. An ethical dilemma occurs when a conflict exists between core ethical values, between "right and right," with no one clear
ethical choice (Wilkins and Walker, 1993). Making ethical decisions requires the
ability to make distinctions between competing choices and often necessitates a
structured procedure to ensure that all members have an opportunity to provide
input.

Various models exist for guiding ethical decision making, but the Josephson
Model works well for coalitions (Josephson Institute on Ethics, 2003). According to
the model, principled decision making is based on six values that cut across time,
culture, politics, religion, ethnicity, and other human divisions. They are especially
useful in developing and maintaining coalitions that value diversity, because they
have common meaning for members who differ in age, gender, ethnicity, socioeconomic level, educational background, or other characteristics. These core ethical
values (the "Six Pillars of Character") are trustworthiness, respect, responsibility,

fairness, caring, and good citizenship (responsible participation in society). The decision-making model is used to help clarify the coalition's needs and values as members discuss the answers to the ten questions presented here in order to analyze an actual ethical dilemma or a case study:

- What is the problem or goal?
- Who are the stakeholders?
- What are the options or choices?
- What are the potential consequences of each option?
- Is there a right versus wrong situation to address?
- Is there an ethical dilemma (right versus wrong) to resolve?
- Which values or principles (six pillars of character) are involved?
- How will you rank them?
- What will you decide?
- Why?

When coalition members understand the factors that impact one another's decision making (for example, personal versus organizational benefit, long-term versus short-term time frames, loyalty to one's own group), addressing ethical decision making becomes easier (Wilkins, Tremethick, Walker, and Meier, 1999).

RESOLVING CONFLICT

Another internal process that must be initiated to ensure smooth internal coalition functioning is conflict management. Coalitions ask members to create a balance among their personal agendas, their organizations' missions, and the coalition's mission and goals. Though this balance is achieved much of the time, sometimes controversy develops into conflict. If unresolved, this tension can hamper the efforts of some or all the partners to reach their common goal.

Mizrahi and Rosenthal (1993) argue that conflict is an inherent characteristic of partnerships. Conflict may arise between the partnership and its priorities for social change or among partners concerning issues such as loyalty, leadership, goals, benefits, contributions, and representation. Conflict has been shown to lead to staff turnover, avoidance of certain activities, and difficulty in recruiting members (Kegler, Steckler, Malek, and McLeroy, 1998b).

In their book, *Reaching for Higher Ground in Conflict Resolution*, Dukes, Piscolish, and Stephens (2000) present an original approach to group problem solving and conflict transformation, demonstrating the value of setting up and maintaining deep commitments and broadly shared expectations as an integral part of effective group process.

"Higher ground" is a metaphor for behavior that brings a group out of conflict. It is an environment where people treat each other as they themselves wish to be treated and come to new understandings about their shared work, their relationships, and their collective potential. Reaching higher ground means developing effective conflict resolution strategies and skills and exercising the leadership needed to guide others to this principled and promising place.

However, Dukes, Piscolish, and Stephens (2000) argue that conflict can actually benefit coalitions because it identifies problems that otherwise might remain hidden; improves understanding of the issues that led to the conflict; creates innovative solutions by forcing new ways to conduct business; strengthens relationships by demanding long-term engagement; improves standards, regulations, and policies; engages interested parties who may formerly not have been involved; and builds the coalition's capacity to appreciate and deal with differences.

They further agree that coalitions should respond to conflict in three ways. They must (1) prevent unnecessary conflict by building strong relationships within and outside of the coalition, based upon clear and shared understanding of roles, purposes, and meeting processes; (2) prepare for conflict by anticipating that differences will occur and developing ground rules and a covenant, or process for handling such differences; and (3) transform conflict by developing the capacity (shared knowledge, skills, commitment) to resolve conflict as it occurs. Conflict transformation can actually strengthen the coalition and build capacity. Research shows that conflict transformation results from effective coalition planning and contributes to goal attainment (Mayer and others, 1998). A diagnostic tool is found in Exhibit 7.5.

Types of Conflict

In a coalition, each partner organization has its domain, or field of operation, with human and material resources, goals, and tasks related to the goals. According to the exchange theory of organizational relations, when these community partners form relationships, they agree to exchange resources (Zald, 1969). The domains of organizations can overlap and lead to several types of conflict.

Conflict over goals. Although general goals of participating organizations seem mutually dependent, a particular strategy for joint action is perceived to work against the interest of one of the intended partners or against another limited goal. For example, a teen pregnancy prevention coalition may refuse to collaborate with a community recreation center because they feel the center would devote more resources to preschool programs than to working with at-risk teenagers.

Conflict over resources. Community partners may compete over proposals, requests for public or private funds, shared staff, supplies, or facilities. Sometimes partners are denied resources or given unequal shares. At other times, partners might disagree over the amount of resources that should be used for a collaborative effort. For example, two coalition partners might apply to the same community foundation for an implementation grant.

Exhibit 7.5. Conflict Resolution Capacity Inventory.

If astute observers of your coalition were to evaluate it, how would they respond?

KEY

1 = Always/Definitely/Strongly Agree
2 = Usually/Probably Agree
3 = Generally/Maybe/Neutral
4 = Sometimes/Rarely Disagree
5 = Almost Never/We have a big problem/Strongly Disagree

1. My coalition handles conflict effectively.

$$1 \quad 2 \quad 3 \quad 4 \quad 5$$

2. Differences are viewed and used as an opportunity to learn and grow.

$$1 \quad 2 \quad 3 \quad 4 \quad 5$$

3. My coalition provides support for resolving conflict when it escalates in a harmful way.

$$1 \quad 2 \quad 3 \quad 4 \quad 5$$

4. Minority opinions that challenge the leadership or mainstream ideas are sought out and encouraged.

$$1 \quad 2 \quad 3 \quad 4 \quad 5$$

5. Conflict in my coalition is handled directly and face-to-face without people going behind one another's backs.

$$1 \quad 2 \quad 3 \quad 4 \quad 5$$

6. My coalition has developed an effective system for addressing conflict productively.

$$1 \quad 2 \quad 3 \quad 4 \quad 5$$

7. Participants in the coalition have sufficient skills and knowledge to address conflict productively.

$$1 \quad 2 \quad 3 \quad 4 \quad 5$$

TOTAL SCORE: _____

Evaluating the Conflict Resolution Capacity Inventory: How Did Your Coalition Do?

7–12   CONGRATULATIONS! Your coalition is very effective at preventing and transforming conflict. Keep up the good work! You may want to offer assistance to other coalitions.

(continued)

Exhibit 7.5. Conflict Resolution Capacity Inventory. (*Continued*)

13–18	You are doing pretty well! Give yourself some well-deserved credit, and realize the only way for you to improve is through continued work. To keep improving, consider finding a consultant who can help you work through your coalition issues.
19–23	You are on the right track but may need some more attention. It may be that the will is there, but the know-how is weak. Or it may be that the knowledge is fine, but the will is weak. Depending on which you think is holding you back, you may want to seek a consultant or you may wish to seek special training for your coalition.
24–28	Your coalition has a shaky grasp of conflict prevention and resolution and needs a major transformation in its approach.
Above 28	Major culture or attitude issues need to be addressed before any coalition work is attempted.

From E. Franklin Dukes, 2000. *Reaching Higher Ground: A Guide for Preventing, Preparing for and Transforming Conflict for Tobacco Control Coalitions.* pp. L1–L2. San Francisco: Tobacco Technical Assistance Consortium. Reprinted with permission.

Conflict over geography. One partner feels it provides services to or represents interests of an area exclusively. Allowing another partner to work in the same area could suggest that the first partner is not doing its job, cause duplication of effort, or confuse the priority population. For example, two coalition partners might propose adult literacy programs in the same neighborhood.

Conflict over methods. Partners generally agree on goals, but one feels the proposed approach will be ineffective or counterproductive to its own interests. Similarly, one partner may feel it has ownership over a strategy or program that another partner plans to use. For example, the coalition proposes an educational approach to smoking cessation, whereas one partner favors a legislative advocacy approach; or the American Lung Association has held a legislative breakfast annually to gain endorsements for its clean indoor air legislation, but now the coalition proposes to host its own legislative breakfast on behalf of all of its partners.

Conflict over identity or public perception. One partner feels that the proposed collaboration would change how the public views its organization (for example, as less powerful or more [or less] conservative) or feels threatened by the potential success of another partner. For instance, a middle school partner with a high percentage of overweight and obese students may feel threatened by a coalition project that focuses on gathering body mass index data for all schools in the district.

Conflict over personalities. A representative of one partner organization personally dislikes another member. Mizrahi and Rosenthal (1993) argue that coalition work should be approached as a conflict resolution model, which requires managing effectively four dynamic tensions: mixed loyalties, autonomy of coalition versus accountability to members, coalition as means versus an end, and unity versus diversity.

Conflict over mixed loyalties. Coalition members have a commitment both to the coalition and to their own organizations, which can produce tension between altruism and self-interest. Coalitions may compete with member organizations for resources, organizational time, and energy. Confusion may also exist as to which "hat" coalition members are wearing when they participate in coalition activities. This tension can be overcome by designing activities that do not threaten the networks of member organizations; being sensitive to issues or positions that compromise members' credibility or funding; avoiding direct competition with member organizations; and agreeing on which activities members can do in the name of the coalition versus those that they do on their own.

- *Autonomy versus accountability.* A coalition must have enough autonomy to take independent action and enough accountability to its member organizations to retain their support and its credibility. To balance this tension, ongoing communication needs to occur between the coalition, its members, and their organizations. Coalitions also must clarify how to integrate new members into the organization, who the coalition represents, and when and how members will be involved in critical decisions and activities.

- *Means versus model.* A coalition can be a means to accomplish a specific social change goal as well as a model of sustained interorganizational collaboration. When a coalition is concerned about being a model, it emphasizes internal coalition development, member commitment to the coalition, and coalition building over social change goals. Coalitions concerned about being a means to accomplish certain goals provide minimal structure, avoid process issues, promote participation only to produce results, and tolerate or work through differences. Effective coalitions try to strike a balance between process and goal orientation.

- *Unity versus diversity.* Coalitions need enough unity to act together, yet enough diversity to be representative and accomplish their goals. Too much unity can stifle creativity and lead to competition among members for turf, access to resources, and visibility. Increasing diversity may slow a coalition toward achieving its goals because it takes time to develop trust and good working relationships.

General Conflict Resolution Strategies

On the positive side, controversy and conflict create a high level of interest and energy. When properly dealt with, conflict allows different ideas to emerge, enables members to learn more about each other and think differently about an issue, and fosters new solutions. On the negative side, conflict can create frustration and discomfort that causes members to stop listening, retreat into "camps" to protect themselves and become polarized (Rebori, 2000). Researchers believe that people have preferred ways of dealing with conflict based on a combination of personality and experience. The five prevalent styles are Competing, Compromising, Accommodating, Avoiding, and Collaborating, as featured below (Rebori, 1998b):

Competing. Competing behavior represents high concern for self and low concern for another. Strategically, members fight for their interests at all costs. Even if they win one issue, the conflict may resurface at another time.

Compromising. Compromising behavior attempts to balance concern for self and other, whereas collaborating behavior signifies high concern for self and other. Each member gives a little; however, neither may get what is actually wanted. Compromising is the most common way to deal with conflict.

Accomodating. Members give in to the one(s) that disagree with them.

Avoiding. Avoiding behavior represents neither interest. All ignore the conflict and hope it goes away.

Collaborating. Both sides of the conflict listen and learn from one another (interest-based bargaining). Out of increased understanding, they create a solution that works best for all.

Coalition members may respond to conflict differently, but with awareness and practice, they gain the ability to choose how to respond to conflict. Exhibit 7.6 provides a table to help coalition members understand these different conflict styles. Depending on the specific situation, any one of these styles may be appropriate. For example, if the conflict is likely to go away if ignored or if it is not critical to the coalition, an *avoidance* strategy such as diverting attention might work. If the issue is very important, a forcing or *competitive* strategy such as insisting or persuading may be a better strategy. However, because success in a coalition depends on achieving cooperation between several partners, *compromising* or *collaborating* strategies such as welcoming differences or bargaining are usually the best approach, regardless of personal opinions about the conflict. Dukes, Piscolish, and Stephens (2000) suggest that coalitions develop "principled negotiation," which includes focusing on interests, not positions; separating people from the problem; inventing options for mutual gain; and developing objective criteria.

Conflict Management Skills

Several skills can become part of a coalition's toolbox for managing conflict. Exhibit 7.7 provides a continuum of conflict resolution approaches to help a coalition develop its own conflict resolution system. Other types of conflict management techniques that are primarily preventive include: active listening, checking emotions, separating people from the problem, focusing on interests rather than positions, and reframing (Fisher and Ury, 1991; Rebori, 1998).

Listen actively. Listening involves more than simply hearing the words spoken; it requires active involvement that includes understanding, acknowledging, and responding. Listen for content, meaning, and feelings. To make sure that what the person has said is understood, summarize or paraphrase what was heard,

(Text resumes on page 211.)

Exhibit 7.6. Understanding Differing Conflict Styles.

FORCING: High assertiveness/Low affirmation   *"We're doing it my way. . . ."*

Strategies: Discourages disagreement, persuades, is firm, sets limits and consequences, cites policy, insists, repeats, controls, and is inaccessible.

Source of power: From position, role, and control of resources.

Benefits: Speed, decisiveness, protection of innocents, preservation of important values, stability.

Costs when overused: Destroyed or hierarchical relationships; loss of cooperation; atrophy of gifts in others; anger, depression, and diminished self-respect in others; stagnation.

COLLABORATING: High assertiveness/High affirmation   *"My preference is . . . but I'm interested in your views."*

Strategies: Asserts self while also inviting other views, welcomes differences, jointly lists strengths and weaknesses of all views, cooperates in seeking additional information.

Source of power: From trust, skill ability, goodwill, creativity.

Benefits: Trust and mutuality in relationships, high cooperation, creativity and growth, others blossom and develop new gifts, energy and joy.

Costs when overused: Fatigue and time loss, distraction from more important tasks, analysis paralysis.

COMPROMISING: Medium assertiveness/Medium affirmation   *"I'll meet you halfway. . . ."*

Strategies: Urges moderation, bargains, splits the difference, finds a little something for everyone, meets people halfway.

Source of power: From moderation and reasonableness.

Benefits: Relatively fast, enables the show to go on, provides a way out of stalemate, readily understood by most people, builds atmosphere of calmness and reason.

Costs when overused: Mediocrity and blandness, possibly unprincipled agreements, likelihood of patching symptoms and ignoring causes.

AVOIDING: Low assertiveness/Low affirmation   *"Let's not make a big deal out of this."*

Strategies: Withdraw, delay or avoid response, divert attention, suppress personal emotions, be inaccessible, be inscrutable.

Source of power: From calmness, silence, noncooperation, being above it all.

Benefits: Freedom from entanglement in trivial issues or insignificant relationships, stability, preservation of status quo, ability to influence others without doing anything.

Costs when overused: Periodic explosions of pent-up anger, slow death of relationships, residue of negative feelings, stagnation and dullness, loss of accountability, sapped energy.

(continued)

Exhibit 7.6. Understanding Differing Conflict Styles. (*Continued*)

ACCOMMODATING: Low assertiveness/High affirmation *"Okay, whatever you say. . . ."*

Strategies: Agree, support, acknowledge error, give in, convince self it's no big deal, placate.

Source of power: From relationships or approval of others.

Benefits: Wins approval and appreciation of others, freedom from hassle (in the short run at least), self-discipline of ego.

Costs when overused: Frustration for others who wish to collaborate, resentment and depression, stunted growth of personal gifts, over-dependence on others, denies others benefit of healthy confrontation.

From E. Franklin Dukes, 2000. *Reaching Higher Ground: A Guide for Preventing, Preparing for and Transforming Conflict for Tobacco Control Coalitions.* pp. 81–82. San Francisco: Tobacco Technical Assistance Consortium. Reprinted with permission.

Exhibit 7.7. A Continuum of Approaches to Conflict.

This continuum of conflict resolution approaches is typical of what a coalition might develop for its conflict resolution system.

	Face-to-Face Discussion (Positive Confrontation)	Informal Conciliation	Mediation	Voluntary Arbitration	Enforcement (Legal or Administrative)
Conflict Prevention					

Low Cost ←   ↔   →   High Cost

Conflict Prevention

Needs:
- Legitimate, effective governance with support of substantial proportion of coalition
- Sensible, understandable bylaws and rules
- Efficient, well-run, and well-attended coalition meetings
- Decision making by consensus for most important issues

Face-to-Face Discussion (Positive Confrontation)

Needs:
- Strong shared expectations (aspirations, principles, and ground rules for behavior) within the coalition that direct communication is normal and positive
- Good communication skills and commitment among participants to use them
- Goodwill (social capital) developed via history of productive meetings and activities

Exhibit 7.7. (*Continued*)

Informal Conciliation

Needs:
- Shared expectations within coalition that conciliation is normal and positive
- Steering Committee member or selected volunteer with time and skills to intercede
- Institutional support for the conciliation process

Third-Party Mediation

Needs:
- Positive expectations within the coalition that mediation is normal and useful
- Formal authority and specification for use of mediation within bylaws or other relevant rules
- Institutional support and (possibly) funding for mediation process
- Access to mediators (professional mediators or perhaps a program of well-trained and experienced volunteers)

Voluntary Arbitration

Needs:
- Formal authority and specification for use of arbitration within bylaws or other relevant rules
- Institutional support and (likely) funding for arbitration process
- Access to professional or (rare) volunteer arbitrator

Enforcement (Legal or Legislative)

Needs:
- Formal authority and specification for use
- Institutional support
- Financial and personnel resources

From E. Franklin Dukes, 2000. *Reaching Higher Ground: A Guide for Preventing, Preparing for and Transforming Conflict for Tobacco Control Coalitions.* p. Q1. San Francisco: Tobacco Technical Assistance Consortium. Reprinted with permission.

and work to understand where the conflict lies. Although it does not necessarily mean agreement, acknowledgment lets the other person know he or she has been heard and understood.

Keep emotions in check. Another important skill in managing conflict is to monitor emotions, both your own and others'. It may not be possible to change emotions, but you can change how you respond to them. Venting emotions during a conflict is helpful as long as you focus on the problem or conflict itself and do not direct negativity toward any person. Using ground rules can provide guidelines for constructive venting and help prevent verbal attacks. During intense conflict, some people's emotions may dominate their actions. If this occurs, call for a break from the discussion; those involved in the conflict can use the restroom, get a drink of water, go outside, or breathe slowly to regain focus.

Separate people from the problem. In every conflict, the substance of the problem and the human relationships may become entangled. One technique for separating people from the problem is to think in terms of perception, emotion, and communication. Understanding how conflict is perceived opens the door to a possible solution. As stated earlier, keeping emotions in check and understanding the emotions or feelings of those involved in the conflict are important. Actively listening to and understanding the other person's concerns will help you understand the conflict. Deal with people as fallible and the problem on its merits, paying attention to the underlying interests behind the conflict.

Focus on interests, not positions. Understanding the difference between interests and positions is critical to managing conflict. A position is a stance that has been decided upon, and an interest is the underlying cause of that position. For every interest, several possible positions exist that could satisfy it. Most people simply adopt the most obvious position and entrench themselves. However, they should look beyond positions for underlying interests. Sometimes an alternative position can be found that meets everyone's interests.

Reframe. Reframing means reinterpreting a statement into a problem-solving plan. For example, if someone is shouting, instead of simply viewing that person as disrespectful, reframe your perception of him or her as having limited skills of expression. In addition, help the other person reframe the conflict into a problem by asking for advice. Being asked for advice is flattering and provides an opportunity for the other person to become educated about the problem. Another helpful tactic for reframing is to ask the person why or what makes a solution fair. When verbally reframing, questions should begin with *How, Why, Why not, What,* or *Who.*

Turfism

Turfism is a special kind of conflict that coalitions may face when members perceive that their goals are incompatible or their relationships are threatened. These perceptions lead to "turf protection," as organizations decide to defend their domain rather than share with another organization (Ross, 1989, p. 172). The term "turf" comes from street gang terminology, where each gang has its neighborhood, or "turf," in which it operates and which it defends against other gangs. Turfism is the noncooperation or conflict between organizations with seemingly common goals or interests (Peck and Hague, 2005). While securing resources that are needed to reach goals, the partners may develop overlapping domains that make them reluctant to honor the expected exchange and which may lead to a turf battle (Levine and White, 1961). If power is the ability to control needed resources, then the degree of power surrendered or gained by competing organizations is the trigger that escalates turf protection to a turf battle.

Turf battles are related to the perceived effect on power and occur when one partner perceives the other as a direct competitor for resources that are not likely to be shared; one partner perceives a "marginal cost" to the proposed cooperation in money, time, or energy greater than perceived benefits of collaboration; one partner feels the exchange will be unequal; one partner is not flexible in changing its mission, goals, and tasks to adopt the proposed course of action; partners lack knowledge about or mistrust other partners (Levine and White, 1961; Ross, 1989; Zald, 1969).

In a coalition setting, turf is more complex than merely two sides fighting for their own personal gain. Turf battles can signify that a coalition is strong and "demonstrate that the issues the coalition encompasses, the specific approaches it undertakes, and the decisions it makes are all worth fighting over" (Cohen and Gould, 2003, p. 4).

Types of Turf Issues That Coalitions Face. Turf battles can be either *covert* or *overt* (Cohen and Gould, 2003). Covert struggles can only be resolved after the elements of the conflict are brought out in the open. Overt battles tend to be more straightforward; however, even seemingly overt turf struggles (for example, over money) can have hidden elements, such as a past conflict or a difference in values. Turf struggles vary "depending on what's at stake, on the individuals competing, and on how explicit the battle is" (Cohen and Gould, 2003, p. 6). Turf within a coalition is usually considered to involve two coalition members, but four different types of conflict have been described, each with its own dynamics (Cohen and Gould, 2003, p. 6; Mizrahi and Rosenthal, 1993):

Coalition member versus coalition member. Conflicts around leadership, decision making, and personality or style are common. Tensions regarding resources and recognition are often not only related to coalition work but may also be related to past competition, for example, for influence or funding.

Coalition members versus coalition. Conflicts here may be related to unshared goals, division of benefits, contributions, commitments, and representation. As the coalition's visibility increases, opportunities for funding increase. Competing for the same pool of resources is the most frequent and difficult turf struggle for coalitions and their members.

Members versus lead agency. As the coalition's visibility increases, the lead agency may acquire resources instead of individual partners. The lead agency may be more visibly linked to the larger coalition and can benefit much more than other partners, which may lead to resentment.

Coalition versus population or institution it wishes to influence. The coalition often may struggle to gain credibility, legitimacy, and power within the community it intends to serve.

Avoiding and Resolving Turf Battles. First and most important, coalitions must recognize that conflict will occur, mixed loyalties are unavoidable, and balancing unity and diversity is demanding (The Advocacy Institute, 2005a). Coalitions can prevent potential conflict by developing clear purposes and goals; ensuring appropriate representation and understanding of roles; planning and conducting effective meetings; and building consensus for coalition decisions and coalition work (Dukes, Piscolish, and Stephens, 2000). Partners will have different goals, ideologies, organizational styles, levels of power, commitments to objectives, expectations of results, and financial and in-kind resources (The Advocacy Institute, 2005e). However, in the long-term, avoiding turf battles is easier than having to deal with them. Rather than denying or suppressing these natural differences, the coalition must create ways to integrate members' passion for social issues and their work into the overall coalition effort (Cohen and Gould, 2003). Here are ten specific tips to avoid turf battles adapted from Peck and Hague (2005), The Advocacy Institute (2005e), and Kretzmann and McKnight (1993):

1. Recognize that a coalition's goals are never fully compatible with each of its partner organization's goals. Each partner must be ready to compromise or modify its commitment to specific goals and to help other partners adjust as needed.

2. Understand each partner's constraints such as the process required for formal support, the tactics the partner feels comfortable using, and the ability to adopt new issues.

3. Spend sufficient time clarifying coalition goals and developing each member's commitment to them. The coalition should establish consensus on its "domain" of action and how partners' resources are related. The stronger the sense of common mission, the more likely that partners will work well together.

4. Delegate responsibility for tasks according to each partner's skills and capabilities.

5. Clearly relate community needs to the potential available resources in order to build momentum and synergy. Being capacity- or resource-centered rather than problem-centered is critical for coalitions that operate in a small geographic area.

6. Explore the relationship between the potential partner and the coalition to ensure that a good match exists between their missions and goals.

7. Keep everyone informed and communicate extensively before coalition meetings with critical agenda items (for example, elections, strategic planning, budget) to elicit potential sources of disagreement and ensure eventual consensus.

8. Make key decisions as a whole group to give partners a stake in carrying out the coalition's actions.

9. Develop active work groups to increase interaction among members who might need clarification and discussion of issues that does not normally occur in coalition membership meetings.

10. Promote effective communication methods (verbal and nonverbal, oral and written) that make mutual understanding, compromise, and consensus more likely.

Group conflict has two basic dimensions: substantive and affective (Guetzkow and Gyr, 1954). Substantive refers to conflicts primarily related to task, such as the turf battles described above that relate to goals, methods, resources, and geography. Affective conflicts relate to emotional or interpersonal relations, such as turf battles related to identity or personality (Ross, 1989, p. 139). To effectively resolve a conflict, the coalition must identify whether the conflict is substantive or affective. If the dispute is *task-related,* the coalition should use an orderly problem-solving process (described earlier in this chapter) to arrive at a workable solution, and improve communication and active listening during and between meetings. Alternatively, they should ask the steering committee to recommend a course of action or negotiate a compromise.

Tension within a coalition may not always be generated by turf. The propensity of some individuals to create struggles and conflicts may be related to character or personality; some people are naturally argumentative. In instances where turf is not the issue, strategies for resolving turf issues simply will not work. To resolve these kinds of *affective* conflicts, the coalition should try to relate the conflict to a task issue to defuse emotions, keep the focus on the whole group rather than on the partners involved in the disagreement, and have a conflict management process in place (Ross, 1989, p. 172).

Effective Turf Management Tips. Instead of instructing members to "leave turf at the door," a more realistic approach acknowledges that turf issues will challenge the group and that individual interests must be balanced against the greater good. Cohen and Gould also offer ten tips for coalitions to effectively manage turf issues (2003, pp. 7–9).

1. *Acknowledge potential turf issues.* Before forming a coalition, have honest conversations with participants about the history of relationships among potential members and their organizations. Based on this information, the lead agency can determine which people are best suited to join the coalition. Choose coalition representatives who are problem solvers and who hold jobs where working together is beneficial.
2. *Talk details.* Coalition members should be encouraged to openly discuss their reasons for being at the table and share information about their respective organizations. Initially, and any time new members are recruited to the coalition, allow time for a discussion of these questions:

    - What is the core mission of your organization?
    - Who are your key members?
    - What strategies are used to reach your goals?
    - What are your funding sources? What activities might threaten or enhance this funding base?

3. *Shape collective identity.* Members must be invested in the coalition's success and see how the work of their own organizations fits into the larger vision of the coalition. To fulfill members' needs for recognition and foster a sense of collectivity, allow *all* members to represent the coalition at meetings, in the media, and at political gatherings; encourage members to assume leadership roles in work groups; and rotate the hosting of coalition meetings among the various member organizations.

4. *Make fair decisions.* The group should be able to discuss the impact of a proposed action on each partner organization to assure that the decision has real support from the membership. The decision-making process should be based on majority support and must be consistently applied. However, sometimes consensus must be used to make sure that no groups feel left out by the coalition's approach. As described earlier in this chapter, consensus is defined as what the majority supports and everyone can live with. When consensus cannot be reached, the coalition must decide how to move on.

5. *Seek funding for coalition coordination.* All members must help sustain the coalition. They should develop plans for how needs will be shared and new resources will be acquired and distributed. All members may not want or be able to contribute financial support, but they should be expected to offer ideas, data, or in-kind support (for example, materials and volunteer time).

6. *Reward members and celebrate successes.* Because coalitions rely on volunteers who have other professional responsibilities, they must provide benefits (for example, solidarity, appreciation, evidence of impact) that exceed costs (for example, time and frustration) in order to reduce turnover and maintain momentum.

7. *Build bridges.* Coalition members are people, not just representatives of organizations. If you create a friendly, respectful atmosphere, offer refreshments, and encourage members to socialize and enjoy one another, they will be more productive. Create work groups to promote closer working relationships and personal satisfaction among members.

8. *Remind participants of the big picture.* When turf issues arise, certain neutral members are indispensable because of their role or professional identity (for example, survivors or those affected by the issue, youth, leaders from faith-based groups). These members, who are removed from the turf issue and dedicated to the coalition's fundamental cause, can re-motivate the members of the coalition and remind them why the coalition formed in the first place.

9. *Make struggles overt.* Acknowledge that conflict exists and discuss its potential causes. Lead agencies must be nondefensive and alert to turf battles between a member and the coalition or lead agency (or both). The chair or a neutral member may also meet with members individually if he or she feels that the methods of dealing with turf issues are not working.

10. *Encourage flexibility.* Leaders must create an open environment where members feel comfortable with diverse perspectives and dealing with conflict. Those who use humor and ground rules, understand group dynamics and group process, and are honest, focused, decisive, flexible, and inclusive, may be more able to create this type of environment.

COALITION SPOTLIGHT: VIRGINIANS FOR A HEALTHY FUTURE

As of 2002, Virginia's excise tax on tobacco products had not changed for thirty-five years, when it had been *lowered* due to fears that the 1964 Surgeon General's Report would reduce tobacco consumption and therefore harm tobacco farmers. For some,

Virginia's position as the state with the lowest tax in the nation at 2.5 cents per pack was a source of pride. For public health advocates, this low figure was both an embarrassment and an opportunity. Raising the cost of tobacco products by increasing the tax would lead to a decrease in numbers of those who use those products. But Virginia's health advocates knew that getting an increase through the General Assembly would require navigating a minefield of potential opposition from powerful tobacco companies, low-tax advocates, and farmers and other tobacco workers. Furthermore, conflict within the tobacco control coalition about how much of a raise was needed and how it would be spent could derail the unified effort that would be required for a raise to have any chance at all.

The tobacco control coalition adopted a multi-tiered strategy to build consensus for its campaign. Leaders invited representatives from other health, education, and environmental advocates to participate in early planning sessions well before any major decisions were made, so these other interests were able to participate in a meaningful way in setting goals and crafting strategy. They secured funding from the Department of Health to pay for the services of an independent facilitator so the leadership would not be dominating meetings. Major decisions about the campaign were made by consensus—that is, all members of this larger coalition had to agree before the coalition would take any action in the coalition's name. Such decisions ranged from the name of this new coalition, Virginians for a Healthy Future, and its campaign slogan, *"From 2.5 Cents to Common Sense,"* to the amount of increase that would be sought. Members openly discussed how they would address any conflicts within the coalition in the future. And they divided their campaign into two components, with the first step being to secure an increase, leaving the determination of how any such increase might be spent for later. They invited other participants as interest grew, taking care to make sure that the coalition was open to potential allies. Promoting this sort of openness, despite concerns that opposition groups would have sufficient time to organize, added to the coalition's legitimacy.

This consensus was sufficiently strong and widespread to weather an entire year's wait when the coalition's lobbyist advised a one-year delay in submitting the legislation. The results were impressive and a testimony to the power of working through differences by carefully building consensus: first, an excise tax increase of 20 cents per pack in September 2004 and an additional 10 cents in July 2005. Second, a 10 percent tax on tobacco products other than cigarettes that also went into effect in September 2004. Finally, a Health Care Trust Fund was created, with money raised from excise taxes on tobacco products to be deposited in this fund and used solely to provide health care services, including tobacco prevention.

SUMMARY

Effective communication is a skill that can be learned and improved upon with practice. Through the process of communication—sending and receiving messages— coalition members can develop understanding and respect for one another, share information, challenge each other to think differently, and find the best possible solutions to key issues around which the group has formed.

Coalition studies have shown that the influence participants have in making decisions is vital to a partnership and is related to increased satisfaction and participation as well as reporting more benefits that are positive. Coalitions often encounter problems that interfere with effective decision making, such as vague or inconsistent goals and procedures, long meetings, unequal group involvement and commitment, group conflicts, low communication and literacy skills, different communication styles, extreme power differences, and poor memory of the group's past. Methods of decision making can include making no decision, using an appointed decision maker, majority rule, or consensus. Specific techniques such as multi-voting and prioritizing can enhance decision-making skills.

Problem solving is related to decision making and has seven major steps: defining the problem, identifying and defining the root causes, generating alternative solutions, evaluating the alternatives, selecting the best solution, implementing the solution, and evaluating the solution.

Conflict is an inherent characteristic of partnerships and has been shown to lead to staff turnover, avoidance of certain activities, and difficulty in recruiting members. Conflict may arise between the partnership and its priorities for social change or among partners concerning issues such as loyalty, leadership, goals, benefits, contributions, and representation.

Turfism is a specific kind of conflict and four different types have been described, each with its own dynamics: coalition member versus coalition member, coalition members versus coalition, members versus lead agency, and coalition versus population or institution it wishes to influence.

Four different types of conflict resolution strategies have also been described: (1) accommodation, where members give in to the one(s) that disagree with them; (2) compromise, where each member gives a little, but neither may get what they actually wanted (the most common way to deal with conflict); (3) competition, where members fight for their interests at all costs, and even if they win one issue, may find the conflict resurfaces at another time; and (4) collaboration, where both sides of the conflict listen and learn from one another (interest-based bargaining) and out of increased understanding, create a solution which works best for all.

QUESTIONS FOR REVIEW

1. What behaviors can be used to reduce roadblocks to communication?

2. What factors lead to poor decision making? How can they be overcome?

3. Describe at least two methods that can lead to better consensus in coalitions.

4. What are the most common causes of conflict in coalitions and how can they be dealt with?

RESOURCES

General

Community Anti-Drug Coalitions of America. National Coalition Academy (contact Mark Yanick, Training Manager at myanick@cadca.org or (800) 54-CADCA). Leader Mentor Program (contact Amy Wiley at awiley@cadca.org or (800) 54-CADCA, ext. 240).

Decision Making

Joseph and Edna Josephson Institute on Ethics is a public-benefit, nonpartisan, nonprofit membership organization. Since 1987, the Institute has conducted programs and workshops for over 100,000 influential leaders including legislators and mayors, high-ranking public executives, congressional staff, editors and reporters, senior corporate and nonprofit executives, judges and lawyers, and military and police officers. Their training seminars are well known, especially *Ethics in the Workplace.* Address: 9841 Airport Blvd., Suite 300, Los Angeles, Calif. 90045. Tel: (310) 846-4800; fax: (310) 846-4858; http://www.josephsoninstitute.org/MED/MED-intro+toc.htm

Community Leadership Guide: Building Blocks to Improve Your Community. http://www.unce.unr.edu/publications/EBPubs/EB0103/default.htm

Conflict Resolution

International Association for Public Participation (IAP2) is an association of members who seek to promote and improve the practice of public participation in relation to individuals, governments, institutions, and other entities that affect the public interest in nations throughout the world. IAP2 carries out its mission by organizing and conducting activities to serve the learning needs of members through events, publications, and communication technology; advocating for public participation throughout the world; promoting a results-oriented research agenda and using research to support educational and advocacy goals; and providing technical assistance to improve public participation. Tel: (800) 644-4273; http://www.iap2.org/

Association for Conflict Resolution (ACR) is a professional organization dedicated to enhancing the practice and public understanding of conflict resolution. ACR represents and serves a diverse national and international audience that includes more than 6,000 mediators, arbitrators, facilitators, educators, and others involved in the field of conflict resolution and collaborative decision making. Anyone interested in the field of conflict resolution is welcome to join. ACR is organized by committees, regional chapters, and special-interest sections. It offers an annual conference and several publications on conflict resolution and collaborative decision making. http://www.acrnet.org/about/index.htm

Community Building Institute (CBI) was founded by William Potapchuk to help communities improve the way they conduct public business and be more inclusive, more collaborative, and more effective. CBI believes that efforts to build vibrant, sustainable, and healthy communities must involve citizens and a wide array of public and private institutions to achieve real change. CBI works directly with communities as well as with federal and state agencies and national foundations in efforts that serve multiple communities. It offers a wide range of services that are often bundled to support the needs of the client. These include providing facilitation and mediation services; providing training and technical assistance and creating peer-to-peer learning environments; assisting public agencies with the development of strategies to become more collaborative; engaging in research and reflective practice, and assisting with program implementation and design. A set of tools is currently under construction at www.communitytools.net/cbi.

EffectiveMeetings.com is an online resource center designed to provide useful information about meetings in the form of articles, tips, and quizzes. It was published as an online magazine for two and a half years, but content has been reorganized and the site has been converted to a resource center, where readers can easily access all the information they need to hold more effective meetings. If you have any questions or comments about Effective-Meetings.com, including those on article submissions and content suggestions, please e-mail guru@effectivemeetings.com. If you would like a press kit or further information about this online resource center, please contact SMART's public relations department: SMART Technologies Inc. Tel: (403) 802-2556; fax: (403) 228-2500; e-mail: pr@smarttech.com; http://www.effectivemeetings.com/features/index.html

Mediation Information and Resource Center has a comprehensive website sponsored by the International Academy of Mediators. Free articles, videos, access to mediators by state, extensive section on community-related mediation. http://www.mediate.com/

The Conflict Resolution Information Source (CR Info) is a free online clearinghouse, indexing peace- and conflict resolution-related web pages, books, articles, audiovisual materials, organizational profiles, events, and current news articles. It also provides recommended readings, overview essays on key topics, and summaries of books and articles. The education section includes a "build your own" virtual textbook system, an Internet-based conflict research-training program, extensive links to resources on professional training, and a network of people working in conflict resolution-related fields. A set of conflict resolution frequently asked questions is also included. Address: Conflict Research Consortium, University of Colorado, Campus Box 580, Boulder, Colo. 80309. Tel: (303) 492–1635; fax: (303) 492-2154; http://members.aol.com/Ethesis/mw1/adr4/links.htm

Publications

Dukes, E. F. *Reaching Higher Ground: A Guide for Preventing, Preparing for and Transforming Conflict for Tobacco Control Coalitions*. San Francisco: Tobacco Technical Assistance Consortium, 2000, pp. K1–K2. Available at http://www.cme.hsc.usf.edu/coph/immcoal/Duke%20Manual.pdf

Highly recommended book that will guide your coalition in preventing and resolving conflict.

Dukes, E. F., Piscolish, M. A., and Stephens, J. *Reaching for Higher Ground in Conflict Resolution: Tools for Powerful Groups and Communities.* San Francisco, Calif.: Jossey-Bass, 2000.

Fisher, R., Ury, W., and Patton, B. *Getting to Yes: Negotiating Agreement Without Giving In*, 2nd Edition, Boston: Houghton Mifflin, 1992.

Kritek, P. B. *Negotiating at an Uneven Table: Developing Moral Courage in Resolving Our Conflicts.* San Francisco, Calif.: Jossey-Bass, 1984.

Ury, W., Brett, J., and Goldberg, S. *Getting Disputes Resolved: Designing Systems to Cut the Costs of Conflict.* San Francisco, Calif.: Jossey-Bass, 1988.

Innes, J. Evaluating Consensus Building. In L. Susskind, C. McKearnon, and S. Carpenter (eds.), *Consensus Building Handbook.* Thousand Oaks, Calif: Sage, 1999.

CHAPTER EIGHT

Coalition Infrastructure

A journey of a thousand miles must begin with a single step.
—Lao Tzu, 600–500 B.C.E.

An effective coalition is primarily an effective organization. Each coalition has its own unique structure, culture, and level of development. Researchers estimate that half of all new coalitions will not survive their first year. Even though most organizers and enthusiastic members would rather spend time generating ideas and implementing programs, dealing early on with the structural development of the coalition will pay long-term dividends.

Establishing internal administrative structures and governance processes is a cornerstone of partnership development (Edwards and Stern, 1998). The structure of the coalition should fit its goals and resources and be no more complex than necessary. Organizers should feel free to be innovative and let the form of the coalition follow its function, not just imitate the structures of other familiar organizations. Members should feel free to change the coalition's structure if it is not serving the purposes for which it was created. In short, a coalition should have a dynamic, flexible, and responsive structure. Certain elements that are developed within the coalition help ensure its effectiveness and durability, such as vision and mission statements, action plans, role or job descriptions, bylaws and guidelines for operation, steering committees, work groups, and written records (agenda, minutes, rosters, and reports).

How the coalition is governed matters. Sometimes coalitions can be so democratic that little order exists and the progress is very slow (Garza, 2005). Community health partnerships often suffer from governance and management problems associated with interorganizational relationships in general and health care challenges specifically (Bazzoli and others, 2003; Mitchell, and Shortell, 2000). External market and regulatory factors beyond the control of the partnership, the availability of local community resources to support efforts, the scope and intensity of tasks associated with an initiative, expansion of the partnership, and the balance of work between partners and paid partnership staff make good management and governance extremely important in these partnerships. Leaders and staff must learn to recognize and anticipate dependency on others, acknowledge that most tasks will be more complicated than imagined, focus on priorities, and learn to be adaptive and creative within a dynamic environment (Bazzoli and others, 2003). Although one cannot point to any single governance structure as the "right" model, evaluating whether the governance structure is working is essential.

FORMALIZED RULES AND PROCEDURES

Formalization, or the degree to which rules, roles, and procedures are formally structured, often results in the routine implementation of the organization's operation. Early research with voluntary agencies showed that when organizations were more formal, the investment of resources and exchanges among agencies, satisfaction with the effort, and commitment of organizations were greater (Marrett, 1971; Schermerhorn, 1981; Andrews, 1990). Goodman and Steckler (1989) found that the more routinized operations become in an organization, the more likely they are to be sustained. Neighborhood block organizations that were more structured and task oriented (in other words, had more officers, committees, bylaws, meeting agendas, and minutes) remained active longer than less structured organizations (Chavis, Florin, Rich, and Wandersman, 1987).

Studies of formal structures show that the more structured and task-oriented the coalition, the more effective the coalition is perceived to be by members and staff (Butterfoss, Goodman, and Wandersman, 1996; Florin, Mitchell, and Stevenson, 1993; Foster-Fishman and others, 2001; Gottlieb, Brink, and Gingiss, 1993; Rogers and others, 1993). Administrative tasks, such as producing minutes and other materials that inform members, were the glue that made it possible for multiple, diverse partners to work efficiently together and maximize their synergistic effect (Lasker, Weiss, and Miller, 2001).

COALITION VISION AND MISSION STATEMENTS

A coalition must clearly define its vision and mission and assure that the goals derived from them reflect the self-interests of various member organizations as well as more altruistic goals for the common good. A clear vision and mission help generate support and awareness for the organization, identify partners, reduce conflict, and minimize time costs and distractions from appropriate actions (Butterfoss, Goodman, and Wandersman, 1993; Fawcett, 1999; Herman, Wolfson, and Forster, 1993; Holder and Reynolds, 1997; Johnson and others, 1996; Nezlek and Galano, 1993; Roussos and Fawcett, 2000).

By developing open lines of communication, members can learn to appreciate and bridge different agendas. Developing task groups or work groups is one way to deal with the many interests of a diverse coalition while keeping focused on the overarching mission of the coalition. The process of developing the mission and vision may be as critical as the product. Representative involvement in planning may help build and sustain future participation, whether or not the original mission was mandated by a funder or developed from community-identified issues (Roussos and Fawcett, 2000). Further, periodic review and revision of the mission (if needed) may help coalitions adapt and respond to new community concerns (Roussos and Fawcett, 2000). What is missing in many coalitions is a clear framework that establishes common language and expresses how the community sees itself and how it approaches its problems. Having a common framework and vocabulary enables members to talk about the problem, share a common understanding, and decide what is expected and how to proceed.

SWOT Analysis

Before developing the guiding vision and mission of the coalition, members must develop a shared understanding of the community. Conducting a SWOT analysis is one recommended way to develop a better understanding of the existing *strengths, weaknesses, opportunities,* and *threats* that a coalition may face in its formative stages. The *strengths* are the internal factors that allow a coalition to take advantage of opportunities or reduce barriers; *weaknesses* are internal factors or challenges that stand in the way of a coalition taking advantage of opportunities or reducing barriers; *opportunities* are external factors that allow a coalition to take action, build membership, or improve the community's health; and *threats* are external factors that stand in the way of accomplishing goals, sustaining momentum, or assuring long-term survival. By involving prospective members in identifying these factors, a coalition has already begun to flesh out the organizing statements that will lead to action. A nominal group process or brainstorming session may be used to elicit these strengths, weaknesses, opportunities, and threats. Then the words and phrases can be combined to form a draft vision statement for members to further edit and refine.

Vision Statements

Vision statements provide a picture of the desired future described in the present tense, as if it were happening now (Campbell, Divine, and Young, 1990). Essentially, *vision statements* are inspiring and uplifting images that are understood and shared by community members (Bryson, 1989). They are broad enough to include diverse viewpoints and easily communicated. Two types of vision statements are developed—image and impact statements. An *image vision* describes the way members want the community and other organizations to see the coalition over the next several years. Here is an example:

> The _____ Coalition is an inclusive and diverse group of individuals and organizations dedicated to improving the health and well-being of families in _____ community. Our members are energetic and committed, and believe that health problems can be solved by working together. We achieve positive outcomes by cooperating across communities and by using sound judgment, data, and resources to implement innovative and effective strategies.

An *impact vision* describes the concrete impacts that members want the coalition to have over the next several years. An example of an impact vision follows:

> The _____ Coalition believes that every child in _____ community has the right to good health and a high quality of life. We seek to actualize this right by improving access to comprehensive, coordinated health care; mobilizing community resources, agencies, and institutions to action; calling together community members to address key health issues; and advocating for children and families.

A visual chart that promotes group thinking and appeals to visual learners and members with low literacy could be constructed in a group setting. The plan would provide easy reference to overarching coalition concepts to guide further planning and would lend itself to train-the-trainer approaches (Grove Consultants International, 2005). A similar tool and process could easily be developed by coalitions with few monetary resources.

Mission Statements

A mission statement describes the purpose of the collaboration, or the fundamental reason for its existence: what the coalition is going to do and why. It is useful for current members, staff, and people who know nothing about the organization. An organization's mission statement should capture what the members intend to do as a total group to achieve the organizational vision. An effective mission statement is concise—it gets the point across in one brief sentence. Finally, a mission statement should be inspirational and inclusive and should not limit the community sectors or strategies that may be involved in coalition projects (David, 1991). An example of a good mission statement follows:

> _____ is a community partnership to promote health and injury prevention among infants and children in _____ community through community planning and action.

Slogans or Bylines

A slogan or byline is a short, catchy phrase that is used to brand the coalition or market it to the public. It is often used as a brief mission statement that appears in campaigns, logos, and on printed coalition material and products. An example is, *"Immunize to save lives."* Chapter Twelve will focus on developing coalition goals and objectives as part of an action plan and as part of an overall strategic planning process.

ROLES AND JOB DESCRIPTIONS

In Chapters Five and Six, the roles of staff, leaders, and members were described, and samples of job descriptions were provided in the exhibits. Written job descriptions confirm the value that a coalition places on ensuring that participants have clear roles in the coalition and that their time is used effectively. Participants should have time to review their role descriptions and clarify any issues that arise during the review. Role descriptions should be made available as part of the coalition bylaws. Exhibit 8.1 provides a sample role description for steering committee members.

Exhibit 8.1. Steering Committee Role.

Steering commmittee is responsible to the coalition.

Job Description

- Serves as representative governance entity for coalition
- Serves as clearinghouse for coalition to connect information from work groups to each other and to coalition as a whole
- Drafts annual coalition goals and objectives
- Develops issues for structured discussion and decision making that arise during coalition or work group meetings
- Schedules and coordinates training sessions and annual retreats
- Reviews and edits coalition reports and documents
- Makes decisions for coalition between regularly scheduled coalition meetings. Such urgent response items will be limited to those concerning funding opportunities with short deadlines, unexpected legislative actions, or issues that are inappropriate for open decision making due to their sensitive nature, such as conflicts among key partners.
- Appoints nominating committee for annual elections
- Develops coalition meeting agenda with staff assistance
- Represents coalition in the community (with staff assistance)
- Consults with coalition coordinator as needed
- Deals with members and staff fairly, sensitively, and confidentially
- Promotes collaboration, conflict resolution, and decision making
- Is open to diverse opinions and points of view

Time Commitment

- Approximately two hours per month
- Attends steering committee and coalition meetings and major coalition activities
- One-year availability

Qualifications

- Ascribes to coalition mission, goals, and bylaws
- Possesses strong leadership and organizational skills

ORGANIZATIONAL CHARTS

Organizational charts are tree diagrams that illustrate the relationships among staff, departments, and divisions in an organization. These charts clarify relationships and identify the key players (for example, staff and chair) or entities (for example, steering committee and work group) within the coalition. They are drawn as either horizontal or vertical trees, with labeled geometric shapes representing the various units of the organization and connectors representing the relationships among the shapes, (see in Figures 8.1 and 8.2).

Following are some tips for creating effective organizational charts:

- The design of the organizational chart should represent the organization's personality. Vertical charts represent hierarchy, whereas circular charts or horizontal charts that omit the connector lines de-emphasize it. An inverted chart makes a statement about the importance of those at the bottom.

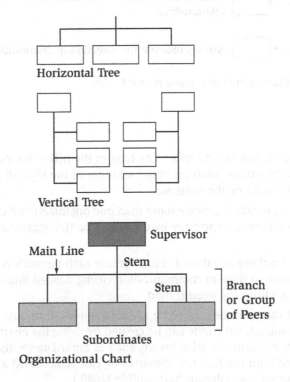

Figure 8.1. Horizontal and Vertical Organizational Charts.

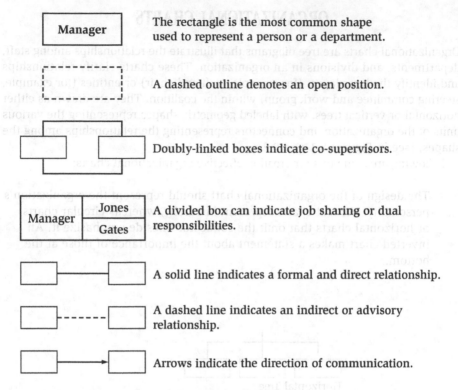

Figure 8.2. Key Components of Organizational Charts.

- The size of the box should reflect the rank of the office. Boxes lower in the tree should be smaller than (or equal to) those at the top. All boxes at the same level should be the same size.

- For large organizations, create more than one organizational chart or focus on a subsection company by drawing a partial organizational chart.

- For a functional organizational chart, include each person's responsibilities, and add informal lines of communication (using dashed lines) to reflect the interactions within the organization.

- A polished chart can be created by adding graphics or photos in place of the boxes. Organizational charts can be created by using the chart function on PowerPoint or using special software, such as SmartDraw®, that can be downloaded from the Internet. (SmartDraw can be accessed at http://www.smartdraw.com/specials/orgchart.asp?id=31686.)

An example of an organizational chart for a coalition is shown in Figure 8.3.

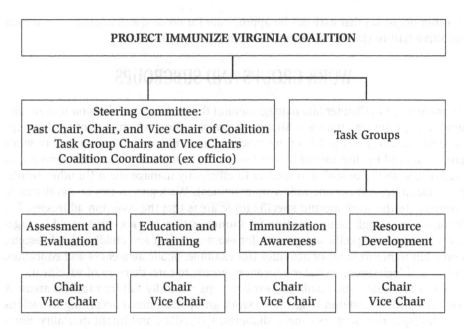

Figure 8.3. Organizational Chart of a Statewide Coalition.

STEERING COMMITTEES AND GOVERNANCE

A common approach to governance in a coalition is the formation of an executive or steering committee composed of officers of the coalition (chair, vice-chair, secretary-treasurer), chairs (and even vice-chairs) of action-focused work groups, and, perhaps, at-large members elected from the coalition. The steering committee may develop from the organizing group that originally convened the coalition, or it may evolve from a deliberate attempt by members and leaders to set up a democratic form of governance that makes equal representation more likely. If the coalition has more than twenty-five members, setting up a steering committee to research issues, present alternatives, and make decisions of a time-sensitive nature is advisable (Sofaer, 2001). The steering committee should plan to meet three to four times per year: once for orientation and training purposes, once or twice for networking and linking work groups, and at least once for strategic planning and coalition evaluation.

Even though steering committee members are elected to represent coalition members, care must be taken that the steering committee does not exert undue influence on decision making or take over the rights of individual members. The best course of action is to outline the role of the steering committee (see Exhibit 8.1) as well as the roles and responsibilities of staff, leaders, and officers (see Exhibits 5.1–5.5 in Chapter Five). The coalition must also identify the types of decisions that can be made without the coalition members' vote or consent. These "crisis decisions" may include funding opportunities with short deadlines, unexpected legislative actions, or other decisions that may not be appropriate for broad dissemination due to their sensitive nature (for example, conflicts among key partners).

WORK GROUPS AND SUBGROUPS

As we learned in Chapter Six, management of the coalition and division into smaller work groups are key strategies. Sharing the work among committees or work groups of approximately ten to fifteen members is most efficient. The number of work groups should be determined by the number of topics that the coalition covers, as well as the ability of staff and leaders to efficiently manage them (in other words, plan, facilitate, and execute follow-up activities). Work groups can be developed to concentrate the work around specific topic areas that the coalition addresses. For instance, in a single-issue coalition for immunization, work groups could be organized to focus on specific age groups (for example, infant and childhood, adolescent, and adult immunization) or activities (for example, public awareness and education, policy and legislation, provider education, access to care, delivery of vaccines).

For a multiple issue coalition, work groups naturally fall into topical areas. A minority health coalition might have work groups organized according to various health disparities, such as cancer, diabetes, HIV/AIDS, and infant mortality. Similarly, an injury-prevention coalition might organize its work groups around poison prevention, playground safety, fire safety, and motor vehicle safety. For statewide coalitions or rural coalitions spread over one or more counties, work groups might be divided geographically, with each one covering similar topics for a specific community or geographic area. Ultimately, each coalition should divide its work rationally and in ways that are efficient and manageable. Providing rosters of work groups and their members, as well as listservs, can increase cohesion and internal member-to-member communication.

Work groups can be organized on an open membership basis, where a core of members is maintained from year to year, and members rotate off as desired or new members are added as they show interest. However, some coalitions start each year with a clean slate of committees, which is known as zero-based committee structure (Bobowick, Hughes, and Lakey, 2001). All committees are abolished annually, and only the ones still needed are re-created. An evaluation process allows the coalition to reassess the composition and redirect the focus of the work group, if necessary. By using this approach, stagnation can be avoided, and the coalition is perceived as more flexible and future-oriented. Additionally, leadership opportunities are more frequent, and changes in leadership are not threatening (Bobowick, Hughes, and Lakey, 2001).

If work groups grow larger due to the interest and commitment of new members, they can convene as whole groups and then subdivide into task groups that meet to accomplish specific tasks in a time-sensitive manner. If, for example, a work group is convened around access to clinical care, then one task group could focus on performing a needs assessment, while another could organize a training seminar for providers. Chapter Six covered the basics of team building for creating more effective and responsive work groups.

BYLAWS AND GUIDELINES FOR OPERATION

Bylaws are the formal, written rules by which an organization defines its purpose and the practical details of how it operates and governs itself. They should outline the group's official name, purpose, requirements for membership, officers' titles and responsibilities, elections, and how and when meetings should be conducted. Bylaws enable members to determine what rules they can all agree upon and abide by, and yet should allow for modifications as the organization grows and changes. These rules ensure stability, continuity, and structure, especially during rapid growth or when not many longtime members are still present to advise newer members. Bylaws also help ensure that the organization does not operate beyond the scope of its original purpose.

Bylaws should be written when the organization forms; when it must clarify its purpose, elections, or other operational matters; when it changes its purpose or the way it operates; or when it applies for nonprofit status (Community Tool Box, 2003). Coalitions often write bylaws that contain more information than necessary. Amending bylaws requires a formal action and vote of the membership. Bylaws serve as the legal guidelines of the organization, and nonprofit organizations must file them with the secretary of the state in which the group is incorporated or registered. Sometimes, bylaws are mistakenly called "standard operating procedures" or "policies and procedures," but those govern day-to-day operations and are not enforceable by law.

Having bylaws can be useful to any coalition or partnership, regardless of its size or purpose. Members need guidelines for accepted behavior within a particular coalition. Bylaws limit members from going in separate directions with different agendas; help ensure equality, fairness, and consistency; and reduce problems like conflict of interest, misdirection of focus, or lack of productive activity (Heimlich and Dresbach, 2004). This checklist (adapted from McConnell, 1997a) provides a starting point for improving the collaborative process in developing bylaws:

- Do bylaws give the final power to members? Or to a steering committee or executive board?
- If bylaws give power to a steering committee, do they provide ways for members to bring business before the committee to consider?
- If the board has power, do bylaws allow members to bring up new business at an annual meeting or other general membership meetings?
- Do bylaws provide for the majority to rule?
- Do bylaws protect rights of the minority and absent members by requiring a two-thirds vote to amend them?
- Do bylaws provide for fair and equitable ways to nominate and elect officers and steering committee members? Do bylaws provide for a nominating committee and nominations from the floor?
- Do bylaws allow all members who wish to serve on committees the opportunity to serve?

- Do bylaws allow new members to be active immediately in the organization, or do they provide for a probationary period?
- Do bylaws set the month and day for all meetings and for proper notification?
- Do bylaws set a reasonable quorum requirement so that meetings can be held?
- Do bylaws provide for a way to withdraw from the organization, an office, or a committee assignment?
- Do bylaws provide for a way to fill a vacancy?
- Do bylaws provide for a way to remove someone from office or a committee appointment if he or she is not performing the assigned duties?
- Do bylaws provide for a way for members to call a special meeting?
- Do bylaws provide for a way for members to propose amendments to the bylaws?

Determining exactly how the coalition will operate and recording those decisions can keep things running smoothly, provide the answers to tough questions, save time and deliberation, and help the coalition define its mission and structure itself to correspond to that mission (Community Tool Box, 2003). Although they may not solve all problems that arise in a partnership, bylaws provide a process to address problems or concerns.

Before beginning, a coalition must think about whether bylaws are needed and what purpose they will serve. For nonprofit organizations, bylaws are actually legal documents that the organization is responsible for upholding. The following ten steps serve as a guide for writing clear, useful bylaws.

1. *Gather examples of the bylaws of similar organizations for reference.*
2. *Decide by whom and how the bylaws will be written and approved.* Will the staff, officers, steering committee, or some combination of these groups write the bylaws? Decide up front whether portions of the bylaws will be approved by consensus or whether each part will have to be agreed upon unanimously. Choose one person to be in charge of writing up the first draft and making additional changes; or if the bylaws are long or complex, divide up writing tasks to have two or more people write particular sections.
3. *Draft the bylaws.* The group that will approve the bylaws should develop an outline before writing begins. Depending on how much is already known about the operation of the organization, the first draft may be easy for one person to complete or may require a group to work through together.

Although bylaws should be custom made for the coalition, the following essentials should be included in the bylaws. Alter these as needed, and understand that bylaws do not have to be arranged in this order or include the same components. (See Exhibit 8.2 for a sample of coalition bylaws.)

(*Text resumes on page 238.*)

Exhibit 8.2. Sample Coalition Bylaws: Texas Oral Health Coalition.

ARTICLE I
NAME

The name of this organization shall be the Texas Oral Health Coalition, or the "TOH Coalition."

ARTICLE II
MISSION

It shall be the mission of the TOH Coalition to promote oral health across the lifespan.

ARTICLE III
GOALS

The goals of the coalition are to
- Spearhead statewide public education efforts.
- Support statewide professional education.
- Facilitate and support partnership formation among community groups, local health departments, businesses, and other agencies throughout Texas.
- Inform and advocate policy issues relating to childhood and adult oral health.

ARTICLE IV
MEMBERSHIP

The coalition shall be an organization of volunteers consisting of individuals and organizations from the state of Texas who are representative of various community segments.

Section 1. Structure. The coalition will be made up of these groups:
1. The General Coalition Membership
2. The Steering Committee
3. The Work Groups and Task Groups

Section 2. Roles
1. Coalition Chair
2. Coalition Vice-chair
3. Work Group Chair
4. Work Group Vice-Chair(s)
5. Work Group Members

(continued)

Exhibit 8.2. Sample Coalition Bylaws: Texas Oral Health Coalition. (*Continued*)

Section 3. Recruitment

1. Recruitment of Coalition Organizations and Members

   Any interested organization may designate a representative to join the coalition, as long as he or she adheres to the mission of the coalition. If that representative cannot attend a meeting or leaves the organization, the organization is committed to send another representative in his or her place. The recruited organization agrees to commit in-kind contributions of financial resources, staff time, or other services to the Coalition.

2. Recruitment of Work Group Members

   Initially, individual volunteers shall choose which Work Group they wish to join. Once the Work Group has been formed and the Chair for each Work Group has been designated, the Chair must approve additional members to any Work Group. The number of Work Group members may vary to meet the need of the Work Group's current project.

Section 4. Term of Membership

Members will agree to serve a one-year term. Members may renew membership indefinitely.

Section 5. Vacancies

Vacancies of the Steering Committee arising from expired terms shall be filled by annual election from candidates nominated; unexpired terms may be filled by affirmative vote of a majority of members present at a regularly scheduled meeting. In case of vacancies of members due to non-attendance, the appropriate TOH Coalition organization will appoint a new representative.

Section 6. Resignations

Notice of resignations shall be made in writing to the respective chair.

ARTICLE V
OFFICERS, STAFF, AND DUTIES

Section 1. Coalition Officers

The officers of the Coalition shall consist of a Chair and Vice-Chair who shall be elected annually by the Board from a list of nominees submitted by the Nominating Committee. Offices will be filled by nominees receiving the majority vote. The Chair and Vice-chair will serve a minimum of one-year terms, and they may be renewed.

The Chair of the Coalition shall preside over meetings of the Coalition, serve as Chair of the Steering Committee, and serve as ex-officio member of all committees. The Vice-Chair of the Coalition shall preside over meetings in the Chair's absence. The Coalition Vice-Chair will be knowledgeable in the business of the coalition

Exhibit 8.2. *(Continued)*

in order to assume the role of the Chair in the event the Chair is unable to complete a responsibility or term. The Coalition Vice-Chair shall perform other duties as directed by the Chair.

Section 2. Work Group Officers

Each Work Group shall have a Chair, Vice-Chair, and Recorder. The Work Group Chair and Vice-Chair shall be selected by a vote of the membership of the respective Work Groups. The offices will be filled by nominees receiving the majority vote. Work Group Chairs and Vice-Chairs will serve a minimum of a one-year term, and they may be renewed.

Chairs of Work Groups shall preside over their respective Work Group meetings and serve as members of the Steering Committee. The Chairs shall perform all duties incident to the office. Vice-Chairs of Work Groups shall preside over their respective meetings in the absence of the Chairs. They also will be knowledgeable in the activities of their Work Groups in order to assume the responsibilities of the Chair in the event of his or her inability to complete a responsibility or term. The Vice-Chairs shall perform other duties as directed by the Chair.

Section 3. Coalition Coordinator

The TOH Coalition Coordinator shall serve as staff to the Coalition. The coordinator is nonvoting and provides support and assistance to help meet coalition objectives and guide all aspects of the Coalition.

Section 4. Records

All officers shall turn over all official materials to the TOH Coalition Coordinator within thirty days of departure from office.

> **ARTICLE VI**
> **STEERING COMMITTEE, WORK GROUPS, AND SPECIAL COMMITTEES**

Section 1. Steering Committee

The officers of the Coalition, the past Chair of the Coalition, and the Chairpersons of each Work Group shall constitute the Steering Committee. The Steering Committee shall act for the Coalition between meetings of the Coalition.

Section 2. Work Groups

The Coalition will form Work Groups to include, but not limited to these:

- Preventive Services
- Oral Health Education and Awareness
- Surveillance
- Access to Care

(continued)

Exhibit 8.2. Sample Coalition Bylaws: Texas Oral Health Coalition. (*Continued*)

Section 3. Nominating Committee

The Nominating Committee shall consist of one member from each Work Group and the Coalition Coordinator. The Committee will convene in November and present a slate of nominees to the Steering Committee for January elections.

ARTICLE VII

MEETINGS

Section 1. Regular Meetings

1. Regular meetings of the Coalition shall be held quarterly or as needed.
2. Regular meetings of the Work Groups shall be held quarterly. Additional meetings of the Work Groups will be scheduled by members of the respective Work Groups.

Section 2. Special Meetings

Special Meetings and their stated purpose can be called by the Coalition Chair, Steering Committee, or by written request of four members of the Coalition. Special meetings may include a planning retreat.

Section 3. Quorum

One-third of the membership of the Coalition shall constitute a quorum at Coalition meetings. A majority of the Steering Committee shall constitute a quorum at Steering Committee meetings.

Section 4. Open Meetings

All meetings of the Coalition, Steering Committee, and Work Groups shall be open.

Section 5. Correspondence and Notification of Meetings

1. Minutes from each meeting (and handouts for absent members) will be mailed within one week after the meeting.
2. Agenda and meeting notices will be mailed out to members at least one week prior to that meeting. Members are reminded to RSVP so that an accurate count for lunch and printed materials can be obtained. Staff should be notified if members wish to invite guests to the Coalition meetings.

Section 6. Meeting Agenda

1. Members may contact the coordinator and add to the meeting agenda up until one week before each meeting. "Emergency" items can be added until the time the meeting begins.
2. Time will be provided at the end of the meeting (10 minutes) for questions and comments.

Exhibit 8.2. (*Continued*)

Section 7. Evaluation

Regular evaluations of the Coalition shall be conducted to maximize the effectiveness of the Coalition and its meetings.

ARTICLE VIII
PARLIAMENTARY PROCEDURE

Section 1. Rules of Order

1. The Chair will moderate meeting. Members must be recognized in turn by the Chair.
2. The Chair has the authority and responsibility to "keep the meeting moving" by cutting discussion short. Side conversations should be kept to a minimum.
3. Members should be open to the diversity of membership. Questions and constructive comments should not be criticized or ridiculed.

Section 2. Conflicts and Decision Making

1. Conflicts that arise during or between meetings will be negotiated by the Chairperson or Coalition Coordinator.
2. Decisions will be made by a consensus of members present. If a consensus cannot be reached, a vote will be taken and a decision made. Decision will be by a simple majority of members present when a quorum exists.
3. In the absence of a quorum, decisions that are critical to Coalition functioning will be made by consensus of all members (in other words, absent members will be polled by phone).

ARTICLE IX
DISSOLUTION

The coalition's property and money will be turned over to Texas Department of Health if it dissolves.

ARTICLE X
AMENDMENT TO BYLAWS

These Bylaws may be amended at any regular Coalition meeting by a majority vote of those present, provided that the amendment has been submitted to members in writing ten days prior to the meeting.

Source: Author.

Article I. Name of the coalition. The official name of the coalition is stated. If other names are used to refer to the coalition, these should be mentioned also. The name of the organization is usually indicated in bylaws with the words, "This organization shall be known as . . ." or, "The official name of this organization is. . . ."

Article II. Mission or purpose of the coalition. Clearly defining the purpose helps the coalition to stay focused. Members must decide whether the primary purpose is service, social, political, or other, and whether the coalition will focus on a single issue or set of issues, a geographic area, or a specific population. These decisions should be reflected in the coalition's vision and mission statements.

Article III. Goals of the coalition.

Article IV. Membership. This explains the members' rights and limitations. Any required fees, attendance requirements, and circumstances in which membership can be revoked are stated. If honorary memberships are allowed, the particulars are included here.

Article V. Officers, staff, and duties.

Governing structure. State who reports to whom in terms of the overall governing structure. The bylaws will explain that the coordinator is hired and overseen by the steering committee, for example, but will not detail to whom other staff members report or what their duties will be. The coordinator is responsible for the day-to-day operation of the coalition.

Officers. Outline the coalition's officers, with correct titles, terms of office, and required duties.

Electing and vacating offices. If an office is elected, describe the succession of leadership, the voting procedure, and how that officer is removed from office. If an office is appointed, state who makes the appointment.

Work groups. Describe the standing work groups (ongoing), how special task groups that exist for the duration of completing a specific task or project will be formed, how work group chairs will be chosen, and how members will be appointed to those work groups.

Decisions. State how decisions will be made and how many members and officers are required for quorum (the number that must be present for official business to take place). Quorum can be a percentage of total or paid membership, a specified number, or a majority of members present at a regular meeting.

Dues. If dues or fees are to be assessed, include here the means, rate, and when they will be collected.

Article VI. Meetings. Explain how often meetings will be held, in other words, whether the coalition will meet regularly or only as needed. The bylaws should explain who has the authority to call meetings, how the notice of upcoming meetings must be given to members, and any special or annual meetings. Include the contents, due dates, and responsibility for annual reports here.

Article VII. Steering committee, work groups, and special committees. Describe the role of the steering committee, number and type of members, terms of office, meeting times, quorum, and how members will be appointed or selected. Name and describe the work groups and any other special committees (for example, nominating committee)

Article VIII. Parliamentary authority. Describe the meeting procedures (in other words, use of Robert's Rules of Order, prerogatives of the chair, who gets the floor, and so on). For most coalitions, an action agenda, modified parliamentary procedure, or consensus replaces Robert's Rules of Order.

Article IX. Dissolution clause. State what happens to property and money if the coalition dissolves.

Article X. Amending bylaws. Explain the rules concerning how bylaws are changed, the procedure for changing them, and the time requirement for the prior notice. State who can propose amendments or call for a complete revision of the bylaws and the vote requirement to amend or revise the bylaws (usually by a two-thirds vote).

4. *Meet as a group to discuss proposed bylaws.* Well in advance of the meeting, provide copies of the proposed bylaws to the group that is going to review and edit them, so they will have time to reflect and have their questions, issues, prospective changes, or concerns ready. This will not only save time but also make it more likely that errors or ill-considered bylaws will be caught and that the final version will reflect the group intent. Get together and go over the bylaws. Carefully review each article and section individually, and consider whether the bylaws are fair and democratic. Do they distribute the power in the organization in a fair way? Do they allow members a real voice in how the organization is run?

5. *Note and discuss any changes, voting when necessary.* Depending on how long and complex the bylaws are, this may take more than one meeting.

6. *Complete and approve final draft.* Make sure that people get copies ahead of time. If the whole membership votes on the bylaws, send a letter or e-mail explaining the history of the bylaws (who wrote them and the process used), and include a reply form for the member to return indicating approval or disapproval. A suspense date to receive the votes should be stated, and tallies are based on either the whole membership or the number of votes received. Another option would be to designate a meeting at which the bylaws will be voted on and give the membership written notice about the meeting in advance. Make all the agreed-upon changes to the bylaws, and meet again to go over the final draft. When everyone is satisfied that the changes have been made correctly, vote to approve them. The date that the final draft was approved should be on the bylaws in all future copies.

7. *Distribute copies of bylaws.* All officers, members of the steering committee, and members should have copies of bylaws. Make copies available to anyone who wants them.

8. *Use bylaws.* Bylaws are not worth much if they are not used. If the coalition has a parliamentarian—an officer or consultant who gives advice on parliamentary procedure and ensures that meetings are run smoothly—then he or she can help remind people whenever the coalition, its officers, steering committee members, or regular members act in a way contrary to the bylaws.

Otherwise, make sure that officers keep bylaws in mind when doing the coalition's business. A copy of bylaws should be on hand any time that official organizational business is conducted so that if questions exist about how to proceed, they can be consulted. If situations arise that are not addressed in the bylaws, consider amending them.

9. *Periodically review and amend bylaws.* Meeting as a group to review the bylaws and, if necessary, amend them will ensure that the steering committee, officers, and members remain familiar with them. It also will allow members to gauge whether the bylaws accurately reflect the direction of the coalition, and whether changes or clarifications should be made due to events that have occurred since the bylaws were written. Significant growth of the coalition, a shift in focus, or a reorganization of the coalition are a few examples of the types of change that may necessitate a review and possible revision of the bylaws. Bylaw amendments can be suggested to the steering committee at any time by anyone.

COALITION MEETINGS

Meetings are a necessity for coalitions and other organizations. Approximately 11 million meetings occur in the United States every day, and the average professional attends sixty-two meetings per month (MCI Conferencing White Paper, 1998, p. 3). Research also indicates that over 50 percent of this meeting time is wasted (Nelson and Economy, 1995, p. 5). Assuming each of these meetings is one hour long, people lose thirty-one hours per month in unproductive meetings, or nearly four work days. Most professionals who meet on a regular basis admit to daydreaming (91 percent), missing meetings (96 percent), missing parts of meetings (95 percent), bringing other work to meetings (73 percent), and dozing during meetings (39 percent) (MCI Conferencing White Paper, 1998, p. 10).

Unproductive meetings lead to widespread negative effects, such as longer, less efficient meetings with fewer results, the need for additional meetings to accomplish objectives, frustration, less time for people to get their own work done, and costs to the organization from wasted work time. In *The Strategy of Meetings*, Kieffer (1988) suggests that the skill to manage a meeting is one of the most critical management assets. "Most professionals have had no real training in devising and managing an effective meeting; in fact, most professionals do not recognize the enormous impact their meetings have on their organizations and their careers" (p. 13). Durable coalitions have frequent meetings and a well-established system of communication to keep staff and members informed (Andrews, 1990).

The first requirement in planning any meeting is to have a clear understanding of its purpose and outcomes and to determine whether it is necessary (Kayser, 1990). One way to clarify aims is to imagine the meeting is over and ask, *What do I hope will have happened?* Second, all coalition partners should understand the fundamentals of an effective meeting (for example, clear goals and agendas) and how to achieve their goals every time they meet. Coalition staff and members must understand the value of improving meeting effectiveness and learning appropriate techniques. If new behaviors are expected and reinforced, members will try to achieve and follow the norms. Third, coalitions should begin to take advantage of new technologies during meetings. Computers, LCD projectors, and interactive whiteboards give participants access to computer-based information so they can share data and save information that will enhance group collaboration. Once back in the workplace, members can use e-mail to communicate information to others. Finally, some coalitions are adopting videoconferencing to communicate and meet across distances.

Presented here is a coalition-meeting checkup that can help diagnose trouble spots in the meeting process (Office of Quality Improvement, 2002). If the coalition can answer *yes* to most of these questions, then the coalition meetings are more likely to be effective:

- Do coalition members feel that meetings are a good investment of their time?
- Do members usually stay on track during meetings?
- Is member participation balanced during most of the meetings?
- Are meetings usually well facilitated?
- Do meetings usually begin and end on time?
- Do members share responsibility to assure that meetings are effective?
- Do members consistently accomplish meeting objectives?
- Do members regularly take the time to evaluate what is or is not working in meetings?
- Are meetings uninterrupted (for example, by cell phones or people coming and going)?
- By meeting's end, are members pleased by their accomplishments and ready to follow up on action items?

Meeting Basics

Effective meetings, whether they are for coalitions or businesses, have many elements in common. To promote an atmosphere of equality, meetings should be held on neutral territory. Rotating the meeting site can promote collaboration as long as the logistics are clearly communicated (Cohen, Baer, and Satterwhite, 2002). Nelson and Economy (1995) offer seven tips for chairing effective meetings:

1. *Spend sufficient time preparing and clarifying the meeting's purpose.* Set goals and objectives, develop agenda, and identify desired outcomes. Invite the right people, set expectations with presenters, give advance notice (at least one week—longer for special meetings), and provide any needed reading materials in advance.
2. *Use effective meeting methods.* The chair should introduce himself or herself, thank people for coming, establish ground rules, and introduce participants.

She or he should review the proposed agenda, briefly explain each item and time limit, and ask for any questions. This provides structure and communicates that the meeting has a schedule and goals that must be accomplished. Following the agenda, taking minutes, and establishing a *parking lot* (a written record of unfinished discussion items or items that are off the agenda) are other important meeting procedures.

3. *Involve as many people as possible during the meeting.* Draw in the talents of the group, ask silent people for their opinions, call on a variety of people, and do not allow nonstop talkers to monopolize the discussion. The more perspectives that are involved, the better the group's decisions will be. Make an effort to involve all participants to move them from passive to active roles. Address disruptive behavior early by reinforcing relevant ground rules or refocusing the meeting.

4. *Make sure everyone understands what is going on.* Frequently clarify and summarize what is happening to show consideration for participants and maintain meeting focus. Help the group come to agreement; the facilitator should step into the discussion only when necessary.

5. *Remember—time is important.* A meeting that runs longer than two hours (unless unique circumstances exist) will lead to frustration and fatigue. Set time limits for agenda items, select a timekeeper, and keep the meeting moving.

6. *Assign action items.* When action items arise from the meeting discussion, immediately assign a responsible individual and due date for each action item. Revisit the parking lot as well, and assign follow-up items, if needed.

7. *End meeting with summary action items and assignments.* Take five minutes to review the outcome of each agenda item as well as the action items list. This ends the meeting on a note of accomplishment and reminds attendees who is responsible for what after the meeting adjourns. Review the meeting process as well. Ask the group what went well during the meeting and which areas need improvement, and try to improve on them at the next meeting. Afterwards, distribute meeting minutes within one week, and incorporate periodic checkpoints for long-term assignments.

Timing of Meetings

Coalitions often wonder how often or at what times they should meet. The best times for meetings are early (8–10 A.M.) or late (3–5 P.M.) in the workday. Many coalitions find it useful to meet during the lunch hour because this time does not detract as much from their regularly scheduled meetings. Which day of the week is less critical, although Mondays and Tuesdays are generally busy for most professionals and therefore days to avoid. Fridays tend to be good days for larger meetings or those with longer time frames (two to four hours), such as general membership meetings, planning meetings, workshops, and retreats. Coalitions should not meet more frequently than once a month; if members are separated by distance, then quarterly meetings are sufficient (Cohen and others, 2002). Generally, one-and-a-half- to two-hour meetings work best (Cohen and others, 2002). The key is to ask members about convenient meeting times and experiment to find the best time for each work group.

Chairs (or facilitators) and participants should commit to starting and finishing meetings on time. Intolerance for tardiness will set a standard for the group, and participants will likely conform if expectations are well defined and enforced. Keeping meetings on time is every member's responsibility. The chair should state that meetings will begin on schedule and that all participants should be on time. The chair should begin the meeting at the scheduled time. Even if the meeting starts late, it should still finish on time. If business is unfinished and the chair wishes to extend a meeting, he or she should ask the participants whether they are willing and able to remain to finish the agenda item being discussed. Participants should review the agenda before the meeting, arrive ten minutes early to allow time to deal with unexpected issues, ask only relevant questions during the meeting, and leave when the meeting is supposed to end.

When planning the agenda, members should decide whether splitting the meeting into two shorter meetings would be more appropriate than one long meeting. Studies have shown that the average person can pay attention in a meeting for approximately twenty minutes before becoming fidgety, starting to daydream, or working on other projects. A change in speakers or mediums (PowerPoint presentation to roundtable discussion) may be enough to refocus participants. After ninety minutes in a meeting, a deterioration in attention and participation often occurs. The maximum time spent in a meeting without a ten- to fifteen-minute break should not exceed two hours.

Scheduling breaks allows participants to get a beverage or snack, use the restroom facilities, or return phone calls. Breaks help participants stay focused and productive, and reduce distractions caused by people wandering in and out of the meeting room. During the break, participants can discuss comments without interrupting the meeting with side conversations or note writing. A break makes it easier for the chair to bring the meeting back to order and remind participants about remaining on schedule. At the start of the meeting, the chair should let participants know about the number and timing of breaks and the location of refreshments, restrooms, and phones. Before the break, he or she should remind participants about the time for reconvening, and then stick to it.

Ground Rules

Ground rules are agreements about expected behavior in meetings. The purpose of ground rules is to clarify the group's norms about how team members will interact in order to prevent or reduce misunderstandings and disagreements. Each coalition should create its own ground rules by group consensus. All groups violate their own ground rules sometimes, and the chair or facilitator should remind the group of them. Ground rules should be posted; each member should have a copy; and they should be reviewed and updated periodically. Lippincott (1994) provides a basic template for procedural ground rules:

- Arrive on time and plan to stay for the entire meeting.
- Send a substitute if you cannot attend.
- Be prepared for meetings.

- Keep discussion to agenda items.
- Turn cell phones and pagers to vibrate.
- Minimize side conversations
- Be realistic when accepting tasks.

Ground rules can also define collaborative behaviors or expectations (Susskind, 1999), such as treating other members with respect, even in the face of disagreement; focusing on interests and ideas, not positions or solutions to the problem; counting all ideas, even wild ones; encouraging everyone to participate; and assuring that everyone follows the ground rules. One critical ground rule is how decisions will be made. Agreeing on how decisions will be made can avoid later disputes about whether key decisions were made properly.

Meeting Process

When an agenda item is introduced at a coalition meeting, most work groups go into open discussion and continue until it is time to move on to the next topic. This type of process can lead to lengthy meetings, unclear outcomes, and frustration. Meetings can be more productive and members more engaged, however, if the meeting time is divided into different formats that enhance participation.

Two types of meeting techniques are brainstorming and creating a parking lot (Lippincott, 1994). Brainstorming was described in Chapter Seven. A *parking lot,* or *idea bin,* allows discussion to stay focused on the agenda item and stores ideas for consideration at an appropriate and convenient time. The parking lot consists of one or two blank sheets of easel pad paper where ideas that are unrelated to the current topic are written, or "parked." The chair or any member should feel comfortable about suggesting moving an unrelated item to the parking lot when he or she feels discussion is getting off track.

Meeting Roles

Most meetings require participants to fill at least these three roles: recorder, who takes notes on paper, laptop, or flip chart; timekeeper, who reminds leader when time is almost up for a given item; and leader, who convenes and facilitates the meeting and keeps the discussion and decision-making process moving. Meeting tasks for the chair or facilitator usually include the following:

- Start meeting on time.
- Ensure quorum (if required).
- Review agenda and revise, if necessary.
- Keep discussion focused on agenda items.
- Encourage full participation.
- Help group come to decisions.
- Summarize decisions.
- Agree on action items, point person, what needs to be done, and when.
- Draft rough agenda for next meeting(s).
- Evaluate the meeting.

Sometimes coalitions decide to hire a professional outside facilitator rather than using an internal person. For groups that meet regularly (for example, project teams, staff groups, and work groups), consider training several people in the skills of facilitation, and rotate the job. However, for critical strategic planning and problem-solving meetings and retreats, engaging a professional facilitator is recommended.

Separating chair and facilitator roles will help ensure that at least one person is focused on group process issues, such as staying on the agenda and keeping people involved. Coalitions may decide to develop facilitators within their organization or use outside consultants or facilitators. The International Association of Facilitators (www.iaf-world.org), the Innovation Network (www.thinksmart.com), and the National Speakers Association (www.nsaspeaker.org) are sources for professional facilitators. Coalitions should request references before hiring. Hawkins suggests that effective facilitators should possess the following skills and traits (1992, p. 80):

- Effective facilitators know the dynamics of group process and are skilled in using techniques to keep the group task-focused, encourage creative thinking, build consensus, and keep all members involved. Good facilitators know how to create and maintain an open and safe environment for group members and can recognize and deal with disruptive behaviors.

- Skilled facilitators should be neutral during a meeting and should never advocate a point of view, regardless of their expertise and opinions on a particular subject.

- Listening and observation skills are essential for facilitators. They should listen and watch for content, body language, and other feedback as well as anything else that impacts the group. Facilitators must be aware of two levels of meetings: what is discussed or decided (content) and how the group functions (process).

- Effective facilitators are tactfully assertive, disciplined, and have a sense of humor. They should intervene when the meeting veers off the subject or stalls.

Common Meeting Challenges

Starting and ending on time. Well-planned and organized meetings normally start and end on time. However, if most of the time a coalition's meetings tend to start late and run over, it is important to understand why. Some reasons might be that time was not managed well throughout the meeting; priority items were not dealt with first; the group went off topic too many times; discussion time for agenda items was underestimated, or too many items were planned; or the group has a history of going over its adjournment time. Here are a few strategies that can help coalitions end their meetings on time:

- Start the meeting on time. Ending on time is a lot easier if the meeting begins on time.

- Appoint a timekeeper to provide feedback to the group regarding the use of allotted time for each agenda item.
- If the chair wishes to extend a meeting another fifteen minutes, he or she should ask the group whether they are willing to remain to finish the business at hand.
- In planning meetings, make sure end times are stated. If attending a meeting that does not have a stated adjournment time, ask the leader to assign one.
- Track meetings. Do most end on time? Be clear that the aim is to do so.
- Set a stop watch to alert members to the start of the meeting.
- If members are not used to starting on time, give fair warning in a separate communication that the meeting will start on time.
- Schedule fifteen minutes to socialize before the start of the meeting.

Difficulty making decisions. Some meetings seem to drag on as group members struggle to reach consensus and make decisions. The responsibility for coming to decisions rests squarely with the chair or leader. Some common reasons why groups seem unable to make decisions are that goals and outcome are not made explicit for the discussion topic; some participants become sidetracked on peripheral issues; the consequences of not deciding are negligible; and people are philosophically divided on issues. The following strategies can help a group reach consensus and make decisions more efficiently:

- Create expectations with actionable agenda items that clearly convey what is expected.
- Use prioritizing tools, such as nominal group process, multi-voting, and zero to ten rating (these methods were discussed in Chapter Seven).
- When participants reach an impasse in decision making, go back to the initial question or purpose of the activity and restate it.
- Ask which alternatives are supported by data.

Questioning decisions already made. Issues that were discussed and decided on in previous meetings sometimes reemerge, which can be discouraging for the group. Reasons for rehashing decisions may be that people were not aware that a conclusive decision was actually made regarding a specific issue; they recall that a decision was made, but the record of it is not available; or dominant participants pushed through a decision in a previous meeting, and silent participants decide now to voice their concerns.

A group leader can do several things to prevent or derail the rehashing of previous decisions. For groups that meet regularly, a secretary or recorder should be responsible for keeping meeting notes, agendas, and supporting documents in one place, where they can be easily referenced during the meeting. Leaders should also use decision-making and prioritizing techniques that involve everyone, including less verbal members.

Preferring to deal with small issues. When meetings focus only on immediate issues, larger issues may be ignored. The following strategies may be used to structure meetings:

- During the coalition's annual strategic planning session, decide which meetings will be devoted to broad topics.
- When creating the agenda, include at least one discussion item that focuses on something important, but not urgent.
- Allot time for topics based on their significance—larger issues should be put on the agenda first, followed by other business.
- Invite leaders with broad responsibility for key issues (such as steering committee members) to attend selected meetings to provide a context for understanding and discussion.

Key persons not attending. When key partners do not attend meetings, decisions may be made that are later questioned and not implemented as hoped. Without some regular interaction, partners become isolated, making collaboration and cooperation more difficult. Here are some strategies to encourage key persons to attend meetings:

- Diagnose the problem by understanding why people are not attending. The chair may ask a few of the non-attendees, in a non-threatening way, why they do not come. He or she might say, for example, "We've been missing your ideas at the meetings. Is it a bad time for you, or are the meetings themselves the problem?" or, "I'd like to have more members attend work group meetings. Do you have any thoughts on what I could do as chair to boost attendance?"
- Make sure real work is done so that meetings are worth attending. If meetings are used primarily for announcements and information sharing, then e-mail or newsletters may be better ways to communicate.
- Communicate the expectation that meetings will be real work sessions and most productive if everyone attends.

Follow-through on tasks is lacking. The effectiveness of meetings can be measured in terms of their outcomes. If no follow-through occurs on action plans, tasks, and decisions, then the value of having meetings at all is questionable. These techniques can lead to more effective follow-through after meetings:

- Use action items in the minutes so that members can see in writing what action is required of them and by when.
- Appoint responsible persons for each action item to ensure that a goal is moving forward.

• Set deadlines to stimulate action, and then check on progress at least once before the next meeting.

Dominant members taking over the meeting. Most groups have one or two people who tend to dominate the discussion. If discussions are open and rambling, they are likely to be dominated by highly verbal individuals. Dominant participants often stifle collaborative problem solving and creativity among participants, but they also frequently have good ideas that deserve consideration. The following methods can be used to direct the energies of dominant participants in a non-threatening way so that others have opportunities to contribute

• Pose thought-provoking questions to structure the discussion. For example, instead of asking, "What do you think of this plan?" the facilitator might ask, "What strengths of the plan would you not want to lose, or what weaknesses cause you concern?"

• Plan some small group work so that highly verbal individuals are in a smaller group. Quiet people are much more likely to speak up and participate in smaller groups. The more people who participate, the less opportunity meeting dominators have to take over the meeting.

• Recap what the dominator said, then explicitly invite alternative views.

• Take the dominator aside at the break and say, "Even though you are very knowledgeable about this topic, other people may want to contribute to the discussion. If you provide all the information, these other people are going to have a hard time participating."

Nonparticipating members. Quiet members may be reticent by nature or may fear that their opinions will be ridiculed or dismissed. Or they may not be comfortable speaking if they do not know everyone, or may not care about the issue at hand. The following strategies may help engage everyone:

• Ask people to create name tags and table tent cards for themselves so that members and participants get to know one another.

• Pick a question that most people can address, and early in the meeting, ask each person for their responses.

• Give people five minutes to write down their ideas or thoughts in a silent brainstorm before opening the general discussion.

• Break into small groups or pairs to discuss aspects of an issue before opening the general discussion. Be sure the issue to be discussed is clear, and then ask groups for their responses.

• For a special meeting, such as a planning retreat, create a timeline on the wall of the meeting room. Ask members to mark with their initials when they joined the organization and to jot down what was happening in the world at the time. This gives new members a sense of the history of the group, allows longtime members to be recognized, and invites shy people to participate.

- The chair may discuss in private with the quiet individual the importance of everyone's ideas and then encourage the person to share his or her thoughts within the meeting.

- By visually recording all the ideas in a brainstorming session, the chair emphasizes the value of everyone's contributions and helps stimulate participation. Delaying a critique of the brainstormed ideas until all have been listed can also be a powerful motivator for quiet participants.

Agenda

The agenda communicates important information such as the topics for discussion, the presenter or discussion leader for each topic, and the time allotted for each. Agendas are valuable because they clarify the objectives so people understand the meeting's purpose and tasks, and provide direction and focus—items can be checked off during the meeting as they are covered. Let participants know in advance what will be discussed so they have an opportunity to prepare an effective contribution.

The format for the agenda can take several forms, but at the least it should include the logistics for the meeting (in other words, the date, time, place, and facilitator's name); a statement of the main purpose of the meeting (or whether it is a regular or special meeting); the mission and goals of the work group or coalition as a reminder of the work focus; the agenda items, person responsible for presenting, and time planned for each item; and dates and times for the next meeting and any other upcoming special meetings or events. To create an effective agenda, the coalition coordinator should follow several steps:

1. Send a postcard or e-mail notifying members of the meeting, its goal, and logistics (for example, when and where it will be held). Ask those invited to respond, indicating whether they can attend. Emphasize that you expect and need them to attend, especially when they accept the invitation.

2. Ask members who request an agenda item to submit it no less than two days before the meeting and to suggest the amount of time they will need to present it.

3. Once agenda requests are submitted and a draft is prepared from action items from the last meeting, hold a phone conference with the work group or steering committee chair to approve or edit the draft. Then prepare a tabular or bulleted agenda with the headings *Agenda Item*, *Presenter*, and *Time*, making sure that each agenda item is directly related to the goals of the meeting. If an inappropriate request is made, suggest an informational e-mail to work group members or recommend that this agenda item be discussed in another meeting.

4. Place the most critical or time-consuming items at the top of the agenda so that people will be encouraged to arrive on time and will have more energy to give these key items their full attention.

5. Be realistic about the amount of time allocated to each item. Do not cram an unrealistic number of agenda items into the meeting, or members will feel overwhelmed and unable to focus. When people accept a ninety-minute meeting, they expect to be finished in that amount of time. Scheduling more discussion time and finishing ten minutes early is better than exceeding the set meeting time.

6. Send the agenda the day before the meeting to remind members of meeting goals, location, and time. Phone reminders are effective, especially if attendance has been less than ideal.

7. Review the agenda and its desired outcome(s) at the start of the meeting to help members focus and develop shared expectations, and set the tone for the meeting.

Minutes

Content of the minutes. Minutes should contain a record of what is done, not what is said. A person reading the minutes should understand what was accomplished at the meeting. Exhibit 8.3 lists the details that should go into the minutes (Robert McConnell Productions, 1996; Robert's Rules of Order, 2000, pp. 458–466).

Form of the minutes. Minutes should be carefully reviewed for accuracy, spelling, and grammar before putting them in their final form—either handwritten into a bound, page-numbered book or electronically archived. Some recommend putting headings such as *Reports of Committees, Reports, Old Business,* or *New Business* at the top of each new paragraph or subject. Some put a title or summary beside each paragraph so that later, people can easily find for a certain topic. For community coalitions, minutes can be less formal and should be easy to read. An example of a tabular format for minutes is included as Exhibit 8.4. This format makes review of the minutes rapid, easy, and therefore more likely to be done.

Parliamentary Procedure

Whenever people meet to make decisions, some formal rules are usually adopted to democratize and facilitate the process; these rules often include some form of parliamentary procedure. More than 1.375 million nonprofit organizations and thousands of local, state, and regional governmental bodies exist in the United States, and people spend 35 to 50 percent of their organizational life attending or conducting meetings (Robert McConnell Productions, 1997b). Further, American adults belong to an average of six organized groups and many other informal organizations (Robert McConnell Productions, 1997b).

Parliamentary procedure should not be a raw use of power but should involve using good judgment instead of rigid rules, and should be used for carrying out the will of the group. Vigilant Interaction Theory argues that the manner in which group members talk about the problems, options, and consequences facing the group affects the way they think about them, which in turn ultimately determines the quality of

(Text resumes on page 255.)

Exhibit 8.3. What Coalition Minutes Should Contain.

1. Name of organization, date, time, place of meeting, and kind of meeting—regular or special.

2. The presence of regular presiding officer and recorder (or names of their substitutes), as well as those members present.

3. What action was taken on the minutes of the previous meeting (approved as read or corrected). Corrections should be recorded in the minutes of both meetings—in the minutes where the mistake is found and in the minutes of the meeting where it was read. For example, "The minutes of the July 3rd meeting were corrected to read 'the balance in the treasury is $500,' and minutes were approved as corrected." The recorder would then correct the July 3rd minutes by drawing a line through the mistake, writing above the mistake "$500," and initialing it.

4. The reports of officers, chairs, standing committees, and special committees are given, as well as what action was taken, if any. Some minutes give the treasurer's report or only the beginning and ending balances, and some include a brief summary of committee reports. When minutes are approved, the word "approved" and the recorder's initials and approval date are written below the minutes.

5. The final wording of all motions with amendments incorporated and what happened to each motion—was it adopted, lost, referred to committee, tabled, or withdrawn? The name of the maker of the motion is put in the minutes and, in some groups, the person who seconds the motion is included. Secondary motions that were adopted are also placed in the minutes.

6. If a vote is taken during the meeting, the votes on each side should be recorded in the minutes (unless the organization has a rule stating otherwise).

7. When recording nominations and elections, the names presented by the nominating committee are named first in the minutes, then those nominated from the floor. The number of votes each nominee received should be recorded in the minutes as well as the terms of office.

8. Important announcements. For example, if the meeting place and time is different for each meeting, and the chair announces where and when the next meeting will be, it is recorded in the minutes.

9. If a guest speaker attends, the name of the speaker and program are written in the minutes. No effort should be made to summarize points given by the speaker.

10. Minutes are closed with the signature and title of the recorder and the time of adjournment.

Source: From "Minutes" in *Parliamentary Internet Newsletter,* 2(4), 1996. Reprinted by permission of Robert McConnell Productions.

Exhibit 8.4. Sample of Tabular Meeting Minutes.

PROJECT IMMUNIZE VIRGINIA (PIV) Steering Committee Meeting—October 4, 2005
Virginia Department of Health (VDH), Division of Immunization, Richmond, Virginia

Attendance: ___, ___ Health District; ___ Center for Pediatric Research/PIV; ___, VDH, Division of Immunization; ___, VDH, Division of Immunization; ___, PIV; ___, ___ Health District; ___, ___ Health District; ___ Hospital; ___ Foundation

Topic	Discussion	Action or Follow-Up
Who's Who on Steering Committee	PIV's Steering Committee currently consists of chairs and vice chairs from each work group and general coalition, VDH and PIV staff. Sarah announced group will begin meeting four times per year—two face-to-face meetings and two conference call meetings. Two members-at-large, who are not members of PIV but are politically savvy and influential people, will be invited to join SC via phone call and follow-up letter. Members-at-large enhance Committee by lending specific leadership and expertise to any decisions made. Following individuals or category types are suggested: • Dr. ___, physician champion from ___, active with American Academy of Pediatrics and imm. registry legislation • Dr. ___, private physician from ___ Health District, founder of ___ Foundation • ___, pediatric nurse practitioner from ___ • Health Systems and Hospitals, in other words, ___ • Parent advocates • School nurses • Newly-elected Governor's spouse—possible spokesperson for PIV	**Jim**—will contact Dr. ___. **Joyce**—will contact Dr. ___. **Sarah**—will contact ___. **Brenda**—will locate a contact for school nurses.
Membership Recruitment	Recruitment letter will be drafted inviting new VDH immunization nurses to join PIV and will be co-signed by Jim and PIV Chair. Community members will receive invitation letter co-signed by PIV Chair and Coordinator. Representation from following organizations will be sought: • American College Health Association	**Sarah**—will draft recruitment letter for Jim's approval and compile list of contacts.

(continued)

	• Kiwanis and Rotary state chapters • Area Agency on Aging • Military • Women, Infants, Children (WIC) • Healthy Childcare Virginia • Primary Care, Rural Health, and Free Clinic Associations • CHIP of Virginia (contact ____ for a recommendation) • Success by Six • Virginia Cooperative Extension/Virginia State University	**Sylvia**—will send Sarah contact person for Rotary Club and AAA in Fredericksburg.
PIV 10-Year Review and Where Do We Go From Here?	PIV convened Planning Retreat in November 2001 and performed SWOT analysis that listed PIV's internal strengths, weaknesses, and external factors that present opportunities and threats. Most issues are applicable today—More opportunities were identified by Steering Committee: **Offer assistance in developing local coalitions.** Local coalitions extend PIV's influence throughout state. Ideally, each of five health regions in Virginia should have immunization coalition. PIV could offer state-level training and training at local sites on coalition building. **Convene focus groups/advisory groups to home program ideas and marketing materials.** ____ University students are developing marketing materials for PIV. The goal is to have the electronic files on the PIV website so materials can be downloaded. **Raise public awareness about vaccine safety.** Enlist help of parent advocate or senior citizens to remind public that vaccines prevent disease to counteract negative press stories. **Put a face on immunization.** Find immunization spokesperson—we need to locate the right person to deliver our message.	**Sarah**—will work with VDH to post print materials on PIV's website.
Leadership Responsibilities, Needs, and Training	Leadership training to be held during first SC meeting following work group and coalition elections. Strategies on how to facilitate meetings and improve member participation during meetings to be discussed. New member orientation and reorientation will be held twice a year, prior to coalition meeting. As new people register for meeting, they will be invited to come early for orientation.	**Sarah**—will prepare an orientation and reorientation program for new members and leadership.

Exhibit 8.4. Sample of Tabular Meeting Minutes. (*Continued*)

Topic	Discussion	Action or Follow-Up
Coalition Structure	• Quarterly meetings will continue. Next year's October meeting will be first week of October to avoid scheduling conflicts with flu clinics. • Coalition chair and vice chair will share meeting facilitation responsibilities by taking turns presiding over first and second halves of meeting. • Recapping of work group activities after lunch at end of coalition meetings is too long. Groups will be asked to only report out action items and needs for assistance from other members. Chair or vice-chair of each work group will be responsible to report for consistency. • Meetings will run on time even if majority of group is late to arrive.	**Chair**—present recommendations to members at Oct. 21 meeting.
Announcements	• ___ Health District was selected to pilot-test immunization information system for private sector physicians. VA will use ___ Immunization Registry software, which is currently employed in twenty-two states. Based on one-year pilot, Virginia will institute a Virginia Immunization Information System (VIIS) that will go online in VFC practices. • Overall, federal funding for programs is expected to be reduced 5–8 percent. • ___ is sponsoring resolution to ban all vaccines that contain thimerosol—seeks patron in Virginia.	**Jim**—will keep PIV updated on pilot results.
Upcoming Meeting	October 21, American Lung Association of Virginia, Richmond. Celebrate PIV's 10th Anniversary! Meeting adjourned 12:30 P.M., _____, Recorder.	

final choices they make as a group. Because parliamentary procedure is designed to direct discussion within a group, it affects the way members think about problems, options, and consequences. Thus it positively or negatively affects vigilance or critical thinking. Invocation of the rules may enhance leadership, promote good judgment, carry out the will of the group, determine decision rules, instigate strategies, and resolve or incite conflict.

A study by Weitzel and Geist (1998) provides insight into how parliamentary procedure is selectively used in community groups and functions as a set of rules that influences the communication process. The study found that wide variation exists in the correct use of parliamentary procedure by community groups, and it is not well understood by members, even though many claim to have adopted it as a way to make decisions. Errors included incorrectly introducing and seconding motions; improperly recording, approving, and correcting minutes; and voting violations. However, group communication was not prohibited by lack of skills (in other words, an able chair facilitating decision making), and most groups were satisfied by just accomplishing their business, without concern for correct adherence to parliamentary procedure. Parliamentary procedure was used only when needed to achieve the group's goals and to facilitate efficient discussion and decision making, while protecting members' interests.

COALITION SPOTLIGHT: CONDUCTING EMPOWERING MEETINGS

One coalition adopted a *Transformation for Health* approach for its meetings, based on Paulo Friere's (1973) concept of critical consciousness or empowering individuals to define issues for themselves, while learning to appreciate one another's perspectives. In this way, members structured their coalition meetings to encourage people to share and have meaningful input. For example, the meeting facilitator posed a question without giving answers, allowing for momentary silence before a group dialogue began. Early on, the coalition also developed and implemented a *Ground Rules for Group Operations,* given to new members, that outlines coalition structure. Their philosophy is "nobody knows everything, everybody knows something." They have learned that when participants feel heard and when their opinions are solicited, they feel empowered to take ownership of the process and outcome. Monthly coalition meetings also usually have an interactive exercise tied to current projects, such as the secondhand smoke point-and-counterpoint activity during their clean indoor air ordinance campaign. This keeps members engaged in the meetings.

This approach was used again when the coalition developed its mission and vision statements; even with forty-five members participating, only part of one meeting was needed to accomplish these potentially time-consuming and divisive tasks. Members were asked to develop draft statements before the meeting, post them, and share and defend them verbally during the meeting. A nominal group process was used to arrive at consensus. This local coalition was instrumental in the passage of an amended 100 percent smoke-free clean indoor air ordinance for public and work places (including restaurants). They reported no significant conflict within the coalition, which they credit in large part to the effective dialogue and listening model they have adopted.

Contributed by E. Franklin Dukes, Ph.D., University of Virginia Center for Conflict Negotiation (letter to the author, February, 2006)

SUMMARY

Each coalition has its own unique structure, culture, and level of development. The more structured and task-oriented the coalition, the more effective the coalition was perceived to be by members and staff. A coalition should be flexible and responsive, with useful governance and management structures that help ensure its effectiveness and durability, such as vision and mission statements, action plans, role or job descriptions, bylaws and guidelines for operation, steering committees, work groups, and written records (agenda, minutes, rosters, and reports). The details of each of these structures are covered in this chapter.

QUESTIONS FOR REVIEW

1. What is the value of vision and mission statements for coalitions?
2. Why are organizational charts and role descriptions needed for coalitions?
3. How can steering committees and work groups lead to goal and outcomes identification?
4. Discuss several meeting problems and their solutions.

RESOURCES

BoardSource®: Building Effective Nonprofit Boards, although technically not a coalition site, has resources that can be easily adapted. Formerly the National Center for Nonprofit Boards, it has practical information, tools and best practices, training, and leadership development for board members of nonprofit organizations worldwide. Through their highly acclaimed programs and services, BoardSource enables organizations to fulfill their missions by helping build strong and effective nonprofit boards. BoardSource provides resources to nonprofit leaders through workshops, training, and an extensive web-based database; governance consultants who work directly with nonprofit leaders to design specialized solutions to meet an organization's needs; comprehensive selection of material on nonprofit governance, including a large selection of booklets, books, videotapes, and audiotapes; and a biennial conference for approximately 700 board members and chief executives of nonprofit organizations from around the world. BoardSource is a 501(c)(3) nonprofit organization. Address: 1828 L Street, N.W., Suite 900, Washington, D.C. 20036-5114. Tel: (202) 452-6262 or 877-89BOARD [(877) 892-6273]; fax: 202-452-6299; http://www.boardsource.org/QnA.asp?Category=9

The Grove Consultants International has taken its pioneering work in visual planning and organization change and seeded it worldwide. The tools and services are organic in their design and delivery, and adaptable to each person's needs. They offer help in leading an organizational process, communicating a critical message to an organization, or becoming an adept team leader. The Grove provides *Guide You* consulting and design services, *Teach You* public and in-house workshops, and *Help You Do It Yourself* products. Tel: (800) 49-GROVE; http://www.grove.com/about_us/about.html

Community Tool Box (CTB) provides over 6,000 pages of practical information to support work in promoting community health and development. This website is created and maintained by the Work Group on Health Promotion and Community Development at the University of Kansas in Lawrence, Kansas. Developed in collaboration with AHEC/Community Partners in Amherst, Massachusetts, the site has been online since 1995, and continues to grow. The core of the Tool Box is the topic sections that include practical guidance for different tasks necessary to promote community health and development, such as sections on leadership, strategic planning, community assessment, grant writing, and evaluation. Each section includes a description of the task, advantages of doing it, step-by-step guidelines, examples, checklists of points to review, and training materials. The resources of the CTB are organized by activity, such as *Learn Skills* (see the Table of Contents); *Plan Work* (see *Toolkits* for "16 Core Competencies" in doing the work); *Solve Problems* (see *Trouble Shooting Guides* for common dilemmas, questions for analysis, links to topic sections); and *Connect with Others* (see online forums, ask a question of an advisor, and find links to other online resources). Part D, *Developing a Strategic Plan, Organizational Structure,* and *Training System* (Chapters Eight through Twelve) is helpful for coalitions. This part of the Tool Box contains information about developing a strategic plan (for example, vision, mission, action plan), organizational structure (for example, bylaws), hiring and training staff, recruiting and training volunteers, and providing technical assistance. http://ctb.ku.edu/tools/en/tools_toc.htm

Partnership Tool Kit: Public Health Excellence Through Partnership, by Sarah Olson, in the National Center for Health Marketing's Division of Partnerships and Strategic Alliances at the Centers for Disease Control and Prevention (CDC). The recently released Draft Version 1.0 was developed for CDC staff to provide guidance and resources to maximize their partnership efforts, as a key strategy for reaching their goals and achieving CDC's mission. This 300+ page resource is highly indexed to facilitate identification of the right tool needed for a task. Included in the tool kit is a rationale of why partnerships are important, characteristics of successful partnerships, a 5-step process, tips for working with specific sectors (for example, business, healthcare, education, faith-based organizations), relevant theories, policies, and additional resources, checklists and templates. Once feedback on this version is received, Version 2.0 will be developed and made available widely to CDC and to outside partners on the CDC website.

Parliamentary Internet Newsletter, by Robert McConnell Productions: Your Parliamentary Resource, is a newsletter for all interested in learning about better meeting procedures and preserving democracy in small groups, organizations, churches, schools, and government organizations. The information is easy to understand, and an e-mail service is available to answer questions concerning problems with meetings or procedures. It is based on *Robert's Rules of Order, Revised,* 1990. Accessed February 22, 2006. Contact drvideo@comcast.net, or see the website: http://www.parli.com/newsletter/index.htm

PART THREE

SUSTAINING
EFFECTIVE COALITIONS
AND PARTNERSHIPS

CHAPTER NINE

Marketing the Coalition and Its Agenda

If one advances confidently in the direction of his dreams, and endeavors
to live the life which he has imagined, he will meet with a
success unexpected in common hours.
—Henry David Thoreau, *Walden*, 1854

For organizations such as coalitions and partnerships, sustainability might be defined as maintaining health benefits achieved through the program, continuing program activities within an organizational structure, and building the capacity of the surrounding community. Several sustainability strategies appear to be critical: *resource development*, or ensuring that coalitions and their partners develop financial and material resources to maintain programmatic efforts; *institutionalization*, or integrating programs and services into existing organizations; *systems and policy change*, or making formal changes to improve the way business is conducted; and *capacity building*, or increasing the community's ability to bring about or maintain change (Shediak-Rizkallah and Bone, 1998).

A recent study found that sustainability must be considered from the start as a planning principle, should guide membership recruitment, and depends on ongoing communication and relationship building (Friedman and Wicklund, 2006). Further, Friedman and Wicklund advocate using data to demonstrate success and funding coalition infrastructure to promote sustainability.

We have already discussed in Chapter Six how recruitment provides the coalition with a foundation for maintaining its operations in the future. In this chapter, we will focus on how self-promotion of the coalition, or marketing, and resource development contribute to sustainability. In Chapter Fourteen (evaluation) we will see how providing data on coalition accomplishments builds support from partners, funders, and the entire community.

MARKETING OR PROMOTING THE COALITION

If coalitions are to survive, they must continually market themselves, their products, and services. *Marketing* is the process by which an organization presents itself as valuable so that other organizations or individuals are willing to make an exchange to be part of that organization (Dowling, O'Donnell, and the Wellington Consulting Group, 2000, p. 42). Novelli describes the process of marketing as offering benefits that an identified group of potential consumers will pay a price for and be satisfied with (1988, p. 7). Marketing may help a coalition build a positive image, recruit members, or attract funders. Besides marketing for promotion, a coalition may also use marketing to convince people and organizations to change their behavior. In this chapter, we will focus on the process of marketing the coalition itself; in Chapter Thirteen, which covers interventions, we will apply social marketing and media advocacy concepts and skills to promote the coalition's agenda and programs.

Most nonprofit organizations, such as coalitions, misunderstand the concept of marketing. For many coalition directors and steering committees, it is a source of uncertainty and anxiety. To sell its agenda and purpose, a coalition must learn to market itself to its community. Many coalitions are stretched thin and manage to accomplish tasks only on a day-to-day basis. Maintenance is difficult enough, and precious little time is available to promote the coalition and what it does. However, investing time and resources in doing so may sustain the coalition in the future. The questions in Table 9.1 serve as a guide in deciding whether a coalition should spend more time marketing (Civicus, 2005). If most of the questions elicit a positive response, the coalition probably should do a better job of promoting itself.

DEVELOPING AN EFFECTIVE ORGANIZATIONAL MESSAGE

Once the coalition has decided that it should do a better job of promoting itself, the next step is to focus on how it communicates its essence as an organization. Here the assumption is that the coalition has already developed its vision and mission statements, goals and objectives, and a number of strategies to accomplish its aims (see Chapter Eight). One of the most important requirements for marketing the coalition to potential funders, volunteers, and other supporters is a clear, consistent, effective description—an organizational message that communicates the coalition's unique purpose, scope of activities, and priority population. The organizational message should be accurate and effectively stated, communicating to funders what the coalition is, what it does, and why it is a vital force in the community. It is longer than a mission statement (a few paragraphs, but no more than one page) and might be considered a consolidation of the coalition's vision, mission goals, and strategies. When it accompanies a letter of inquiry about funding or a proposal, the message encourages the funder to learn more about the coalition. When the message is included as part of a newspaper article on a coalition project, it might attract new

Table 9.1. Do We Need a Promotion Plan for Our Coalition?

	No	*Yes*
When someone asks about the coalition and gets a description, does that person say, "Never heard of it"?		
Does the coalition tend to do promotions in an improvised, knee-jerk way?		
Does the coalition have limited resources of both time and money?		
Are important opportunities to promote the coalition missed?		
Is the coalition relatively new so that not many people know about it?		
Has the coalition changed what it does since it began, but not communicated this change widely?		
Does the coalition operate in a competitive environment?		
Do other coalitions do similar work and get more secure funding?		
Do members feel that promotion work is a waste of time and the coalition should move on to "real" work?		
Does the coalition do work that more people should be aware of?		
Does the coalition have a profile in the community?		
Is there a possible beneficiary group that is unaware that the coalition exists?		
Should the coalition raise funds?		
Should the coalition attract more members?		
Should the coalition attract steering committee members?		
Should the coalition be more visibly accountable?		
Does the coalition project a less than positive image?		

Source: Civicus, 2005. From *Promoting Your Organisation* by CIVICUS: World Alliance for Citizenship Participation. Reprinted by permission of CIVICUS, www.civicus.org

volunteers and partners to the coalition's efforts. A sample organizational message is included below for the Mosaica Center for Nonprofit Development and Pluralism.

> Mosaica, the Center for Nonprofit Development and Pluralism, is a values-based multicultural nonprofit organization that provides tools to other nonprofits to build just, inclusive, and thriving communities and societies (Mission Statement). Since its inception in 1994, Mosaica, the Center for Nonprofit Development and Pluralism, has provided organizational development assistance to more than one hundred local, regional, and national nonprofit organizations in the United States. In keeping with Mosaica's mission, most are led by or serve communities of color. Mosaica provides a wide range of services for boards, staff, and volunteers within these organizations, including organizational assessments and strategic planning, resource development planning, fundraising capacity building, program design and delivery, personnel management, community organizing and advocacy, program evaluation, and coalition building. Mosaica helps strengthen nonprofits so they can provide high-quality services and advocacy and be sustainable, well-run nonprofit organizations that strengthen their communities and help the United States live up to its ideals.

According to Mosaica, the Center for Nonprofit Development and Pluralism (2005), an organizational message should

Provide a clear understanding of the coalition's purpose or mission. Why does it exists and what are its long-term goal(s).

Provide basic information about the coalition's legal status or affiliation. Is it an independent nonprofit organization with its own tax-exempt status or a project of a larger organization? Was it initiated by, or is it associated with, some other organization that may be known to funders?

Clearly define the coalition's service area or priority population. Is it national in scope, or does it serve a particular geographic area (for example, a specific city or region of the country)? Does it focus on a particular group or subgroup—for example, people with HIV/AIDS, refugee and immigrant families, children or youth of a particular age, women, or persons from a particular racial or ethnic group?

Clearly describe the coalition's scope of activities or program focus. Does it provide direct services, training, advocacy, public education, or some other function? Does it focus on a particular program area, such as asthma, women's issues, or primary health care?

Explain what is unique about the coalition. Is it the only one of its kind, the only one in the community, the only one using a certain approach, or the only one with its kind of structure?

Make the reader want to learn more about the coalition. The content and preservation of the message should be effective.

Be clear and understandable. The message should

- Be specific (for example, "Provide health care, tutoring, and sports activities for African-American youth to help them be healthy and do well academically and socially").
- Avoid clichés and vague terms, such as *empowerment* and *holistic approach.*
- Use active verbs.
- Explain any acronyms or names that have meaning to the coalition or community, but not to an outsider, in order to provide a positive message that is likely to be remembered.

Provide summary statistics and historical information about the coalition membership. This will help the reader understand the organizational message in context.

Use the message consistently in promotional material and proposals. You may need to tailor wording for different audiences and emphasize different aspects of the coalition, especially if the coalition is seeking support for a particular project. Using consistent content and key words helps increase visibility and communicates a clear message to outside groups.

DEVELOPING A BUSINESS PLAN

The organizational message can now be expanded into a more ambitious document called a *business plan.* A business plan is a written document that describes how a business intends to operate and why it is expected to be successful. Just as the organizational message informs the community or a specific audience about what the coalition is, the business plan takes this process a step further, formalizing that description in order to develop material resources for the coalition. It is a *selling* document, designed to convince outside backers to support the venture. Even though most community coalitions do not think of themselves as businesses, adopting a business-like mindset will help them to accrue needed resources to market themselves and their agenda. A coalition should create a business plan when it is considering a particular business venture and is unclear about the details; wants expert feedback or advice on its specific ideas; or must attract outside donations, grants, supplies, or moral support (Berkowitz, 2005).

A business plan should be written clearly and persuasively in ten to thirty pages, with color graphics (an executive summary or shorter version can be created for other promotional purposes). The Community Tool Box provides examples of business plans and recommends that the following elements be included (Berkowitz, 2006b):

Cover page. This page includes the title, coalition name, and contact information. The title should reflect the nature of the plan and appeal to the intended audience.

Table of contents. Each section of the plan is listed with page numbers.

Executive summary. This one- to two-page section should entice the reader to finish reading the whole document by succinctly presenting the coalition's purpose, what it wants, and why. It should communicate the coalition's vision of the future, establish its credibility, describe its product(s) or service(s), the need for them, and how they will be sold, and should outline key action steps. The request for funds or support should be reasonable and defensible.

Coalition description. This section describes the coalition's location, size, history, goals and objectives, activities, accomplishments, financial support (if any), and unique features.

Management. This section details the coalition's key leaders (steering or executive committee), members, and staff, and their qualifications, as well as provides a roster.

Products or services. The coalition's products or services are described here, including special features, such as cost and quality. Photographs, drawings, brochures, and catalogues are helpful. Special permits, licenses, or regulations that the coalition holds should be listed. Finally, previous awards, customer support, endorsements, and expert testimony should be highlighted.

Market Information. Explain the coalition's market or consumer base, in other words, the number of potential consumers, their characteristics (for example, demographics), and where they are located. Show that enough consumers will use or buy the coalition's product or service to justify projected sales. Document why, based on data and research, potential consumers will become actual consumers. If the coalition has conducted pilot studies or tested model programs or products, provide results here. Describe how the coalition plans to reach the intended market and how consumers will find products or services (for example, where and how they will be advertised and sold; what, if any, discounts, contests, free samples, or tie-ins with other local happenings will be used). Offer contingency plans, in case such strategies fail.

Competition. The coalition's products or services may have been sold before, are being sold now, or both. Profile the competitors and provide reasons why this product or service is superior to theirs, or at least document that enough consumers will demand the coalition's competing product or service.

Operations. Describe the production process and location, staffing, whether production occurs now, how production will be scheduled or supplied, other subcontractors or vendors, outside regulations, labor and maintenance considerations, service or product delivery, quality control, contingencies, and assessment and assurance of consumer satisfaction. Include a flowchart that summarizes operations.

Finances. Provide historical data from selling the product or service (if any), income projections, projected sales costs broken down by category, projected profits, financial assumptions which justify your projections, available cash and assets, and additional cash needed to operate the business well. The budget should describe exactly how the requested funds will be used.

Timelines. Create a timeline with key completion dates.

Appendices. Provide supporting information to strengthen the plan, such as management qualifications, letters of endorsement, and details of market research.

COALITION BRANDING: LOGO AND NAME

Social marketing is a new idea for most nonprofits. Consequently, *branding* is a marketing concept that coalitions and partnerships are just beginning to embrace. A *brand* is a name, term, sign, symbol, design, or a combination of these designed to identify the goods and services of one organization and differentiate them from those of competitors (Social Marketing Institute, 2000b). The American Marketing Association calls a brand "a promise"—a promise of value and a promise to deliver. Branding usually involves at least a name and logo, recognized by the consumer, that "underscores the organization's value and consolidates its identity" (Social Marketing Institute, 2000b, p. 7).

Brands are critical because they help motivate a larger segment of the priority audience. A brand can enhance a product's image and visibility in a way that changes customer perception of the organization that created it (Ramirez, 2005). Powerful causes, like those espoused by community coalitions, need powerful brands. Branding should influence the entire coalition; staff and members should use the logo whenever possible to reinforce the coalition's identity and mission.

Deciding on a name and logo for the coalition are activities that can engage members and lead to early outcomes or "quick wins." A consensus method or contest can give each member an equal voice in the decision. Of course, a public relations firm may produce a more professional logo or more catchy name, but the social capital that is built by a do-it-yourself process is valuable. Coalitions should keep in mind the best names and logos are simple, easily recognizable and understandable, and can be easily reproduced in one- or two-color print. A good rule of thumb is to imagine what the logo and name would look like on a tee-shirt or banner.

Mascots can be another visible way to promote the coalition and its messages. A person dressed as a cartoon character or animal can use humor to pique people's interest in a campaign. For Project Immunize Virginia, Tracker the Hound (Virginia's state animal) travels the state promoting the coalition and its message to children, adolescents, and adults: "Stay on track—get your shots." Local immunization coalitions purchased their own Tracker costumes to use for local promotions. Tracker interacting with children is a good photo opportunity for local news media.

PROMOTIONAL MATERIALS

Promotional materials may be used to promote the main goals of the coalition, its programs, and the involvement of community members. The materials should be clear, easy to read, and stay on message. Printed materials can be readily created on a personal computer and then professionally printed if resources are scarce (see the following section on brochures). Fliers can be great recruitment tools to get the message out at local events. Even though they are an inexpensive way to market programs, fliers should be aesthetically pleasing and carefully laid out. Black print on colorful paper is one way to cut costs.

Give-away promotional items with the coalition's logo and slogan prominently displayed can also be useful—sometimes community partners are willing to pay the cost for such items because they tangibly reflect the partners' involvement. Consider using balloons, balls, Frisbees, bibs, cups, pencils, pens, notepads, and pocket calendars—the possibilities are limitless.

Brochures

If a coalition wants to be credible and look like it means business, it needs printed literature. People want the convenience of printed material to take home and read at their leisure. A coalition's brochure is often the most important part of its marketing communication toolkit. A coalition can direct potential members and partners to its website, but a brochure is a handy way to highlight the coalition's products or services and next steps for contact. Although it should be brief, the brochure must provide enough information about these products or services, while it conveys the right feeling about the organization and its leadership. To create an effective brochure, ask the following questions (OnLine PR and Marketing, 2006):

- What is the purpose of the brochure?
- Who is going to read it?
- What is the demographic profile and interest level of the people who may read it?
- How many people do you expect to receive it?
- What style of brochures do you like?
- What can you afford per piece?
- Who approves the final piece?
- When must the material be completed?

Once all of these questions are answered, assess any existing in-house visuals (such as photography, line drawings, illustrations). If nothing is suitable and the budget allows, commission new photography; or rely on stock photography or graphics. Write one paragraph containing the message to be conveyed. If the coalition then reviews, revises, and agrees with the message, the brochure will work better. Exhibit 9.2 provides summary information on the content of a brochure. Following are twelve tips on writing a brochure that will support the coalition's marketing efforts (About Business and Finance, 2006; OnLine PR and Marketing, 2006; Stock Layouts, LLC, 2006).

1. *Know what the reader wants.* Write the brochure from the reader's point of view. Given the nature of the coalition's work, a reader will have many questions he or she will want answered before joining the coalition. The brochure should answer these questions in a logical sequence, following the reader's train of thought. A good way to organize key points is to write down the questions that a potential member might have and the answers the brochure might supply.

Exhibit 9.2. Brochure Content Worksheet.

Use this worksheet to help you prepare the copy for your brochure.

- Describe your coalition.

- List the benefits of coalition membership.

- Describe the features of the coalition's product(s) or service(s).

- Describe what distinguishes your product or service from others like it.

- Include member or client testimonials or quotes.

- List any special offers.

- List the coalition's contact information: name, address, phone, fax, website, and e-mail.

Source: Adapted from StockLayouts LLC. Brochure Writing Tips. Accessed July 17, 2006. http://www.stocklayouts.com/downloads/Brochure-Writing-Tips.pdf

2. *Motivate the reader to look inside.* The cover must give the reader a compelling reason to open the brochure. An eye-catching cover will engage readers and guide them to look inside at its contents. Think of benefits, thought-provoking statements, and questions that will motivate the reader. Add a little pizazz that tells the reader there is something of interest inside—an exclusive invitation or a free report, for instance.

3. *Be bold.* If you can use one large photo to tell the story instead of several smaller ones, your message will have more impact and be easier to understand.

4. *Keep the message simple.* Make the brochure easy to read. Use a fourth- to sixth-grade reading level and a lot of white space. Divide the copy up into easy-to-read sections with straightforward subheadings. Give necessary directions to guide readers from page to page. All headlines, graphics, photos, and charts should have a purpose. If pictures or clip art are included, do they inform the reader or are they irrelevant?

5. *Describe the product.* Highlight the benefits of the coalition and its services right away. Be direct and to the point. Keeping the message simple does not mean it must be shallow. The brochure should have substance. If you are impassioned by the coalition's products or services, the reader will want to learn about these benefits and how others have gained from using them in the past. Consider including testimonials to add a real-life touch.

6. *Make it a keeper.* Design the brochure not only to advertise and promote the coalition but also to be worth keeping. Putting helpful tips, information, and how-to's in the brochure will encourage the reader to keep it, refer to it, or pass it on to others.

7. *Alter the shape.* Be creative enough to make a brochure unique in size and shape, to stimulate interest among readers. Try tall and slim, square, oblong—the only limitation is imagination and budget.

8. *Make it one-on-one.* An experienced speaker talking to a large audience will pick out a face in the crowd and talk to that face. This connection allows the speaker to make the talk more personal than if he or she were merely addressing a mass of faces. Similarly, the words in the brochure should use this technique and zero in on one imaginary single person.

9. *Add atmosphere.* Make sure the brochure does not sound aloof. Involve the reader in sharing your feelings. Add a little spice by including feature writing with clear and vivid descriptions, and avoid being too plain or passive.

10. *Make it easy for people to contact you.* Include the coalition's address, phone number (and toll-free number, if applicable), e-mail address, fax number, website address, directions, and a map.

11. *Call potential partners to action.* A good way of ending the brochure is by asking readers to take some action. Go for the close, rather than leaving the reader wondering what he or she should do. Potential members and partners are more likely to join the coalition when they are told how much they are needed.

12. *Personalize it.* If the brochure will be mailed in response to potential member or partner requests, accompany it with a personalized cover letter. Make sure recipient has a reason to open the envelope by imprinting it with a statement such as, "Enclosed is the information you requested."

Newsletters

Quarterly one- to two-page newsletters are another way to market the coalition's accomplishments. With the advent of listservs and mass e-mails, an electronic newsletter is timely and informative. The newsletter may include highlights from coalition events, reports from the work groups, a calendar of upcoming coalition activities, individual or member organization "spotlights," topic-related news or breakthroughs, and calls to action. Scanned color photos add a nice touch and personalize the publication. See Exhibit 9.3 for a sample coalition newsletter. The same tips that were given above for brochures apply to newsletters. In addition, the following tips apply (Search Engine Marketing, 2006):

Give readers concrete, useful information. Such information could be details of forthcoming events, useful websites, and how-to tips. Try not to exceed seventeen words per sentence, and strive for a good mixture of sentence lengths.

Use an acknowledgment box. Creating a good newsletter depends on plentiful and reliable sources. An acknowledgment box that lists contributors can be used to reward people for helping and to encourage others to participate.

Welcome reader feedback. After creating a newsletter, look for reader feedback. Watch to see how people scan your publication, and talk with a few readers after each issue is distributed. Do a formal readership survey on a regular basis to track what is happening.

Give your URL. Once the newsletter is created, ensure that the sender's name is your website and not the name of an individual in the company who created the newsletter. First-time readers will recognize your company and respond to it but might dismiss an e-mail from a stranger as SPAM.

Exhibit 9.3. Tracker Talk.

Tracker 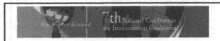 Talk

January 2006   Vol. 5, No. 1

PIV Marks 10th Birthday

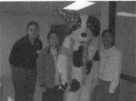

Tracker was ready to party at PIV's 10th Birthday celebration during the October 21, 2005 meeting. Pictured above are Old Dominion University Nursing Students Jennifer Gelardos, Lindsey Kopf, Agnes Agustin, and Bonnie Skopal (aka Tracker).

Project Immunize Virginia commemorated its first decade of accomplishments during the October 21st general membership meeting at the American Lung Association of Virginia. A slide show highlighting PIV's major events and programs over the past 10 years was presented. PIV has the unique distinction of being one of only two immunization coalitions in the country that are supported by their state's immunization program. Jim Farrell recalled that prior to PIV he never had a positive experience with coalitions and then went on the record as saying that PIV is the best investment he ever made.

PIV owes its success to the work of all of the dedicated, diverse and creative members through the years. 2006 is on track to being another productive year promoting timely immunizations across the lifespan. In fact, Oprah Winfrey may have had PIV in mind when she said "When I look into the future, it's so bright it burns my eyes."

Call for Abstracts for 7th National Conference on Immunization Coalitions

The 7th National Conference on Immunization Coalitions will take place August 9-11, 2006 at the Hyatt Regency Denver at the Colorado Convention Center. It is hosted by the Colorado Influenza and Pneumococcal Alert Coalition. The conference offers training on how to create, lead, and sustain effective coalitions for ALL health related issues. It provides participants with examples of field-tested programs, which can be implemented in their own communities and the opportunity to network with professionals who have designed and implemented those successful programs. This year's conference theme, *On Higher Ground*, will address coalitions as agents of social change, the elements of a successful coalition, and social and ethnic diversity in public health initiatives.

Abstracts are being sought in the following topic areas: Partnerships and Collaborations; Social Marketing/Health Education; Fundraising; Media and Public Policy Advocacy; Event Planning; Cultural Competency; Evaluation; New Vaccines; Immunization Registries; Pandemic Influenza Planning and Response; Vaccine Safety; Vaccine Supply and Delivery Challenges; and Provider Relations. Abstract applications must be received electronically, no later than February 28, 2006.

To submit an abstract online, go to:
http://www.seeuthere.com/survey/m2c666-163085121572

Mark Your Calendars for 2006

- ☑ PIV Quarterly Meetings – January 20, April 7; July 14; October 6
- ☑ 40th National Immunization Conference – March 6-9, Atlanta, GA
- ☑ National Infant Immunization Week – April 22-29
- ☑ Hepatitis Awareness Month – May
- ☑ National Adolescent Immunization Awareness Week – June 4-10
- ☑ National Immunization Awareness Month – August
- ☑ 7th National Conference on Immunization Coalitions – August 9-11, Denver, CO
- ☑ National Adult Immunization Awareness Week – September 24-30

(continued)

Exhibit 9.3. Tracker Talk. (*Continued*)

Childhood & Adolescent Immunization Schedule Revised for 2006

The CDC, AAP, and AAFP have released the 2006 U.S. Recommended Childhood and Adolescent Immunization Schedule. Some of the changes to the previous childhood and adolescent immunization schedule, published in January 2005, are as follows:

- The importance of the hepatitis B vaccine (HepB) birth dose has been emphasized.
- Tdap is recommended for adolescents aged 11-12 years who have completed the recommended childhood diphtheria and (DTP/DTaP) vaccination series and have not received a tetanus and diphtheria toxoids (Td) booster dose.
- Meningococcal conjugate vaccine (MCV4), should be administered to all children at age 11-12 years as well as to unvaccinated adolescents at high school entry (age 15 years).
- Influenza vaccine is now recommended for children aged 6 months and older with certain risk factors
- Hepatitis A vaccine is now universally recommended for all children at age 1 year (12-23 months).
- The catch-up schedule for persons aged 7-18 years has been changed for Td.

To access a ready-to-print (PDF) version of a two-page 2006 schedule, go to:
http://www.aafp.org/PreBuilt/immunization_child2006_engl.pdf

From the IAC Express #574

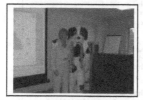

Tracker and Fran Butterfoss celebrate PIV's 10th Anniversary

New Leadership for 2006

PIV Chair: Ed Arnsdorff, GlaxoSmithKline
PIV Vice Chair: Deborah Bundy-Carpenter, Central Shenandoah Health District

Childhood Workgroup:
Chair: Alfreda Brown, Chesterfield Health District
Vice Chair: Sylvia Newport, Rappahannock Health District

Adolescent Workgroup:
Chair: Kim Spruill, Virginia Pharmacists Association Foundation
Vice Chair: Laura Newell, GlaxoSmithKline

Adult Workgroup:
Chair: Terry Hargrove, American Lung Association of Virginia
Vice Chair: Jayne Gilbert, Chiron Vaccines

CONGRATULATIONS NEW LEADERS!

An Election Day Tradition: Virginians like to Vaccinate and Vote

PIV partners once again implemented the Vaccinate and Vote program across the Commonwealth on Election Day 2005. Below is a synopsis of the results.

Petersburg: 289 flu shots were administered primarily to patients age 65 and older, from 8:00 a.m. until 3:00 p.m., at the Petersburg Health Department. Volunteers distributed 150 influenza informational flyers at 3 polling locations.

Roanoke & Salem City: Volunteers distributed educational materials at all polling locations in Roanoke City and most locations in Salem City. Two clinics were held from 7:30 a.m. until 5:00 p.m., with a total of 1,135 flu shots administered.

Waynesboro, Staunton & Augusta County: Flu vaccine flyers were circulated at 35 polling sites while shot clinics were held in Staunton, Waynesboro and Verona. Although clinics were scheduled to be open from 7:00 a.m. until 7:00 p.m. in all three locations, they all had to close early because the vaccine supply was depleted! A total of 1,211 flu shots were given.

Richmond: Volunteers distributed informational brochures at 7 polling locations. Vax and Vote partners administered a total of 80 flu shots at the 31st Street Baptist Church clinic. Due to supply limitations, the additional clinic scheduled was cancelled.

Results from Rotavirus Studies Announced

The New England Journal of Medicine released results of two international vaccine studies for rotavirus on January 4, 2006. The study found that the RotaTeq® vaccine, developed by Merck, prevented 98% of illness from severe forms of the intestinal virus. Dr. David Matson at Eastern Virginia Medical School's Center for Pediatric Research led the U.S. portion of the study. GlaxoSmithKline's vaccine showed an 85% prevention rate. Infants in the GlaxoSmithKline study were mostly from low and middle-income families in Latin America, while the Merck study's subjects were mainly from the United States and Finland.

Rotavirus usually strikes children under 5 during the winter months and causes 70,000 hospital admissions and 250,000 visits to emergency rooms in the United States per year. Worldwide, the virus annually causes 2 million hospital visits and 500,000 deaths. In poor, underdeveloped countries, prompt treatment is not always available and dehydration in babies is often fatal.

Researchers closely monitored the incidence of bowel obstruction that caused the previous vaccine to be removed from the market. Children who received RotaTeq® showed a lower incidence of the bowel obstruction than the control group.

The Food and Drug Administration advisory committee has recommended that the federal agency approve the vaccine for marketing, possibly making it available as early as this summer. The vaccine is given in 3 oral doses, 4 to 10 weeks apart.

From a report in the Virginian-Pilot January 5, 2006

Center for Pediatric Research
855 West Brambleton Avenue
Norfolk, VA 23510
757-668-6435
http://www.vdh.state.va.us/imm/piv.asp

Websites

Unfortunately, the promotional materials just described are sometimes dated almost as soon as they are published. One way to avoid unnecessary rewrites and printing costs is to develop a website for the coalition. Although initial costs for setup and ongoing costs for management are significant, these services may often be donated or offered as in-kind resources by member organizations. Students or interns might even establish the website to fulfill an educational requirement. More and more, websites are no longer a luxury but are needed to help coalitions function effectively and network widely. Websites can be separate sites or incorporated under the existing website of the lead agency or a member organization. As with all written materials, the website should be professionally executed and hold the reader's attention. All member organizations should be asked to include a link to the coalition's site on their own organizations' websites as well. The following items should be considered when designing the coalition's website (The Advocacy Institute, 2005a; Lynch and Horton, 2001).

Website planning. People are the key to successful websites. To create the site, the coalition will need content experts, writers, graphic designers, technical experts, and a small working group of coalition and community members. Although the people who will actually use the coalition's website will determine whether the project is a success, those very users are the people least likely to be present and involved when the site is designed and built (Lynch and Horton, 2001). The work group must function as an active, committed advocate for the users and their needs. Involve real users, listen and respond to what they say, test the designs with them, and keep the site easy to use— and the project will succeed.

The work group should develop a website plan identifying two or three goals as the foundation of the coalition's website design (Lynch and Horton, 2001). The plan should also include strategies for designing the site; a timeline for the design, construction, and evaluation periods; and specific measures (quantitative and qualitative) of how success will be evaluated. Building a website is an ongoing and dynamic process—the budget must cover long-term editorial management and technical maintenance. The following questions can be used to guide website development (Lynch and Horton, 2001):

- What is the mission of the coalition?
- How will creating a website support that mission?
- What are the two or three most important goals for the site?
- Who is the primary audience for the website?
- What do you want the audience to think or do after having visited the site?
- What web-related strategies will be used to achieve those goals?
- How will you measure the success of the site?
- How will the coalition maintain the finished site?

The priority audience. The next step is to identify the potential readers of the coalition's website so that the site is structured to meet their needs and expectations. Establish who the priority audience is, and create a tone in all materials on the website that will communicate best to that audience (The Advocacy Institute, 2005a). The knowledge, background, interests, and needs of users will vary from tentative novices, who need careful introduction, to expert users, who become irritated if access to information is delayed. A well-designed site should accommodate a range of users' skills and interests.

Group critiques. Once the coalition has agreed on the website plan, establish consensus on the overall design approach for the website. Group critiques are one way to explore what makes a website successful (Lynch and Horton, 2001). Work group members should bring their lists of favorite sites to the critique, introduce their sites, and comment on the successful elements of each design. In this way, members will learn one another's preferences and skills, and begin to build consensus on the experience the coalition's audience will have at the finished site.

Content inventory. Content development is the hardest, most time-consuming part of any website development project. Once the website's mission and general structure are established, assess the coalition's existing content resources, and make a detailed outline of its needs (Lynch and Horton, 2001). Then the group can concentrate on areas that are short on content and avoid wasting time on areas with existing resources. A clear grasp of content needs will also help the group develop a realistic schedule and budget for the project.

Site specification and production issues. A good site specification should define the content scope, budget, schedule, and technical aspects of the website (Lynch and Horton, 2001). The best site specifications are very short and to the point, with bulleted lists for the major design or technical features planned. The finished site specification should contain the goals statement from the planning phase, as well as the structural details of the site. One way to manage the overall scope of the site content is to specify a maximum page count in the site specification. A page count reminds everyone involved of the intended scope. If a member wants to add pages, he or she must nominate other pages to remove or obtain an increase in the budget and schedule to account for the increased work involved. Changes are fine, as long as everyone is realistic about the impact of potential changes on the budget and schedule. The coalition should be able to answer the following questions before beginning website construction (Lynch and Horton, 2001):

- What is the budget for the website?
- How many pages will the site contain? What is the maximum acceptable count for the budget?
- What special technical or functional requirements are needed?
- What is the production schedule for the site, including key milestones and dates?
- Who are the vendors and what are their responsibilities?

Site design. Although people will notice the graphic design of the web pages right away, the overall organization of the site will have the greatest impact on their experience. The main organizing principle in website design is meeting users' needs. Many make the mistake of using websites to describe their organizations, and only secondarily do they offer the services, products, and information the average user wants. Ask the priority audience what they want, and display those items and services prominently on the home page.

Page design. The organization of graphics and text on the web page can simplify navigation, reduce user errors, make it easier for readers to take advantage of the information and features of the site, and make their interactions with the website more enjoyable (Lynch and Horton, 2001). Content should be structured for skimming and easy updates; readers are already in information overload and are unlikely to read everything on the page, no matter how important (The Advocacy Institute, 2005a). Break information down into chunks and make it easy to skim wherever possible. Keep language and technology clear, simple, and consistent.

Without the visual impact of shape, color, and contrast, pages are boring and will not motivate the viewer. Dense text without contrast and visual relief is also hard to read on personal computers. But without depth of content, pages with a high graphical content disappoint the user by offering a poor balance of visual sensation, text information, and interactive hypermedia links (Lynch and Horton, 2001). The website's organization, graphic design, and content are essential to convince the priority audience that the site offers timely, accurate, and useful information. Although creating web multimedia (combining text, graphics, sounds, and moving images) is tempting, it is often safer to use technology that works for the great majority of users (Lynch and Horton, 2001).

Tracking, evaluating, and maintaining the site. The aesthetic and functional aspects of a website need constant attention and updating. Someone must be responsible for coordinating new content, maintaining graphic and editorial standards, and assuring that the programming and linkages of all pages remain functional (Lynch and Horton, 2001). Any site can become stale. Also, if the coalition disappoints the audience by not providing working links, that audience will be difficult to attract back.

Detailed web server logs are the key to quantifying the success of a website. Logs track how many people saw the site over a given time, how many pages were requested for viewing, what pages were the most popular, what brands and versions of web browser people used to view the site, and the geographic location of site visitors (Lynch and Horton, 2001). By analyzing these quantitative data, site success can be determined. The usefulness of the site logs depends on what the coalition asks of the server and the webmaster who maintains it.

Coalition Spokespersons

Who speaks for the coalition? Attracting a spokesperson to deliver the organizational message is a critical step in getting the word out about the coalition and its goals. Coalitions often look for a trusted and credible leader from within their ranks. They may even use this role as a reward for volunteer services rendered on the part of loyal members and leaders. The key question for coalitions to consider is, *Who is the best person to represent our organization and deliver our message?* Most often, the best candidate is *not* the respected physician, researcher, public health director, social services director, or teacher. Instead coalitions might ask the question, *Who is well-known, respected, and even admired by those in the priority population?* Chances are that the list of names that are derived from that one question will include many people who are neither members of the coalition nor know much about it. However, they may be local or national celebrities who are charismatic, persuasive, and could potentially reach those in the intended audience. A local newscaster, elected official, NASCAR driver, or entertainer may provide the needed cue to action, inspiring people to notice the coalition or change their behavior. For example, Willard Scott, former weatherman on NBC's *Today* show and advocate for the elder generation, agreed to serve as spokesperson for Project Immunize Virginia's annual influenza campaign. He knew nothing about the coalition prior to his involvement, and even less about influenza, but he did know how to connect with an audience. When he stared into the camera and said, "Make sure *you* live to be a hundred—get your flu shot," and when he donned a birthday hat to appear on posters bearing the same message, people listened. Immunization rates rose 22 percent among Virginians over sixty-five years old.

SUMMARY

To assure sustainability, coalitions must continually market themselves, their products, and their services. Once a decision is made to improve its promotional activities, coalitions must begin by developing an effective organizational message that communicates its unique purpose, scope of activities, and priority population to potential members, funders, and the greater community. This message then becomes part of the coalition's business plan, a document that describes how it intends to operate and why it should be successful. The plan is used to accrue needed resources and to market the coalition and its agenda. Coalitions use a number of promotional strategies to communicate who they are and what they do. Names, logos, mascots, incentive items, and communication tools, such as websites, brochures, and newsletters are all used to develop the coalition's *brand*—the goods and services that differentiate it from other competing organizations, coalitions, and partnerships.

QUESTIONS FOR REVIEW

1. Should a coalition have to promote itself?
2. Does self-promotion detract from a coalition's advocacy and service roles?
3. How can the coalition members be involved in creating promotional materials? How can the priority audience be involved?

RESOURCES

CIVICUS is an international alliance dedicated to strengthening citizen action and civil society throughout the world. The site offers extensive toolkits for fundraising, media advocacy, action planning, budgeting, and evaluation. www.civicus.org

Service Corps of Retired Executives (SCORE), with more than 500 chapters nationwide, provides free counseling, workshops, and seminars for small businesses. SCORE is sponsored by the Small Business Administration and is on the web at http://www.score.org.

Publications

Bangs, D. H., Jr. *The Business Planning Guide: Creating a Plan for Success in Your Own Business*, 7th ed. Chicago, Ill.: Upstart Publishing Company, Inc., 1995. This book includes sample business plans, documents, and a comprehensive list of references. Call for a catalog at 1-800-235-8866.

Herron, D. B. *Marketing Nonprofit Programs and Services: Proven and Practical Strategies to Get More Customers, Members, and Donors.* San Francisco, Calif.: Jossey-Bass, 1997.

Lynch, P. J., and Horton, S. *Web Style Guide: Basic Design Principles for Creating Web Sites,* 2nd ed. New Haven, Conn.: Yale University Press, 2001. Accessed July 21, 2006. http://www.webstyleguide.com/process/plan.html. This text (and segments available online) is a valuable tool for any coalition embarking on the adventure of building a website. Information is practical, detailed, and comprehensible for the novice.

Siegel, M., M.D., and Doner, L. *Marketing Public Health: Strategies to Promote Social Change.* New York: Aspen Publishers, Inc., 1998.

CHAPTER TEN

Funding, Resource Development, and Sustainability

He that is of the opinion money will do everything may well be suspected of doing everything for money.
—Benjamin Franklin

Lack of money is no obstacle. Lack of an idea is an obstacle.
—Ken Hakuta

Whereas private, for-profit corporations have large promotional budgets and modest behavioral expectations (for example, a 1 percent market share growth), nonprofit organizations have high expectations and limited resources (for example, conquer hunger in America with $1 million) (Social Marketing Institute, 2000c). One thing is certain: nonprofit organizations and coalitions must have or obtain the human and financial resources to do collaborative work. Collaborative efforts need financial resources to operate the coalition and implement new programs (Roussos and Fawcett, 2000; Foster-Fishman and others, 2001). However, funding itself does not ensure longevity and effectiveness. Some coalitions have succeeded in accomplishing their goals with little or no outside funding, and other well-funded coalitions have failed (Wolff, 2001a). A coalition must constantly ensure that its agenda is driven by its mission and goals, not by its funding. A coalition can do some activities with minimal funding, as long as member organizations are willing and committed to its vision and work.

Fund-raising is the proactive process of marketing the critical services an organization provides to the community and generating financial support for these services (Anderson and Adams, 2000). By seeking a variety of resources, coalitions are better able to recruit members, retain member commitment to the effort, successfully sponsor or implement programs, and sustain themselves over the long haul (Foster-Fishman and others, 2001, p. 255). Multiple funding also helps alleviate undue influence by a single funding source when coalitions are heavily involved in advocacy efforts. Diversified funding can stabilize a coalition and ensure its survival, but it often leads to more administrative work and the need to comply with a variety of regulations. Securing multiple funds requires staff time, an established identity, documentation of organization history and data, credibility, and leverage (Smith and Seik, 2000).

SOURCES OF COALITION FUNDS

Funds to operate the coalition can come from many sources. Membership dues, line items in the lead agency's budget that pay for staff and basic operating expenses, community donations, partner financial and in-kind contributions, grants, and contracts are typical revenue sources. Most successful coalitions develop a funding portfolio that is diverse and flexible. Obviously, contract and outright donations are preferable to grants that may or may not be secured, but a mixture of both keeps members engaged and interested in the finances of the organization. Over $174 billion was donated to U.S. charities in 1998. Of that, 77 percent came from individuals, 10 percent from foundations, 8 percent from bequests, and 5 percent from corporations (Anderson and Adams, 2000, p. 1). Philanthropy is a big business, and nonprofits should pursue these resources with a business-like strategy.

SUSTAINABILITY

Planning for financial sustainability is just one part of the coalition's plan for institutionalizing. It helps the coalition to focus on its real mission, not just on day-to-day survival (Brinckerhoff, 1996); to become more competitive in its field; and to assist in transitioning when current funding is depleted. *Sustainability* refers to the coalition's capacity to support and maintain its activities over time; it depends on whether the coalition raises money for and coordinates joint projects or services, as well as coordinates existing programs of its members, or whether it only shares information and ideas. Sustainability usually connotes financial stability and resources (cash and in-kind). Rarely, a coalition can be sustained without cash funding if its primary activities require active member participation rather than staff or cash funding. Funding alone does not make a coalition sustainable; it must fulfill a continuing purpose and be effectively managed and governed.

Coalitions must decide whether their work is short or long term and whether their mission and vision require a sustainable coalition or the development of sustainable activities that members or other institutions can eventually assume. Coalitions bring together diverse organizations and individuals around a common vision, creating synergy that would not exist if the members worked independently. Sometimes the coalition should be sustained because of its capacity to share information, develop innovative ideas, and encourage coordination and cooperation among members. Sometimes it should continue because of its ability to raise funds for projects and services that cannot be funded or implemented as effectively by individual organizations. And sometimes it should continue only until systems have been changed and collaboration among its members is institutionalized. A coalition often operates under the umbrella of a lead agency rather than existing as an independent nonprofit. Its sustainability is closely linked to the ongoing commitment and involvement of both its membership and its fiscal sponsor.

SOCIAL ENTERPRISE

One way to think about the diversity of resources that promote sustainability is to consider a different kind of business model for the revenue-generating function of partnerships and coalitions. *Social enterprise* is a relatively new concept that has emerged in social and philanthropic circles and may hold great promise for community health purposes as well. Social enterprises are organizations that provide moneymaking goods or services *and* are linked to a social mission, so-called "double-bottom-line" businesses (Social Enterprise Magazine Online, 2003).

Social enterprise includes the contribution(s) any partner or organization makes toward social improvement, regardless of its legal form (nonprofit, private, or public-sector). It recognizes that nonprofit organizations and corporations can individually and collaboratively generate significant social value. Three types of social enterprises exist:

Social purpose businesses are nonprofit, for-profit, public/private, or some combination of the three (for example, affirmative businesses that provide permanent jobs for specific populations or mission-driven businesses that deliver housing and food services directly to their clients.

Earned income businesses have an indirect impact on a social need (for example, thrift shops or the Newman's Own food brand).

Business partnerships are collaborations between nonprofits and for-profits (for example, community development corporations) (Social Enterprise Magazine Online, 2003). Sullivan Mort, Weerawardena, and Carnegie propose four key dimensions to a social entrepreneurship: a mission to create better social value; unity of purpose and action in the face of complexity; an ability to recognize opportunities to create better social value for participants; and decision making that is marked by risk taking, a proactive stance, and innovativeness (2003).

Furthermore, social entrepreneurship has many aims that are similar to those that coalitions espouse, namely:

- Building social capital to improve the quality of life in economically disadvantaged communities.
- Identifying assets and unmet needs and generating solutions with affected populations.
- Partnering with local governments, businesses, faith-based communities, charities, and other community institutions.
- Implementing ambitious projects with minimal resources.
- Recognizing, encouraging, and employing skills from different faiths, cultures, and backgrounds.
- Utilizing unrecognized or neglected human and physical resources (skills, expertise, contacts, buildings, equipment, open spaces) in creative ways.

SOCIAL ENTREPRENEURS

Social entrepreneurs are the equivalent of business entrepreneurs, mainly operating in the nonprofit sector to create innovative solutions to social problems. They act as change agents to take advantage of missed opportunities and improve systems by inventing new approaches that change society for the better (Social Enterprise Magazine Online, 2003). While a business entrepreneur might create a new industry, a social entrepreneur comes up with new solutions to social problems and implements them widely. Social edntrepreneurs are often role models who recruit local changemakers and show them how to channel their efforts to accomplish more than they believed was possible. Bill Drayton, an expert in this arena, describes social entrepreneurs as "relentless in the pursuit of their vision, people who simply will not take no for an answer and who will not give up until they spread their ideas as far as they possibly can" (Bornstein, 2004, p. 23).

Social entrepreneurship is not new. Consider the following examples: Vinoba Bhave (founder of the Land Gift Movement that redistributed more than 7,000,000 acres of land to India's poor); Mary Montessori (developed the Montessori approach to early childhood education); and John Muir (established the National Park System and Sierra Club) (Bornstein, 2004).

FUNDING CHARACTERISTICS

Few coalitions or partnerships are able to produce enough funds through income-generating activities to fully support programs or direct services. However, sometimes a coalition with an information-sharing and coordination purpose can be self-sustaining because its members provide the in-kind or cash resources needed to support its efforts. To be sustainable as an organization, a coalition should have all the following characteristics (Mosaica, 2005c). Even if the coalition does not require external funding, it still should have those characteristics not directly related to funding (numbered 4–10 here).

1. *Diversity in funding sources.* The coalition is not dependent for its survival on any single type or source of funding. It obtains funds from a variety of sources, such as in-kind contributions from members, government agencies, foundations, corporations, or small businesses; individual contributions; income-generating ventures; membership dues; community fund-raising events; and fees for service.
2. *Ability to generate funds internally.* The coalition is not completely dependent on external donations or grants, but receives significant in-kind support from its lead agency, partner organizations, or both. Sometimes membership dues are also an important source of internal support. If the coalition operates programs, it may raise funds through fees for services, third party payments (for example, Medicaid or other health insurance reimbursements), income-producing ventures, or other efforts that do not depend on philanthropy.

3. *Multi-year funding.* The coalition has some multi-year grants or contracts and does not have to raise the full amount of its budget each year.

4. *Involvement in significant activities that address continuing needs.* The coalition is engaged in activities that address long-term community concerns and are likely to be considered worthy of continuing support over many years.

5. *"Program" capacity.* The coalition is effective and can demonstrate positive results or outcomes that justify its existence. Member organizations also collaborate to provide high-quality information or services.

6. *Adherence to clear values or operating principles.* The coalition is guided by shared values that are reflected in its priorities, strategies, and day-to-day operations.

7. *Core leadership with strong commitment.* The coalition has a leadership team (for example, steering committee, staff, members) that is committed to the coalition, keeps it focused, resolves conflicts, and carries out its work.

8. *Management capacity.* The coalition has sound financial and program management policies and procedures, and staff who consistently implement them. It develops and maintains appropriate management roles for its lead agency, subcontractors, and steering committee.

9. *Constituency or support group.* The coalition has individual and organizational members who value and support its work and speak out on its behalf. The coalition benefits from the solid member constituencies of its partner organizations.

10. *Power and influence.* The coalition is respected and credible because of its members, work, and demonstrated values, enabling it to influence others. The coalition is able to get community decision makers to consider the recommendations of its leadership and perhaps even influence public policy.

Achieving and maintaining sustainability is a continuous task. The coalition must address community concerns and capitalize on community assets. Shared vision and values, effective activities, sound management, involved partners, and active and informed governance all help to build the capacity for sustainability. If the coalition requires funding, these factors are key elements in developing and maintaining strong relationships with donors, which in turn contribute to successful fund-raising. Sustainability requires diversification of funding sources and the capacity to generate funds or in-kind resources through its membership and activities.

TO INCORPORATE OR NOT?

A coalition generally operates as a *not-for-profit,* or *nonprofit, organization*—that is, it has no owners; its governing body (steering committee) assures that its work benefits the public good; and, if any of its activities make money, that money goes back into the work of the organization (BoardSource, 2002a, p. 2). Once a coalition forms, the question of its nonprofit status is often central to its ability to apply for grants and receive tax-exempt status.

Coalitions often begin by using the nonprofit status of their lead agencies as a protective umbrella. A possibility may also exist to work out collaborative arrangements with more than one agency to receive funds and administer them for a program that benefits the coalition and its partners. These arrangements help avoid many complexities of establishing a separate framework. They may work well for the entire life of the coalition or may eventually lead to competition or conflict. If conflict or competition occurs, the coalition may decide to seek its own nonprofit status. The advantage of incorporation is that a clear identity is established for the coalition; the disadvantage is the need to establish and follow operating rules and procedures that are more formal.

All nonprofits are exempt from federal corporate income taxes. Most are also exempt from state and local property and sales taxes. Nonprofits are, of course, not exempt from withholding payroll taxes for employees, and they are required to pay taxes on income from activities that are unrelated to their mission. Most formal membership organizations have 501(c)(6) or 501(c)(4) status, which allows them to lobby without limit. Organizations like coalitions and boards that serve the general public tend to be 501(c)(3) public charities, with limited lobbying allowance but with the ability to accept deductible donations (BoardSource, 2002b). Charitable organizations are allowed to lobby, provided the activity is insubstantial in relation to the overall organization, and they must report their lobbying expenditures to the IRS. Charitable organizations are not allowed to participate in or attempt to influence political campaigns; if they do, they risk losing their tax-exempt status. However, charities may engage in voter education activities during political campaigns, including getting statements from candidates, conducting public forums, giving testimony on party platforms, and providing issue briefings for candidates (BoardSource, 2002c).

Coalitions and nonprofit organizations must have well-developed structures and operating procedures in place to be effective. Good governance begins with helping these organizations become legally and financially sound, while complying with federal, state, and local requirements for nonprofits.

Coalitions should be aware of two main obstacles to incorporation. The first is the time, effort, cost required to incorporate, and the ongoing cost for fiscal reporting. To incorporate, the coalition must designate someone to act on its behalf. If the group is seeking a start-up grant, an agency can be designated to do this, and the grant can cover the costs. The process of incorporation takes approximately six months and is best done with the assistance of an attorney, whose fees may run $2,500 dollars or more, unless his or her services can be retained *pro bono*.

The second issue to consider is that the legal structure of incorporation makes it necessary to *formally* disband the coalition if it chooses to cease operations. This involves additional effort, sometimes some costs, and can create some negative publicity for member organizations if the media interprets disbanding as a sign of failure. Exhibit 10.1 provides a checklist to guide coalitions through the steps to become a 501(c) (3) organization (BoardSource, 2002a). Exhibit 10.2 provides a reference chart for the most common tax-exempt organizations.

Exhibit 10.1. Checklist to Become a 501(c)(3) Charitable Organization.

❑ **Determine the purpose of the coalition or partnership.** Every partnership should have a written mission statement and goals that describe its reason for being.

❑ **Form a steering committee or executive board.** A steering committee can translate the ideas behind the coalition into practice through planning and fund-raising. As the coalition matures, the nature and composition of its steering committee may also change.

❑ **File articles of incorporation.** For nonprofits that want to incorporate, the requirements for forming and operating a nonprofit corporation are governed by state law. Contact your secretary of state or state attorney general's office.

❑ **Draft bylaws.** Bylaws should be drafted and approved by the coalition early in its development. An attorney experienced in nonprofit law can review your bylaws for appropriateness.

❑ **Develop a strategic plan.** The strategic planning process expresses a vision of the coalition's potential. Outline the steps necessary to work toward that potential, and determine the staffing needed to implement the plan. Establish program and operational priorities for at least one year.

❑ **Develop a budget and resource development plan.** Financial oversight and resource development (for example, fund-raising, earned income, membership) should be described in a resource development plan and budget.

❑ **Establish a record-keeping system for the coalition's official records.** Corporate documents, minutes, financial reports, and other official records must be saved for the life of the coalition.

❑ **Establish an accounting system.** Good stewardship of the coalition's finances requires an accounting system that meets current and future needs. Regular audits by a certified public accountant may be required.

❑ **File for an Internal Revenue Service (IRS) determination of federal tax-exempt status.** Nonprofit corporations with charitable, educational, scientific, religious, or cultural purposes have tax-exempt status under section 501(c)(3)—or section 501(c)(4)—of the Internal Revenue Code. To apply, obtain application form 1023 and publication 557 (detailed instructions) from the local IRS office. The application is a legal document—an attorney can help prepare it.

❑ **File for state and local tax exemptions.** According to state, county, and municipal law, apply for exemption from income, sales, and property taxes with the appropriate revenue department.

Exhibit 10.1. *(Continued)*

❑ **Meet requirements of state, county, and municipal charitable solicitation laws.** Many states and county and city local jurisdictions regulate organizations that solicit funds. Compliance involves obtaining a permit or license and filing an annual report and financial statement. Check with your state attorney general's office, state department of commerce, state or local department of revenue, or county or municipal clerk's office.

❑ **Obtain an employer identification number from the IRS.**

❑ **Register with the state unemployment insurance bureau.**

❑ **Apply for a nonprofit mailing permit from the U.S. Postal Service.**

❑ **Obtain directors' or officers' liability insurance.**

Adapted with permission from www.boardsource.org. BoardSource, formerly the National Center for Nonprofit Boards, is the premier resource for practical information, tools, and training for board members and chief executives of nonprofit organizations worldwide. For more information about BoardSource, call 800-883-6262 or visit www.boardsource.org. BoardSource © 2006. Text may not be reproduced without written permission from BoardSource.

DEVELOPING THE COALITION BUDGET

Why is it critical that a coalition or partnership develop a budget? Some reasons are that a budget helps clarify coalition goals, provides a realistic picture of finances to formulate a spending plan, provides required information to potential funders, and helps staff and members maintain fiscal control of the organization (Rabinowitz, 2006). Budgets also compel members of the organization to use funds efficiently; provide accurate information to adjust, analyze, and evaluate programs and activities; and can provide a historical reference to be used for future planning (University of Nevada Cooperative Extension, 2005b).

Budgets are usually developed for each financial (or *fiscal*) year, which often corresponds to that of a coalition's lead agency or its major funder. A budget consists of the following parts (Rabinowitz, 2006):

- *Projected expenses,* or the amount of money the coalition expects to spend in the coming fiscal year, broken down into categories, for example, salaries, rent, and other office expenses

- *Projected income,* the amount of money the coalition can reasonably expect to take in for the coming fiscal year, broken down by sources, for example, grants, contracts, fund-raisers, memberships, and sales of products

- *Interaction of expenses and income,* or how funds are broken down for specific positions, activities, or items in each grant and contractual arrangement

- *Adjustments* that reflect reality as the year goes on, or how estimates are converted to actual expenses and income

Exhibit 10.2. Tax-Exempt Organization Reference Chart.

1986 Tax Code	Description of Organization	Nature of Activities	Form #	Annual Return Form Number	Contributions Allowable
501(c)(3)	Religious, educational, charitable, scientific, literary, public safety testing, fostering national or international amateur sports competitions, prevention of cruelty to children or animals organizations	Activities implied by description of organization	1023	990 or 990EZ	Yes, generally
501(c)(4)	Civic leagues, social welfare organizations, or local employee associations	Promotion of community welfare; charitable, educational, or recreational	1024	990 or 990EZ	No, generally
501(c)(5)	Labor, agricultural, or horticultural organizations	Educational or instructive, to improve conditions of work or products of efficiency	1024	990 or 990EZ	No
501(c)(6)	Business leagues, chambers of commerce, real estate boards, and so forth	Improvement of business conditions	1024	990 or 990EZ	No
501(c)(7)	Social and recreational clubs	Pleasure, recreation, social activities	1024	990 or 990EZ	No
501(c)(8)	Fraternal beneficiary societies and associations	Lodge providing for payment of life, sickness, accident, or other benefits to members	1024	990 or 990EZ	Yes, if for certain 501(c)(3) activities
501(c)(9)	Voluntary employees beneficiary associations	Providing for payment of life, sickness, accident, or other benefits to members	1024	990 or 990EZ	No
501(c)(10)	Domestic fraternal societies, lodges, and associations	Devoting net earnings to charitable, fraternal or other specified purposes. No life, sickness, accident benefits to members	1024	990 or 990EZ	Yes, if for certain 501(c)(3) activities

Source: Adapted from IRS Publication 557: Tax Exempt Status for Your Organization. (1997). Accessed July 18, 2006. http://www.muridae.com/nporegulation/documents/exempt_orgs.html

Before the actual budget is constructed, the coalition must decide what it will spend money on in the coming year. According to the Community Tool Box, asking the following questions will assist coalition leaders and staff in this process (Rabinowitz, 2006):

- What activities or programs will best advance the coalition's mission and can be accomplished with the income and resources it has or can foresee having?

- How many staff positions will it take to run those activities or programs? How much money will be needed for hourly wages, salaries, consultant fees, and benefits, and from what sources will it come?

- What else will be needed to run the organization and its activities—space, supplies, equipment, phone and utilities, insurance, transportation, and so forth?

STEPS IN THE BUDGETING PROCESS

The steps for completing the budget process follow (Rabinowitz, 2006).

1. *Estimate coalition expenses.* To create a budget, the coalition will have to estimate expenses for the coming fiscal year. For some expenses, actual figures are available (for example, rent and salaries); for others, estimates will have to be guessed or based on the previous year's expenses (for example, telephone and utilities). The *projected expense* is the sum total of the following:

   - *Estimated yearly expense totals of the absolute necessities of the organization.* These include but are not limited to salaries or wages, listed separately by position; fringe benefits for employees, separated by position (generally 12 to 15 percent of salary); rent or mortgage payments; utilities (heat, electricity, gas, water); phone service; Internet server costs; and insurance (liability, fire, and theft).

   - *Estimated expenses for things needed to conduct coalition activities.* Most items here will probably be tangible: program and office supplies (for example, paper products, software, educational materials); program and office equipment, defined as items that last for than three years and cost more than a set amount (for example, $5,000, which would include even computers and copiers); and repairs or service contracts for printers, copiers, and fax machines.

   - *Estimated expenses for anything else the coalition is obligated to pay or cannot do without.* This might include loan payments, consultant services (for example, CPA for annual audit, program consultants, evaluators); printing and copying; transportation (for example, mileage fees for staff and volunteers, vehicle upkeep, parking); and postage and other mailing expenses.

   - *Estimated expenses for things the coalition would like to do or have in the coming fiscal year.* These wish-list items might include new staff positions, programs (including staff, supplies, space to run them), and equipment.

2. *Estimate coalition income.* Once the coalition decides what it wants to spend, it must determine whether it can afford to do so. The *projected income* is the sum of the following items:

- *Actual or estimated amounts expected from known funding sources,* which may include federal, state, or local government agencies; private and community foundations; United Way; religious organizations; corporations or other private entities; and individual donors.
- *Estimation of funds the coalition might raise.* Fund-raising efforts might include community events (for example, a raffle), more ambitious events (for example, a benefit golf tournament), media advertising, or phone or mail solicitation. The coalition might also raise funds by charging membership fees or fees for services, or by selling products.
- *Estimate amount from investments, endowment income, annuities, or interest income* (for example, from a certificate of deposit or from a money market or checking account).

3. *Create a budget spreadsheet.* The projected expenses and income are the foundation of preparing an annual budget. To be useful, however, the budget must be efficiently organized. The easiest way to do this is by using a spreadsheet, or grid, in which columns represent funding sources and rows represent expense categories. A spreadsheet allows assignment of restricted funds to the proper categories, providing the ability to see at a glance how much money is available for any given expense. Although a spreadsheet can be prepared by hand, a computer spreadsheet is easier to use because it is self-adjusting; when figures in cells are changed, the totals change as well. Software is available, from simple spreadsheet programs (for example, Microsoft Works®) to accounting programs designed specifically for nonprofit organizations. Table 10.1 provides a sample budget spreadsheet.

Table 10.1. Coalition for a Healthy Future Spreadsheet.

	Department of Public Health	United Way	Membership	Department of Welfare	Totals
Salaries	$30,000	$5,000	$2,500	$21,000	$58,500
Fringe	6,000	1,000	500	4,200	11,700
Supplies	700	300	0	500	1,500
Equipment	3,500	2,500	0	0	6,000
Travel	400	150	0	600	1,150
Utilities	500	200	0	500	1,200
Insurance	800	200	0	400	1,400
Rent	4,000	500	0	3,000	7,500
Totals	$45,900	$9,850	$3,000	$30,200	$88,950

Once the grid is constructed, total expenses can be compared to total income. Different strategies can be used to adapt to the following scenarios:

- *The budget is balanced.* Even though projected expenses and income are approximately equal, make sure that they can be used as planned, in other words, that enough money is available in each of the projected expense categories, given the restrictions on funding. If not, several things can be done: obtaining permission from the funder to change the budgeted categories; reassigning some expenses from one category to another; or rethinking priorities to come in line with the budget (Rosenthal, 2006).
- *A surplus exists.* Options available in this instance are to invest or bank the leftover money to save for emergencies; improve working conditions within the organization, in other words, raise salaries, add a benefit package, or buy items that the coalition has not been able to afford; add positions or start a new program or initiative; make a long-term capital investment; or partner with other organizations to achieve a goal that none could have accomplished alone (Rosenthal, 2006).
- *A deficit exists.* Options available to make up the gap in the budget are to use savings or investments from prior years; raise additional money through grant writing, fund-raising efforts, and increasing fees; collaborate with another organization to share the costs of services, personnel, or materials and equipment; cut expenses by reducing some costs, for example, use less electricity and supplies, monitor phone use, try to get donated items, renegotiate insurance or Internet services, or find cheaper space; or eliminate some items from the budget that are not essential to coalition operations, remove programs, or reduce staff positions (Rosenthal, 2006).

4. ***Create the budget document.*** Once an accurate, balanced budget is drawn up for the next fiscal year, it becomes the basis for the coalition's finances during that period. Most coalitions review their budgets on a regular schedule (for example, once a month) and revise them to keep them accurate. Funders are usually willing to adjust budgets over the course of a year, as coalitions realize that they need more or less money in particular areas. Some grants allow for adjustments in line items of up to a certain amount (10 to 20 percent is common) without any discussion, and most can be adjusted in larger amounts with a funder's permission. At any time during the fiscal year, the budget should illustrate whether any gaps in funding exist and where they are, what should be done to close them, and whether any expense category is overspent or underspent. The budget should also allow transfer of money from one category to another for unexpected developments. Referring to the previous spreadsheet, a simple budget is shown in Table 10.2.

A short budget narrative can also expand each category to show how various estimates were obtained. For example, the salary item might look like Table 10.3. (A summary of the steps is provided in Exhibit 10.3.)

Table 10.2. Coalition for a Healthy Future for Fiscal 2010 (July 1, 2009, to June 30, 2010).

Expenses:

Salaries	$58,500.00
Fringe	11,700.00
Supplies	1,500.00
Equipment	6,000.00
Travel	1,150.00
Utilities and phone	1,200.00
Insurance	1,400.00
Rent	7,500.00
Total expenses	**$88,950.00**

Income

Department of Public Health	$45,900.00
United Way	9,850.00
Membership	3,000.00
Department of Welfare	30,200.00
Total income	**$88,950.00**

Table 10.3. Salaries.

Salaries

Director or coordinator: 40 hours a week × $16.70 an hour × 52 weeks	$35,180.00
Health educator: 30 hours a week × $14.95 an hour × 52 weeks	23,320.00
Total salaries	**$58,500.00**

FUND-RAISING

For most coalitions and partnerships, fund-raising is often seen as a lesser priority. However, no organization can function without money, and fund-raising is essential for providing the resources for community activities. The roles of coalition members and leaders in raising funds from outside sources vary by size and type of coalition. In small partnerships, the coalition coordinators or directors are the primary fund-raisers. They research potential funders to learn about grant guidelines and priorities, grant history related to community-based organizations and specific program areas, typical grant size, contacts, and deadlines. They also

Exhibit 10.3. Developing and Managing the Coalition's Budget.

Developing the Budget

- Begin preparations a month or more prior to the end of the fiscal year.

- Prepare an outline of the coalition's planned activities for the coming year.

- Determine available funds (carry over monies, cash on hand, savings, and so on).

- Do careful studies of possible funding sources, such as fundraisers.

- Estimate expected income and when it will be available.

- Get price quotations on certain expenditures (members can help with this task).

- Rank in order which activities are the wisest expenditures of funds.

- Decide how much of the budget should be allocated to highest priorities.

- Negotiate as necessary; eliminate or limit certain expenditures.

- Revise, cross-reference, and assemble these figures into final budget.

Managing the Budget

- Set and maintain a minimum cash balance.

- Formulate general policies and procedures to achieve objectives and maintain accurate accounting.

- Keep an accurate log of financial transactions in a coalition spread sheet.

- Review and balance budget at least quarterly.

- Control costs—allow only approved expenditures.

Source: University of Nevada Cooperative Extension, 2005a. Adapted from *Community Leader's Guide* developed cooperatively by: Community Colleges of Spokane, Institute of Extended Learning and Washington State University Cooperative Extension. Reprinted with permission.

usually prepare fund-raising proposals and supporting documents, and keep records of information about and contacts with potential funders, including requests for funding, proposals, and letters. Some coalitions retain volunteer fund-raisers who assume some of those major responsibilities for fund-raising. However, raising funds is one way that coalition members can demonstrate their enthusiasm about the coalition and its programs.

Smith and Siek (2000) offer the following tips that practitioners and fundraisers can follow in their fieldwork

- Network to keep informed about what's going on and to develop connections with others.
- Have someone in the coalition assume the task of tracking available opportunities.

- Consider hiring someone to do the work of writing grants, especially if he or she is willing to work at least partly on commission. Find a local professional with background in grant writing to review grant proposals for form and content; follow his or her advice.
- Successful fund-raising depends upon being in the right place at the right time, not always on the actual merits of you proposal. Stay connected with possible funding sources and have action plans developed so that the coalition can be ready to move quickly when the right opportunity presents itself.
- Get to know local politicians (legislators) well enough so that they return calls, and make sure that they and other politicians understand the issue and its importance.
- Diversify funding, so the coalition isn't completely dependent on any one form of support.
- Stick to the mission and keep doing what the coalition does best; then the community will know what the coalition is all about, and it will help in creating a local base of support.

The Resource Development Team

A resource development team, a subgroup of the steering committee, or a temporary task force can be formed to help obtain resources to help the coalition thrive, ease the transition from one source of funding to another (such as at the end of a grant period), and locate money or goods from many different sources. This group is ideally formed when the coalition begins, but the need for the group becomes more apparent when funding is uncertain or when the coalition lacks needed resources to implement planned activities.

Active, committed, knowledgeable members and leaders who are willing and able to speak publicly on behalf of the coalition are essential to fund-raising efforts. Funders tend to view coalition member involvement in requesting funds as evidence of the organization's credibility and community support. Because such volunteers are not paid for their efforts, funders see their help as proof of their belief in the organization and its accomplishments. No matter how committed or competent coalition staff may be, funders may view them as motivated by the need to raise money to cover their own salaries.

In most coalitions, members can identify funders, especially those with whom they have personal or professional contact and those who make solicitation visits or assist with fund-raising events. Foundation or corporate funders are more likely to meet with coalition representatives with whom they are personally acquainted; individual donors often contribute specifically because they are asked by a friend, colleague, or acquaintance whose opinion they respect (Mosaica, 2005b, p. 5). The best solicitation team is the coalition director or another key staff member *and* a chair or member of the resource development team. Staff may be more knowledgeable about the details of coalition programs and operations, but members often are better able to describe the coalition in context of community needs and assets (Mosaica, 2005b, p. 5).

Coalition member participation in annual campaigns and other individual solicitation efforts is also critical. The most likely coalition donors are coalition members themselves; other active volunteers; current donors; and individuals with strong links to the coalition, lead agency, staff, or coalition program. Coalitions do not usually conduct effective, large-scale mail solicitation campaigns; they are more useful in identifying and directly approaching potential donors. A coalition volunteer is effective in selling the organization in a personal solicitation, because he or she has passion and a deep understanding of its work and importance (Mosaica, 2005a, p. 3).

The Resource Development Plan

Fund-raising requires preplanning and organization; it generally cannot be done well in response to a crisis. The coalition should first develop a well-structured *case statement* that provides the rationale of a fund-raising effort, grant proposal, or capital campaign. The case statement makes a case for a specific program or project, or for general operating support. It focuses on a problem that must be fixed and explains the coalition's proposed resolution.

Like other coalition projects, effective fund-raising also requires a well-thought-out *resource development plan* that provides short- and long-term objectives, strategies, and action steps to get and keep financial resources. This type of plan should include project needs; current and required resources; potential matching and funding organizations or individuals; the amount that will be requested from each organization, individual, or funding source; and how it will be requested (as well as by whom and when) (Nagy, 2006). The resource development plan is essentially a work plan that lists tasks and time deadlines and divides responsibilities and tasks among staff and volunteers.

The plan should be comprehensive and guide the coalition through fund-raising activities for at least a one-year period. It should include obtaining direct funds through new and continuing competitive grants and contracts from public sources (for example, CDC, NIH, health departments), national organizations, foundations, and corporations; and it should cover raising funds in the community through special fund-raising events or individual donations.

Different funding sources provide different types of support. For example, government agencies usually will not provide general support but will provide project money. Foundations and corporations will provide general support, but their larger grants are usually for specific types of activities and projects with defined objectives. They will usually allow grant funds to be used to pay the share of administrative costs associated with the project, if that is part of the budget. Funds that are raised from community donations and fund-raisers are usually used for a specific purpose, such as starting a new program.

Resource Planning Steps

The plan should be created early in the life of the coalition and be revised annually. Coalition members, leaders, and staff should first consider what the coalition truly needs and wants in terms of financial sustainability. For example, just because the coalition conducted a certain program in the previous year, should it sponsor it again or should a new partner organize it? Let members and funders know about plan development, as they may have suggestions that the resource development team would not have considered; this also helps build trust and mutual respect. Resource development planning involves several steps (Nagy, 2005; Mosaica, 2005a, p. 7):

Examine the organization and its resources. Figure out where the coalition is, where it wants to be, and what it needs to get there. Self-evaluation should be done annually and should include feedback from both external and internal sources and from everyone connected with the organization. A coalition that is experienced in resource development will be able to raise more resources than one that is just beginning to diversify its funding base. To arrive at a feasible fund-raising goal, assess the personnel, skills, materials, and procedures that the coalition already has, and identify what should be developed or strengthened.

Successful coalitions should be able to manage a variety of resources. Start within the coalition, determine its needs, and then identify available resources in the community at large. Looking at the coalition's past performance (three to five years of donor records) and current resources will provide the best picture of its strengths and weaknesses. This process will also clarify the funding mix and identify the amounts contributed by foundations, corporations, local businesses, individuals, and government agencies (federal, state, and local). Most importantly, the assessment will help the coalition to build on its strengths, identify and pursue new opportunities, measure success, and refine fund-raising techniques (Anderson and Adams, 2000). Resources fall into four main categories, sometimes independent of one another and sometimes interconnected: money, people, goods, and services (Smith and Siek, 2002).

- *Money.* The importance of money to nonprofit organizations is obvious. Eighty-six percent of Americans, representing all ages, incomes, occupations, and education levels, give to one or more charitable organizations. Ninety percent of donations are from individuals; 10 percent come from foundations and corporations (Smith and Siek, 2002, p. 2). Although corporations and foundations may be the source of some large, one-time donations, individual giving adds staying power. In addition to donations, the other sources of money are investment income; membership dues; earned income from businesses, goods, and services; government grants and contracts; and program-related investments.

- *People.* People resources are persons giving their time free of charge, for a small fee, or for payment by a third party on a coalition's behalf. People may volunteer their services, or employers may give release time to employees to work on worthwhile community efforts. The resource potential of people is boundless; the challenge is to figure out how to use the most people, in a collaborative way, to the coalition's best advantage.

- *Goods.* Any personal property, excluding money and securities, is a good. Goods are a vital noncash resource for any coalition and can be used to complement other resources. Sometimes in-kind or noncash contributions of goods can cover the entire cost of a service or staff person; sometimes they can be used creatively with other funding. Types of in-kind goods include office furniture and equipment, office supplies, space (including maintenance fees and utilities), equipment, and furniture. With grants, in-kind resources must be documented carefully for audits. Some alternative arrangements for in-kind goods are used or surplus goods, new products and merchandise, loaned goods, and goods purchased cooperatively with another group.
- *Services.* Services are often grouped with goods as in-kind contributions and may include construction and renovation, printing, transportation, public relations and promotion, recreational activities, and clerical assistance. However, most services are not tax deductible. Some coalitions deduct the time used in performing community service as a normal business expense. Most organizations that provide services to coalitions usually do it free or at a discount.

Evaluate the coalition's current financial status. Find out what financial resources and expenses the coalition has—in other words, how much money is currently available, where it is from, how it is used, and how much is expected in the future, as well as how much debt the coalition has. This information should be in the annual budget, but should be verified to ensure that everyone working on the resource development plan understands it. Determine how much money the coalition *needs.* Construct a bare-bones budget and list what the coalition is doing now that is essential to its mission and what the coalition *should* be doing. Consider both programmatic and staff costs in determining this base amount, and consider the expenses that are independent of programs (for example, office rental and utilities). Decide what activities can be cut, if any.

Then decide how much money the coalition *wants.* Think about long-term goals—if money were not a problem, what would members want to see happen? Ask staff, members, and leaders to recommend ideas that are worth pursuing. What resources will it actually take to accomplish these goals? Are more or better-trained staff needed? More space? Even if the coalition did not add any new work or programs, it might need printers, computers, or an administrative assistant. Estimate first-year costs and long-term three- to five-year costs.

Set fund-raising objectives. How far is the coalition from its goals? On an annual basis, how much money will be needed in the next five years to reach these goals? Once the coalition's capability is assessed, it must decide how much funding it can reasonably count on receiving at this point. Set specific and realistic funding objectives, both short- and long-term. For example, a short-term objective might be increased funding next year for two more positions.

Long-term funding goals might include the development of an endowment or buying office space. Base the coalition's objectives on answers to the following questions:

- How much money do we need to continue operating *current* programs?
- How much more is needed to start one or more *new* programs or to *expand* current ones?
- Of the total amount needed for current and existing programs, how much is already received, committed, or very likely to be received?
- How much still must be *raised* by a program or another type of activity?
- How much should be allotted for new programs and administrative or operating costs for core activities?
- Is the total amount a *reasonable* goal, given past experience and success in raising funds? If not, what new programs or expansion should be delayed, and what is the revised goal?

Decide on available funding possibilities and strategies. Many different ways to obtain resources are feasible for coalitions: leveraging shared positions and resources, becoming a line item in an existing organization's budget, incorporating activities and services in organizations with a similar mission, applying for grants, using existing personnel resources, soliciting in-kind support, fundraising, using third-party funding, developing a fee-for-service structure, acquiring tax revenues, securing endowments and giving arrangements, establishing membership fees and dues, developing a business plan, creating a for-profit corporation to help pay for the nonprofit side, or having programs adopted by other partner organizations (Community Tool Box, 2005a). Of the total amount needed, how much could be raised from federal or foundation grants and contracts and from corporate and individual donations? What cost-reduction strategies can be identified to obtain in-kind assistance with services, equipment, materials, or other parts of the budget? Then decide which funding possibilities to follow up on, based on which ones fit the coalition's mission, are easiest to do, are most likely to succeed, and whether they would change what the coalition normally does. Strategize how to get what the coalition wants. Decide whom to work with to implement the coalition's funding strategies.

Find out what potential donors want and how the coalition can give it to them. For instance, many donors want recognition; some want to spread their interests in the community; and others just want to feel good about what they are doing. Traditional philanthropy spreads available resources widely to as many agencies as possible, often resulting in single-year, program-oriented grants that do not build organizational infrastructure. *Venture philanthropy* is a new concept that has grown out of the desire for individuals and foundations to strengthen the capacity of charitable organizations. It focuses on building the capacity of grantees (organizations) by using multi-year grants and focused technical assistance. Its donors look for entrepreneurial potential within organizations and outcomes that are focused on programs, as well as organizational sustainability (Social Enterprise Magazine Online, 2003).

Draft the resource development plan. This draft should incorporate all of the information compiled so far, including the coalition's current financial situation (budget), long- and short-term financial goals, strategies to use to carry out those goals, timeline with specific actions, and a one-page executive summary at the beginning of the document that summarizes the whole plan. Specifically, the plan should

- Identify tasks and activities needed to achieve the objectives and list them in chronological order.
- Specify criteria that will be used to decide when each task or activity is completed.
- Indicate who will have primary responsibility for each task or activity and what other individuals, partners, or work groups will help with each one.
- Specify a timeline by which each task or activity will be completed.

The resource development plan may be created as shown in Table 10.4 (Mosaica, 2005a, p. 10):

Table 10.4. Resource Development Plan.

Task or Activity	Criteria	Who Is Responsible	Deadline
Set up resource development task force.	• Include at least one staff member, two coalition leaders, and two members. • First meeting held.	Steering Committee chair and coalition director	January 1
Provide fund-raising training for steering committee	Eighty percent of steering committee attends training	• Director sets up training. • Chair promotes attendance.	February 15
Prepare general support proposal	Proposal written and approved by steering committee	Coalition director and staff	September 30

(continued)

Table 10.4. Resource Development Plan. (*Continued*)

Task or Activity	Criteria	Who Is Responsible	Deadline
Design annual campaign plan	Plan prepared and approved by steering committee	Director and resource development task force chair	November 15
Identify ten potential new donors	Ten donors with addresses are identified	Resource development task force chair	January 30

Staff members, coalition members and leaders, key community leaders, current funders, and consumers should review the plan and suggest improvements. Allowing those who will be involved in implementing the plan opportunities to change it makes it theirs. People are more willing to work and support what they helped to create.

Implement the plan. Implementation will be a joint effort of the steering committee, staff, the resource development team, and the coalition.

Monitor and evaluate progress. Planning is ongoing, changes with the coalition, and must be constantly revisited. Once the resource development plan is completed and approved, it becomes the work plan for fund-raising efforts. Review it regularly and change it as needed.

OBTAINING CORPORATE, FOUNDATION, AND GOVERNMENT GRANTS

Sometimes a coalition can do excellent community work with very little money or no money at all. Organizing a meeting, holding a social event, getting local policies changed—these and similar community actions are either cost-free or come with very modest price tags. Money can become an actual drawback because it requires record keeping and management, and can cause competition among partners.

Should coalitions apply for grants? Grants enable the coalition to do work it might never do otherwise. In many situations, grants are desirable; in some, they are essential. Grants are an excellent way to generate money, but not the only way. As stated previously, the resource development plan should include other sources of income as well.

When should coalitions apply for grants? Eventually, every community coalition decides to extend its scope of activities to start a new project or expand an existing one, and cannot cover this in the existing budget. The coalition may be aware of a foundation or agency that funds the type of initiative that is envisioned, or perhaps the coalition has been invited to apply for a grant award. These and other reasons may make it enticing for the coalition to submit a grant application. However, before that happens, the coalition and its leadership should decide if this is the best course of action.

What are the reasons for and benefits of applying? (Berkowitz, 2006b). What are the coalition's long-term program goals and how would this grant promote them? What are the tangible benefits in addition to the dollars obtained—increased collaboration, improved services, or access to care? Is the coalition applying to compete, to gain recognition, or just because grant funds are potentially available? Can the coalition do the same work as well, or almost as well, without grant money? What will the money be used for? Is a grant the best or only way to do what the coalition wants to do? Are there other (and perhaps better) ways of getting the needed money? What are the consequences of not starting or discontinuing a program?

What is the feasibility of grant seeking? (Berkowitz, 2006b). Could the time needed to prepare the application be better spent doing something else? Is the proposed intervention or project realistically within the capability of the coalition and its partners? What are the realistic chances of success? Are personnel prepared to work to produce a quality grant proposal? Is the funding period conducive to the accomplishment of coalition objectives?

What are the challenges of grant-seeking? (Berkowitz, 2006b). The lure of funds has its price in conditions and restrictions, such as limitations on eligibility, constraints on the manner in which the community is served, qualifications required of staff, and prescribed methods of reporting activities (Smith and Siek, 2002). Moreover, the potential for conflict always exists between the funder's need for control and the organization's requirement for autonomy (Smith and Siek, 2002). Cash flow is another problem related to reimbursement, because delays usually occur between submitting the first invoice and actually receiving funds. The coalition should be sure it wants to implement the proposed project, because a commitment is incurred if a grant is secured. Finally, responding to application guidance can be extremely time-consuming because of the required forms, assurances, attachments, format and length requirements, and limitations.

Developing the skills to prepare successful, competitive applications requires organization, planning, attention to detail, and practice. Because public- and private-sector funding is increasingly being awarded through this process, developing the staff capacity to respond effectively can be an excellent long-term investment for a community coalition.

Identifying and Researching Grant Funding Sources

The first step in the grant-seeking process is to learn about the types of support available and then focus on the type of support desired. Three main sources of grants exist: federal, state, and local government agencies; foundations; and private businesses and corporations. Grants are offered for different purposes—some offer start-up, or seed, money, whereas others offer ongoing support. Grant awards vary in amount. The amount should be matched to the coalition's needs, and more than one source can be applied to simultaneously. Some funders have geographic preferences as well as restrictions. Usually, coalitions are better off applying to nearby agencies. A good approach is to find out which foundations have given grants in the coalition's region to proposals similar to the coalition's planned proposal.

Federal, state, and local government agencies. The federal government has sources of information for grant seekers about available program grants for federal and state agencies, such as the Centers for Disease Control and Prevention (CDC), the Office of Minority Health (OMH), Health Research Services Administration (HRSA), or state and territorial departments of health. Grants from these and other agencies may be found in the *Federal Register*, published each weekday. Requests for Proposals (RFPs) are being listed online more frequently, and grant proposals are now often being accepted online (see www.grants.gov). Listservs are often used to disseminate RFPs.

Foundations. Three major types of foundations offer grant-funded opportunities for coalitions: independent, community, and corporate foundations (Anderson and Adams, 2000). The best approach is to identify initially a core of foundations that match the coalition's interests (see the Foundation Center under Resources at the end of this chapter). *Independent foundations* usually have giving guidelines that target areas of interest and types of support available, as does the Annie E. Casey and Robert Wood Johnson Foundations. *Community foundations* are funded by gifts from multiple donors and public entities, and are generally limited to a specific geographic area. For example, influential citizen-funded and not-for-profit conversion foundations for hospitals and insurance companies are good sources of coalition-related grants at the local level. Agencies such as the American Heart Association, American Lung Association, and American Public Health Association also offer grant opportunities for states and localities.

Business and Corporations. In addition to direct donations, many private corporations fund coalitions and other community-based organizations. These charitable entities, or *corporate foundations* (for example, the Kellogg and Ford Foundations), also have grant guidelines that drive their grant-making efforts. Retail organizations (for example, Target, Wal-Mart, Ben and Jerry's Ice Cream) and manufacturers (for example, Merck, GlaxoSmithKline, Eli Lilly) have set up foundations that offer grants to community groups like coalitions. Funding community partnerships can improve an organization's image as a good neighbor. Corporations realize that resources are scarce, and they are usually interested in helping communities to be more healthy. Corporations are more likely to give money if they know the community at large is also supportive of the coalition's efforts. The key to grant seeking with private corporations and businesses is to build relationships and make them an integral part of the coalition and its activities. Invite representatives from industry and small businesses to sit on the steering committee. Recruit volunteers from local businesses to fulfill their community service goals by working on coalition activities. Offer to employees at the local factory such services as application assistance for state-sponsored child health insurance (The Ohio State University, 2002).

With this in mind, narrow the field to one or more sources and make sure the funding agency offers grants in the coalition's area of interest. Then investigate the leading prospects. Before applying to a foundation or granting agency, the coalition should learn as much as it can about each funder, and call for information or visit the websites of funding agencies. Almost all foundations and corporate entities that accept public applications will send application guidelines and forms. Many websites include an annual report, a grants list, or both, which will provide more information about the funder's organization, its goals, whom it has made recent grants to, and in what amounts. Each foundation and granting agency does business in a different way, and guidelines often vary. Some foundations ask for a full application up front; others ask for a short letter that describes the proposal and, after screening, may request more information. Some first want to know the applicant's credentials; others are primarily interested in their ideas. Some want detailed budgets, whereas others ask for them later. Because proposal-writing details are somewhat different from source to source, doing homework can save time in the long run.

Contacting the Funder

Many potential grantees wonder whether it is acceptable to contact the funding agency before, during, or after an application for funding is submitted. Even though guidelines are usually clear, asking additional questions by telephone is a good idea. Some funders discourage face-to-face meetings, whereas others are more open to them. If the guidelines do not prohibit a pre-application meeting, the coalition should consider making the request, because it may get answers to lingering questions that will help improve the application, clarify what to emphasize and what to tone down, and prevent wasted time. The coalition will also have made a personal contact, and perhaps the staff person may volunteer some information, not explicitly covered in the RFP or guidelines, that may affect the final form and focus of the proposal. Foundations appreciate those who take the time to gather the facts, and might even recognize their names when their proposal comes up for review. Personal contact does not have to be initiated by the grant writer; a well-connected friend or coalition member who knows a program officer at a local foundation could contact the foundation on the coalition's behalf. This is helpful if the grant writer has recently relocated or is promoting an untested idea.

Building Support for the Grant Proposal

Most funders want to know that proposals have community support, because part of their mission is to serve the community. Sometimes the support is already available and sometimes it must be actively cultivated. A good way to build support for new ideas is to circulate a concept paper and ask for feedback. This validates whether community members are interested in the idea, gets others actively interested, makes it easier to get formal letters of support for a future application, and provides constructive feedback about the proposal (Berkowitz, 2006a). Forming a working group (perhaps as a subgroup of the resource development team) to plan and write the grant application is also a good way to build support. Even if they are not experts, others may have attractive content ideas, good strategic thoughts, specialized knowledge, and the support the coalition needs to get the job done (Berkowitz, 2006a).

The group may only meet a few times, unless the application is lengthy. Group members can apportion tasks, for example, data gathering, making contacts, drafting, and editing the first and later drafts. When the coalition does have a proposal draft, find an outside expert(s) in the field who is willing to review it and provide commentary. The expert could be knowledgeable about the grant's content area or about how foundations (particularly the potential funder) work.

The coalition must demonstrate awareness of who has done similar projects and show that appropriate partners have been engaged to assure that the project will have enough support for completion. It should choose partners wisely because money can change previous trusting, valued relationships, and consider carefully the choice of partners and whether to include them in the budget if funding is received, to assure buy-in and commitment. Grant reviewers expect collaboration and feel safer when their money is invested with solid partners.

Requests for Proposals

Federal, state, and local government agencies, as well as most foundations, typically use an application guidance or request for proposal (RFP) process to ensure open competition for funding. The range of eligible applicants varies. Some competitions are open to profit-making and nonprofit entities; public agencies may also be eligible. Some competitions are limited to public or nonprofit organizations; minority or disadvantaged businesses; small businesses; or in some cases minority-controlled nonprofit organizations, universities, or consortia.

If funding is made available under specific legislative guidelines, and because the government has a responsibility to make the opportunity to apply for funding widely available, an RFP provides a way to obtain applications that meet legislative requirements and are submitted in a similar format, facilitating the review of a large number of them. Federal agencies can make noncompetitive grants, though they represent a small proportion of total federal funding and require extensive internal justification. Nonprofit organizations can sometimes obtain public funding through unsolicited proposals, based on discussions with potential funding sources. If the coalition is asked to submit an unsolicited proposal, it should take advantage of the excellent opportunity but remember that funding is by no means assured. A complicated process is required to justify *sole source* awards, that is, grants or contracts awarded without a funding competition.

Sometimes only one grant, cooperative agreement, or contract will be awarded, as when an agency wants to have a program evaluated or needs a single national technical assistance contractor to assist local grantees involved in a particular category of program, such as injury prevention. In other cases, multiple awards are given, such as regional and national grants to minority-controlled organizations under the CDC HIV Capacity-Building Initiative (CBI). In such situations, several coalitions in various parts of the country may receive grants or cooperative agreements from a federal agency to carry out related projects with particular priority populations. Grants may be made on a regional or neighborhood basis or without regard to location.

Limitations on allowable activities or population groups, as well as required program components, are typically specified in the RFP. An RFP also includes specific information on how proposals will be evaluated, often with a particular number of points allotted to each major component of the proposal. When there is a single award in a particular funding category, the RFP is usually very detailed and defines a specific work scope. When multiple awards are expected, more flexible guidelines are provided, allowing various types of activities as long as they contribute to a specific set of goals and focus on one or more specified populations (Mosaica, 2005b, p. 3). City and state agencies typically use RFPs not only for funds raised through their own tax revenues but also for pass-through and block-granted federal programs.

Large national foundations, such as the Robert Wood Johnson Foundation and the Kellogg Foundation, have used competitive RFP processes in awarding grants involving HIV/AIDS and substance abuse prevention, and children's health. The Pfizer Foundation used an RFP process for its Community Health Ventures Program, as has Johnson & Johnson for its health outreach and access grants. More often, however, private sources wait for potential applicants to find them, and then they make their funding guidelines and application procedures available—increasingly on their websites as well as in written documents. They indicate funding priorities, specify the kinds of information that must be included in a funding proposal, and set deadlines for submission of proposals.

Proposal Timelines

A grant proposal is often a labor-intensive undertaking that requires a commitment of resources devoted to producing a fifteen- to fifty-page document (sometimes even longer) in a relatively short time. When an RFP is released by an agency, the deadline for proposal submission is frequently only a month away, so coalitions must prepare to work hard for a few weeks to develop a grant proposal, keeping in mind that this finite period of hard work might potentially provide multiple years of funding.

Writing a Grant Proposal

Coalitions should not be intimidated by RFP rules and instructions—anyone who is organized, diligent, and has a good idea can write a proposal. Grant writing is a skill that improves with practice. Each grant becomes a resource of ideas and already-written sections for the next grant. The RFP should be read carefully, and key elements, such as the deadline for submission, mailing address, and number of copies to be submitted, should be highlighted as it is read (a one-page checklist of all required items is usually included). Colleagues or others who are committed to secure funding for the coalition's project can be asked to help with the writing process itself. The coalition should contact the agency soliciting grant proposals for samples of previously funded proposals, or ask one of the awardees for a copy of theirs. It should ask how the awardee's application was organized and packaged, and how much detail and documentation went into each section. Such a model is a useful reference point when a coalition is unclear how to proceed.

Reviewing Process for Competitive Grant Applications

Understanding the review process helps the coalition prepare a competitive application. Most RFPs are prepared and disseminated to encourage eligible organizations to compete for funding. Using a standardized review process (usually involving an external review panel of individuals who do not work for the funding agency), the funder selects the organization(s) it believes will best meet the program's purposes.

Coalitions should understand the review process of those they are asking for money. When foundations hire grant reviewers to evaluate proposals, they require them to use the RFP as the basic measure of comparison, assigning a specific number of points to each section of the grant. Grant reviewers will quickly exclude all proposals that do not follow or clearly address the required guidelines. A frequent error is trying to sell a project on its merits instead of following the RFP instructions (Community Tool Box, 2006).

Proposals may be evaluated by staff of the funding agency, outside reviewers, or a combination of the two. The trend is toward using outside panels as the primary reviewers, with staff doing second-level review of applications that are scored above a certain level by the initial reviewers. Review panels include three or more individuals who do not work for the funding agency and who have appropriate credentials and experience related to the program for which funds are being allocated.

A major problem with outside review panels has been the underrepresentation of minorities and community people, and an overdependence on researchers and academicians (Mosaica, 2005b, p. 5). In addition, reviewers from the West and East Coasts have tended to be overrepresented, and reviewers from the Midwest, the South, and rural areas, underrepresented. As a result, review panels may contain few individuals knowledgeable about the special problems and needs of African Americans, Latinos, Asians and Pacific Islanders, or Native Americans (Mosaica, 2005b, p. 5). However, some agencies are making serious efforts to include minority group members, consumers, and community-based organization staff on their review panels.

A representative from the coalition might be a reviewer in a program competition for which the coalition did not submit a proposal. Or he or she might be asked to read proposals in a different category or region from the one for which the coalition submitted a proposal. Serving on a review panel can help coalitions understand reviewer and funder expectations in order to strengthen future grant applications.

In general, reviewers consider the following overall merits of the proposals (Mosaica, 2005b, p. 4):

- *Technical quality.* Has the applicant documented the need for the project in the proposed locality and among the priority population? Are the objectives appropriate, significant, and feasible? Is the work plan practical and workable? Are the strategies innovative, or do they represent business as usual? Is the evaluation plan of high quality and feasible? Is the project creative and potentially replicable? Several different review criteria may address technical quality, such as problem, goals, objectives, methodology, work plan, and evaluation.

- *Skills and related experience of staff and organization.* Do the organization and proposed personnel have the capacity to carry out the project, based on resumes, job descriptions, past experience, and relationships and agreements with other organizations?

- *Cost and appropriateness of budget.* Is the total cost within guidelines and reasonable, given the work to be done. The best technical proposal and most capable staff and organization may not be funded if projected costs are very high or the budget is poorly prepared. Less highly rated proposals may be favored if their proposed costs are lower (Mosaica, 2005b, p. 5).

Letters of Intent

Some funders may initially ask for a brief two- or three-page letter of intent (LOI) that describes the coalition and its objectives; the problem to be addressed; the proposed solution; documentation of the coalition's ability to carry out the objectives; the budget requested and financial needs associated with the request, including evidence that the effort will not rely solely on the funder's support; and the evaluation that will be conducted to demonstrate that funding has made a difference. The LOI (in business letter format) should provide sufficient information to demonstrate eligibility and capacity to implement the project.

Initial screening of the LOI may be done to ensure that the applicant is eligible. Sometimes, technical review of the program concept, and applicant experience and capability are used to screen out some groups so that the number of full proposals will be reduced. In this case, the coalition may prepare a full proposal only if the LOI is approved. Sometimes, an LOI is voluntary and used by federal agencies to anticipate how many applications and in what mix to expect, as well as to set up review panels.

The Grant Application

Generally, all funding organizations expect an organized proposal of planned activities and expenditures. The process of preparing proposals for government funding depends on the funder. Although different programs may require different formats for the proposals, grant applicants should be prepared to include the following standard sections in their proposals: cover letter; title page and abstract; statement of the problem, needs, or issue; project description (goals, objectives, methods, and activities); evaluation plan; budget request and budget justification; applicant qualifications; future funding plans and plans for sustainability; and appendices. Each section is discussed in detail here:

Cover letter, title page, and abstract. The *cover letter* should be on agency stationery and signed by the appropriate organization official. It should be one page and describe the coalition's interest and capacity to successfully implement the proposed project. The coalition should strive for an enthusiastic and positive tone, and summarize the project, designating a contact person for any further questions.

Typical *title pages* include the project title, name of the coalition or lead agency submitting the grant, agency address, name of the prospective funder, beginning and ending project dates, and the total amount requested.

An *abstract* is a one- or two-page summary of the problem, need, or issue that should include proposed project aims, methods that will be used to implement and evaluate the project, and a final paragraph describing the coalition's or agency's capacity (expertise and resources) for carrying out the proposed project. It should also describe how the project dovetails with the RFP. This beginning summary should interest the reader in what is to follow. First impressions and a memorable name, like *Kids Count*, can make a difference to funders who plan to promote the project. The abstract is the key part of any proposal, and it should solidify the impression that the coalition knows what it wants to accomplish and how. What the coalition plans to do with the funder's money must be simply and powerfully stated; the abstract may be the only part of the proposal that is read.

Statement of problem, need, or issue. This statement must get the reviewer's attention and make a strong case for the need for funding. It should document the issue to be addressed (using statistics, graphs, and charts as well as text, if including them will make the coalition's needs statement more persuasive); describe contributing factors of the issue, causes of the problem, or the circumstances creating the need; and identify current approaches or solutions, based on a review of the literature. The statement should use existing data sources to document the problem or argue that such statistics are lacking. United States census data is collected every ten years from over 115 million housing units across the country, and it includes geographic, demographic, and socioeconomic information (http://www.census.gov). Many state and national organizations and agencies publish statistics about special populations on their websites.

Consideration should be given to whether this grant proposal will build upon existing efforts, introduce an innovative strategy, or both. Some reviewers may be searching for an innovative approach to a problem that has been well documented, but not yet effectively addressed.

Project description. Once the need for funding is documented, the coalition must present the details of program implementation. This section should guide the reviewer step by step through the activities needed to accomplish the goal(s) in a way that will continue to engage his or her interest. Furthermore, this description will be referred to often over the course of program implementation. Even if program staff changes over time, the project description should provide a road map for anyone to follow. It includes goals and objectives, methods or activities for addressing the identified problem or need, and a timeline for completing each activity. The coalition should tie itself to a major health issue and position the proposal as a model program, making the overall benefit of the project clear—that a problem shared by many communities will be addressed, and a replicable model that can be used to broadly share solutions may result.

Goals and objectives. In this section are the goals and objectives for the proposed project. (See Chapter Twelve for a description of how to write goals and objectives as part of an action plan.) Goals are two or three broad statements with a projected long-term, ideal outcome. For each goal, develop numerous corresponding *objectives,* or specific statements that will indicate to the reviewer exactly the goals to be achieved.

Methods. The methods section describes in detail how goals and objectives will be carried out over the course of a project. The tasks should be sequentially ordered and cohesive. A flowchart of the sequence of events is advisable, in addition to the required timeline.

Timeline. The timeline includes the tasks to be accomplished and the sequence for developing them according to the months, quarters, or years of the grant period. All activities in the timeline will shape the budget request. Timelines can help to define tasks and monitor progress so that midcourse corrections can be made (McDermott and Sarvela, 1999). All timelines are similar in that they consist of rows on the left-hand side of the chart that represent the tasks or activities to be completed, while columns represent periods of time (such as yearly, quarterly, or monthly). A task development timeline is used most often by coalitions and community groups, and it provides a detailed, sequential list of activities and their projected dates of completion (Anspaugh, Dignan, and Anspaugh, 2000). The Gantt chart accomplishes the same purpose; it uses different width lines to indicate projected progress (wider line) versus actual progress (thin line) across boxes, thereby providing an indication of progress made toward completing tasks (Timmreck, 2003). The timeline is meant to be used for planning purposes and may be revised later. Some activities will be dependent upon the completion of prior activities, and multiple items may have the same completion date.

Evaluation plan. The evaluation plan clarifies objectives so they are measurable, helps refine or revise program approaches, and provides information about the relative costs and effort for tasks, so activity and budget adjustments can be made in future years of funding. It also helps the funder assess whether objectives were met and whether the program's benefits (for example, outcomes) justify the cost of implementation. The plan details how process and outcome objectives will be measured, how data will be collected and analyzed, what results are expected, and how many people are expected to benefit.

Two main types of evaluation are used: process and outcome. Most likely, a combination of both approaches will be implemented, depending on the types of objectives drafted. *Process evaluation* assesses the implementation of a program, emphasizing activities to be completed. *Outcome evaluation* assesses the short- or long-term impact of a program. Objectives may be evaluated as follows: not accomplished, partially accomplished, accomplished, or exceeded. Evaluations can be complex, time-intensive aspects of a program. Unless the coalition can afford to budget for an evaluation consultant, the evaluation plan should be designed within the strengths and limitations of program and staff resources.

Budget request. Once the goals and objectives, methods, and evaluation plan are drafted, the foundation for the *budget request* is laid. The proposal should be limited to fewer, more attainable goals instead of promising more than the coalition and budget can deliver. Most projects underestimate funding for staff and technology support. Varying degrees of detail are required in an estimated budget, and funders usually provide budget forms and instructions. Make sure the budget does not exceed the maximum amount stated in the RFP and that the funds proposed in the narrative, line-item budget, and budget justification text match. If required to submit budget projections for multiple years, the coalition should allow for a cost-of-living raise in staff salaries and inflation for supplies, utilities, and other line items. If a coalition is inexperienced with a proposed activity (for example, conducting focus groups), it should talk with someone who has done this to learn how much to budget. Common budget line items include these:

- *Staff salaries* are listed in a budget as FTEs, or "full time equivalents." A person working a forty-hour week will be listed at 1.00 FTE, and the actual amount for salary requested in the budget will be 100 percent of the proposed salary for that position. The FTE equivalents and salary amounts are adjusted for part-time positions.
- *Fringe benefits* may include social security tax (nonprofit agencies are exempt) and benefits such as medical, dental, disability, life insurance, and retirement plans, which are calculated as a percentage of staff salaries.
- *Indirect costs (or overhead)* are used to compensate the lead agency or coalition for housing or sponsoring a project. Indirect costs may be provided by the coalition's funding agency, but if so, they are allocated as a fixed percentage of the direct costs of the grant.
- *In-kind line items* do not add any costs to the project because they are paid for or absorbed by the grant applicant. In-kind services might include paying for rent or a portion of an administrative staff person's time.

Budget justification. The budget justification describes the need for each budget item requested. In one or two sentences per budget line item, the total line item reached for each item must be specifically indicated; funders do not like to see cost estimates but expect the true anticipated costs.

Applicant qualifications. This section of the proposal is used to convince reviewers why *this* coalition should be funded. Although reviewers often do not need to be convinced that a health issue is important and timely, they have limited funds to award. What makes *this* approach or strategy and *these* qualifications better than the competitor's? The coalition or agency must describe its mission, history, and existing experience, emphasizing agency strengths and contributions to the field or community in the topic area for which funding is requested. Links to community partners and other resources should be highlighted and letters of support from those collaborators obtained for inclusion in the appendices.

Future funding plans and plans for sustainability. Many projects disappear after grant funding is gone. Federal or state agencies often expect a long-term plan for the self-sustainability of a project because funding at the federal or state level may only be available for a limited time or until elections bring in new legislators with different fiscal and policy priorities. Some programs require a match of funding from the beginning. For example, in a two-to-one match, the coalition will be required to contribute matching funds of two dollars for every dollar awarded. Funders will want to know how grantees' matching funds will be provided and sustained.

Many initiatives must be in place for years if they are to have a long-term impact on outcomes, such as health status indicators. Therefore, if a funder can only afford to cover a chronic health issue like obesity for a limited time, it may want to know obesity-prevention efforts will be continued in the community over the *long* term. Funders rarely subsidize projects beyond three years and prefer to rotate resources, because needs are always greater than dollars available in any year. They also want to avoid any long-term personnel costs, usually in the fringe benefit area. Even if the coalition is unable to guarantee that its proposed program will be self-sustainable, it should make a good case for sustainability and describe a plan. It should also define a strategy and timeline for building the revenue-generating part of this project (for example, by outlining whether and how fees will be charged for services provided, and how materials developed during this grant will be marketed and sold, membership dues instituted, and *new* grants or contracts developed).

Appendices. Appendices provide supplemental, supporting information that does not belong in the body of the proposal. These may include a marketing or dissemination plan graphic; volunteer recruitment flowchart; graphic timeline of proposed activities (in addition to a description in the narrative); an evaluation instrument (for example, questionnaire); educational or printed materials; biosketches or curriculum vitae of key project personnel, steering committee members, and consultants; and letters of support or memoranda of agreement.

One-page letters of support, signed by an executive director of the collaborating or supporting agency, should be submitted on official letterhead from each agency that has been proposed as a partner. These can be drafted by a grant writer, but make sure that each letter is unique to the working relationship and shared interests of the partner and the coalition. Highlight the significance of the proposed relationship in the context of goals and objectives, and summarize the partner's capacity and strengths for addressing the issue considered.

Dealing with Rejection

Even if the proposal is excellent, it may not be funded for reasons that might have little to do with the coalition's actual proposal. For example, the funder may have only a limited amount of money to give; another application may have come closer to a foundation priority; political considerations may have intervened; or the budget may have been too high (Berkowitz, 2005a). But coalitions should take the opportunity to learn from rejection. If the application is rejected and written feedback is not provided, the coalition should call the funder and ask what could have been done to improve the proposal, thus keeping the door open to a positive future working relationship. It should consider resubmitting a revised proposal or pursuing other ways to resolve health issues with fewer resources. The planning and grant-writing process allows coalitions to resubmit their ideas elsewhere. Often project partners get so committed to the proposal that they are willing to seek other sources of funding. Seasoned grant writers recycle and reuse paragraphs from successful grants. The same grant should not be submitted to multiple funders at the same time; however, it can be changed slightly so multiple-funded grants mesh together instead of creating duplication (Berkowitz, 2005a).

Improving Competitive Applications

The task is to design a project that meets community needs and fits the priorities and capability of the coalition, while being fully responsive to grant requirements. Steps to award-winning proposals and common mistakes that are made in submitting proposals are presented in Exhibits 10.7 and 10.8. The following fourteen steps should guide any coalition through the grant process and improve the competitiveness of any proposal in response to an RFP (Mosaica, 2005b, pp. 6–10):

1. ***Read the guidance very carefully.*** Read first for general content, checking to see that the RFP calls for projects that are consistent with the coalition's mission and capabilities. Be sure that the coalition or lead agency is eligible to apply for funding, and find out how broad the competition will be. Is it only

---

Exhibit 10.7. Elements of Award-Winning Grant Proposals.

The number of grant proposals submitted outweighs the number of grants available. What elements will ensure that your grant proposal is superior?

- Following all directions!
- Well-organized, integrated, easy to comprehend proposal sections (good layout and graphics, and so forth)
- Well documented problem statement
- Previous experience in the area of the identified need, problem, or issue
- Community involvement in the planning process
- Problem, need, or issue explicitly addresses the funder's priorities
- Feasible goals, measurable objectives
- Appropriate yet innovative strategies for addressing the need, problem, or issue
- Realistic timeline for accomplishing proposed activities
- Budget is realistic and justifies how funds will be spent
- Potential for the program to become self-sustainable (when applicable)
- A sound evaluation plan that focuses on methods, data, and results

---

Berkowitz, B. (2006b). Apply for a Grant: The General Approach. Lawrence, KS: Community Tool Box. Accessed January 4, 2006. http://ctb.ku.edu/tools/EN/sub_section_main_1300.htm

Exhibit 10.8. Common Mistakes in Grant Applications.

These common mistakes are unrelated to a proposal's content but nevertheless make it less competitive.

- **Failure to follow application instructions.** The application does not follow requirements on margins, type size, or page limitations, and is declared nonresponsive and returned unread.

- **Missing component.** A required component (for example, budget justification) is missing. The funder may or may not give the applicant a chance to provide the information.

- **Narrative not in specified order or sections misnamed.** The narrative does not follow the specified order or uses different section titles; reviewers have trouble locating required information.

- **Misplaced or missing content.** Required material is put in the wrong section of the narrative or is omitted altogether. Reviewers do not find required information, and the proposal loses points.

- **Failure to use preferred terminology.** The application uses terminology that differs from the RFP. Thus it does not seem to be written specifically for this funder and funding opportunity, and it loses points.

- **Missing references.** Data are used without citations or references to indicate their source and appear questionable to some reviewers, so the application loses points.

- **Focus inconsistent with review criteria.** The proposal does not exceed the maximum number of pages, but the allocation of pages to sections is inconsistent with the RFP. Too many pages are spent on sections that are worth few points and too few pages address key sections, so the proposal loses points in those sections.

- **Unclear narrative or poor editing.** The application contains typos, incorrect sentence structures, or other evidence of limited editing or lack of quality control. Reviewers assume that carelessness in writing the proposal may portend lack of care in implementation, and the applicant loses credibility.

- **Weak or nonmeasurable objectives.** The application does not include measurable project objectives, or the objectives address process objectives when outcome objectives are required. The application may lose points for the work and evaluation plans because they are based on objectives.

- **Weak evaluation plan.** The evaluation plan does not provide a specific, practical plan for determining whether tasks are completed and results (outcomes) are accomplished. The plan is vague, without specific outcome indicators or steps to be followed. Overall, it is unclear whether the applicant has the capacity to plan and conduct the evaluation.

(continued)

Exhibit 10.8. Common Mistakes in Grant Applications. (*Continued*)

- **Inconsistencies in the application.** The application has a narrative, a separate work plan chart, and a budget. Perhaps different people prepared these major sections and time to review them properly was limited, so they disagree or are inconsistent. Some aspects of the methodology are not reflected in the work plan, and some staff mentioned in the narrative are not listed in the budget.

- **Budget problems.** The budget does not add up, has costs in the wrong sections, or does not include a budget narrative. Even if the proposal narrative is clear and effective, the budget gives the impression of having been done quickly and carelessly, and the application loses credibility.

- **Application arrives late.** The application is not postmarked on the deadline date or does not arrive by the specified time deadline; therefore, it is returned, unopened, to the applicant.

Source: Mosaica, 2005b.

for other nonprofit organizations, or are public and for-profit organizations included as well? See whether a cash or in-kind match is required and whether the funding agency will provide full project funding. After the initial review, read the guidance again and *mark* key information. Use marginal notes to highlight priorities, objectives, preferred methods, and activities that are *not* fundable. If the RFP is not read carefully, some information or component that is required may be omitted, and the proposal may be judged nonresponsive and not considered (applications often include a checklist to prevent this).

2. *Review the section that explains how to prepare and organize the proposal.* This usually describes the proposal outline or format to be followed and what information should be included in each section. Read it carefully, then re-read and underline key information. Identify the proposal outline that is to be followed, and note whether page limitations are specified. The current trend is to limit the length of applications, including appendices. Again, failure to follow instructions may result in the application being returned without review.

3. *Carefully study the "Evaluation Criteria" (or similar section), which explains how applications will be evaluated and often numerically scored.* This section provides an outline for a desirable proposal. Whatever the format, the RFP usually indicates the maximum number of points that may be awarded for each proposal component or the percent of total points allowed for that component. Study the point scales carefully; they usually include a description of the factors to be rated to help preparers focus time and effort in composing the application. Sometimes no numerical scores are provided, but the RFP will state that the proposal will be judged on a specified set of factors. Most often, they are provided in priority order, with the most important factors listed first. Sometimes reviewers will look for specific information in a particular section, and if they fail to find it, will assume that it was excluded and give no points, even if the information is located in another section.

4. *Once the RFP is thoroughly read, prepare an outline of the application.* Be sure that the format is the one required or suggested in the RFP and that the subsections contain all the information needed to meet the scoring criteria. When constructing the outline, include the required components for each section and subsection. Use the *same terminology* as the RFP throughout the narrative to improve the application's score, because it implies a familiarity with the funder, its priorities, and the preferred terminology of the program area.

5. *Review the cost information.* With most programs for which multiple awards are projected, activities may be funded at a level lower than the amount requested in the original proposal, so the budget amount is not usually critical. Propose a reasonable budget that is within the maximum permitted and allows all activities specified in the work plan to be implemented. Some RFPs will indicate an *average* or *maximum* grant amount. Do not propose a budget that is well above the average unless a compelling reason exists for higher costs. Where a single award, or a small number of awards, is expected, cost may be a major factor in who gets the grant.

6. *If unanswered questions arise once the RFP is reviewed, e-mail or call the identified contact within the funding agency and ask for clarification.* Most RFPs list contact persons within the funding agency who may be approached with questions. Contact *only* those persons identified (no one else in the agency is supposed to talk to applicants during the application process). Make a list of questions before contacting these individuals, so that all the information can be obtained through a single telephone call or e-mail; many other potential applicants may also ask questions. Agencies often identify two contacts for assistance: one from grants management to provide answers to grants management or cost-related questions and one from the appropriate program branch to provide program-related information or technical assistance.

7. *Develop a work plan for preparing the application.* This helps identify all the tasks required to prepare the narrative and to collect and organize the information needed for the application (for example, letters of support (LOSs) from partner organizations, letters from prospective staff or consultants, epidemiologic, or demographic data). Develop a work plan with tasks, activities, responsibilities, and time deadlines, and go over it with the grant application team. Make sure the division of labor and the deadlines are agreed upon, especially if the application is prepared in collaboration with other organizations whose capability and cost information must be collected and integrated with those of the applicant agency. Collect statistics, resumes, LOSs, and other data as early as possible. Most applications require the use of federal forms that can be downloaded from a website or obtained from the agency, but allow time to get them. Sometimes key personnel (or at least the project director) must be identified by name and must provide resumes. This may mean talking to nonstaff persons and obtaining permission to use their resumes or biosketches, with the understanding that if the grant or contract is awarded, they will be offered positions. The resumes should reflect the skills required by the application. Sometimes job descriptions can be substituted for resumes, but proposals are always stronger if the project director and other key staff are identified by name and their resumes provided.

8. *Assign writing sections of the proposal.* If possible, have one person do the narrative and another, the capability and back-up materials. If responsibility for the narrative must be divided, one person should write the needs statement and the other, the methodology and work plan. The fewer writers, the better. On the other hand, involve as many knowledgeable people as possible in meetings to discuss the proposal, agree on objectives, and come up with a detailed content outline. Be strict about deadlines for drafts.

9. *Ensure that all sections are reviewed, revised, and fit together well.* Have one person responsible for final editing, reviewing, and ensuring that all support material is prepared. With planning ahead of time, the draft proposal may be sent to someone outside the organization for review.

10. *Once objectives and the work plan have been developed, prepare the budget.* Have a target figure in mind, do a rough budget, and then review. If inexperienced in budget preparation, enlist the help of someone else skilled in budgeting. Generally, the best approach is to first prepare a budget, using the agency's standard budget format to be sure that no cost categories are omitted, and then to revise the format to fit the funder's requirements. If the initial budget is higher than the maximum allowable, and cutting it may mean that the project cannot be accomplished as designed, then modify the work plan and scale back objectives until the budget is reasonable. Balance the proposal's need to get a high score on personnel and capability with the need to keep the cost reasonable, but do not propose personnel or a work plan that cannot be implemented effectively.

11. *Finish preparing the application at least one or two days before the deadline.* Allow for broken copiers and support staff that may be ill. Go over the completed application package very carefully and be sure all RFP requirements are met.

12. *Make sure to meet the RFP deadline.* That means mailing the proposal or delivering it to the funder by a particular time and date, or the application will be refused or returned unopened. Save the certified mail receipt until the return receipt card is received from the funder.

13. *Once the application is submitted, have the team debrief to learn from the experience.* The team should talk about problems encountered and how to minimize them in the future.

14. *If not funded, request reviewer comments or a debriefing on the coalition's application.* The federal government is required to provide such information, usually by mail, and it will help improve the coalition's next competitive application.

COALITION SPOTLIGHT: ARKANSAS ORAL HEALTH COALITION

Although prevention and treatment for oral disease has improved, thousands of Arkansans continue to experience dental pain and dysfunction. Arkansas mirrors the nation in that oral disease remains pervasive among some groups within the population. Dental caries (tooth decay) continue to be a major problem for many children, with 61 percent of third-grade children having experienced tooth decay and 31 percent having untreated decay. Thirty-four percent of Arkansans aged sixty-five or older have lost all their teeth, compared to 23 percent nationally.

The Arkansas Office of Oral Health has utilized a statewide oral health coalition, supported by funding from the Centers for Disease Control and Prevention (CDC), to begin to address the oral disease problems in Arkansas. Smiles: AR, U.S.™ is a statewide partnership of more than thirty member organizations whose mission is to improve oral health for Arkansas residents. Since its formation in 2000, this coalition has continued to grow and has played a key role in five annual Arkansas Oral Health Summits and in the development of the state oral health plan (revised in 2001).

One influential coalition partner is Delta Dental of Arkansas, the state's largest administrator of group dental benefits, serving 2,000 Arkansas-based employers and more than one million employees and their families. Since 2002, Delta Dental has made a significant commitment (more than $600,000) to funding projects oriented toward improving oral health education, prevention, and treatment, especially for the neediest. The coalition has served the critical role of assessing need and informing partners like Delta Dental how they can best help implement promising projects that are likely to lead to successful health outcomes. Some examples include Teeth on the Go©, an oral health education kit distributed to every public and private elementary school (kindergarten through second grade) in the state; Language Line Services, a free language translation service for all Arkansas dental offices; University of Arkansas College of Dentistry Scholarships ($115,000) to ensure ongoing, quality dental care for the state; Future Smiles, a program of school-based oral screenings, dental sealants, dental health education, and partnerships with dental professionals; and twenty-two grants to community dental care organizations that provide care for low-income persons. The coalition representative from Delta Dental acknowledged that before becoming part of the coalition, his organization "had heart, but not always the expert knowledge of what programs would work best in the community" (Mouden, personal communication). The coalition "helped us find the right niche and put us in touch with a network of experts" (Mouden, personal communication) who could help us implement feasible and effective programs, like Future Smiles. That collaboration has even led to the first-ever elementary school dental clinic in Arkansas, the Future Smiles Dental Clinic at Wakefield Elementary in Little Rock.

Even though Delta Dental probably would have contributed funds to promote oral health and dental treatment, their relationship with the Arkansas Oral Health Coalition, Inc., made successful outcomes likely. The programs were well targeted to the priority populations that needed services and were offered as part of a total continuum of programs and services supported by both public health and private sectors. As a measure of mutual respect and collaboration, the coalition named Delta Dental CEO Ed Choate as 2003's Oral Health Humanitarian of the Year. The coalition also nominated Delta Dental for the Arkansas Community Foundation's 2004 Outstanding Philanthropic Corporation award in the midsize business category, which they won.

An effective state coalition can facilitate successful, well-funded statewide oral health prevention and treatment programs. The grant funds and technical support and training offered by CDC made coalition infrastructure development possible and encouraged collaboration from a diverse group of partners, including organizations that variously promote access to care, reductions in health disparities, interfaith alliances, and dental insurance. Collaboration provides mutual benefits for the coalition, its partners, and the state as a whole. The coalition receives funding and resources that make sustainability more likely. Formalizing the coalition through incorporation and obtaining Internal Revenue Service (IRS) nonprofit status has also allowed the coalition to receive other, tax-deductible donations. The partners achieved their organizational missions and received recognition for philanthropy. Finally, the state and its citizens benefited from needed programs and services. With key partners and a solid coalition in place, the Office of Oral Health is prepared to lead oral health infrastructure development efforts in Arkansas and serve as a model for other states.

Contributed by Lynn Douglas Mouden, DDS, MPH, Director, Office of Oral Health, Division of Health, Arkansas Department of Health and Human Services, 2006.

SUMMARY

By seeking a variety of resources, coalitions are better able to recruit members, retain member commitment, sponsor or implement programs, and sustain themselves long term. *Sustainability* refers to the coalition's capacity to support and maintain its activities over time. Resources to sustain the coalition are available from four main sources that work together and independently: money, people, goods, and services. Coalition funds can be obtained from membership dues, the lead agency, community donations, partner financial and in-kind contributions, grants, and contracts. The coalition can convene a resource development team to help develop a long-term plan that will make fiscal health and sustainability more likely. Tips for fund-raising and submitting competitive grants and contracts are highlighted.

QUESTIONS FOR REVIEW

1. Identify at least four resource development strategies that can be used by coalitions to ensure sustainability. Discuss the pros and cons of each strategy.
2. What is the value of involving coalition members and leaders in fund-raising for the coalition?
3. What are the four main kinds of resources that coalitions have and how can each be developed to ensure financial security and sustainability?
4. What are the key elements that make an application for grant funding more competitive?

RESOURCES

Educational Technology Grants and Grant-Writing. http://www.nand so onorg/grants/index.html

Foundation Center is a national clearinghouse that provides a catalogue and CD-ROM with major sources of information about private and corporate foundations. The online directory of grants available requires a subscription fee for access to thousands of grant opportunities. The Center also has a cooperating network of ninety library reference collections in all fifty states, Mexico, and Puerto Rico, and publishes *The Foundation Directory* as well as many specialized directories available in most libraries. Address: Foundation Center, 888 Seventh Avenue, New York, N.Y. 10106. Tel: (212) 620–4230 or (800) 424–9836; http://fdncenter.org to locate state branches.

Grantsmanship Center offers nationwide training programs and an excellent set of reprints. *The Grantsmanship Center Magazine is* a quarterly newsletter that contains articles and how-to information on fund-raising, program planning, and nonprofit management. Free subscriptions are offered and back issues are available by e-mail. Address: P.O. Box 17220, Los Angeles, Calif. 90017. Tel: (800) 421–9512; http://www.tgci.com/

Publications

Brice, H. J. *Financial and Strategic Management for Nonprofit Organizations.* Englewood Cliffs, N.J.: Prentice-Hall, Inc., 1987.

Catalog of Federal Domestic Assistance addresses preparation for and writing of grants. http://www.cfda.gov/

Chronicle of Philanthropy is for the prospective grant writer. This biweekly newspaper is the most useful periodical in the field and the best source for staying up to date on foundation activities nationally, especially for activities of larger foundations. Each issue lists grants made by foundations and upcoming application deadlines, as well as general articles on grant writing and fund-raising. *The Chronicle Guide to Grants,* affiliated with *The Chronicle of Philanthropy,* is a computerized search service that lists foundations in certain categories, and foundation grant awards by type. Address: 1255 23rd Street, N.W., Washington, D.C. 20037. Tel: (800) 347–6969; for details on *The Chronicle Guide to Grants:* (800) 287–6072.

Coley, S. and Scheinberg, C. *Proposal Writing.* Newbury Park, Calif.: Sage Publications, Inc., 1990.

Hall-Ellis, S. D., and others. In F. W. Hoffman (ed.), *Grantsmanship for Small Libraries and School Media Centers.* Englewood, Colo.: Libraries Unlimited, 1999.

Internet Nonprofit Center publishes the *Nonprofit FAQ,* a resource about nonprofits and their work provided by participants in online discussions. Grants and grant writing are just one of the categories. Join the nonprofit discussion listserv on the website: http://www.nonprofits.org/ or http://www.rain.org/ mailman/listinfo/nonprofit.

Mosaica: The Center for Nonprofit Development and Pluralism provides organizational development assistance to nonprofit organizations and a range of services that include organizational assessments, strategic planning, resource development planning and fund-raising capacity building, restructuring support, financial management and oversight, program design and delivery, personnel management, volunteer activities, community building and organizing, advocacy, program evaluation, and coalition building. Downloadable resources include *Nonprofit Organizations: The Basics and Operating Principles for Boards of Directors of Nonprofit Organizations,* and *Resource*

Development. Address: 1522 K Street, N.W., Suite 1130, Washington, D.C. 20005. Tel: (202) 887–0620; fax: (202) 887–0812; mosaica@mosaica.org

National Science Foundation (NSF) is an independent federal agency created by Congress in 1950 "to promote the progress of science; to advance the national health, prosperity, and welfare; to secure the national defense. . . ." With an annual budget of about $5.5 billion, NSF funds 20 percent of all federally supported basic research conducted by U.S. colleges and universities. In fields such as mathematics, computer science, and the social sciences, NSF is the major source of federal backing. Address: 4201 Wilson Boulevard, Arlington, Va. 22230. Tel: (703) 292-5111, (800) 877-8339, (800) 281-8749; http://www.nsf.gov/funding/research_edu_community.jsp

Nonprofit Resource Center includes many helpful links, including foundation sites and management advice for administrators, board members, and volunteers of nonprofit organizations as well as people who are considering forming a nonprofit organization. http://not-for-profit.org

Nonprofit Online News delivers news of the online nonprofit community and is free by e-mail. http://news.gilbert.org/

OhioLine. Ohio State University Extension, OhioLine provides access to fact sheets, bulletins, and other educational materials covering a wide array of subjects such as agriculture, natural resources, family and consumer sciences, community development, partnerships, 4-H clubs, and youth.

Ohio Literacy Resource Center provides links to grant writing information and funding information on the Internet. http://literacy.kent.edu/Oasis/grants_funding.html. It also provides links to Grantshotline.com (http://www.grantshotline.com/), a newsletter about funding for education, local governments, and law enforcement.

Philanthropy Journal Online is an electronic publication of the *Philanthropy Journal of North Carolina.* Its searchable site offers news on fund-raising, volunteers, foundations, and more. http://gort.ucsd.edu/newjour/p/msg02367.html

Philanthropy Links furnishes links to Philanthropy Research Centers. http://www.lib.msu.edu/harris23/grants/zphilres.htm

Virtual Foundation is an online philanthropy program that supports grassroots initiatives around the world. Screened projects are posted on the website, where they can be read and funded by online donors. http://www.virtualfoundation.org/

Mutz, J., and Murray, K. *Fundraising For Dummies,* 2nd ed. Foster City, Calif.: IDG Books Worldwide, Inc., 2000. A fun-to-read, straightforward, yet detailed, guide to the art and science of raising money for nonprofits. It covers all the changes in tax law, philanthropy in general, and the business environment since 2001. It provides information on developing a fund-raising plan, conducting donor research, cultivating major givers, writing grant proposals, online donations and fund-raising, new rules for faith-based organizations, finding and training volunteers, and direct mail.

PART FOUR

COALITIONS AND PARTNERSHIPS IN ACTION

CHAPTER ELEVEN

Community Assessment

*The relevant question is not simply what shall we do tomorrow, but
rather what shall we do today in order to get ready for tomorrow.*
—Peter Drucker, writer, management consultant,
university professor, 1909–2005

Before coalitions can begin work to achieve their mission and goals, they must work to become grounded within their communities. The first task is to focus on issues that resonate with the community. If the issue is mandated by a grant or contract, the coalition must engage the community and develop awareness of and support for the issue by framing it within the context of the community. The type of issue that is chosen or mandated will affect the makeup of the coalition and its scope of work.

Next, the coalition must determine the priority population that will be the focus of its intervention and projects, and figure out how to meaningfully involve this group in its efforts. The best way to involve the priority community and the institutions and organizations that serve them is to conduct a community assessment with a specific concentration on the health issues the community faces. The SWOT analysis, discussed in Chapter Eight, is an assessment of the strengths, weaknesses, and opportunities that the coalition demonstrates in relation to its community. Assessments usually rely on several methods of gathering and analyzing data, creating data reports, and disseminating the results of the assessment. Each facet of community assessment will be covered in this chapter. The strategic and action plans that detail how the coalition will use the assessment data are the subject of Chapter Twelve.

CHOOSING COALITION ISSUE(S) THAT RESONATE WITH THE COMMUNITY

Kretzmann and McKnight (1993) set forth powerful arguments for building healthy communities from the inside out, while recognizing that each community possesses a unique combination of assets upon which to build its future. The reasons for rejecting a need- or problem-based approach are clear: viewing a community as problem-ridden is demoralizing for residents, reinforces stereotypes among outsiders, fragments efforts to provide solutions, and directs funding primarily to service providers instead of residents (Kretzmann and McKnight, 1993, p. 4).

There are compelling reasons for using an asset-based approach. First, evidence indicates that significant community development takes place only when community members are committed to invest themselves and their resources in the effort. Second, in light of recent budget constraints, significant help from outside the community is unlikely (Kretzmann and McKnight, 1993, p. 5). The key to empowered, healthy communities is to locate available assets, connect them with one another to maximize their effectiveness, and engage local institutions, organizations, and other partners in the effort. Although the authors did not specifically name coalitions as a necessity, their vital role in the process of community development should not be missed.

In the ideal world, all coalitions and partnerships for health promotion and disease prevention would be formed in response to issues that were chosen by the community in question. This community-development approach is the model most likely to lead to sustained coalition efforts that respond to dynamic environmental conditions. The coalitions would be resource-rich, broad-based, multi-issue partnerships that shift priorities as community conditions mandate.

However, most communities do not find themselves in this situation during the first decade of the twenty-first century in America. Instead, they are reeling from a shift in federal and state priorities that has drastically cut direct funding for local services and programs. Health education and clinical and research services are no exception. The expectation is that faith-based institutions, community-based organizations, and voluntary agencies will pick up the slack and partner with health departments, hospitals and health care providers, social service agencies, and academic institutions to promote health and prevent disease. Resources are scarce, volunteers are few, and the health issues that communities face are complex and costly. Coalitions have become a popular strategy out of necessity.

Preferably, any assessment should begin with the community, gathering viable partners and having them self-assess their resources and identify the health issues on which they would most like to focus. This is preferable to searching for outside resources to find a community or coalition interested in working on a specific health issue. However, a compromise approach uses community assets to focus on an identified health issue(s) within the community. Lofquist's (1983) prevention model focuses on the strengths and assets of community members and associations, their skills and social capital (McKnight and Kretzmann, 1984), and civic participation

(Putnam, 1995). The principles of this asset-based model emphasize the immediate social community in which participants reside as the context for intervention; the strengths represented by human diversity, or "participatory inclusiveness"; expandable, renewable, sustainable, and environmentally benign resources; and program accountability and evaluation (Schmidt, 1998).

Issue identification, whether sparked from an outside funding opportunity or from within the community itself, is only a starting point. The involvement of a community coalition in developing a plan of action to improve health is the first step that partners commit to as they work to transform the community and themselves. Success in improving one set of health outcomes can be used as a springboard and capacity builder for tackling larger issues or ones that emanate solely from the community.

Kahn (1991) suggests that coalition members ask themselves the following set of questions before they decide to focus on a particular issue:

- Will the coalition be able to impact the issue—in other words, is it solvable and winnable?
- Will the issue build a coalition to the extent that members will be involved?
- Will the issue unite people and motivate them to act upon it?
- Will the issue affect a sufficient number of people and create a critical mass to warrant a coalition?

See Exhibit 11.1 for a checklist that coalitions can use for choosing a problem or issue.

FRAMING THE ISSUE TO BUILD SUPPORT

A coalition initiative will compete with other obligations that community partners face and may invite potential costs and risks as well. Partners must perceive a payoff and the promise of positive change in order to embrace the coalition issue as a priority. Some issues such as concerns about children, safety, healthy housing, threats to natural resources, and concerns and fears about health or disease have global appeal in motivating communities to participate in coalition efforts (Mattesich and Monsey, 2005).

Recognition or awareness of the issue as important. Recognition of an issue can occur from inside or outside the community. A concerned citizen or pastor of a local church may identify the issue, or someone outside the community, such as a local health department employee or a state legislator, may do so. However, successful coalition efforts are more likely to occur in communities where residents recognize the need for some type of collaborative initiative and take ownership. Community residents must perceive that the health problem or issue exists, that it is important enough to warrant their attention, and

Exhibit 11.1. Checklist for Choosing Coalition Problems or Issues.

To compare issues and choose the best one(s) for your coalition to focus on, use this checklist of questions, or have your coalition adapt it or develop their own criteria. For each potential issue, place a check mark under *Yes, No,* or *Unsure.* If an issue receives an *unsure* answer, then coalition members must do further research to clarify it.

Will the issue (or resolving the problem) . . .	Yes	No	Unsure
Result in a real improvement in people's lives?			
Give people a sense of their own power?			
Build strong, lasting organizations?			
Raise awareness about democratic rights?			
Change power relations?			
Be worthwhile?			
Be winnable?			
Be widely felt?			
Be deeply felt?			
Be easy to communicate and understand?			
Provide opportunities for people to learn about and be involved in policies and decisions?			
Have clear advocacy targets?			
Have a clear, feasible time frame?			
Be nondivisive among potential partners and priority population?			
Build accountable leadership?			
Be consistent with community values and vision?			
Provide potential for developing resources and raising funds?			
Link local issues to regional, national, or global issues?			

Source: Adapted from Bobo, Kendall, and Max, 2001, pp. 24–28.

that it affects enough of their residents to encourage self-interest in participation (Mattesich and Monsey, 2005).

Building community ownership of the issue. Once it is recognized as important, the next step is building community ownership of the issue. By designing coalitions where citizens are engaged from the start, community ownership is built in right away in a bottom-up fashion (Wolff, 2001a). Creating community ownership requires a different approach in how the coalition is initiated and in how power is shared. Community members must be involved in first defining the issues and then identifying solutions and strategies. As Kaye and Wolff put it, "There are no greater architects of solutions than those who are experiencing the problem" (1995, p. 102). These authors acknowledge that practitioners and professionals bring invaluable information and skills for developing programs and strategies to the coalition table, but grassroots community members know how to engage the community to market those programs to reach high-risk populations. Finally, community members must be given the tools and resources to implement programs and strategies, rather than having their creative ideas used by professionals.

Few studies explain how partnerships prioritize issues and set agendas, but most coalitions engage in a process of discerning the most important community issues, whether by formal health assessments or surveys (Roussos and Fawcett, 2000).

CDC's Community Coalition Partnership Programs for the Prevention of Teen Pregnancy (CCPP) provides a good example of how a community identified its priorities and views regarding teen pregnancy prevention and framed the coalition's approach accordingly (The National Campaign to Prevent Teen Pregnancy, 2003). In many communities, issues like crime, substance abuse, and unemployment were higher on the agenda than preventing teen pregnancy. Furthermore, communities were polarized, with some partners favoring an abstinence-only approach and others wanting to include information about contraception as well.

By framing the issue of preventing teen pregnancy within a broader youth development philosophy, coalitions provided a "big tent" that helped recruit new partners and bring together advocates of an abstinence-only approach with those wanting more comprehensive approaches (The National Campaign to Prevent Teen Pregnancy, 2003, p. 10). Organizations and constituencies focused on other issues could join these coalitions with broader issues that included their priorities as well as others. Confident that their concerns would be addressed, organizations were motivated to join the coalitions. Groups with strong views about the issue were reassured that the coalitions would not promote a single approach but instead would encourage diverse strategies. The goal was to define teen pregnancy prevention in such a way that the broadest array of potential coalition members could embrace the effort. Usually, staff and founding members first framed the issue of teen pregnancy prevention. Then, as new members joined the coalition, discussion ensued and the approach was redefined. Once community assessments were conducted and the community's views were known, the issue was often reframed again.

The California Healthy Cities and Communities Project promoted increased community capacity within their partnerships and communities by sharing principles of broad community engagement and emphasizing a noncategorical assets approach, rather than focusing on predetermined problems and needs. The most visible evidence of increased capacity included leadership, mechanisms for participant interaction and dialogue, interorganizational and social networks, skill building, and leveraged resources (Kegler, Norton, and Aronson, 2003). Community capacity was also found to be an important precondition and facilitating factor for the community-development process.

IMPACT OF THE ISSUE ON THE COALITION

The issue(s) that a coalition chooses to work on can also have an impact on the coalition itself. If the coalition is formed with a prevention focus, then it might be a stretch to include a specific disease issue. For example, a coalition formed to promote healthy nutrition and fitness might be derailed if it became entrenched in issues related to improved management of diabetes. Likewise, a coalition that focuses on improving access to primary care services for children would have to seriously consider taking on a pregnancy prevention program for teens. As coalitions mature, they are faced with many difficult decisions about whether to focus on single versus multiple issues; expand geographically, in other words, from one neighborhood to an entire city, to a region; focus on health promotion versus disease prevention and management activities; focus on educational activities versus advocacy efforts or service provision; or expand the age range, or ethnic or racial groups of interest.

As the recognition of coalition efforts and respect in the community increases, these decisions occur more frequently. Likewise, the promise of new resources and the clamor by potential partners for attention to their issues may compromise a coalition's original intentions. The coalition must carefully define its vision, mission, goals, and objectives to ensure that each of the above decisions matches those parameters. Coalition members and leaders should be jointly involved in deciding the coalition's direction. It is best for a coalition to proceed slowly and use evaluation results to inform its choices concerning issues that it can resolve most effectively.

PRIORITY POPULATIONS

Closely related to the impact of the issue is how priority populations are chosen for intervention. If the coalition is formed around priorities for senior citizens, then the funding and choice of issue should logically follow. The term *priority population* as opposed to *target population* is used here deliberately. In public health epidemiology, we are inured to the word *target* because we generally use it to describe a population or vector of interest. However, in coalition and community building, the term can be dehumanizing and demeaning. No person or group of people would like to be "targeted" or described as the "target" of an intervention. Instead, consider how the term *priority* changes the focus to one that is positive, caring, and energizing. The meaning and the work are transformed by substituting the term *priority population* for the more generally used *target population*. Brown (1984) suggests a set of questions that can help coalitions decide who makes up the priority population for any coalition effort:

- Who is directly affected by the issue?
- Who has similar interests or concerns?
- Who has a vested interest in the outcome?
- Who might be threatened by the outcome?
- Who is respected or powerful in the community?
- Who has acted on this issue in the past or might in the future?
- Who can help you reach other potential members?

For instance, the pregnancy prevention partnerships that were previously described (CCPP) found that before they could recruit coalition members, they had to lay the groundwork by defining the boundaries of the community and identifying the priority population to be served (The National Campaign to Prevent Teen Pregnancy, 2003, p. 10). CCPP was designed to focus on neighborhoods and population groups with high teen pregnancy rates, but defining neighborhood boundaries was more complex than expected.

Census tract data was used to identify the areas with high teen pregnancy or birth rates, and, when possible, coalitions broke out this data for specific population groups, such as African Americans, Hispanics, and Native Americans. However, relying solely on census tract data divided by zip codes sometimes produced boundaries that did not correspond to actual neighborhoods. Neighborhoods often crossed zip codes, and sometimes several neighborhoods coexisted within one zip code area.

Also, real neighborhoods were typically defined by socioeconomic and racial or ethnic boundaries as well as by physical boundaries, such as bridges, roads, rivers, and train tracks. The solution was to use census tract data as well as physical boundaries and socioeconomic factors to define neighborhoods. The Allies Against Asthma initiative encountered similar issues when coalitions attempted to describe by zip codes neighborhoods with the highest rates of emergency room visits and hospitalizations due to asthma (Butterfoss, Kelly, and Taylor-Fishwick, 2005).

INVOLVING THE PRIORITY POPULATION IN THE WORK

The key to developing community ownership is involving members of the priority population in the coalition's work. When community members who understand the needs, assets, priorities, and dynamics of the community are involved in identifying and prioritizing issues, planning and implementing strategies, and evaluating the results of their endeavors, the strategies are more likely to be effective and well received by the community, and the sustainability of community partnerships is increased (Lasker and Weiss, 2003). Consequently, the continued commitment and participation of key community members is more likely to be sustained over time, and community members are more likely to become involved in similar efforts in the future. For example, coalition members involved in planning comprehensive immunization promotion and asthma management programs for children rated their planning abilities as high or moderately high, agreed that the plan reflected the needs assessment and that it would be effective, and were satisfied with the assessment and planning process (Butterfoss and others, 1998; Butterfoss, Kelly, and Taylor-Fishwick, 2005).

In another example, youth have been integrated into pregnancy prevention and tobacco control coalitions in a variety of ways. They play pivotal roles in carrying out community assessments and presenting the results to their communities. Youth advisory panels are established to provide feedback and to counsel the coalition on strategy and direction. By engaging youth in the process, coalitions learned what teens really think and what strategies might work with their peers. To encourage youth involvement, coalitions offer material incentives, such as gas coupons, money, movie tickets, and food. It should be noted, however, that youth often join coalitions for less tangible rewards, such as the opportunity to form new friendships, express their views, and develop leadership, teaching, training, and other related skills.

AN ASSET-BASED APPROACH TO COMMUNITY ASSESSMENTS

A community assessment is a type of evaluation that tries to understand the context of a coalition by fully describing the priority community (as defined by the coalition). Such assessments are often called *needs assessments* in public health, but because coalitions should aspire to use an asset-based approach, the term *community assessment* is used here to refer to the realistic appraisal of a community's strengths, assets, and challenges (Kretzmann and McKnight, 1993, 2005). A community assessment involves evaluating the current situation in the community, reaching value-based judgments regarding the preferred or desired situation, and prioritizing local concerns.

An assessment is usually performed in the beginning stages of a coalition's development in order to better understand the community and to determine how the coalition can best address the local community's concerns and problems. However, both communities and coalitions are dynamic and develop over time. As a continuous understanding of the community's strengths, needs, resources, and makeup is critical, regular (yearly or biannual) assessments of the community will help any coalition be more proactive, responsive, and effective. The acquisition of some information drives the need to obtain more information.

A community assessment often begins by identifying the community's problems and weaknesses instead of its assets (Besser, 1995). A problem orientation forces a community to focus on what is wrong, ignore what is right, overlook valuable internal resources, and view themselves as recipients and consumers instead of producers (Kretzmann and McKnight, 1993). It defines vision according to what others expect and depends upon available new programs or potential employers. Outside funders expect communities to demonstrate that they have a serious problem (worse than in other communities) to be eligible for financial support. Kretzmann and McKnight (1993) further suggest that communities must look inside themselves to find direction and resources and that outside resources will be used more effectively if the community is invested and mobilized.

Asset-based community assessment begins by examining four areas to determine community strengths (Kretzmann and McKnight, 1993):

- An inventory is taken of the gifts, skills, and capacities of community members, including those who are often overlooked, for example, youth and children, the elderly, the mentally challenged, or low-income groups.
- A list is generated of neighborhood associations, church groups, bowling leagues, parent–teacher organizations, support and self-help groups, and civic and fraternal groups. Names of their officers and members, as well as their mission statements, are obtained.
- Formal institutions, such as schools, churches, private businesses, government agencies, hospitals, and retirement communities, are examined for their strengths and resources.
- Local physical characteristics, such as geographic features and resources, buildings, housing, transportation, and utility systems, are evaluated.

Once community assets are recognized, community members can be involved in creating a vision for the future and an action plan to realize that vision. An asset-based orientation emphasizes the importance of building and sustaining relationships among all coalitions and other groups, associations, and institutions. Research consistently shows that friendship ties between people form the basis for community spirit and persistence in the face of threats (Besser, 1995); therefore, a coalition that focuses on assets and rebuilds local relationships is more likely to develop a strong community.

A community assessment may assess the demographic characteristics, risk and protective factors, or the types of prevention and treatment programs, practices, and policies that exist within the community. Coalitions have to decide several issues in advance of conducting the assessment, namely, the boundaries of the assessment (defined geographically or by age, income, or racial or ethnic groups); area(s) to be served by the coalition; organizations that have similar interests and whether they will be supportive or competitive; available resources; whether the coalition's actions will be seen as intrusive; the specific questions about the health issues; and whether other issues are considered to be more urgent by the community.

Hancock and Minkler (2005) also distinguish between conducting *a community health assessment,* which focuses on health status, versus conducting a *healthy community assessment,* which focuses on positive health status and low levels of disease, as well as the community's commitment to improve the health, well-being, and quality of life of its members. A community health assessment is only one component of a healthy community assessment (which includes ten other components such as a clean, safe environment, a thriving economy, and a rich cultural heritage) (Hancock and Duhl, 1986).

BENEFITS AND CHALLENGES OF CONDUCTING ASSESSMENTS

Coalitions can accrue many benefits by conducting community assessments. The coalition can use these data to assess strengths, prioritize real needs within the community, ensure that efforts are not duplicated, and understand the resources that exist to implement desired programs, practices, and polices. A community assessment can also help determine resource gaps that must be filled to accomplish coalition goals. The gap between what *is* and what *should be* may help the coalition establish objectives for programs, select the strategy a program might use, or design or modify the program. Community assessments also can be used to evaluate progress in reducing a discrepancy or gap, similar to the way data from pre-tests and post-tests are used (Archer, Cripe, and McCaslin, 2005).

As the assessment is conducted, coalition members and staff come into contact with influential leaders, youth, and members of the clergy and business community, who may join the coalition's future efforts by becoming partners, providing resources, or offering to host a program or event. Thus the assessment is an important community mobilization tool in itself. Involvement of local leaders in the assessment lends credibility to the project in the wider community, and involvement of community residents helps to legitimize the coalition at the neighborhood level. Finally, collaborating to conduct these assessments helps identify similar personnel, facilities, equipment, and funds in other organizations and agencies, generates support for the cause, and increases clout with potential funders and policy makers (Archer, Cripe, and McCaslin, 1992).

Following are some other benefits that communities can realize from conducting assessments, according to the National Highway Traffic Safety Administration (U.S. Department of Transportation, 2001):

Community assessments make projects defensible, fundable, and measurable.
Coalition members can use community data to explain and defend their activities by describing their relationship to the actual problems. Members can also demonstrate the basis for their plan when they request participation or monetary assistance from government agencies, corporations, foundations, or other funders. Assessment data is often the basis for determining the efficacy of the program and may lead to subsequent funding.

Community assessments target resources. An assessment enables a coalition to use resources more effectively because solutions are targeted at the real causes of the problem. As resources for most coalitions are scarce, results can be achieved without wasting funding or time.

Community assessments can reenergize existing efforts. A new or improved initiative, identified by the assessment, can generate fresh perspectives and energize partners to become active again. Enthusiastic coalition members are crucial in obtaining funding and media attention, and advocating for legislative change.

Community assessments can help garner media attention. Media attention on an issue often unites a community to take action. The data should convince the media that the issue is worth covering. Newspaper and television coverage can raise awareness that an issue is serious and demands attention. This awareness makes it easier for a coalition to attract members, obtain funding, and make systems change.

Community assessments provide opportunities for reflection. By reviewing assessment data, the coalition can generate new ideas and alternatives, and decide whether to start new programs, improve existing ones, or replicate the ones that are working well. Existing programs or activities need reexamination to determine whether changes in the community make the effort relevant.

Community assessments involve coalition members in meaningful activities. Coalitions that engage partners in the design and execution of the assessment secure their support and commitment to the coalition's work. Assessments also give members opportunities to express their views and experiences and help collect data from other community members.

The challenges of conducting community assessments are similar to those encountered when engaging in any intense collaborative activity. Extra effort and increased meeting times are usually required; responsibilities may not be clearly determined and shared; and hidden agendas and turf battles may emerge when resources to conduct the assessment are scarce (Archer, Cripe, and McCaslin, 1992). To decrease problems, the coalition should involve members as much as possible in the assessment, stress how assessment data are crucial for obtaining funds from public and private sources, and make assessment findings public at an event that acknowledges partners' contributions.

CONDUCTING THE ASSESSMENT

A comprehensive community assessment usually includes collection and analysis of data, a policy review, and a review of current programs, activities, and resources. Before beginning a needs assessment, the coalition must come to agreement on what is going to be assessed, what data are already collected and known, what further data are needed, how and by whom that data will be collected, and how and by whom it will be analyzed.

Although no right way has ever been agreed upon for conducting a community assessment, Witkin and Altschuld (1995) provide a three-phase process for conducting community assessments, from pre-assessment, to assessment, to post-assessment. Based on these phases, the following eight steps appear to be critical:

1. Determining the assessment's purpose and scope
2. Defining the assessment's goals and objectives
3. Selecting the approach and methods for collecting data
4. Designing and pilot-testing the instruments and procedures
5. Preparing a timeline and budget
6. Collecting the data
7. Analyzing the data
8. Preparing and disseminating a report of findings
9. Evaluating the assessment's merit and worth

Each step will be expanded upon during the rest of this chapter.

Determining the Assessment's Purpose and Scope

Key stakeholders and key decision makers should decide first whether a community assessment is necessary and appropriate. The coalition must also consider whether the assessment is being done to generate awareness, to satisfy a mandate, as part of a funding process, as an aid in decision making, or to promote a specific action plan. Finally, stakeholders will want to know how extensive and resource intensive the assessment will be.

Defining the Assessment's Goals and Objectives

What type of information is needed: demographic, awareness, attitudinal, or behavioral? Who is the priority audience? Is the coalition concerned about those who are currently served or the total community? If categorical funding does not dictate what health problems should be addressed or if an assessment has not been conducted for a long time, then coalition planners must collect a wide range of data, compare the importance of multiple health problems, and set priorities. If the coalition plans to focus its assessment on an identified health issue (perhaps in response to categorical funding from a federal source), then it will be important to determine the prevalence of the issue, the population it most affects, the high-risk subpopulation, economic costs, and trends over time (McKenzie, Neiger, and Smeltzer, 2005, p. 89).

Selecting the Approach and Methods for Collecting Data

Does the needed information exist or is more data collection needed? If the type of information that is needed is not available, then it must be collected. Common methods that coalitions use for gathering information about the community and its partnerships include the following (Phillips, 1997; Taylor-Powell, Rossing, and Geran, 1998):

- Written survey (handout, telephone, fax, mail, e-mail, or Internet)
- Interview (individual or key informant and group; structured or semi-structured)

- Public or community forum
- Observation (windshield tours, Photovoice, and critical incident reporting)
- Document or content analysis
- Case study
- Group assessment (structured brainstorming, Nominal Group, or Delphi Processes, all of which elicit and rank priorities, set goals, and identify problems)
- Role play, dramatization
- Expert or peer review
- Portfolio review
- Testimonials and storytelling
- Hypothetical scenarios
- Developing community health indicators (CHIs)
- Geographical, asset, and concept mapping
- Neighborhood and community profiles
- Pile sorting (respondents freely categorize items and reveal perceptions of a domain)
- Free-listing (method to elicit a complete list of all items in a cultural domain)
- Social network diagramming
- Simulation, modeling
- Debriefing sessions
- Photography, drawing, art, videography, and photonovella
- Diaries or journals
- Logs, activity forms, and registries.

Butler and Howell note that the "quality of information about a community is only as good as the technique or combination of techniques used. A single technique may be too narrow in the information it provides; using too many methods may be costly in terms of time and dollars" (1980, p. 4). For most assessment activities, these techniques can be successfully used in concert with one another. For example, the Key Informant Approach and the Nominal Group Technique can be employed to generate the types of questions to be included in a formal survey of the community.

Selected approaches should be based on the nature and extent of information needed by the coalition to assess the current situation, size, and characteristics of the priority population(s); the coalition's relationship with the priority population(s); and the level of resources available for securing such data (for example, time frame, number of people involved in collecting and analyzing data, financial assets). Some methods involve little or no contact with the community (for example, neighborhood profiles and review of extant data); others are observational and involve minimal contact (for example, windshield tours and asset mapping); and still others are interactive (for example, focus groups, surveys, interviews) (Hancock and Minkler, 2005). A selected sample of methods commonly used by coalitions and partnerships, as well as their advantages and disadvantages, follows.

Neighborhood and community profiles. Census data and other sources of secondary data can be used to describe the demographic, social, health, and economic characteristics of a community. Data can be compiled on the quality of housing and the incidence of crime as well as on income, employment, health status, education, and other social and economic indicators of well-being. These profiles can also draw on interviews with community leaders and residents, observations from windshield surveys, published reports of the community's social and health status, and historical records of how it has dealt with the health issue in question.

The advantages of creating community profiles are that the data are often readily available and do not require time and undue expense to obtain. However, the data may not be in a usable format; in other words, the neighborhood data may be broken down by one unit of analysis and the coalition needs by another (for example, data is available by region of the city, but zip code data is needed). Other disadvantages are that the data may not be properly cleaned or checked for accuracy, may be out of date, or may only be accessed by authorized users. For instance, hospitalization data may be collected at the state level, but data on hospital admissions to the emergency department may only be available on an individual hospital basis. Likewise, prescription claims data may be available for Medicaid and Medicare recipients, but not for self-pay or private insurance users. Coalition members for key institutions are valuable links to accessing needed data sources. Coalitions should also be aware of the tendency to "drown in data" and should try to focus on useful secondary data.

Standardized tests (physiological, knowledge, achievement, attitudinal, or psychological). These tests can be used to measure participants' health and mental status, knowledge, attitudes, beliefs, or behavior. Written pre- and post-tests can help determine what participants need to learn in a program and then measure the outcomes of what was actually learned. Systematic observations of behavior can be conducted and compared to standardized indices for coding observations. Client–patient satisfaction surveys can be used to rate existing health services or reactions to a program. Health surveys can measure general health (including items on physical, emotional, and social function), mental health and depression, and disability status. Screenings can be done to measure blood pressure, serum cholesterol, genetic markers, and urinary byproducts of nicotine, steroids, and other drugs. Although physiological measures can provide clear quantitative data for analysis, the accuracy of measurement instruments, skill of those taking the measurements, and confounding variables related to environmental conditions or the individual on whom measurements are taken are disadvantages of these methods (Butterfoss, Francisco, and Capwell, 2000).

Development of community health indicators (CHIs). Coalitions can also work with community partners and residents to develop community health indicators (CHIs), quantitative and qualitative measures that indicate the health status of a community over time (Bauer, 2003). Qualitative measures might include the number of nonsmoking restaurants or the availability of nutritious snacks in school vending machines in the community. Quantitative measures might include the percentage of children who are overweight or obese in the school district or the percentage of adults who are over age sixty-five in nursing homes and have had their flu shots.

Good community indicators should reflect health determinants (for example, air quality) as well as process indicators (for example, education and civil rights) (Hancock, LaBonte, and Edwards, 1999). Hancock and colleagues (1999) note that the relevance of CHIs for community members and policy makers is increased when they make sense to people, measure an important health determinant or characteristic that people care about, and carry social and political "punch." By categorizing the indicators and testing their importance through querying community members via interviews, focus groups, or Nominal Group Process in small group settings, CHIs can help coalitions mobilize the community and select issues of importance to focus on.

Document review. Records kept for purposes that are directly or indirectly related to the program being evaluated can provide valuable information. These data include insurance or pharmacy claims data, enrollment or attendance records, transportation routes and scheduling, media PSA airing, or financial records necessary to conduct cost analyses (Tyler Norris Associates, 1997). Internal documents (such as mission statements, organizational charts, annual reports, activity schedules, funding proposals, portfolios, proceedings, policies or legislation, curricula, and promotional literature) are another helpful source of evaluation data. They provide information about the history, philosophy, goals, and outcomes of a particular project and the level of program development or maturity.

Reports can detail how the project began, how it is currently organized, what it claims to do, how it intends to reach its objectives, the nature of its target population, and what efforts are being made to achieve sustainability (W. K. Kellogg Foundation, 1994, p. 83). Promotional literature, such as brochures and flyers (or the lack of them), can help a coalition assess program outreach. Logs and diaries provide insights into project activities, staff relations, key events, and changes in the program over time. Minutes of meetings give information on attendance, dominance and other role relations, planning, and decision making. This method is used often because of the low cost and ease of accessing information (especially by searching databases available on state and government websites). However, sometimes, extant data are unavailable, inconsistent, or difficult or costly to obtain. Further advantages and disadvantages of this method are covered in Table 11.1.

Table 11.1. Advantages and Disadvantages of Observations and Document Review.

Observations

Advantages	Disadvantages
Can collect highly credible, first-hand data about what actually happens	Needs credible, well-trained observers
	Presence of observers may alter what occurs
Permits understanding beyond what can be obtained through interviews	
May provide unanticipated information	Time-consuming to develop instruments, guidelines, and to train observers
Provides outside perspective	Time-consuming to schedule and conduct multiple observations

Document Review

Advantages	Disadvantages
Saves time and effort of developing data-collection instruments	Sensitive information may be missing, dated, unreliable, or incomplete
Data can be collected in a relatively unobtrusive manner.	Accessing existing documents may require substantial effort, due to ethical or legal constraints
Efficiency of time and resources	
Credible because information was gathered as events occurred	Examining documents, extracting data can be time-consuming and costly
	Need to train reviewers and validate reviews to assure reliability and accuracy
	Cannot obtain information about relationships or interactions

Source: Adapted from Butterfoss, Francisco, and Capwell, 2000. From "Choosing Effective Evaluation Methods," by F. D. Butterfoss, V. T. Francisco, & E. M. Capwell in *Health Promotion Practice, 1*(4), 307–313. Copyright © 2000 by Sage Publications, Inc. Reproduced with permission of Sage Publications Inc. via Copyright Clearance Center.

Observations. One way to collect information is to observe the activities of staff and participants in community-based programs. Observation may indicate strengths and weaknesses in operations and suggest ideas for improvement. Information gathered through observation will help program planners formulate questions that can be used in interviews or surveys; examine the physical and social setting, staff and consumer characteristics, group dynamics, and formal and informal activities; become aware of aspects of a program that may not be consciously acknowledged by participants or staff; learn about issues that program staff or participants are unwilling to discuss; and observe how activities evolve over time (W. K. Kellogg Foundation, 1995, p. 73).

More unobtrusive evaluation measures are useful when interaction with the priority population could alter the accuracy of the evaluation information obtained. Observations allow us to obtain information about what actually occurs from different perspectives (Martin and Pear, 1992). Observations can range from quantitative tabulation of actions to qualitative field observation of complex social interactions. Examples of quantifiable observations are counting infants who wear seatbelts in car safety seats or noting the length of time patients wait in a clinical setting (Bernard, 1998). A considerable amount of information can be gained about what actually happens, not just what is reported, by training interviewers to use a carefully developed instrument. Photographs and video recordings allow other members of the evaluation team to observe these behaviors. Even the most passive, unobtrusive observer is likely to affect the events under observation. Here are some points to consider when doing observations for assessment or evaluation purposes (W. K. Kellogg Foundation, p. 74):

- Establish goals for the observation, but be prepared to modify them on site if needed. Develop instruments to record observations efficiently, so observers can concentrate on what is happening on site. If these instruments do not work well, modify them.

- If time is limited and the project occurs over multiple sites, concentrate on collecting data that are most useful. Decide how observation can be used to complement or corroborate the data collected from other sources (for example, surveys, interviews, focus groups).

- Systematically observe diverse participants at many sites at various times on different days.

- Set aside time to discuss observations with the evaluation team to help put the observed events in context and gain a better understanding of what happened.

For coalitions, the advantage of observational approaches is that they help identify community problems, resources, and details about neighborhoods, such as the places where priority populations assemble. These methods also provide opportunities to discuss the coalition's plan and project(s) with residents and to recruit them to the coalition. They are not costly to implement, the only expenses being mileage and disposable cameras. And by involving students from local colleges, as well as members, coalitions can easily use them to jump-start the action phase of work.

One disadvantage is that a coalition must provide for the personal safety of its surveyors or observers in neighborhoods where the crime rate is high. The safety of these individuals will be promoted if they are wearing clothing with the coalition's logo prominently displayed, have identification that connects them to the coalition, and carry a flyer or short description of the project. Observers also may encounter linguistic and cultural barriers when their backgrounds differ from those of neighborhood residents. Further advantages and disadvantages of these methods are found in Table 11.1.

Windshield tours or surveys. A specialized observation technique called windshield tours offers coalitions an opportunity to obtain a hands-on view of the community. By driving or walking through neighborhoods, observers can inspect the physical, geographic, social, and economic characteristics of an area (Quinn, 2000). Observations must be made at different times of the day and different days of the week to fully capture the life of the community. A windshield tour is not a research method in the formal sense, but the coalition can develop a standard form for reporting observations by adapting existing forms. Alternatively, observers could just take free-form notes. Observers are urged to drive or walk through the community with open eyes and minds, and record their first impressions, in other words, what they see, hear, smell, and feel by observing (Eng and Blanchard, 1991). Here is a list of some observations that could be made:

- Biophysical elements: housing (type, variety, availability, condition), grocery stores, restaurants
- Education: schools, libraries
- Religious and expressive: churches, synagogues, other places of worship
- Politics: county courthouse, jail, city hall
- Transportation: condition of roads, availability of public transportation
- Recreation: availability and accessibility of recreational facilities, who participates
- Topography and geography: major features, obstacles, physical barriers
- Economy: worksites, signs of unemployment
- Interaction: locations where people congregate
- Health and medical care needs: hospitals, nursing homes, health-related businesses, pharmacies
- People: ethnic groups, ages, genders

Asset mapping. A windshield tour may lead to the process of identifying the assets of institutions, organizations, groups, and even individuals that exist in your community. The coalition can create an asset list, with members assisting by adding and drawing upon community resources such as these (Community Toolbox, 2005): yellow pages and community directories, lists of businesses from the Chamber of Commerce; published and unpublished lists of organizations from the library or town hall; other print sources, such as local and regional newspapers and community newsletters; bulletin boards in community gathering places; community calendars on cable television; and friends and colleagues who may know of other informal groups and organizations.

The list of assets can be broken down in several different ways, for example, alphabetically, geographically, or by function, size, public or private membership, or governance. The list could also be mapped to visually clarify the patterns (coined *asset mapping* by Kretzmann and McKnight, 1993). One mapping method is to use a street map of the community from the local planning department and to mark the locations of community institutions, groups, and organizations with symbols or colored pushpins. This makes patterns stand out; for instance, some parts of town have many different types of associations and some have few. This type of mapping can also be done with computer software programs that create overlays by placing one kind of map over another. Finally, resources can be diagrammed graphically to show the *linkages* among different types of assets.

Photovoice. Windshield tours can also be combined with Photovoice techniques that capture the findings from the visual assessment on camera (Wang and Burris, 1994, 1997; McDonald, Sarche, and Wang, 2005). Coalition and community members are given cameras and asked to photograph everyday health and work activities and realities. Then they engage in critical dialogue about the pictures and their context by asking the following questions (McDonald, Sarche, and Wang, 2005, p. 338; Shaffer, 1983):

- What do you see here?
- What is really happening here?
- How does this relate to our lives?
- Why does this problem, concern, or strength exist?
- What can we do about it?

The ultimate goal of Photovoice is to reach policymakers with heartfelt issues in order to obtain funding for new and existing community-based programs to improve health and welfare.

Critical incident technique. This technique involves collecting brief, written, factual reports of actions in response to explicit situations or problems (Witkin and Altschuld, 1995). An incident is considered critical when the action taken contributed to (1) an effective outcome in which it helped to solve a problem or resolve a situation; or (2) an ineffective outcome in which it partially resolved a problem, but created new problems or a need for further action. Critical incident reports may be written by qualified observers, participants who took action, or both.

Public forums. Public forums are used to gather data concerning issues and community needs from a wide range of residents. The coalition or one of its members sponsors a series of public meetings (forums) where participants discuss the issues that face the community, the priority needs, and what can be done about them. In conducting a public forum, broad questions such as those presented here serve as the basis for group discussion:

- What are the most important issues facing this community?
- What has been done to address these issues in the past?
- Where have we failed in our attempts to address these issues?

Public forums are most useful where specific issues are being addressed. A strategically located place, geographically and socially acceptable to all segments of the population and conducive to openly exchanging ideas, is selected for the initial meeting. The purpose, date, and place at which the forum will be held are publicized, using flyers and the media to encourage all members of the community to attend. Special invitations may be extended to other key informants.

The coalition should organize and conduct the first meeting. After stating the objectives and ground rules, the facilitator poses the prepared questions to the audience. Open discussion and interchange of ideas is encouraged. A recorder is responsible for documenting the ideas and suggestions presented at the meeting. If the meeting is effective, topics and directions for possible future forums will emerge, and the coalition can assemble an ad hoc committee of participants to plan the next meeting. The names of all the participants should be collected so they may be contacted before the next forum. Listening sessions are similar to public forums, also used to build community involvement in the assessment process, but are generally smaller.

Community forums offer a flexible way to elicit opinions from a wide range of people and enhance communication between providers and consumers of services and programs, and are inexpensive and easy to implement. They provide a quick, intensive picture of community concerns, give community issues broad visibility, and suggest questions that need further study (Carter and Beaulieu, 1992, pp. 4–5). However, the burden is on the sponsoring coalition and its members to encourage wide participation—forums require good leadership and advance organization. Although poor turnout is disappointing, a large turnout may prevent everyone from speaking and force time limits for each speaker. Forum participants may actually represent a variety of vested interest groups that use the sessions as a vehicle to publicize their grievances about local organizations or agencies; if these forums are not well facilitated, only vocal minorities will be heard (Carter and Beaulieu, 1992, p. 5). Finally, forums may generate more questions than answers and lead to unrealistic expectations.

Interviews. Oral questioning and recording by interviewers provides a way to verify and complement the information collected through observations (Bailey, 1996, p. 79). The knowledge gained from interviews also helps coalitions understand hard-to-measure concepts such as community participation, empowerment, and cohesiveness (W. K. Kellogg Foundation, p. 81). Phone surveys, such as the Behavioral Risk Factor Surveillance Survey, allow evaluators to question individuals who may be dispersed geographically. Face-to-face interviews—reaching individuals in their homes or workplaces, as is done by the U.S. Census Bureau—can derive more qualitative information about people's opinions, attitudes, or judgments. Because interviews provide in-depth and detailed information, they can be telling as to whether a program was implemented as originally planned and, if not, why and how the program has changed. This information helps policymakers and administrators understand how a program actually works and is useful for program replication.

Individual or key informant interviews. The purpose of key informant or opinion
  leader interviews is to collect information from community members who,
  because of their professional training, expertise, or affiliation with particular
  organizations or agencies, are in a prime position to know the issues and
  have special insights about their community or a particular health problem.
  These interviews also may provide information about perceptions of community needs that can guide program planning. Typical key informants might
  be elected officials (for example, mayors, county commissioners, state
  legislators), institutional representatives (for example, religious leaders,
  bankers, public safety officials, and school, hospital, and social service administrators), public service organization leaders (for example, Chamber of
  Commerce and Kiwanis Club), professionals in specific service areas (for
  example, physicians, lawyers, school faculty), or volunteer leaders (for example,
  chairs of parent–teacher and civic associations). In some cases, informal
  neighborhood or youth leaders can provide unusual perspectives.

Interviews provide coalitions with contextual feedback about their issue; the
available resources, assets, and services that address the issue; and recommendations for action. By conducting these interviews, the coalition will benefit from
diverse viewpoints, establish relationships within the community, build community
awareness of the project, and even recruit new participants to the coalition. These
interviews may range from semi-structured (with questions and leading probes for
further questioning) to unstructured (with a few very general questions that participants are invited to expound on), depending on the needs of stakeholders. Advantages and disadvantages of key informant interviews are found in Table 11.2.

First, the coalition must construct a brief interview form that elicits specific information about the key informant's demographic background, as well as perceptions or
attitudes about community strengths or needs (for example, the local economy, education, health services). The coalition must ask what is currently being done to meet
those needs and what should be done about unmet needs (Carter and Beaulieu, 1992,
p. 2). Then a list of key informants is compiled by name, and coalition staff, members,
or volunteers conduct interviews.

Key informant interviews are used often because the interview frameworks are
easier to develop than surveys; they save printing and data analysis cost; and they
can be conducted by community volunteers, which builds citizen and organizational
awareness and involvement. Qualitative interviews also establish rapport with
respondents to provide insider opinions, different perspectives, and rich information. The disadvantages of this approach are that results may be biased. To represent the whole community's perspective, the results should be combined with data
from other methods. Additionally, the persons who might provide the best
information may not hold visible positions in the community or wield enough power
and influence to be selected as informants.

The *snowball technique* is used to reach those individuals who may be omitted
using the traditional approach, but who are informal community leaders (Carter and
Beaulieu, 1992). In this technique, five individuals who hold official positions in the

Table 11.2. Advantages and Disadvantages of Surveys, Interviews, and Focus Groups.

Written Surveys

Advantages	Disadvantages
Can be answered anonymously	In mailed surveys, intended respondent may not be the one who completes it.
Can be administered to many people simultaneously; can be mailed	Difficult to persuade people to complete and return questionnaires
Allow respondent time to think before responding	Not all questions may be answered.
Impose uniformity by asking all respondents the same questions	Limited by simplicity of questions needed for the general public
Risk the least social desirability bias	Potential self-report bias
Are considered highly credible	Difficult to obtain results from open-ended items; respondents may be unable to express themselves easily
Are relatively easy to administer and complete	
Generate large amounts of data for aggregation and computer analysis	Time and expertise needed to develop valid and reliable instruments
	If survey is too short, data may be too general; if too detailed, respondents may be discouraged.

Interviews

Advantages	Disadvantages
Can obtain information from those who have difficulty reading, or understanding English	Costly to arrange for interviews for non-English speaking interviewees
	Time-consuming
Respondent has opportunity for free expression to reveal attitudes and feelings.	Difficult to reach intended respondent; respondents can screen calls
Higher response rate than mailed survey	Interviewer can influence responses due to dissimilarity with respondent (age, gender, race) or skill in interviewing
Nonverbal behaviors can be observed and recorded in face-to-face interviews	

Table 11.2. (Continued)

Focus Groups

Advantages	Disadvantages
Interview framework easy to design	Data more difficult to analyze
Require fewer respondents than surveys	More than one group is needed for reliability; difficult to access priority groups
High face validity	
Socially oriented; more natural environment	Nonquantitative; not representative
	Less control compared to individual interview
Can provide fast, low cost results	

Source: Adapted from Butterfoss, Francisco, and Capwell, 2000. From "Choosing Effective Evaluation Methods," by F. D. Butterfoss, V. T. Francisco, & E. M. Capwell in *Health Promotion Practice, 1*(4), 307–313. Copyright © 2000 by Sage Publications, Inc. Reproduced with permission of Sage Publications Inc. via Copyright Clearance Center.

community are selected and asked to name five to ten individuals who may be knowledgeable about community issues. The individuals most frequently mentioned by these key informants are asked to complete the same interview. If time and resources permit, these persons identify another five to ten people who they believe are knowledgeable about the issue(s). When the same names begin to reoccur, the process is at an end, and the most frequently mentioned persons are interviewed.

Permission must be obtained from interviewees if the interviews are to be tape-recorded. If recording makes interviewees uncomfortable, notes can be taken and other impressions recorded immediately after the interview. People may be interviewed individually or in groups. If concern exists about maintaining anonymity or ensuring that informants feel free to express unpopular ideas, people should be interviewed individually. This also allows the coalition to compare different perspectives, which is useful when the topic is sensitive. When confidentiality is not an issue and the coalition wants to obtain a range of opinions on a topic, a group interview is preferable.

Nominal Group Process. Nominal Group Process gathers information in a face-to-face non-threatening atmosphere. This technique takes advantage of each person's knowledge and experience, and is useful in generating and clarifying ideas, reaching consensus, prioritizing, and making decisions on alternative actions (Delbecq, Van de Ven, and Gustafson, 1975; Adler and Ziglio, 1996). If a large number of participants are involved in a Nominal Group Process, participants are divided into small groups of six to twenty. Group members write their individual ideas on paper, and then each person discusses his or her ideas. All ideas and concerns are listed on a chart or board, where they are discussed, clarified, and evaluated by the group. Then each person assigns priorities by silent ballot; ballots are tallied and a decision is reached.

The advantages of using Nominal Group Process in community assessments are that it expands the data obtained from surveys or existing documents and can generate surveys that are more specific. It engenders many ideas quickly and allows for a full range of thoughts and concerns from a diverse group. Nominal Group Process gives all participants an equal opportunity to express opinions and ideas. Finally, this process stimulates creative thinking, effective dialogue, and clarification of ideas, which may lead to actual conclusions. This process is difficult to implement with large groups unless many facilitators are trained in advance. The facilitator is a critical catalyst who must be flexible, encourage agenda building, keep assertive personalities in check, and respect all ideas and concerns. Just as in key informant interviews, participants may not represent all community subgroups, and follow-up surveys, observations, or document analyses may be required.

Delphi Technique. The Delphi Technique generates ideas without requiring face-to-face interaction (for example, by mail or e-mail), although it also can be used in small group settings. More structured than the Nominal Group Process, the Delphi Technique uses a series of questionnaires and summarized feedback reports from preceding responses in an iterative fashion (Delbecq, Van de Ven, and Gustafson, 1975). This approach can be used by coalitions when they must generate and clarify ideas, reach consensus, prioritize, or decide among alternatives. A questionnaire is created that identifies the problems, causes, solutions, and actions surrounding a specific issue. It is distributed to a sample of respondents who each independently generates ideas in response to the questions and returns the completed questionnaire. The responses are summarized and a second questionnaire is created that asks the same respondents to prioritize or rank input from the first round. The process is repeated until general agreement is reached. A final summary is prepared and sent to respondents.

This process promotes an exchange and subsequent rethinking of opinions and priorities after respondents evaluate the group's input. It is inexpensive, confidential, and relatively free of social pressure. In addition, it promotes information sharing, can be used to resolve conflict, and provides "a broad analytical perspective" on local issues and concerns (Carter and Beaulieu. 1992, p. 7). This approach can be time-consuming and requires good writing skills. Because it calls for consensus, extreme but innovative options may be eliminated.

Focus groups. Another popular collective interview technique is the *focus group*, where six to eight individuals are led in a structured discussion on a specific topic, such as a local health concern (Krueger, 1994). Unlike a random sampling of the population, the participants in a focus group are generally selected because they share certain characteristics (such as having specific health problems), making their opinions relevant to the assessment. In responding to a specific interview guide, participants share their beliefs and experiences in a way that would not be feasible in other methods.

The key characteristic that distinguishes focus group interviews from other kinds of group interviews is the insight and data produced by the interaction between participants (Morgan, 1997, p. 12). Participants ask questions of each other, trade viewpoints, and reconsider their own understanding of common experiences. Attendees often find the experience rewarding and empowering because their opinions are valued. A focus group enables coalitions to gain a larger amount of data in a shorter time than observation does. Focus groups are particularly useful when power differences exist between the participants and decision makers or professionals, or when the language and culture of particular groups or the degree of consensus on a given topic is of interest (Morgan and Krueger, 1993).

Focus groups can be used to assess feasibility of a community program, to evaluate the administration of or participation in a program, or to assess its impact (Krueger, 1994). They are widely used for many purposes, such as developing educational programs for HIV (Munodawafa, Gwede, and Mubayira, 1995); gathering information to use in developing community action plans for promoting immunization or asthma management in children (Butterfoss, Houseman, Morrow, and Rosenthal, 1997; Butterfoss, Kelly, Taylor, and Fishwick, 2005); or understanding how media messages are processed (Kitzinger, 1995).

One disadvantage of focus groups is that the moderator has little control over the interaction other than keeping participants focused on the topic (Morgan, 1997). Besides their unpredictable nature, focus groups can be difficult to assemble. Moreover, representation is not assured, and those who are not articulate and confident, or who have communication problems or special needs, may be discouraged from participating. Finally, focus groups are not fully confidential or anonymous, because the material is shared with others in the group. Other advantages and disadvantages of focus groups are found in Table 11.2.

The recommended number of people per focus group is usually six to ten (Krueger, 1994), and sessions last from one to two hours. Usually, one session is held with several groups, but sometimes the same group meets several times (Kitzinger, 1994, 1995). Recruitment can occur by word of mouth, through key informants, by advertising or poster campaigns, or through existing social networks. Incentives (such as expenses, gift vouchers, or presents) often promote better participation.

Neutral locations are best in order to avoid possible negative or positive associations with a particular site or building. Otherwise, sessions can be held in a variety of places, for example, people's homes, rented facilities, or where participants hold their regular meetings, if they are members of a pre-existing group (Krueger, 1994). Participants should feel comfortable with each other; meeting with others who seem to share a similar understanding about an issue is more appealing than meeting with those perceived as holding significantly different views (Morgan, 1997).

The role of the focus group moderator is to clearly explain the purpose of the group, help people feel at ease, and promote interaction among participants. From an ethical standpoint, he or she should clarify that participants' contributions will be shared with the others. Participants should be encouraged to keep confidential what they hear during the meeting; in addition, participants' identities must be protected after data is collected.

During the session, moderators stimulate debate by asking open questions or by challenging participants, to draw out differences. Sometimes they must probe for details, move the conversation forward when it drifts or stalls, or refocus the discussion. Moderators must ensure that everyone gets a chance to speak but avoid favoring certain participants or giving personal opinions that may influence participants (Krueger, 1994). They must be good listeners and nonjudgmental in order to build trust and increase the likelihood of open, interactive dialogue. A note taker is also recommended to record nonverbal activities and manage the recording equipment.

Surveys. Surveys are used to collect information from a sample of the broad community, priority population, or program participants. Responses to specific questions are used to ascertain priority issues and community needs. Surveys may be conducted by personal or telephone interview, or in a self-completed questionnaire administered in person or by mail (Berg, 1998). Questionnaires can vary in length and may contain open-ended or closed items, or both. Open-ended questions provide relatively rich information about a topic by allowing participants to report thoughts, opinions, and feelings. However, sometimes people are reluctant to write down opinions, or the survey may be time-consuming to complete (and also to analyze).

Unlike open-ended questions, closed-ended questions provide discrete, multiple-choice responses from which the respondent selects the most appropriate. Closed-ended questions are uniform and easy to administer, complete, and analyze. However, they impose a set of fixed ideas or values, and participants have a limited choice of responses. As a result, they do not allow nuances of meaning that lead to deep understanding.

Some training or experience in the construction of survey instruments and sampling techniques is recommended if they are to be used. Surveys can be administered in many settings. For example, a short patient satisfaction survey on a postcard could be given to clients after clinic visits to rate the quality of their experiences. Written surveys are not advised if respondents have low language literacy; a survey administered by telephone or in person might be more appropriate for this population.

Decisions about how responses will be recorded and analyzed must be made early. After the instrument is developed, it is usually piloted with a test group that provides feedback on clarity, tone, length, and any problems encountered in completing it. Surveys can often be compared in terms of the cost of implementation, time needed for completion, rate of refusal, and the extent and type of staff training needed (Carter and Beaulieu, 1992, p. 7).

Surveys are popular because they elicit responses concerning knowledge, attitudes, beliefs, and behaviors from a *broad range* of respondents in a rapid manner, and instruments can be tested for validity and reliability. Surveys can help coalitions engage community members in their issues, including those who may benefit from programs that are implemented as a result of the assessment.

However, surveys can be costly, and they require time and expertise to draw samples, track results, develop the instrument, train interviewers, conduct interviews, and analyze results. Moreover, response rates may be poor, or respondents may be hesitant to answer certain questions or may provide only what they think are socially desirable answers. Finally, results are obtained at one point in time; attitudes and behaviors can change rapidly due to a variety of intervening factors (Carter and Beaulieu, 1992, p. 8). More advantages and disadvantages of surveys are found in Table 11.2.

Self-completed diaries or logs. Some indicators of interest may be best measured
or monitored by means of diaries. Individuals may use diaries to record
progress on a behavioral management program or subjective responses to given
phenomena. For example, participants might record their daily intake of fruits
and vegetables for a five-a-day program or incidents of injury to toddlers for an
injury-prevention program. More quantitative record-keeping systems also can
be developed to record events that meet pre-established criteria. A good example
is Francisco, Paine, and Fawcett's (1993) system in which coalition members
track and log products, services, resources, media coverage of a community
coalition, and community actions or changes that result from their efforts.

To obtain multiple viewpoints and rich data, coalitions should use a variety of methods to gather data. The methodologies are usually determined by preference, feasibility, cost, and time, but coalition members should have a say in deciding how, when, and why a particular method is chosen over another. This builds buy-in, future participation, and a sense that the data will provide valid results that can be used to further the coalition's aims.

Designing and Pilot-Testing the Instruments and Procedures

Simple instruments are less expensive to produce, distribute, collect, and analyze. If valid and reliable instruments and procedures that have been tested in a similar community with a similar population are available, then the coalition should consider the cost and time savings inherent in not having to create them from scratch. Whether an instrument must be adapted from existing tools or newly created, it should reflect the assessment's objectives and include essential information. Instruments and procedures must be reviewed by a human subjects committee or Institutional Review Board (IRB). Sample surveys and assessment tools are included throughout this text and can also be obtained from other published studies or investigations, as well as from commercial sources. Pilot tests of instruments and procedures should be done to identify and eliminate confusion and mistakes early.

Preparing a Timeline and Budget

These tools keep procedures on track and let coalition members and collaborating organizations know how they can contribute in-kind to make the assessment more cost-effective. See Chapter Ten for budget preparation and timeline construction.

Collecting the Data

Aim for a two- to three-month time frame to promote commitment and keep the assessment on task. Existing relevant secondary data should be collected first. If local data cannot be obtained or does not exist, then coalition planners may need to use state, regional, or national data and apply them to their locality. For example, national or state cardiovascular mortality rates could be used to estimate the number of deaths in a local community based on its population. Primary and secondary data will give the best picture of the community's health, but coalitions must often compromise to use the best data available given the existing constraints.

Analyzing the Data

After collecting data from different sources, coalitions must organize the data by main topics and questions; review the data with their planning needs in mind; determine trends among population groups, services, and resources; identify themes and patterns; and prepare results for presentation to coalition staff, members, and the community at large.

The goal of this step is to analyze the data collected to identify and prioritize the health issues. Whenever possible, coalitions should conduct a formal statistical or content analysis of the data. Even if the results seem obvious, a closer, more objective analysis is preferable to just "eyeballing" the data to discover differences between "what is and what ought to be" (Windsor, Baranowski, Clark and Cutter, 1994, p. 63). Sometimes the health issue is obvious, such as an increase in rates of a particular disease or reduced access to health care services in the community. However, assessments may yield mixed or confusing data. The coalition may have to collect additional data for clarification or ask members of the priority population or other experts to sort out differences that relate to specific community or cultural factors (McKenzie, Neiger, and Smeltzer, 2005).

Who makes the decisions about what to do with the data collected is a key issue for coalitions to consider—the health professional or the consumer? Windsor and colleagues differentiate between service needs and service demands (1994, p. 64). Service needs are health issues and programs that health professionals and planners determine should be provided, based on the analysis of collected community data. Service demands, on the other hand, are those health issues that the priority population feels should be resolved. The best approach may be to identify health priorities based on service needs, but ensure that all interventions are based on service demands (McKenzie, Neiger, and Smeltzer, 2005, p. 90). If coalition and community members are heavily involved in the data-collection process and subsequent validation of the results, they are more likely to agree on the issues and their solutions.

Because most coalitions and communities have limited resources, they must prioritize the identified health issues. Prioritizing can range from rank ordering

Table 11.3. Factors Ranked by Importance and Changeability.

	More Important	Less Important
More Changeable	High priority for coalition focus	Low priority except to show change for political reasons
Less Changeable	Priority for innovative approach	No priority

Source: Green and Kreuter, 1999.

by a group of stakeholders to using one of the decision-making processes, such as Nominal Group Process, discussed in Chapter Seven. Other complex priority rating formulae often used by strategic planners and economists consider the size and seriousness of the problem and the effectiveness of possible interventions, as well as issues of propriety, economics, resources, and legality (Pickett and Hanlon, 1990).

After the health issues are prioritized, the coalition must identify the behavioral, social, and environmental risk factors that are associated with them. For example, if the prioritized health issue is pediatric asthma, then the factors related to asthma may include poor compliance with the medical regimen, lack of access to quality asthma care, and household or other environmental triggers to asthma. Again, these factors would be derived from the data that were collected and analyzed. The coalition's task would be to figure out how to ameliorate these factors to improve asthma management. A two-by-two prioritization matrix (Green and Kreuter, 1999) can be used to rank the identified factors by importance and changeability (see Table 11.3).

The other data that must be analyzed concern the quality, accessibility, and affordability of the existing health services and programs available to the priority population in the community. If these data were not collected formally in the assessment, they can be compiled by networking with coalition partner organizations and stakeholders or by asking the priority population directly in town meetings, forums, or focus groups.

Preparing and Disseminating the Findings

Those who might have the most interest in the results should be identified early and regularly updated throughout the assessment process. Relationships with new potential users also should be cultivated. Presenting data at coalition meetings keeps partners abreast of the findings and involved in the project's activities. Partners' reactions and recommendations give staff and evaluators valuable feedback about what additional information is needed. Before disseminating the findings, the final results should be validated by rechecking the possibility of bias in collecting or analyzing data, conducting a focus group with community stakeholders to get their reaction to the data, and sharing the results with other health professionals and experts outside of the coalition. Such double-checking may avoid surprise and embarrassment later.

In most cases, results are shared with the professional community (for example, service providers and social service agencies, teachers, public health personnel, police), adults, teens, and the media. Findings are also disseminated to politicians as well as to members of the clergy and business community. Sharing the results of the assessment with the community helps to meet several important goals. It raises awareness about the issue, helps to sustain the involvement of existing partners and recruit new members to the coalition, builds trust within the community, and provides a road map for moving forward by informing the coalition's action plan. Once the data-collection part of the community needs assessment is complete, results will more likely be used if the issues that the users perceive as important were addressed and if data were communicated to potential users in a timely and understandable form.

The most common methods for disseminating findings are briefings, group events, and reports. Reports should summarize and highlight the results of the assessment by using graphs and charts to illustrate the findings and should include the following information:

- Incidence and prevalence broken out by zip codes and, in some cases, by race and ethnicity
- Neighborhood and community profiles with attention to assets
- Catalogue of existing programs, services, and resources in the community
- Gaps in community programs, services, and resources
- Prioritized needs
- Recommendations for meeting those needs

Several issues should be considered when preparing assessment findings (Archer, Cripe, and McCaslin, 1992):

- Make the community needs assessment report readable and include an executive summary, logically sequenced and in easily understandable language. To keep the report user-friendly, create several brief documents instead of one long report.
- Prepare multiple reports using a variety of media, because people's preferred methods of receiving information differ. Compact discs and online availability of results increase access to the data and save money. Audiovisual reports presented in press-release format can generate support and highlight the coalition's work.
- List or identify the limitations and alternative explanations to increase the credibility of the process. Include oral reports as well as written documents to engage community members, promote interaction, and generate support of new ideas and insights.
- Keep information relevant, practical, and applicable. Make sure the audience knows why the needs assessment was done, what is now known that was not known before, and how the new information will help the coalition and the community.

Once assessment data are shared and key stakeholders are familiar with the results, the coalition may use the data to determine or refine its mission statement, goals and objectives, and action plan. The plan is more likely to succeed if it is built on accurate needs assessment data.

Evaluating the Assessment's Merit and Worth

After the assessment is completed, coalition members should identify what worked well, what problems were encountered, and how the process could have been improved. The assessment process is one that builds capacity among coalition members and community partners alike to conduct further assessments when needed.

COALITIONS AND ASSESSMENTS: ISSUES AND LESSONS LEARNED

For an assessment to be of the greatest value, it must generate accurate and reliable data; yet coalitions often encounter challenges and barriers when they plan and carry out community assessments. First, coalitions need certain skills to be able to conduct useful assessments. They need skills in designing effective surveys, interview protocols, and focus group questions; determining samples for surveys, interviews, and focus groups; facilitating focus groups; analyzing both quantitative and qualitative data; and writing clear, concise reports based on the data. Coalitions often lack trained staff or a professional research team with this broad array of research and assessment skills.

Second, the data-collection and analysis process can be both time-consuming and expensive. A coalition can easily be overly ambitious in terms of the size and scope of the assessment it undertakes (Wolff, 2001a). A comprehensive assessment that includes multiple methodologies takes considerable time to complete. Coalition and community partners may lose interest in a long-term planning effort that lacks tangible services, programs, or activities. When many people are carrying out the assessment, even more time must also be allotted for training. Expenses include those involved in hiring an evaluator or consultant to design and conduct the analysis, other staff salaries, printing, software programs, and any incentives offered to youth and community residents for participating.

To deal with these barriers, coalitions are reminded to keep a balance between planning and action, in other words, to keep planning efforts action-oriented. For busy community leaders, business representatives, and neighborhood residents, a little bit of planning may be all they want; this is probably even truer for youth (The National Campaign to Prevent Teen Pregnancy, 2003). However, other community partners, such as health administrators and academics, may enjoy planning and find secondary gain in their involvement (employee recognition, presentations and publications, and tenure). Overall, partners need concrete activities. Seeing tangible results from programs can encourage partners to stick with a comprehensive planning effort. Small-scale pilot programs or trainings based on the assessment information can be created to keep partners engaged and demonstrate to the community the seriousness of the coalition's intentions.

Involving community residents in data collection, presentation of data to the community, or both is another strategy for combining planning and action. Before starting an assessment, coalitions should carefully define the scope, budget, staff, and resources available for the effort. Involving coalition partners and residents in a needs assessment may compromise some of the research goals, but wider community buy-in will probably result as well.

COALITION SPOTLIGHT: COMMUNITY ASSESSMENT WITH THE METROPOLITAN BOSTON HAITIAN HIV PREVENTION COALITION

A good example of a community-driven assessment process was the Metropolitan Boston Haitian HIV Prevention Coalition's collection of comprehensive public health data that brought the Haitian community together to reduce HIV transmission rates (Madison, Hung, and Jean-Louis, 2004). The first step was to create a "community of inquiry" through weekly meetings, to assure that valid, reliable data could be collected. This approach does more than just involve people in the assessment process; a community is formed, "bonded by a shared commitment to the evaluation" (Madison, Hung, and Jean-Louis, 2004, pp. S1–S20). The community of inquiry included service providers, consumers, other stakeholders, and evaluators. A safe environment was created in which trust was built and core operating values were established to guide the assessment process.

Early on, conflicting values concerning research were discussed and negotiated. These values formed the basis for procedures, rules, roles, and responsibilities for conducting the research. Then process and outcome measurement criteria were identified, an evaluation plan was designed, data sources were identified, and data-collection methods and responsibilities were decided upon. A survey was developed and the coalition conducted an intensive radio campaign to inform the Haitian community about it, solicit their participation, and have them call in with questions or comments. Survey information also was distributed to churches and businesses in the Haitian community.

Due to this concentrated outreach effort, the community was ready to participate. As a result, 2,719 of 3,500 Haitian households responded to the thirty-minute telephone survey (78 percent response rate). The community-of-inquiry approach provided an opportunity to develop a community-based research culture, which builds trust and respect for research as a tool. The community took pride in its role in the survey and was eager to learn from the results. The coalition learned new skills in conducting assessments that embrace ethnic cultural differences as well as differences in professional practices. Finally, as a full participant in all aspects of the assessment, the community took ownership of the process and responsibility for using the results (Madison, Hung, and Jean-Louis, 2004, p. S1–S240).

SUMMARY

Successful coalition efforts are more likely to occur in communities where residents recognize the need for some type of collaborative initiative and take ownership in order to embrace the coalition issue as a priority, community residents must perceive that the health problem or issue exists, warrants their attention, and affects their neighbors, and that the coalition's initiative promises personal benefits and community changes. The issue(s) that a coalition chooses to work on can also have an impact on the coalition itself. When community members help identify priority populations and issues, plan and implement strategies, and evaluate outcomes, the strategies are more likely to be effective and well received by the community. A community assessment is performed to better understand the community and its assets, and to determine how the coalition can best serve the community in addressing its local concerns and problems. The steps of the needs-assessment process involve identifying community assets, concerns, and the priority populations for intervention; collecting data to answer research questions; analyzing and summarizing the data; and disseminating the result to the community. The common methods that coalitions use to collect community information are neighborhood and community profiles, windshield tours, asset mapping, Photovoice, developing community indicators, key informant interviews, public forums, Nominal Group Processes, and surveys. Each method has its advantages and disadvantages, but most coalitions rely on a combination of methods to gain a comprehensive picture of the health of the community.

QUESTIONS FOR REVIEW

1. What is the difference between a needs approach and an assets approach to community assessment? Is there value in doing both? Why or why not?

2. What are the trade-offs in deciding the coalition's issue a priori versus determining the issue after a community assessment? What constraints favor the former approach?

3. Why should the priority population and coalition members be involved in community assessment and planning? Name two ways that they can be meaningfully involved in this aspect of coalition work.

4. Choose two methods of community assessment and describe the advantages and disadvantages of each.

RESOURCES

Publications

Altschuld, J. W., and Witkin, B. R. (eds.). *From Needs Assessment to Action: Transforming Needs into Solution Strategies.* Thousand Oaks, Calif.: Sage Publications, 1999. This sequel to the authors' 1995 book, *Planning and Conducting Needs Assessments: A Practical Guide,* shows how the results of needs assessments can be transformed into action plans for an organization and includes procedures for facilitating that change. Using real-world examples from various fields, it provides in-depth procedures for analyzing and combining different types of data; prioritizing needs; selecting, designing, and implementing solution strategies; and examining major multiple-method needs assessment studies.

Butler, L. M., and Howell, R. E. *Community Needs Assessment Techniques.* Corvallis, Oreg.: Western Regional Extension, 1980. (http://ext.usu.edu/crd/wrdcpub/). Discusses the purpose of community assessments and guidelines for deciding on methods, and includes a description of thirteen different methods.

Carter, K. A., and Beaulieu, L. J. "Conducting a Community Needs Assessment: Primary Data Collection Techniques." Florida Cooperative Extension Service (CD-27), 1992. (http://hammock.ifas.ufl.edu/txt/fairs/5598). Discusses five main data-collection methods and the advantages and disadvantages of each technique.

Community Resources. *The Knowing Your Community, Showing Your Community Method and Handbook.* Provides a step-by-step method for community residents on how to collect and present information about their communities, and includes tools such as community mapping, elder interviews, neighborhood observation, photographs, and participatory charting. Address: Community Resources, 5131 Wetheredsville Road, Baltimore, Md. 21207. Tel: (410) 448–0640.

Community Tool Box. Identifies community assets and resources for promoting community health and development. Address: Work Group on Health Promotion and Community Development, 4082 Dole Human Development Center, 1000 Sunnyside Avenue, University of Kansas, Lawrence, Kans. 66045-7555. Tel.: (785) 864-0533; fax: (785) 864-5281; e-mail: Toolbox@ku.edu; http://ctb.ku.edu/contact.jsp

Francisco, V. T., Paine, A. L., and Fawcett, S. B. "A Methodology for Monitoring Health Action Coalitions. *Health Education Research: Theory and Practice,* 1993, 8(3), 403–416.

Johnson, D. E., and others (eds.). *Needs Assessment. Theory and Methods.* Ames: Iowa State University Press, 1987. Addresses the theoretical, historical, national, and international dimensions of needs assessments, and discusses their political and social contexts and frequently used methods.

Kretzmann, J. P., and McKnight, J. L. *Building Communities from the Inside Out: A Path toward Finding and Mobilizing a Community's Assets.* Evanston, Ill.: Center for Urban Affairs and Policy Research, Northwestern University, 1993. This is the standard book on how to rebuild communities from an asset-based approach and provides hands-on guidance to assess individuals, associations, and institutions in the context of community economy, community development, and policy. Address: Asset-Based Community Development Institute, Institute for Policy Research, Northwestern University, 2040 Sheridan Road, Evanston, Ill. 60208–4100. Tel: (847) 491–3518.

Langmeyer, D. B. "Sticky Figures: Using a Needs Assessment." Chapel Hill, N.C.: Action Research and Community Health and Development (ARCH), Fact Sheet No. 27, 1993. Summarizes data-collection steps and methods, including social indicators, key informant, community forums, surveys, and Nominal Group Method. http://chtop.com/archfs27.htm

Minkler, M. (ed.). *Community Organizing and Community Building for Health,* 2nd Edition. New Brunswick, N.J.: Rutgers University Press, 2005. The definitive text on all aspects of community building, from theory and models to assessment and implementation techniques, to evaluation.

Rosenthal, B., and Rubel, D. *How to Conduct a Needs Assessment Study in Your Community: A Training Manual for Community Board and Area Policy Members.*

Prepared for the New York City Community Development Agency, 1991. Outlines steps of the needs assessment process; analysis of objectives and outcomes; documentation and analysis of existing conditions; arguing for change; and producing an action strategy.

The National Campaign to Prevent Teen Pregnancy. *Breaking Ground: Lessons Learned from the Centers for Disease Control and Prevention's Community Coalition Partnership Programs for the Prevention of Teen Pregnancy.* Washington, D.C.: Author, 2003. A comprehensive report on the CDC-funded initiative, Community Coalition Partnership Programs for the Prevention of Teen Pregnancy (CCPP). The report details the findings of thirteen communities with higher-than-average teen birth rates. From 1995 to 2002, each site mobilized its community by developing broad-based partnerships; determined the needs of youth in the community as well as the assets and resources available to meet those needs; prepared a community action plan, based on assessment of needs and assets, to establish programs to prevent initial and subsequent pregnancies; and implemented their community action plans and evaluated their effectiveness. Lessons learned and examples abound in this report. http://www.dhs.state.or.us/children/publications/tpp/breakingground.pdf

Samuels, B., and others. *Know Your Community: A Step-by-Step Guide to Community Needs and Resources Assessment.* Chicago: Family Resource Coalition, 1995. Discusses how to assess needs from residents' perspectives, identify assets and resources, set community priorities, establish a community planning team, define community boundaries, and develop a statistical profile. Includes sample surveys, data-collection worksheets, and progress charts, which can be customized using a companion disk. Family Resource Coalition. Tel: (312) 338–0900.

Soriano, F. I. *Conducting Needs Assessments. A Multidisciplinary Approach.* Thousand Oaks, Calif.: Sage Publications, 1995. Provides a short, practical introduction to needs assessments. Includes chapters on planning assessments, assessment methods, reporting the findings, social and cultural considerations, and specific examples.

United States Department of Transportation, National Highway Traffic Safety Administration. *Community How-to Guide on Needs Assessment and Strategic Planning.* Describes the benefits, barriers, and key elements of needs assessment and strategic planning for underage drinking prevention programs. http:// www.nhtsa.dot.gov/people/injury/alcohol/Community%20Guides%20HTML/Book2_NeedsAssess. html#strategic%20plan. Accessed December 16, 2005.

Witkin, B. R., and Altschuld, J. W. (eds.). *Planning and Conducting Needs Assessments: A Practical Guide.* Thousand Oaks, Calif.: Sage Publications, 1995. Provides an advanced analysis of planning, managing, and conducting complex needs assessments. Discusses the stages of pre-assessment, assessment, and post-assessment as well as various methods, including records and social indicators, surveys, interviews, group processes, and causal analysis.

CHAPTER TWELVE

Coalitions and Planning

*What you can do, or dream you can do, begin it; boldness
has genius, power, and magic in it.*
—Johann Von Goethe, 1749–1832

Public health planning is a key step in addressing complex health issues that
require long-term strategies and multiple approaches, such as changes in policy and the environment (Institute of Medicine, 2002a). Clearly, the public
health community assumes that planning is the foundation for program success and
that funds should be allocated for planning (Butterfoss and Dunet, 2005). A familiar
public health approach is for coalitions and other community- and state-based organizations to receive federal funds and technical assistance to support comprehensive planning as a first phase of program development. A coalition may serve as a
convener of a planning group or a partner in a strategic process, or may simply
develop action plans for its community efforts.

Coalitions and their partners continue to be involved in many planning initiatives,
such as Turning Point, Healthy People 2010, and Healthy Communities, as well as comprehensive cancer, tobacco control, diabetes, asthma, and oral health initiatives. Large-
scale prevention efforts, such as HIV Prevention Community Planning and
Comprehensive Cancer Prevention and Control, also encourage community-based planning as an important public health strategy. Several models offer guidance for partnering with the community as part of a community health planning process. A coalition
should choose a model that matches its intended goals and is acceptable to its community partners.

To be effective, coalition plans must be clear to all participants and demonstrate
how goals, objectives, and activities are meaningfully integrated (Foster-Fishman and
others, 2001; Kegler, Steckler, McLeroy, and Malek, 1998b; Roussos and Fawcett, 2000;
Wolff, 2001a). Although intensive planning efforts by coalitions have contributed to

successful implementation (Butterfoss, 1996; Kumpher, Turner, Hopkins, and Librett, 1993; Kegler, Steckler, McLeroy, and Malek, 1998b), many collaborative efforts have failed to produce rigorous plans (Kreuter, Lezin, and Young, 2000). Therefore, coalitions and partnerships must emphasize the importance of comprehensive planning and develop members' skills in this area. An array of public health community planning, health education, and program development models has been developed. Given the broad focus of this text, a summary of each model will be provided, with reference to the primary sources.

PUBLIC HEALTH PLANNING MODELS

PRECEDE–PROCEED, or Predisposing, Reinforcing, and Enabling Constructs in Educational and Ecological Diagnosis and Evaluation; and Policy, Regulatory, and Organizational Constructs in Educational and Environmental Development (Green and Kreuter, 1999), is perhaps the most well-known public health program planning model that builds on the strengths within the community. The model, developed and refined over twenty years, was influenced by the PATCH planning process described here. PRECEDE–PROCEED is composed of nine phases that provide a logical sequence for program planning. To use this model, one begins by identifying the desired outcome and then, by working backward, determines the underlying causes. Once the causes are known, the appropriate intervention(s) can be created and implemented. The first four phases (the PRECEDE portion of the model) include the assessment activities: (1) social, (2) epidemiological, (3) behavioral and environmental, (4) educational and ecological, and (5) administrative and policy-related. The last four phases (the PROCEED portion of the model) include the implementation and evaluation activities: (6) implementation, (7) process evaluation, (8) impact evaluation, and (9) outcome evaluation. Planners can interact seamlessly between the PRECEDE and PROCEED parts of the model as needed.

MATCH, or Multilevel Approach to Community Health (Simons-Morton, Simons-Morton, Parcel, and Bunker, 1988) is an ecological planning model focusing on interventions that use many objectives for programs with a diverse set of individuals and organizations. The MATCH model is composed of five multistep phases: (1) goals selection, (2) intervention planning, (3) program development, (4) implementation preparation, and (5) evaluation.

MAPP, or Mobilizing Action through Planning and Partnership (National Association of City and County Health Officials [NACCHO], 2004), is a planning approach developed by city and county health departments to improve health and quality of life through mobilized partnerships that take strategic action. MAPP has six multistep phases: (1) organizing for success and partnership development; (2) visioning; (3) conducting four assessments that include community strengths, local public health, community health status or epidemiology, and the forces of change (social, political, and technological environment); (4) identifying strategic issues; (5) formulating goals and strategies;

and (6) taking action. This model differs from the previous two models in that it requires local public health officials to work jointly with members of the priority population (consumers) to design and deliver interventions. Thus MAPP is especially appropriate for coalitions and partnerships.

APEX-PH, or Assessment Protocol for Excellence in Public Health (NACCHO, 2004) is a planning and assessment process developed by the National Association of County and City Health Officials in response to the Institute of Medicine's (IOM) *Future of Public Health* report (1988). The report declared that public health departments should systematically collect and analyze data on community health needs. APEX-PH has three phases: (1) organizational capacity assessment (SWOT analysis), (2) community process (collecting and analyzing data), and (3) completing the cycle (development of policies, services, and activities within an implementation plan that includes evaluation).

PATCH, or Planned Approach to Community Health (Kreuter, Nelson, Stoddard, and Watkins, 1985; Green and Kreuter, 1992; Goodman, Steckler, Hoover, and Schwartz, 1993; U.S. Department of Health and Human Services, 2000) was designed, using the PRECEDE model, to strengthen health departments' capacity to plan, implement, and evaluate community-based health-promotion activities that impact priority health problems. PATCH is a team approach in which community members use a consensus method to make decisions about health issues and programs, and actually implement the programs with technical assistance and funding from CDC and their local health departments. The five phases of PATCH are presented as a circular model: (1) mobilizing the community, (2) collecting and analyzing data, (3) choosing health priorities, (4) developing a comprehensive intervention plan, and (5) evaluating PATCH.

Healthy Cities **and** *Healthy People in Healthy Communities* are planned processes that spread from Canada to Europe in the 1980s with support from the World Health Organization (Hancock, 1993). Recent iterations have included the Indiana and California Healthy Cities programs (Kegler, Norton, and Aronson, 2003). Healthy Cities is distinguished by active participation of diverse community partners who work with health professionals to identify and solve health issues. Community values, ownership, and empowerment are key aspects of this planning process. *Healthy People in Healthy Communities* is a community guide that provides a five-step process for Healthy Communities: (1) mobilizing key individuals and organizations; (2) assessing community needs, strengths, and resources; (3) planning for action; (4) implementing the action plan; and (5) tracking progress and outcomes (U.S. Department of Health and Human Services, 2001).

Based on these planning models, some others have emerged that try to blend the common elements of each into a generic model, such as the Community Health Improvement Program, or CHIP (Institute of Medicine, 2002b), and the Six-Step Program Development Chain Model (Sussman, 2001). Other public health planning models address particular public health strategies, such as the CDCynergy model for planning, managing, and evaluating public health communication programs (Centers for Disease Control, 2000b) and Intervention Mapping for designing theory- and evidence-based health-promotion programs (Bartholomew, Parcel, Kok, and Gottlieb, 2001). Still others are focused on planning for a particular public health problem, such as planning for Comprehensive Cancer Control (Abed and others, 2000).

Getting to Outcomes (Chinman and others, 2001; Chinman, Imm, and Wandersman, 2004) is a model that can be used for both planning and evaluating prevention programs, such as those for substance abuse and violence prevention.

GETTING TO OUTCOMES: METHODS AND TOOLS FOR PLANNING, EVALUATION, AND ACCOUNTABILITY (GTO)

GTO was developed as an approach to help practitioners plan, implement, and evaluate their programs to achieve results (Chinman and others, 2001; Chinman, Imm, and Wandersman, 2004). GTO is based on answering ten accountability questions. Addressing the questions involves a comprehensive approach to results-based accountability that includes needs and resource assessment, objectives (identifying goals, target populations, and desired outcomes), science and promising practices, logic models, fit of programs with existing programs, planning, implementation with fidelity, process evaluation, outcome evaluation, continuous quality improvement, and sustainability. By thoughtfully considering the following questions and using practical tools to achieve evaluation objectives, program developers increase their probability of reaching outcomes and demonstrating accountability to stakeholders:

1. *Needs and resources.* What are the needs and resources in the organization, school, community, or state?
2. *Goals.* What are the goals, priority population, and desired outcomes (objectives) for the organization, school, community, or state?
3. *Best practice.* How does this program incorporate knowledge of science and best practice in this area?
4. *Fit.* How does this program fit with other programs already being offered?
5. *Capacities.* What capacities are needed to put this program into place with quality?
6. *Plan.* How will this program be carried out?
7. *Implementation.* How will the quality of program implementation be assessed?
8. *Outcomes.* How well did the program work?
9. *Continuous quality improvement (CQI).* How will CQI strategies be incorporated?
10. *Sustaining.* If the program (or program components) is successful, how will it be sustained?

As can be seen, most public health planning models incorporate a common set of five or six steps, which are summarized in Table 12.1. A distilled version of five

Table 12.1. Summary of Public Health Planning Models.

PRECEDE–PROCEED	MATCH	APEX-PH	MAPP	PATCH	Healthy Communities
Green and Kreuter, 1999	Simons-Morton, Simons-Morton, Parcel, and Bunker, 1988	NAACCHO, 1991	NACCHO, 2001	Kreuter, Nelson, Stoddard, and Watkins, 1985; USDHHS, 2000	USDHHS, 2001
1 Social assessment	Select goals.	Assess organizational capacity.	Organize for success and develop partnership.	Mobilize community.	Mobilize key individuals and organizations.
2 Epidemiologic assessment	Plan intervention.	Develop community Process.	Engage in visioning.	Collect and organize data.	Assess community needs, strengths, and resources.
3 Behavioral and environmental assessment	Develop program.	Complete the cycle.	Conduct four MAPP assessments.	Choose health priorities.	Plan for action.
4 Educational and eco-logical assessment	Prepare to implement.		Identify strategic issues.	Develop intervention plan.	Implement action plan.
5 Administrative and policy assessment	Evaluate.		Formulate goals and strategies.	Evaluate PATCH.	Track progress and outcomes.
6 Implement			Initiate action cycle.		
7 Process evaluation					
8 Impact evaluation					
9 Outcome evaluation					

important steps, which follow Parts II to IV of this text, is presented here. The first step, mobilizing the community, was discussed in Chapters Five through Ten. The last four steps, community assessment, planning, implementation, and evaluation, are addressed in Chapters Eleven through Fourteen. Strategic planning involves similar components: assessing, planning, implementing, and evaluating, as will be detailed in the next section.

THE STRATEGIC PLANNING PROCESS

Most coalitions engage in a one- to two-year assessment and strategic-planning process that is then followed by implementation of the resulting action plan over a three- to five-year period. Kreuter and colleagues (2000) noted that despite good needs assessments and detailed objectives and logic models, written plans were not rigorous. Several studies have examined the quality of action plans and found that they are associated with strong staff and leaders and mobilization of resources, and they contribute to effective implementation of activities (Butterfoss, Goodman, and Wandersman, 1996; Kegler, Steckler, McLeroy, and Malek, 1998b; Kumpher, Turner, Hopkins, and Librett, 1993). Research, however, has failed to show a linkage between effective plans and demonstrable outcomes. Many state health departments that are funded by CDC to implement obesity prevention, diabetes management, and oral health and cancer prevention programs are paying special attention to the planning process, and developing tools and technical assistance to make effective written plans and their implementation more likely (Dunet, Butterfoss, Hamre, and Kuester, 2005).

Strategic planning is valuable because it promotes a sense of community among citizens and other stakeholders; emphasizes thinking about the future; helps coalitions focus scarce resources into areas considered most beneficial by stakeholders; aids in continuity of decision making; promotes relevance as well as efficiency when public services and amenities are weighed; takes into account the community itself and its environment; and helps avoid unpleasant surprises (Strawn, Sumners, and Easterwood, 1999).

Strategic planning is a systematic process by which an organization like a coalition attempts to anticipate and plan as it meets the challenges of a changing environment. It helps the coalition maximize organizational strengths in relation to external opportunities, while countering external threats and addressing internal weaknesses that prevent effective action. Any successful planning process identifies broad issues and defines specific operational procedures. Strategic planning involves several steps: developing a vision and mission for the organization, scanning the environment, identifying strategic issues, selecting goals and objectives, and defining an action plan or steps for accomplishing goals and objectives.

Coalition staff and members often confuse a strategic plan with an action plan. The strategic plan is an overall view of the whole coalition and its assets and liabilities over a longer time frame (five to ten years). The action plan is a short-term plan (one to three years) that focuses on the actions or steps needed to achieve the strategic plan. Annual or biannual revisions of the action plan are recommended as the focus of work, partners, or funding changes.

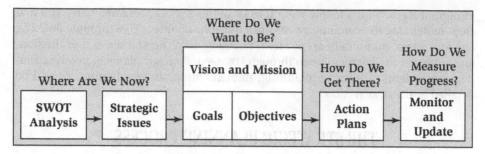

Figure 12.1 Strategic Planning Process.

Source: Figure reprinted with permission from "Strategic planning for local communities and government." *Action* newsletter, Fall 1999, edited by Tom Chesnutt, Extension Tourism Specialist, Auburn, AL: Alabama Cooperative Extension System. Chart by Harry B. Strawn, Extension Economist (retired); and Joe Sumners, Director, and Mike Easterwood, Senior Outreach Associate, Economic and Community Development Institute. All at Auburn University. Used courtesy of the Alabama Cooperative Extension System (Alabama A&M and Auburn Universities).

Essentially, the strategic planning process asks the organization to respond to four questions (Strawn, Sumners, and Easterwood, 1999):

• Where are we now? (assessing)

• Where do we want to be? (planning or strategizing)

• How do we get there? (implementing)

• How do we measure our progress? (evaluating)

The process is depicted in Figure 12.1.

Where are we now? (assessment) Coalitions should analyze local institutions, services, economic conditions, and population trends. The community assessment will provide valuable data for this process. Coalitions may begin by conducting a SWOT analysis, analyzing their Strengths, Weaknesses, Opportunities, and Threats (see also Chapter Seven). For strengths and weaknesses, organizations should examine internal factors that they can control, such as resources (inputs), current strategies (process), and performance (outputs). For opportunities and threats, organizations should look to *external* factors, which the organization does not control, but which, nevertheless, have an impact on the organization. The strategic plan should outline ways to overcome the coalition's weaknesses and counter environmental threats, while ensuring that the coalition takes advantage of its strengths and environmental opportunities.

Where do we want to be? (plan or strategy) After determining where the coalition is now, the next step is to determine where the organization wants to be in the future, a process that involves reaching consensus about what the organization would like to become.

Vision. First, members develop an overall vision for the community in the form of an inspirational statement that reflects their organizational hopes and future aspirations (see Chapter Seven).

Mission Statement. Members then create a clear, succinct mission statement that defines the organization's purpose (see Chapter Seven). The mission statement is based on the coalition's vision of an ideal community and answers the question, *Why do we exist?* Finally, for each strategic issue that is identified, the coalition must develop goals and objectives.

Goals. Goals are broad and general descriptions of desired outcomes that emerge from the mission statement and specify the priority actions for the coalition. They are dreams with deadlines. Goals should be long range and not time dependent. They may be used as mission statements and reasons for forming work groups. Thus if a coalition has four main goals, it may decide to develop four work groups, one to focus on each goal. Work groups can then develop more specific objectives from the goals. An example of a goal is, *To better the knowledge and practices of health care providers in improving patients' self-management of asthma.* Exhibit 12.1 provides an example of mission and vision statements, goals, and objectives by a community coalition's work groups.

Setting goals encourages discussion, reveals differences of opinion, and allows the coalition to move toward consensus. Worthwhile goals should energize the coalition and be attainable within a reasonably short time frame. Discussing goal achievement helps the coalition define the nature of its work with representatives from the community and identify possible funding sources and media opportunities. A goal is directly linked to community needs and assets and is related to a specific accomplishment. Goals can be tested and prioritized according to the following criteria (Meek, 1993):

- *Believable.* The goal must describe situations or conditions that the coalition can achieve.

- *Attainable.* The coalition should be sure it can achieve the goal in the designated timeframe.

- *Tangible.* The goal must be capable of being understood or realized.

- *Win–Win.* The goal must allow all members of the coalition to be successful.

- *Acceptable.* Each member and group in the coalition must understand and embrace the goal.

Objectives. After establishing the mission statement and goals, the coalition should develop at least one measurable and specific objective for each goal. Objectives should challenge the coalition to stretch for significant improvements that are important to members of the community. An objective is a statement of the expected result of an accomplished goal that can

(*Text resumes on page 366.*)

Exhibit 12.1. Sample Coalition Mission, Vision, Goals, and Objectives.

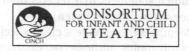

CINCH Mission

Community partnership to promote health and prevent disease among all children in Hampton Roads, Virginia

CINCH Impact Vision

The Consortium for Infant and Child Health (CINCH) believes that every child in Hampton Roads has the right to good health and a high quality of health. CINCH actualizes this right by

- Improving access to comprehensive, coordinated health care.
- Mobilizing community resources, agencies, and institutions to action.
- Calling together community individuals to address key health issues.
- Advocating for children and families.

CINCH Goals and Objectives

Obesity Prevention

Improve nutrition, fitness, and healthy weight maintenance by promoting healthy environments and lifestyle behaviors.

- Increase capacity and commitment within medical community to provide preventive and chronic disease treatment for obesity.
- Collaborate with schools to promote inclusion of obesity prevention education in curriculum, lunch programs, fitness programs, and physical education activities.
- Improve the knowledge, attitudes, and beliefs of individuals and organizations related to nutrition and physical activity through programming delivered by community organizations.
- Advocate for improved community environment and programs to promote nutrition and physical activity.

Immunization

Improve the knowledge and practices of health care providers to eliminate barriers that contribute to under-immunization.

- Increase completeness of private provider immunization records.
- Sponsor immunization update workshops and facilitate immunization education for providers.
- Promote parent immunization education by providers.
- Increase awareness of adolescent immunization recommendations.

Perinatal Health

Promote the birth of healthy infants through community partnerships and collaboration.

Exhibit 12.1. (*Continued*)

Injury Prevention

Promote childhood safety awareness and behavior to reduce unintentional injury, disability, and death.

- Identify and implement strategies to increase public awareness of unintentional injury.
- Advocate for changes in policies and procedure to reduce unintentional injury.
- Increase community capacity to address unintentional injury.
- Promote improvements to the physical environment to reduce unintentional injury.
- Assess community's needs and resources and intervene where gaps exist.

Asthma

- Increase knowledge of and compliance with NIH standards of asthma care among identified providers in high-risk areas.
- Ensure that patients have appropriate medical equipment and supplies needed to manage their asthma.
- Improve communication and management of care among primary providers, patients, families, schools, and hospital emergency departments.
- Increase the quality of care for children with asthma in hospital emergency departments.
- Ensure that all asthmatic children have asthma action plan, appropriate medications, medication form, and equipment at school.
- Establish asthma care coordination in each school division.
- Improve community awareness and response to asthma.
- Empower parents and caregivers to be knowledgeable advocates for their children with asthma.
- Improve environmental quality for children with asthma.

Health Disparities

Reduce health disparities that affect children and families systems in Hampton Roads.

- Promote education and awareness of community health resources and programs.
- Promote access and appropriate utilization of health care and community services.
- Educate families on how to appropriately manage acute and chronic diseases in children.
- Educate the community to reduce health disparities in children, to include poor birth outcomes, diabetes, HIV, mental health, asthma, obesity, access to health insurance, and immunizations.

Child Health Insurance

Ensure that all children have adequate health insurance coverage.

- Advocate for systemic changes to improve enrollment and delivery of state child health insurance programs.
- Increase number of children with health insurance to 100 percent.
- Advocate for improved coverage for health conditions where gaps in coverage exist.
- Increase awareness and enrollment in available health insurance programs.

be measured both quantitatively and qualitatively. Objectives may also be seen as specific and measurable targets for accomplishing goals. A *process objective* measures the accomplishment of tasks completed as part of the implementation of a program. An *outcome objective* measures long-term results, or the impact, of a program. Objectives describe how much of what will be accomplished by whom and by when. Overall, well-written objectives should be SMART (Specific, Measurable, Achievable, Relevant, and Time-Sensitive):

- *Specific.* They tell how much (for example, percentage) of what (outcome of specific activity, program, plan) is to be achieved by whom (person(s) responsible for implementation) by when (time frame, for example, by 2020).

- *Measurable.* Information about the objective can be collected, detected, or obtained from records.

- *Achievable.* Not only are the objectives themselves possible, but the coalition can feasibly accomplish them.

- *Relevant.* The coalition understands how these objectives fit with its overall vision and mission.

- *Time-sensitive.* The coalition has developed a timeline by which they will be achieved.

Several categories of objectives should be written, such as administrative, learning, behavioral, and outcome objectives:

Administrative objectives refer to changes in administrative policies or activities that promote the program. For example, the health department decides to hire two outreach workers to identify children who are living in public housing and are not immunized.

Learning objectives refer to changes in knowledge, attitudes, or beliefs, for example, teaching parents strategies to deal with their children's disruptive behavior.

Behavioral objectives refer to changes in behaviors or practices, for example, encouraging adults to access neighborhood centers to receive annual screening exams.

Outcome objectives refer to changes in health status indicators, such as immunizing 90 percent of adolescents against hepatitis B before they enter college.

A set of objectives developed for the *Healthy People in Healthy Communities Guide* (UDDHHS, 2001) is included as Exhibit 12.2. Once the coalition has developed a mission statement, goals, and objectives, then it is halfway to developing an action plan, described next.

(*Text resumes on page 370.*)

Exhibit 12.2. Health Objectives.

These selected HEALTHY PEOPLE 2010 objectives should apply to community coalitions. (Developmental objectives do not yet have a data system or data set available for measuring how the nation is doing on those objectives. Efforts are under way to develop such data sets and systems.) To make these objectives specific and measurable, add numerical outcomes.

Environmental Health

8-5 Increase the proportion of persons served by community water systems who receive a supply of drinking water that meets the regulations of the Safe Drinking Water Act.

8-11 Eliminate elevated blood lead levels in children.

8-12 Minimize the risks to human health and the environment posed by hazardous sites.

8-15 Increase recycling of municipal solid waste.

8-18 Increase the proportion of persons who live in homes tested for radon concentrations.

8-22 Increase the proportion of persons living in pre-1950s housing that has been tested for the presence of lead-based paint.

Communities

6-12 (Developmental) Reduce the proportion of people with disabilities reporting environmental barriers to participation in home, school, work, or community activities.

7-9 (Developmental) Increase the proportion of hospitals and managed care organizations that provide community disease prevention and health promotion activities that address the priority health needs identified by their community.

7-11 Increase the proportion of local health departments that have established culturally appropriate and linguistically competent community health promotion and disease prevention programs.

8-28 (Developmental) Increase the number of local health departments or agencies that use data from surveillance of environmental risk factors as part of their vector control programs.

18-3 Reduce the proportion of homeless adults who have serious mental illness.

19-18 Increase food security among U.S. households and in so doing reduce hunger.

21-9 Increase the proportion of the U.S. population served by community water systems with optimally fluoridated water.

25-13 Increase the proportion of tribal, state, and local sexually transmitted disease programs that routinely offer hepatitis B vaccines to all STD (sexually transmitted disease) clients.

25-14 (Developmental) Increase the proportion of youth detention facilities and adult city or county jails that screen for common bacterial sexually transmitted diseases within twenty-four hours of admission and treat STDs (when necessary) before persons are released.

(continued)

Exhibit 12.2. Health Objectives. (*Continued*)

25-15 (Developmental) Increase the proportion of all local health departments that have contracts with managed care providers for the treatment of non-plan partners of patients with bacterial sexually transmitted diseases (gonorrhea, syphilis, and chlamydia).

26-23 (Developmental) Increase the number of communities using partnerships or coalition models to conduct comprehensive substance abuse prevention efforts.

27-13 Establish laws on smoke-free indoor air that prohibit smoking or limit it to separately ventilated areas in public places and worksites.

Schools

7-2 Increase the proportion of middle, junior, and senior high schools that provide school health education to prevent health problems in the following areas: unintentional injury; violence; suicide; tobacco use and addiction; alcohol and other drug use; unintended pregnancy, HIV/AIDS, and STD infection; unhealthy dietary patterns; inadequate physical activity; and environmental health.

7-4 Increase the proportion of the nation's elementary, middle, junior, and senior high schools that have a nurse-to-student ratio of at least 1:750.

8-20 (Developmental) Increase the proportion of the nation's primary and secondary schools that have official school policies ensuring the safety of students and staff from environmental hazards, such as chemicals in special classrooms, poor indoor air quality, asbestos, and exposure to pesticides.

14-23 Maintain vaccination coverage levels for children in licensed day care facilities and children in kindergarten through the first grade.

15-31 (Developmental) Increase the proportion of public and private schools that require use of appropriate head, face, eye, and mouth protection for students participating in school-sponsored physical activities.

19-15 (Developmental) Increase the proportion of children and adolescents aged six to nineteen years whose intake of meals and snacks at schools contributes to good overall dietary quality.

22-8 Increase the proportion of the nation's public and private schools that require daily physical education for all students.

22-10 Increase the proportion of adolescents who spend at least 50 percent of school physical education class time being physically active.

22-12 (Developmental) Increase the proportion of the nation's public and private schools that provide access to their physical activity spaces and facilities for all persons outside of normal school hours (that is, before and after the school day, on weekends, and during summer and other vacations).

27-11 Increase smoke-free and tobacco-free environments in schools, including all school facilities, property, vehicles, and school events.

Exhibit 12.2. (*Continued*)

Worksites

7-5 Increase the proportion of worksites that offer a comprehensive employee health promotion program to their employees.

8-17 (Developmental) Increase the number of office buildings that are managed using good indoor air quality practices.

10-6 (Developmental) Improve food employee behaviors and food preparation practices that directly relate to food-borne illnesses in retail food establishments.

20-2 Reduce work-related injuries resulting in medical treatment, lost time from work, or restricted work activity.

20-9 Increase the proportion of worksites employing 50 or more persons that provide programs to prevent or reduce employee stress.

20-11 (Developmental) Reduce new cases of work-related, noise-induced hearing loss.

22-13 Increase the proportion of worksites offering employer-sponsored physical activity and fitness programs.

23-1 (Developmental) Increase the proportion of tribal, state, and local public health agencies that provide Internet and e-mail access for at least 75 percent of their employees and that teach employees to use the Internet and other electronic information systems to apply data and information to public health practice.

26-8 (Developmental) Reduce the cost of lost productivity in the workplace due to alcohol and drug use.

27-12 Increase the proportion of worksites with formal smoking policies that prohibit smoking or limit it to separately ventilated areas.

Access to Health Care

1-6 Reduce the proportion of families that experience difficulties or delays in obtaining health care or do not receive needed care for one or more family members.

3-12 Increase the proportion of adults who receive a colorectal cancer screening examination.

3-13 Increase the proportion of women aged forty years and older who have received a mammogram within the preceding two years.

12-15 Increase the proportion of adults who have had their blood cholesterol checked within the preceding five years.

14-24 Increase the proportion of young children and adolescents who receive all vaccines that have been recommended for universal administration for at least five years.

14-29 Increase the proportion of adults who are vaccinated annually against influenza and pneumococcal disease.

(*continued*)

Exhibit 12.2. Health Objectives. (*Continued*)

Health Communication

11-1 Increase the proportion of households with access to the Internet at home.

11-2 (Developmental) Improve the health literacy of persons with inadequate or marginal literacy skills.

11-3 (Developmental) Increase the proportion of health communication activities that include research and evaluation.

11-4 (Developmental) Increase the proportion of health-related websites that disclose information that can be used to assess the quality of the site.

11-5 (Developmental) Increase the number of centers for excellence that seek to advance the research and practice of health communication.

11-6 (Developmental) Increase the proportion of persons who report that their health care providers have satisfactory communication skills.

Source: United States Department of Health and Human Services, Office of Disease Prevention and Health Promotion, 2001.

How do we get there? (implementation) This step involves developing an *action plan*—a detailed description of how goals and objectives will be implemented. An action plan provides overall direction, fits resources and opportunities, minimizes resistance and barriers, and reaches the priority populations. The action plan describes the specifics of who will do what, by when, and at what cost. The components of a good action plan include these:

- People responsible (by whom)
- Date completed (by when)
- Resources required (costs)
- Action steps or strategies (what will be done)
- Collaborators (who should know, be involved)

A good action plan should include the *strategies* or *activities* that describe how an initiative will reach its objectives and advance the coalition mission. Many types of strategies exist, such as those which provide information or enhance skills (for example, professional conference); enhance services or support (for example, home visitation program); modify access, barriers, or opportunities (for example, mobile van to immunize rural residents); change consequences of efforts (for example, provide volunteer incentives); or modify policies (for example, nursing home vaccination policy).

An action plan also specifies who will be involved (individuals and organizations), the time frame for accomplishment, resources needed (personnel, money, equipment, or other), key milestones, and the expected result(s) or product. The more action-oriented the plan, the better it will be. Without a written plan, it is unlikely that such a diverse set of members—from organizations with different organizational cultures, from communities with different interests and concerns, and with varying levels of involvement—will be able to bring about significant change (Archer, Cripe, and McCaslin, 1992). The action plan "turns strategic planning into strategic management" (Strawn, Sumners, and Easterwood, 1999). Because the action plan tells what the coalition is going to do, it should be distributed in written form to all coalition members and the community where the coalition is looking for support.

How do we measure progress? (evaluating or benchmarking) Each strategic issue should have a corresponding set of benchmarks or measures to evaluate its implementation and accomplishments. Without appropriate measures, coalition members and community stakeholders will not know whether they are accomplishing their goals. Benchmarking assures that clear, objective measurement information is available and that results as well as activities are measured. The steering committee should monitor the plan's progress and continue to involve key stakeholders in a dynamic and evolving process. As goals are accomplished, the committee will be able to develop new tasks or modify existing goals.

Strategic planning can provide a useful framework for making policy-level decisions and designing effective techniques to implement those decisions. The process of aligning an organization with its environment often leads to better decision making, improved communications, unity of purpose, and increased organizational effectiveness (Strawn, Sumners, and Eastwood, 1999). Strategic planning helps an organization to establish a broad long-range perspective, identify strategic issues, and develop short-term goals, objectives, and action steps to address identified issues. Because strategic planning is time- and labor-intensive, it should not be considered as an end in itself that prescribes the coalition's activities and results. Strategic planning calls for staff and community partners to think continuously and act strategically to enhance the coalition's value and effectiveness.

EVALUATING STRATEGIC AND ACTION PLANS
AND THE PLANNING PROCESS

After a coalition's action plan or strategic plan is completed, an evaluation of the planning process as well as the plans that were created should be considered. Most planning models prescribe a planning process rather than articulate the desired attributes of a finished plan that is the outcome of such a process. To date, evaluation instruments have focused on the assessment of planning (Linney and Wandersman, 1991; Valdiserri, Aultman, and Curran, 1995) and methods to inventory or describe the content of community plans (Butterfoss and others, 1996; Centers for Disease Control, 2002). The Plan Quality Index, an assessment tool, is included as Exhibit 12.3.

Tools to assess public health infrastructure or capacity have been developed and disseminated, such as CDC's School Health Index, which provides comprehensive questionnaires that schools can use as self-assessment and planning tools to improve the effectiveness of their health and safety policies and programs (Centers

(*Text resumes on page 378.*)

Exhibit 12.3. Plan Quality Assessment Tool: Plan Quality Index (PQI).

Coalition: _____ Rater: _____ Date: _____ Score: _____

Check all elements of a comprehensive plan that are present in this plan.	
☐ **Needs Assessment Report**	☐ **Activities**
☐ **Goals**	☐ **Target population**
☐ **Objective(s)**	☐ **Timeline**
☐ **Budget**	☐ **Evaluation Plan**

	RATING SCHEME: Check one choice for each component (1–18)
0	**None of this plan component is adequate.**
1	**Approximately less than 20 percent of this plan component is adequate.**
2	**Approximately 20–40 percent of this plan component is adequate.**
3	**Approximately 41–60 percent of this plan component is adequate.**
4	**Approximately 61–80 percent of this plan component is adequate.**
5	**Approximately 81–100 percent of this plan component is adequate.**

COMPONENTS OF ACTION PLAN GOAL(S), OBJECTIVES, AND ACTIVITIES	*Rating (percent adequate)*						Score
	0	1–20	21–40	41–60	61–80	81–100	0–5
1. Needs assessment is comprehensive.							
2. Goal(s) adequately reflect desired outcomes to problems and needs identified in needs assessment.							
3. At least one relevant objective is stated for each goal.							
4. Specific, feasible activities are provided for each objective.							
5. Objectives and activities are logically related to statewide prevention priorities as reflected in a statewide plan or planning process.							
6. Objectives and activities are measurable, to facilitate evaluation.							
7. Specific priority populations are identified for each activity.							

Exhibit 12.3. (*Continued*)

COMPONENTS OF ACTION PLAN GOAL(S), OBJECTIVES, AND ACTIVITIES	*Rating (percent adequate)*						Score
	0	1–20	21–40	41–60	61–80	81–100	**0–5**
8. A timeline is provided for each activity.							
9. The agency, group, or individual who will coordinate each activity is identified.							
10. Sources of coordination and collaboration among community agencies and groups are identified.							
11. New preventive activities are coordinated with existing community programs and activities.							
12. The combined activities form a comprehensive, multilevel community-wide intervention.							
13. A budget that outlines sources of funding and expenses for activities is provided.							
14. The plan is feasible given the human resources and budget.							
15. The evaluation plan is clear and comprehensive.							
OVERALL IMPRESSION OF PLAN							
16. Clarity							
17. Effectiveness							
18. Quality							

Please feel free to add additional comments about plan or planning process on back.
Source: Butterfoss, Goodman, and Wandersman, 1995. Revised Butterfoss, 1996.

Instructions for Using the PQI to Rate Community Coalition Plans

These coalition plans should represent local efforts to achieve statewide prevention goals. They are developmental, and details such as timelines, budgets, and responsibility rosters may not yet be available. Rate each plan against the ideal that each coalition is striving to attain. Work alone on this evaluation and take as long as needed. Do not discuss your findings with other raters as it may influence their judgment.

(continued)

Exhibit 12.3. Plan Quality Assessment Tool: Plan Quality Index (PQI). (*Continued*)

STEP 1: Review *each* entire plan for general content. Refer to the first block of items on the PQI and check whether each component of an ideal plan is present in each coalition plan.

STEP 2: Review each component of the plan and determine whether it is adequately presented. If the component is missing, check 0. Otherwise check one of the 5 scores for each component (1–20 = 1, 21–40 = 2, 41–60 = 3, 61–80 = 4, 81–100 = 5) and put the proper number (1–5) in the score columns at the far right of the tool. If the component is subjective, consider the numbers as representing 1 = poor, 2 = weak, 3 = acceptable, 4 = good, 5 = outstanding.

STEP 3: To determine the percentage of adequacy for each component, review the parts of the plan which refer to that component. For example, look at component 3 (at least one relevant objective is stated for each goal). If only three objectives were adequate, the component would only be 75 percent adequate, so check the column labeled 61–80 percent adequate. Approach each component in the same way. For overall impression components, determine to what extent (percentage) the coalition has suceeded in achieving this component. See the detailed rating system that follows.

Component 1. Is the community needs assessment clear and comprehensive?

This component is scored according to whether the plan includes a complete or summarized assessment of community needs assessment covering
1. Local needs and strengths.
2. Target population(s) and sampling techniques.
3. Survey instruments.
4. Data collection methods.
5. Description of analysis.
Assignment of score is based on both subjective and objective criteria. Score as follows:

0	Blank
1	One of the above elements included
2	Two of the above elements included
3	Three of the above elements included
4	Four of the above elements included
5	Five of the above elements included

Score for Component 1: Points received out of five available in needs assessment part of plan.

Component 2. Do the goals adequately reflect desired outcomes to problems and needs identified in the community needs assessment?

If no goals are included in the plan, check 0. If a needs assessment is included, determine whether the goals address the needs. Each need should have one or more goal. If only three goals are present but five needs are stated, then rate the

Exhibit 12.3. (*Continued*)

component 66 percent, or 6. If no needs assessment is included, rate the goals subjectively, from poor to outstanding.

Score for Component 2: Percent of goals that reflect needs in the action plan.

Component 3. Does each goal have at least one relevant objective?

For each goal, determine if there is at least one accompanying objective. Rate 0 if no objectives are present and 1–5 based on the percentage of goals that have objectives.

Score for Component 3: Percent of goals with an accompanying objective.

Component 4: Are specific, clear activities provided for each goal?

Score this section according to amount of detail in the plan and the extent to which a logical flow of subtasks occurs that will accomplish the overall activity.

1. Bare minimum of tasks, no sequential order
2. Fairly logical progression of tasks, but gaps remain between completion of the tasks and the overall activity or between the tasks themselves
3. Logical progression of tasks, no gaps between tasks and activity, but could be more complete
4. Tasks fleshed out well, but no target groups/numerical targets in either tasks or activities
5. Tasks fleshed out well, identification of either the target group, numerical target, or both in either the task or activity sections

Score for Component 4: Percent of activities that have well developed activities.

Component 5: Are objectives and activities logically related to state prevention activities as reflected in a state plan or planning process?

Review objectives and activities and assess whether they follow logically from the state plan. Rate component as 0 if none of objectives or strategies follow logically from the state plan or 1–5 based on the percentage of objectives and activities that follow logically from the state plan.

Score for Component 5: Percent of activities logically related to the state plan.

Component 6: Are objectives and activities measurable?

For each activity, determine if either the objective or activity can be evaluated. Assess whether each of the following criteria is listed in either the objective or activity.

- Who will sponsor, conduct, or evaluate the activity?
- Who will receive the intervention/benefit?

(continued)

Exhibit 12.3. Plan Quality Assessment Tool: Plan Quality Index (PQI). *(Continued)*

- When?
- What?
- How much?

Give each activity a score of 0–100 percent depending on whether the criteria are met. Then average the scores of all activities to arrive at a mean percentage score.

Score for Component 6: Percent of activities that are measurable.

Component 7: Are specific priority populations identified for each activity?

For each activity, determine if a priority population is listed in either the objective or activity. The priority population is the population or group receiving the intervention—it can include organizations, the general public, or sociodemographic groups. Score each activity as follows:

1   No priority population
3   General priority population (i.e., residents, general public, schools, businesses)
5   Specific or quantified priority population

Then average the scores across all activities to arrive a final score.

Score for Component 7: Points received out of those available given the number of activities.

Component 8: Is a timetable provided for each activity?

For each activity, read the timeline section. Some breakdown of time should occur by quarter or month. If time is not differentiated (i.e., each task lists first quarter, or each task lists Mar–Jan), the timeline is not adequate.

Score for Component 8: Percent of activities with a detailed timeline.

Component 9: Is the agency, group, or individual coordinating each activity identified?

This section is scored according to the level of commitment and responsibility indicated in the respondent section of the action plans. Assess whether each of the following is listed:

- The local coalition or "all" of the action teams
- Specific action teams/task forces
- Local staff
- Each organization or individual listed

Then determine what percentage of activities include at least one of the above coordinators.

Score for Component 9: Percent of activities that identify coordinator.

Exhibit 12.3. (Continued)

Component 10: Community agencies who will *collaborate* in each activity are identified.

Identify the percentage of activities that include the collaborating groups or agencies.
Score for Component 10: Percent of activities that include at least one collaborating agency.

Component 11: Are new preventive activities coordinated with existing community programs or activities?

Identify the percentage of activities that are coordinated with existing programs.
Score for Component 11: Percent of activities that are coordinated with existing programs.

Component 12: Do the combined activities form a comprehensive, multi-level community-wide intervention?

First, rate each activity according to its expected highest level of change.

1 = Individual
2 = Interpersonal
3 = Institutional
4 = Community
5 = Public Policy

Then take the mean of the scores for all activities and use it as your rating.
Score for Component 12: Number of points for all activities. A higher score means that the coalition has activities planned at multiple levels of intervention and are more comprehensive.

Component 13: Is a budget that outlines sources of funding and expenses for activities included?

Review the budgetary references and rate the plan according to the activities that have sources, actual budgets, or both included.
Score for Component 13: Percent of activities that identify budget sources, amounts, or both.

Component 14: Is the plan feasible given the human resources and budget?

The appropriateness of the budget will be assessed for the action plan as a whole. The number of activities per $10,000 will be calculated. Plans will be ranked by activities per $10,000 and locally grouped to reflect their level of ambition given the available resources. Moderately ambitious plans will be scored the highest, with

(continued)

Exhibit 12.3. Plan Quality Assessment Tool: Plan Quality Index (PQI). *(Continued)*

very ambitious scoring the next highest, and low ambition levels scoring the lowest as follows:

1 = 20%	less than 1 activity per $10,000
2 = 40%	1 to < 2 activities per $10,000
3 = 60%	4 or more activities per $10,000
4 = 80%	3 to < 4 activities per $10,000
5 = 100%	2 to < 3 activities per $10,000

Score for Component 14: Total points received out of 5 available for budget.

Component 15: Is the evaluation plan clear and comprehensive?

This component is scored according to whether the plan includes a clear and comprehensive evaluation plan covering these questions:

1. Who will coordinate the evaluation?
2. Are target populations identified?
3. Are methods of assessment identified?
4. How will data be collected and who will do it?
5. How will data be analyzed and who will do it?

The evaluation plan is given one point for each of the elements above and scored 1–5.

Score for Component 15: Total points received out of 5 available for evaluation plan.

TOTAL SCORE: Add each of scores at the far right of the fifteen components and write the sum at the top of PQ1 form. Plans can receive from 0–75 points.

Overall Strength of the Plan

Component 16—Clarity	Component 17—Effectiveness	Component 18—Quality

Rate each component on a report card scale of A–F, corresponding to a subjective evaluation of poor to outstanding.

---

for Disease Control, 2004). On a larger scale, the National Public Health Performance Standards provide a framework for assessment of state and local public health systems (Centers for Disease Control, 2000c). Finally, the State Plan Index (SPI) was developed as part of the evaluation of CDC's Nutrition and Physical Activity Program to Prevent Obesity and Other Chronic Diseases (see Exhibit 12.4 on pages 380–389). SPI provided a tool to evaluate state plans that were developed by state public health practitioners and their community partners, using many different public health planning models (Butterfoss and Dunet, 2005).

In general, communities tend to do well in involving stakeholders; presenting epidemiologic data on disease burden; identifying their goals, objectives, and strategies; and making sure that the plan is disseminated. The more difficult tasks involve identifying resources for plan implementation, evaluation of programs, and integrating strategies with existing community efforts (Dunet, Butterfoss, Hamre, and Kuester, 2005). The exhibits in this chapter include two tools that may be used to evaluate comprehensive coalition plans—the Plan Quality Index (Butterfoss, Goodman, and Wandersman, 1995; Butterfoss, 1996) for community action plans in Exhibit 12.3 and the State Plan Index (Butterfoss and Dunet, 2005) for state-level plans (developed for obesity prevention, but adaptable for other health issues) in Exhibit 12.4.

COALITION SPOTLIGHT: STRATEGIC PLANNING WITH THE DECADE OF HOPE COALITION IN DULCE, NEW MEXICO

A tribal coalition in north central New Mexico cleverly modified the strategic planning process to conform to community cultural norms. Faced with increasing community problems, the Jicarilla Apache formed the Decade of Hope Coalition. Community leaders conceived the coalition as a community-led effort to address concerns about the high rates of both substance abuse and suicide among teens.

The University of Kansas (KU Work Group) was asked to provide technical assistance in strategic and action planning for coalition staff. The aim of this process was to create a vision and mission statement, objectives, strategies, and action plans to address identified community problems. A well-tested Action Planning Guide (Fawcett and others, 1994) provided a framework for creating and adopting a vision statement for a healthy community, and a mission statement of what the community would do and why. The Guide provided specific prompts for potential community changes (in other words, new or modified programs, policies, and practices) that could reduce risk and enhance protection for substance abuse.

Tribal members identified sectors of the community targeted for change by the Decade of Hope Coalition, including tribal and nontribal businesses, religious organizations, public schools and tribal education, tribal government, cultural organizations, tribal police and courts, youth organizations, media, health and service organizations, and native healers. Tribal members identified desired community changes related to substance abuse for each sector, such as banning fights in local bars and developing after-school programs for youth, as well as eighty-five objectives that would lead to those changes. Then coalition members specified who would do what activities by when to reach the action plan objectives. Coalition members and staff reviewed objectives and related accomplishments both informally and formally during monthly coalition meetings.

Three groundbreaking adaptations were made in the usual public health-planning process. First, coalition staff encouraged community members to generate ideas for

(Text resumes on page 389.)

Exhibit 12.4. State Plan Index Assessment Tool.

STEP 1: Review the plan and determine whether each of the sixty items is adequately presented. Measure the plan against the ideal stated in each item. Do not fill in missing details in your mind. The plan should stand on its own as written. If an item is not addressed in the plan, check the box labeled *N/A (Not Addressed)* for that item. Otherwise, check scores 1–5 for each item by using the guide below.

N/A = Not Addressed	Item was not mentioned or included in the plan.
1 = Low quality	The plan mentions the item, but no detail is given. The plan is very far from ideal.
2	Very limited detail is provided, or the plan is generally weak in the quality of information presented.
3 = Partial or variable	The plan addresses the item to some extent. An item scored "3" may also reflect a plan that sometimes reaches an ideal but sometimes also falls far short of ideal on the item. This is a middle-of-the-road score for an item.
4	The plan does a good, solid job in addressing the item. Some key pieces may be occasionally missing, but the item is judged generally adequate.
5 = High quality	For this item, the plan is consistently strong and often close to ideal.

STEP 2: On the State Plan Index Summary Page (last page), assign an overall score for each component as a whole by checking the box for that score in the space provided. This score should be based on your own judgment and assessment. It does not need to be an average of the scores in the category; however, if your overall score is very different from an average of the items, please be sure to comment, using a separate page.

STEP 3: Assign an overall assessment of the whole plan by checking the Overall Score for Entire Plan in the space provided on the State Plan Index Summary Page.

Exhibit 12.4. (*Continued*)

Component A: *Involvement of Stakeholders*	Not Addressed	1 = Low	3 = Variable/partial	5 = High			
	N/A	1	2	3	4	5	
1. Stakeholders in the planning process represent a balance among academic, government, public health, nonprofit, business, and advocacy organizations that represent people affected by obesity.	☐	☐	☐	☐	☐	☐	
2. Department of Health representatives in the planning process included experts in nutrition and physical activity as well as stakeholders with expertise in other chronic diseases.	☐	☐	☐	☐	☐	☐	
3. Leaders from state and community organizations were included in the planning process.	☐	☐	☐	☐	☐	☐	
4. Key stakeholders actively participated throughout the planning process.	☐	☐	☐	☐	☐	☐	
5. Organizations likely to be involved in providing resources and/or implementing the plan were involved in the planning process.	☐	☐	☐	☐	☐	☐	
6. Written endorsement of plan from governor, secretary of health, or other high-ranking state official is included.	☐	☐	☐	☐	☐	☐	
Component B: *Presentation of Data on Disease Burden and Existing Efforts to Prevent and Control Obesity*							
7. Data are presented on disease burden of obesity and chronic diseases related to poor nutrition and physical inactivity.	☐	☐	☐	☐	☐	☐	
8. Epidemiologic data are from reliable source(s) (for example, Behavioral Risk Factor Surveillance System, National Health and Nutrition Examination Survey).	☐	☐	☐	☐	☐	☐	
9. State-level data are provided, including results of state-specific epidemiologic or evaluation studies.	☐	☐	☐	☐	☐	☐	

(*continued*)

Exhibit 12.4. State Plan Index Assessment Tool. (*Continued*)

	Not Addressed	1 = Low		3 = Variable/partial		5 = High
10. Disease burden on subpopulations in state are identified, with special emphasis on diversity related to age, gender, ethnicity, sexual orientation, and income.	N/A ☐	1 ☐	2 ☐	3 ☐	4 ☐	5 ☐
11. Potential facilitating factors and barriers (behavioral, social, environmental, and economic) that contribute to healthy diet and physical activity are described.	N/A ☐	1 ☐	2 ☐	3 ☐	4 ☐	5 ☐
12. A conclusion is stated based on data presented to indicate population(s) at highest risk.	N/A ☐	1 ☐	2 ☐	3 ☐	4 ☐	5 ☐
13. Previous interventions conducted in state to address disease burden associated with poor diet and physical inactivity are described.	N/A ☐	1 ☐	2 ☐	3 ☐	4 ☐	5 ☐
Component C: Goals						
14. Plan relates to statewide effort, not just to selected cities, counties, or regions of state.	N/A ☐	1 ☐	2 ☐	3 ☐	4 ☐	5 ☐
15. Goals reflect needs and efforts of broad sector of organizations, not just state health department.	N/A ☐	1 ☐	2 ☐	3 ☐	4 ☐	5 ☐
16. Goals cover eight- to ten-year time frame.	N/A ☐	1 ☐	2 ☐	3 ☐	4 ☐	5 ☐
17. Goals focus on changing health status indicators within a state (for example, decreasing rate of increase in overweight and obesity).	N/A ☐	1 ☐	2 ☐	3 ☐	4 ☐	5 ☐
18. Circumstances in state expected to have a major influence are described (such as windfall from tobacco settlement, major reorganization of health department, budget crisis).	N/A ☐	1 ☐	2 ☐	3 ☐	4 ☐	5 ☐
19. Plan is not an inventory of existing programs. Plan makes clear that something *new* is gained that is likely to lead to change.	N/A ☐	1 ☐	2 ☐	3 ☐	4 ☐	5 ☐

Exhibit 12.4. (*Continued*)

Component D: Objectives	Not Addressed	1 = Low		3 = Variable/partial		5 = High
	N/A	1	2	3	4	5
20. Objectives are clearly organized.	☐	☐	☐	☐	☐	☐
21. Objectives are logically related to goals.	☐	☐	☐	☐	☐	☐
22. Objectives are related to state's public health goals (such as Healthy People 2010 nutrition and physical activity objectives).	☐	☐	☐	☐	☐	☐
23. Short-term objectives (changes in process) are included.	☐	☐	☐	☐	☐	☐
24. Intermediate objectives (changes in behavior, environment, or policy) are included.	☐	☐	☐	☐	☐	☐
25. Long-term objectives (changes in health status) are included.	☐	☐	☐	☐	☐	☐
26. Objectives include multiple ecological levels: individual, family, institutions, and community.	☐	☐	☐	☐	☐	☐
27. Objectives are SMART (Specific, Measurable, Attainable, Results-oriented, and Time-phased).	☐	☐	☐	☐	☐	☐
28. Objectives are sufficient in intensity to impact health status indicators.	☐	☐	☐	☐	☐	☐
29. Responsibility (a person, position, or organization) is identified for each objective.	☐	☐	☐	☐	☐	☐
Component E: Selecting Population(s) and Strategies for Interventions						
30. Criteria used to designate population subgroups selected for intervention are described.	☐	☐	☐	☐	☐	☐
31. Process of selecting groups for intervention included consideration of social marketing data, social habits, beliefs, and other social data relevant to population subgroups.	☐	☐	☐	☐	☐	☐

(continued)

Exhibit 12.4. State Plan Index Assessment Tool. (*Continued*)

	Not Addressed	1 = Low	3 = Variable/partial	5 = High
32. Assessment of resources and gaps in existing programs relevant to priority population was included in the planning process.	N/A ☐	1 ☐	2 ☐ 3 ☐ 4 ☐	5 ☐
33. Highest risk group(s) (identified in the description of epidemiologic data) are designated as high priority for intervention. If not, justification is presented.	N/A ☐	1 ☐	2 ☐ 3 ☐ 4 ☐	5 ☐
34. Criteria used to select interventions are described.	N/A ☐	1 ☐	2 ☐ 3 ☐ 4 ☐	5 ☐
35. Selection of intervention strategies is based on scientific evidence of effectiveness (for example, strategies recommended in the *Guide to Community Preventive Services* or promising new strategies) and strategies recommended by CDC (decreasing television time, increasing consumption of vegetables and fruit, balancing caloric intake and expenditure, increasing physical activity, and promoting breast-feeding).	N/A ☐	1 ☐	2 ☐ 3 ☐ 4 ☐	5 ☐
36. Strategies fit with characteristics (age, gender, culture, and so on) of population selected for intervention.	N/A ☐	1 ☐	2 ☐ 3 ☐ 4 ☐	5 ☐
Component F: Integration of Strategies with Other Programs and Implementation of Plan				
37. Plan describes how strategies will be integrated with existing programs that focus on chronic diseases, prevention, education, and service delivery.	N/A ☐	1 ☐	2 ☐ 3 ☐ 4 ☐	5 ☐
38. Plan describes how existing or potential partners (government, community-based, faith-based, business or industry, and private organizations) will be involved to implement plan.	N/A ☐	1 ☐	2 ☐ 3 ☐ 4 ☐	5 ☐
39. Ways that partners will be supported in the future (for example, training, technical assistance, and funding) are described.	N/A ☐	1 ☐	2 ☐ 3 ☐ 4 ☐	5 ☐
40. Sustainability of interventions is addressed in the plan.	N/A ☐	1 ☐	2 ☐ 3 ☐ 4 ☐	5 ☐

Exhibit 12.4. (*Continued*)

	Not Addressed	1 = Low	3 = Variable/partial	5 = High
41. Process for updating or revising the plan during implementation is described.	N/A ☐	1 ☐	2 ☐ 3 ☐	4 ☐ 5 ☐
Component G: Resources for Implementation of Plan				
42. Resources needed to implement plan are described.	N/A ☐	1 ☐	2 ☐ 3 ☐	4 ☐ 5 ☐
43. Strategies that will be used to obtain needed resources are described.	N/A ☐	1 ☐	2 ☐ 3 ☐	4 ☐ 5 ☐
44. Sustainability of resources over time is addressed in the plan.	N/A ☐	1 ☐	2 ☐ 3 ☐	4 ☐ 5 ☐
45. Plan identifies who will assume fiscal responsibility (lead agency).	N/A ☐	1 ☐	2 ☐ 3 ☐	4 ☐ 5 ☐
46. Plan describes how funds will be allocated to and from partners to support plan implementation.	N/A ☐	1 ☐	2 ☐ 3 ☐	4 ☐ 5 ☐
Component H: Evaluation				
47. Potential effects on priority population(s) and communities if goals and objectives are met are described in the plan.	N/A ☐	1 ☐	2 ☐ 3 ☐	4 ☐ 5 ☐
48. Short-term indicators (process) to be measured are outlined in the plan.	N/A ☐	1 ☐	2 ☐ 3 ☐	4 ☐ 5 ☐
49. Intermediate-term indicators (behavior, environment, or policy changes) to be measured are outlined in the plan.	N/A ☐	1 ☐	2 ☐ 3 ☐	4 ☐ 5 ☐
50. Long-term indicators (body mass index (BMI), BMI for age, and other health status outcomes) to be measured are outlined in the plan.	N/A ☐	1 ☐	2 ☐ 3 ☐	4 ☐ 5 ☐
51. Stakeholder involvement in ongoing evaluation activities is described.	N/A ☐	1 ☐	2 ☐ 3 ☐	4 ☐ 5 ☐
52. Methods that will be used to collect and analyze evaluation data are described.	N/A ☐	1 ☐	2 ☐ 3 ☐	4 ☐ 5 ☐

(*continued*)

Exhibit 12.4. State Plan Index Assessment Tool. (*Continued*)

	Not Addressed	1 = Low	3 = Variable/partial	5 = High
53. Needed changes in data collection and surveillance systems to support measurement of intermediate and long-term indicators are discussed.	N/A ☐	1 ☐	2 3 ☐ ☐	4 5 ☐ ☐
54. Plan describes regular reporting of evaluation data to stakeholders.	N/A ☐	1 ☐	2 3 ☐ ☐	4 5 ☐ ☐

Component I: Accessibility of Plan

55. Plan is written in clear and understandable language.	N/A ☐	1 ☐	2 3 ☐ ☐	4 5 ☐ ☐
56. Plan is logically organized into sections to make information easy to find.	N/A ☐	1 ☐	2 3 ☐ ☐	4 5 ☐ ☐
57. Plan includes description of intended audience.	N/A ☐	1 ☐	2 3 ☐ ☐	4 5 ☐ ☐
58. Plan is appropriate in content and scope for intended audience.	N/A ☐	1 ☐	2 3 ☐ ☐	4 5 ☐ ☐
59. Plan includes executive summary or other brief summary.	N/A ☐	1 ☐	2 3 ☐ ☐	4 5 ☐ ☐
60. Plan describes how it will be widely distributed (for example, posted on a website).	N/A ☐	1 ☐	2 3 ☐ ☐	4 5 ☐ ☐

State Plan Index Summary Page

Score by Component

Directions: Please assign an overall score for each component and note any comments in the space provided. Attach additional sheets if needed for comments.

	Not Addressed	1 = Low	3 = Variable/partial	5 = High
A: Involvement of Key Stakeholders	N/A ☐	1 ☐	2 3 ☐ ☐	4 5 ☐ ☐
B: Presentation of Data on Disease Burden and Existing Efforts in Obesity	N/A ☐	1 ☐	2 3 ☐ ☐	4 5 ☐ ☐

Exhibit 12.4. (*Continued*)

	N/A	1	2	3	4	5
C: Goals	☐	☐	☐	☐	☐	☐
D: Objectives	☐	☐	☐	☐	☐	☐
E: Selecting Population(s) and Strategies for Interventions	☐	☐	☐	☐	☐	☐
F: Integration of Strategies with Other Programs and Implementation of Plan	☐	☐	☐	☐	☐	☐
G: Resource Development	☐	☐	☐	☐	☐	☐
H: Evaluation	☐	☐	☐	☐	☐	☐
I: Accessibility of Plan	☐	☐	☐	☐	☐	☐
WHAT IS YOUR OVERALL ASSESSMENT OF THE ENTIRE PLAN?	☐	☐	☐	☐	☐	☐

Source: Butterfoss, 2005.

STATE PLAN INDEX COMPONENTS*

A. Involvement of Stakeholders. Early involvement increases the likelihood that stakeholders will develop a sense of ownership in the plan and a commitment to making it succeed. The different experiences and perspectives that partners bring will help ensure that the plan is responsive to the needs of all segments of the population. Each partner brings its own contacts and constituents, widening the base of support for the plan and increasing its credibility across the state. Community planning models emphasize the need for meaningful involvement of stakeholders with some models designed for community-led planning. (See, for example, MAPP[3].)

B. Presentation of Data on Disease Burden and Existing Efforts to Control It. Evidence-based public health practice must include a systematic examination of data on disease burden for population subgroups. Assessing existing resources that address a public health problem identifies opportunities for partnership and the potential to leverage additional resources. The use of reliable data sources lends credibility to the planning process. Evidence-based planning models, such as PRECEED-PROCEED, emphasize the need for data to inform decision making.

C. Goals. Goals provide a vision of what planners intend to achieve. Because planning itself consumes time and other resources, something important should be gained. Goals should unambiguously convey that something new is intended that is likely to lead to

(*continued*)

Exhibit 12.4. State Plan Index Assessment Tool. (*Continued*)

desired change in health status indicators. Tools based on community planning models have been developed to assist in developing goals, including the Community Tool Box.

D. Objectives. Objectives should be specific, measurable, achievable, results-oriented, time-phased, and logically organized. They should be consistent with the overall public health priorities of the state and tied directly to the goals specified in the plan. As with goals, tools that support planning models provide guidance on developing and writing sound objectives.

E. Selecting Population(s) and Strategies for Intervention. Advances in social marketing applied to public health have contributed to the design of interventions better matched to the intended audience. Many planning models, such as CDCynergy, emphasize the importance of understanding a community and the unique attributes of its members before selecting strategies. Setting criteria for a systematic selection of interventions supports an evidence-based approach to public health. Although disease burden may figure prominently among the criteria used to select interventions, other criteria may be even more important, for example, political factors in a community or a subgroup's readiness to change. Documenting the rationale for selecting strategies clarifies the planning group's decision-making process and informs plan implementers who become involved later.

F. Integration of Strategies with Other Programs and Implementation of Plan. Public health partnerships and collaborations are key strategies to leverage limited resources. Often, however, a trade-off with partnerships is less direct control of action steps. Planning for systematic assessment of implementation steps helps ensure that a plan is carried out as designed and provides feedback useful for midcourse correction. Planning models, such as CHIP, may emphasize the need to consider how new strategies can be integrated into existing infrastructure.

G. Resources for Implementation of Plan. A plan may serve little purpose unless planners address how to locate, maintain, and sustain resources needed to implement the plan. Although this step is not often explicitly addressed in planning models, public health practitioners provided many examples of promising new initiatives that terminated because of the lack of resources that could sustain efforts for a time period long enough to achieve intended outcomes. In an era when public health resources are stretched thin, it is important for planners to consider what resources are currently available as well as what would be needed to implement the plan.

H. Evaluation. Virtually every planning model reviewed for this study identified evaluation as an important and useful activity. Some planning models also emphasize the importance of incorporating evaluation into a planning process, such as Getting to Outcomes. As part of planning, measures of success can be identified and systems set in place to monitor progress and identify problems once plan implementation begins.

Exhibit 12.4. (*Continued*)

Because planning groups may disband after a plan is written, planners should identify those who will carry out an evaluation, and the audience for evaluation information.

I. Accessibility of Plan. Just as varied planning models may be used, a written plan may have several different audiences. A good plan should be understandable and useful. As much as possible, the plan should be designed to elicit interest and support in the reader. Early plans should be made for distribution to ensure that the plan is disseminated to those who can contribute to its success.

---

community changes by "meeting them where they were"—in homes, offices, and on the street. Compared to formal planning retreats, many more participants were engaged by using this innovative method. As a result, community members willingly volunteered to bring about changes that many coalitions can only accomplish with intensive staff involvement.

Second, instead of using a written action plan grid (as described on pp. 370–371 of this chapter), the coalition office had a "planning wall" with sticky notes that detailed the proposed changes, dates, and names of the person(s) responsible. The sticky notes with the proposed changes were moved to the "success wall" as they were accomplished. This process was closer to the tribe's oral tradition and was received much better by coalition members than a planning document would have been.

Third, implementers (the change agents) were publicly recognized for their contributions, and the process became an ongoing, celebratory activity. Whenever someone who had not already contributed entered the room (and sometimes even if that person had contributed), he or she was asked to nominate some desirable community change. The Decade of Hope Coalition proved that strategizing and action planning could be fun and productive.

Contributed by Vincent T. Francisco, Ph.D., University of North Carolina, Greensboro

SUMMARY

The assessment process and resulting data become the foundation for the coalition's strategic planning, whereas an action plan is the short-term (one- to three-year) plan for implementing activities that will impact the health issue under consideration. The strategic planning process usually includes a SWOT analysis of the internal and external environment (Strengths, Weaknesses, Opportunities, and Threats), visioning, and developing the coalition's mission, name, goals, and objectives. The action plan usually details the individuals and organizations involved in accomplishing those objectives, the time frame for accomplishment, needed resources (personnel, money, equipment, or other resources), key milestones, and the expected result(s) or product(s). Careful planning helps ensure that community partners will think and act strategically to enhance the coalition's value and effectiveness.

QUESTIONS FOR REVIEW

1. What steps do most of the comprehensive planning models have in common?

2. Which planning model(s) seem most useful for coalition planning? Why?

3. What is the difference between strategic planning and action planning?

RESOURCES

Community Tool Box. *Developing a Strategic Plan.* 2005. Accessed January 15, 2006. http://ctb.ku.edu/tools/en/section_1085.htm. Provides specific examples, directions, and worksheets for developing vision and mission statements, goals and objectives, and action plans.

The National Campaign to Prevent Teen Pregnancy. *Breaking Ground: Lessons Learned from the Centers for Disease Control and Prevention's Community Coalition Partnership Programs for the Prevention of Teen Pregnancy.* Washington, D.C.: Author, 2003. http://www.dhs.state.or.us/children/publications/tpp/breakingground.pdf

United States Department of Health and Human Services, Office of Disease Prevention and Health Promotion. *Healthy People in Healthy Communities: A Community Planning Guide Using Healthy People 2010.* Washington, D.C.: Author, 2001. http://www.healthypeople.gov/Publications/HealthyCommunities2001/default.htm. Accessed July 20, 2006. A guide for building community coalitions, creating a vision, measuring results, and creating partnerships dedicated to improving the health of a community. Includes "Strategies for Success" for help in starting community activities.

United States Department of Transportation, National Highway Traffic Safety Administration. *Community How-to Guide on Needs Assessment and Strategic Planning.* http://www.nhtsa.dot.gov/people/injury/alcohol/Community%20Guides%20HTML/Book2_NeedsAssess.html#strategic%20plan. Accessed December 16, 2005.

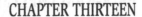

CHAPTER THIRTEEN

Coalition Activities and Interventions

If you always do what you've always done, then you'll always
get what you've always got.
—Moms Mabely, comedian, 1894–1975

Once the coalition has carefully done a community assessment and developed its action plan, the next step is to develop and implement strategies to achieve its goals and objectives. Effective strategies should reflect the values and priorities of the coalition. Moreover, they should build on existing resources, opportunities, and programs in the community. Coalitions are usually judged on the merit of the programs, activities, and services that they provide within their communities. Some coalitions implement programs themselves; some subcontract with organizations outside of the coalition to be the actualizers; and still others stimulate and work with member organizations to execute initiatives that partners have agreed upon. In all of these scenarios, coalitions "play a critical catalyst role in identifying community needs, designing innovative solutions, and mobilizing community support for those efforts" (Foster-Fishman and others, 2001, p. 256).

These programs are more likely to achieve realistic goals and be supported by the community because they use limited resources efficiently, complement existing programs, are culturally competent, provide focus for coalition member work efforts, achieve intermediate outcomes, and promote coalition credibility by addressing community needs in an innovative way (Foster-Fishman and others, 2001, pp. 256–257). This chapter will focus on the phases of program implementation, how to select and implement promising interventions at all levels of the social ecology, and types of interventions, with an emphasis on social marketing and media advocacy strategies. Finally, the ethical and legal considerations encountered by coalitions and partnerships when implementing their strategies will be highlighted.

PHASES OF PROGRAM IMPLEMENTATION

Program implementation involves converting goals and objectives into action (Timmreck, 2003, p. 328) and setting up, managing, and executing a project (Keyser and others, 1997). A good program plan, however, does not always translate into an effective intervention (Steuart, 1993; Steckler and others, 1995). Program evaluations indicate that a disproportionate amount of resources often goes into program planning versus intervening with actual programs, with the programs themselves becoming increasingly less effective as they move from the planning stage to implementation (Steckler, Orville, Eng, and Dawson, 1992; Goodman, Steckler, Hoover, and Schwartz, 1993).

Implementation is generally accepted as consisting of five phases: adopting the program; identifying and prioritizing tasks (that is, the program *logistics* of hiring personnel and procuring materials, equipment, and space); establishing a system of management; putting plans into action; and sustaining or ending the program (McKenzie, Neiger, and Smeltzer, 2005). The fourth phase, putting plans into action, will be the focus of this chapter.

Programs can be piloted, phased in, or initiated all at once. They should go through all three phases in order, as long as time and resources are available. Pilot-testing allows program planners to work out any "bugs" before the program is offered to more people in the priority population and to validate the work completed prior to this phase. The new program should be piloted in a setting similar to the one where it will be implemented and with people similar to those who will eventually use it. The coalition should ensure that the strategies were implemented and worked as planned and that resources were adequate, and participants should evaluate the program (McKenzie, Neiger, and Smeltzer, 2005).

Once the program has been piloted and revised, the coalition should phase it in gradually, to control for quality and avoid being overwhelmed by a large number of participants. Phasing-in can occur by gradually adding more parts of the program, limiting the number of participants, offering it in select locations, or offering it for different levels of ability—that is, beginner, intermediate, and advanced (McKenzie, Neiger, and Smeltzer, 2005). Total implementation should only happen for single programs, such as screenings or lectures, where resources do not allow for pilot programs. Exhibit 13.1 provides a summary of the practical steps involved in developing a program from initial conception to funding.

SELECTING AND IMPLEMENTING
PROJECTS

After a list of potential projects is developed, the coalition should prioritize it, discarding those projects that are not relevant to its core set of goals. For each potential project, the coalition can use the following set of criteria to evaluate feasibility and

Exhibit 13.1. Practical Steps in Program Development.
___

The following steps will help move a program concept to a funded program. Program quality and marketability can be improved by addressing these key concepts.

1. **Community needs assessment:** Assess and review community needs and service gaps—formally and informally—on a regular basis, and also consider crisis needs.

2. **Community assets assessment:** Recognize and continually update your understanding of community strengths, resources, and other assets.

3. **Concept development:** Brainstorm and assess concepts and approaches for meeting community needs, both immediate and long-term.

4. **Program content outline:** Once a promising concept is identified, develop it into a program outline with clear goals, measurable objectives, defined components, implementation tasks, rough budget, and staffing requirements.

5. **Assessment of concept:** Evaluate the proposed program based on formal criteria or informal questions to decide whether to continue developing and marketing it.

6. **Potential funder research:** Identify and research possible funding sources, and then review the program against the missions, funding priorities, and past grants of several potential donors to determine its probable marketability.

7. **Consultation with donors:** Discuss the program concept with one or two supportive donors, particularly those that might be interested in supporting it. Ask for feedback on the program's marketability, including any specific concerns that need to be addressed in the proposal.

8. **Marketability analysis:** Develop a marketability summary for the program to identify the program's strengths and weaknesses. Then decide how to maximize strengths and overcome weaknesses in written and oral presentations.

9. **Proposal preparation:** Prepare a general proposal that includes key points to be made in presenting the project to funders and a targeted proposal or letter of inquiry for specific donors.

10. **Donor meetings:** Meet with potential donors if possible, using your marketability summary to prepare a strong presentation about why they should support the program.
___

Source: Adapted from Mosaica, 2005c.

likelihood of success (Finklestein, French, Variyam, and Haines, 2004; The National Campaign to Prevent Teen Pregnancy, 2003; Rabinowitz, 2003a):

- Does justification for the intervention exist (what is the health concern)?
- What are the intended consequences (will the intervention help resolve the health concern)? What might be the unintended consequences?

- Does this intervention reflect clear coalition priorities, goals, and objectives?
- Is this intervention aligned with the priorities of community partners?
- Does this intervention focus on the appropriate level of influence (for example, intrapersonal, interpersonal, institutional or organizational, or community)?
- Are the strategies based on appropriate theory and constructs?
- Is the intervention within the scope of the staff and partners who will implement it? Is anyone missing whose lack of participation could weaken the whole project?
- Does the intervention integrate with existing ones in the community?
- Is this intervention an appropriate cultural fit for the priority population?
- Is this intervention likely to have early results (for example, within one year) and succeed?
- What types of strategies are known to be effective in dealing with this health issue?
- Is the intervention cost-effective?
- Is the intervention politically feasible?
- How will success be measured and evaluated?
- Will the intervention have a meaningful impact, that is, will it change access or delivery of services, save considerable resources, or maximize the efforts of partners?

After applying the above standards, the list of potential projects may be reduced to two or three that best fit the criteria. To test the viability of the prioritized list, it should be vetted with coalition partners to get their initial reactions. Partners should be actively engaged in brainstorming the details of the projects to see whether they are feasible. To prevent undermining the projects, the coalition must ensure that it has the human and material resources to implement each project; the coalition leadership is committed to support these potential projects; approval or support is obtained from the coalition's lead agency and its partner organizations; staff are aware of and support the projects; and potential barriers to implementation have been assessed. For instance, can the coalition find resources or willing partners to cover project costs? Are coalition partners willing to share information or help implement strategies? Will the time and energy invested in the project pull staff and partners away from other work (Rabinowitz, 2003a)?

The Project Team

Once a project is identified, the next step is to choose the project team. Team membership should be determined by the members' commitment and capacity to implement the project. The persons who will lead the project should be determined, as well as those who will have primary responsibility for other tasks such as marketing, communication, and evaluation. The team must ensure that information about the project and its aims is communicated within the coalition, the lead agency, and the community. As detailed in Chapter Twelve, the coalition should develop an action plan that includes a timeline, a list of deliverables, specific outcomes, and measures that will let the coalition know whether it has achieved those outcomes.

After the project is initiated, the project team should meet on a regular basis to evaluate progress and ensure that the project is on track to reach expected outcomes. In addition to regular meetings, the team should hold a special meeting within a year of the project's initiation to review its progress, examine barriers, and learn from mistakes. If the project is going well, members can celebrate its achievements and perhaps expand it. Because one successful project often leads to another, they may be encouraged to select another project to implement from the original list of ideas. If progress is poor, members should ask themselves whether the project was truly a priority, whether community or coalition barriers interfered, or whether incentives were insufficient to build participation and support (Rabinowitz, 2003b). This self-assessment should be the basis of improving the planning process and the project itself.

Assessing Promising Practices and Interventions

A *practice* is a particular way of doing things, usually involving a single method, whereas an *intervention* is usually a whole initiative meant to achieve an overall result; thus practices are the tools of interventions (Rabinowitz, 2003a). An example of a practice is immunizing eleven- to twelve-year-olds against hepatitis B, because that schedule provides protection when they most need it. However, an intervention chosen to carry out this hepatitis B immunization practice is an integrated program of making contact with adolescents and their parents, enlisting a popular teen role model to promote the program, providing incentives, and ensuring that the entire series of immunizations is administered. Sometimes an intervention with several components may be considered a practice if the program needs all of the components and a given structure to work.

Sometimes, no model exists for what the coalition wants to do. If so, the coalition can base its practices and interventions on theory, a new research idea, or past experience (Community Tool Box, 2003a). The coalition could also discuss the problem with the priority population and the community at large, and develop a practice or intervention that is sensitive to that population's or community's history and culture (Rabinowitz, 2003a).

Quality of life and health in the United States have been improved by the use of practices that were demonstrably effective in randomized controlled trials. Research-proven practices over the past five decades include vaccinating for polio and measles, thereby effectively eradicating these diseases; interventions for hypertension and high cholesterol that have decreased coronary heart disease and stroke by more than 50 percent; and cancer treatments that have improved survival rates from leukemia, Hodgkin's disease, and many other cancers (Partnership for Prevention, 2004). Similarly, guided by knowledge about "what works" from randomized controlled trials over the past ten years, changes in welfare policy have moved many people from welfare into the workforce (Partnership for Prevention, 2004). However, practices that are guided by strong evidence of effectiveness (such as randomized controlled trials) are often difficult to implement and replicate in a community setting.

Coalitions should research whether a program they plan to implement has been tried before and found effective. *Proven interventions* are backed by at least one credible, scientifically rigorous study showing the program improves at least one indicator. Credibility and rigor are determined by how issues such as study design, sample size, use of a reasonable comparison group, achieving a sizeable effect, low attrition, and the program's direct effect on the given indicator are handled (Promising Practices Network on Children, Families, and Communities, 2005). Such interventions have the following factors in common (U.S. Office of Management and Budget, 2004):

- Adequate sample size; few or no systematic differences between intervention and control groups prior to the intervention
- Low attrition and little or no difference in attrition between intervention and control groups
- Outcome data collected and reported for intervention group members who do not participate in or complete the intervention
- After randomization, few or no crossovers between intervention and control groups
- Valid outcome measures, preferably well-established tests, objective, real-world measures, or both (for example, DUI [driving under the influence of alcohol] rates for an injury-prevention intervention)
- Appropriate tests for statistical significance
- Long-term outcome data to judge whether intervention effects were sustained over time
- Corroboration of study resulting in more than one implementation site— preferably similar community settings

Many organizations, agencies, or government departments identify *promising interventions or practices* as those that solve a specific problem or treat a specific condition; address the underlying causes of a disease or health issue; or promote positive health knowledge, attitudes, and behaviors (Rabinowitz, 2003a). Promising programs are backed by at least some direct evidence that the program improves outcomes for participants. However, they may affect intermediate variables rather than direct outcomes, be evaluated with less rigorous methodologies, or contain many caveats about the findings (Promising Practices Network on Children, Families, and Communities, 2005). Promising interventions have the potential to effectively address the issues of concern in a given community. The coalition benefits from others' experiences on how to make the intervention even more effective, but promising interventions may also be untried if they are based on solid criteria.

The Guide to Community Preventive Services (*Community Guide*) is a federally sponsored initiative that provides public health decision makers with recommendations regarding population-based interventions to promote health and to prevent disease, injury, disability, and premature death, appropriate for use by communities and health care systems. The Independent Task Force on Community Preventive Services makes its recommendations based on systematic reviews of topics in three general areas: changing risk behaviors; reducing diseases, injuries, and impairments; and addressing environmental and ecosystem challenges (Briss, Brownson, Fielding, and Zaza, 2004). Systematic reviews are conducted for selected interventions within each health topic and organized as a *chapter*. Within the Community Guide, systematic reviews evaluate the evidence of effectiveness, which is then translated into a recommendation or a finding of insufficient evidence. For those interventions where evidence of effectiveness is insufficient, the Community Guide will provide guidance for further prevention research. However, a determination that evidence is insufficient should not be confused with evidence of ineffectiveness.

The Community Guide is useful because it assures more effective delivery of essential public health services at the local level; assists in refining the approaches to identifying and weighing the evidence; and helps the public better understand the power and reach of public health programs working on their behalf (McGinnis, 2005).

Community-based health-promotion practices and interventions have also been systematically assessed, using categories of effectiveness, plausibility, and practicality (Cameron and others, 2001). *Effectiveness criteria* assess scientific evidence of efficacy, or effectiveness. This evidence may result from outcome or impact evaluations and is classified as positive, insufficient, no evidence, or no positive change found.

Plausibility criteria assess the extent to which a program incorporates these elements: formative evaluation, pilot testing, and process evaluation to ensure practical implementation; clear behavioral objectives and appropriate behavioral principles to ensure that it is conceptually sound and takes advantage of scientifically established principles for inducing change; and sensitivity to adopters' priority issues to ensure that broader community concerns are addressed, namely collaborative approach, visibility, sustainability, community leader support, outreach, community buy-in, and mobilization of community resources.

Finally, *practicality criteria* assess the extent to which the intervention was cost-effective (addressed start-up costs, ongoing implementation costs, reach, and projected longevity); available; and compatible with local practices and policies (supportable, generalizable, adaptable, linguistically and culturally accessible, and able to be evaluated). Practicality criteria also address the extent to which an intervention had the proper expertise needed for implementation.

When looking for promising practices and interventions, coalitions should be aware that an intervention that worked adequately well in one community may, with minor adjustments, work very well in their own communities. On the other hand, something that worked well in one community may not be appropriate for another. The coalition should be clear about which practices and interventions fit its goals and interests, and whether its resources are sufficient to implement them. Coalitions should also seek out examples of promising interventions that did *not* work; they may even find some in their own communities. Information about promising practices and interventions can be obtained through a variety of resources (see websites under Resources at the end of this chapter). Coalitions can network with community members, clergy, service clubs (for example, Rotary and Kiwanis), and businesses, all of which may have knowledge of successful intervention models through their networks. Coalitions can also search the Internet and libraries for promising practices for a given health-promotion issue. State and national advocacy organizations, as well as professional ones, give awards for best practices, feature them at annual conferences, and publish them in journals. Finally, international, state, and federal agencies, as well as foundations and private funders, often list best practices in the programs they fund. Exhibit 13.2 is a self-assessment tool that coalitions may use to search for, and choose, promising practices.

Exhibit 13.2. Self-Assessment to Find or Choose Promising Practices.

A. To search for promising practices for your coalition and community

1. What is the broad area of interest (for example, health promotion or disease prevention)?
2. What specific issue are you working on (for example, substance abuse or obesity)?
3. What population(s) will benefit from your effort (for example, Hispanics, youth, rural groups)?
4. What type of intervention or community change (in other words, change in program, policy, or practice) do you seek? Is it prioritized in your strategic plan?
5. In what sector of the community will this take place (for example, business, youth groups, churches)?
6. Are you interested in an intervention for a high-risk group, a comprehensive approach, or both?

B. To choose promising practices for your coalition and community

1. Does the promising practice meet all of the criteria set by your search?
2. Do community coalitions or other organizations exist that can support the effort?
3. What is the evidence that the promising practice will have some impact?
4. Will you be able to replicate the practice? If not, how will you modify it for your community?
5. What resources or potential resources are available to support the practice?
6. Is the practice compatible with your community's beliefs, attitudes, and values?
7. Have you found examples or stories of the practice in the Community Tool Box or other resources?
8. Have you contacted others who have implemented the practice?
9. How will this promising practice work for you? What would make it successful?

Source: Rabinowitz, 2000. KU Work Group on Health Promotion and Community Development. (2006). "Tool 1: A Self-Assessment To Help You Find and Choose Promising Practices" from *Criteria for Choosing Promising Practices and Community Interventions* contributed by Phil Rabinowitz, with material adapted from Lisbeth Schorr's Common Purpose, edited by J. Schultz & V. Renault. Lawrence, KS: University of Kansas. Retrieved July 17, 2006 from the World Wide Web: http://ctb.ku.edu/tools/en/sub_section_tools_1152.htm

Characteristics of Successful Interventions

One way to approach the search for promising practices and interventions is to look at the general elements of programs that seem to work. First, successful interventions are comprehensive, flexible, and responsive (Schorr, 1997). They address many aspects of an issue and change according to the needs of the participants and the community. Successful programs and interventions change their practices in response to new information, shifts in the community, and the reactions of program participants. By being dynamic, these programs evolve over time, continually striving to be better. According to Rogers (1995), when individuals and organizations adopt a new practice or idea, they often reinvent it, or make it their own, by changing it to meet their particular needs. These *reinvented innovations* work better and are more likely to be adopted permanently because they are better adapted to local conditions and imbued with a sense of ownership.

Second, successful interventions target the underlying causes of problems, have a long-term preventive orientation, and are maintained for as long as it takes to accomplish their purposes (Schorr, 1997). Program effects should last for at least one year beyond treatment, although many programs that demonstrate initial success fail to show long-term maintenance of the effects after the intervention has ended (Center for the Study and Prevention of Violence, 2005). The full impact of an intervention may not occur at the end of treatment; significant improvement may be realized over time, or a decline may result.

Third, successful programs are managed by competent and committed individuals with strong skills in budget and personnel management and communication (Rabinowitz, 2003a). Competent staff are collaborative and willing to experiment and take risks; they also tolerate ambiguity and seek evidence of results. These staff should include people who represent the priority population(s) and are committed to high-quality service and to building leadership and other capacities in the local population. The coalition and lead agency should support them with ongoing education and training. Most important, staff must work to build strong relationships based on mutual trust and respect with program participants (Schorr, 1997).

Fourth, successful programs should have reasonable costs that are less, or at least no greater, than their expected benefits. Expensive programs are difficult to maintain when competition is high and funding resources are low. Implementing expensive programs that will, at best, have small effects is counterproductive (Center for the Study and Prevention of Violence, 2005).

Fifth, successful programs are collaborative both internally and externally (Rabinowitz, 2003a). Internal collaboration refers to the inclusion of both staff and participants in the planning, implementation, and decision making of the program. External collaboration means involving a broad range of partners who have connections to the issues being addressed in order to provide a comprehensive, integrated program.

Sixth, successful interventions build shared purpose among staff and participants to overcome barriers and setbacks (Rabinowitz, 2003a). Core values, such as a passion for the work and social justice, encourage personal development and empowerment among participants.

Seventh, successful programs depend less on their structure and content (that is, how they are conducted) than on the development of relationships that help sustain and support people (Henderson, Bernard, and Sharp-Light, 1999). Policymakers often seek "silver bullets" for solutions to social problems and would like to fund *the* program that can eliminate the problem. However, poor community health outcomes rarely result from a single incident or source. Other supporting structures and institutions *besides* the program must also work to strengthen the community.

Lastly, effective community-based programs contribute to the community as mediating factors or "social-capital builders" (Bruner, 2004). Their broader community impact is missed if they are recognized only for their direct impact on participants. The best interventions are more than a set of strategies; they serve as "community-building anchors" and create opportunities for community members to exercise leadership (Bruner, 2004). Case studies of exemplary programs consistently show these community-based impacts as the most significant (Schorr, 1997).

To satisfy the diverse interests of coalition members, promising practices should involve a mix of community service strategies, research activities, and advocacy actions. This mix can vary at any given time, but effective coalitions learn how to juggle priorities to meet the needs of their members without concentrating on any one activity, which could alienate partners or be seen as competitive. Many coalitions succumb to the trap of becoming a provider of community services that directly compete with those provided by organizational members. Instead, the coalition might think of itself in a variety of roles for stimulating change, including these: an incubator of novel ideas and new ways of conceptualizing public health practice; a vehicle for testing innovative strategies that can, if the coalition is successful, be disseminated to its partners; a model of an academic-community partnership that engages in groundbreaking research; an advocate for the underserved or those experiencing disparities in health; a link that helps new relationships among its partner organizations develop and flourish; and a trainer and technical-assistance provider that builds skills and capacities of its members and the greater community for assessment, implementation, and evaluation. According to the Community Tool Box (Rabinowitz, 2003a), the following steps can assure that promising practices and interventions fit the coalition and community needs and circumstances. All of these steps assume that the coalition and community will be involved in aspects of planning and implementation.

1. Conduct a community-based assessment and planning process to identify the most appropriate and pressing issues for the community.

2. Decide whether the issues will be addressed directly or whether working on their causes will be more effective.

3. Find practices or interventions that have successfully addressed the issues in the way the coalition wants to address them.

4. Change the promising intervention, or parts of it, so that it suits the community's needs.

5. Implement the intervention, making continuous adjustments to fit the community and the priority population.

6. Evaluate progress regularly, understanding that no matter how well any intervention works, it can always be improved.

Implementing Community-Based Strategies

A *strategy* is one of the broad steps in a plan to accomplish a specific goal. Sometimes community activists and coalitions also use the term *tactics* to refer to individual, grounded acts that make up an overall strategy (Community Tool Box, 2005b). Many coalitions are involved in reducing the risk for disease and disability and increasing protective factors. *Risk reduction* means discovering which factors lead to the problem and working to reduce or eliminate those factors; for example, in preventing lung cancer, reducing or eliminating smoking reduces risk (Community Tool Box, 2005b). *Protective factors* help reduce or counteract risks; for example, eating healthy, low-cholesterol food is a protective factor in reducing heart disease.

Effective risk reduction strategies work to increase protective factors in ways that are appropriate for the culture and maturity of the priority population. They are used early in the intervention and make the best use of available time and material resources. Interventions that include more than one strategy are more likely to have an effect on the priority population than those consisting of only one, especially if multiple risk factors are involved (Shea and Basch, 1990; Erfurt, Foote, Heirich, and Gregg, 1990). Furthermore, few people change their behavior after an exposure to a single strategy; multiple exposures, or *doses,* are needed to change most behaviors (McKenzie, Neiger, and Smeltzer, 2005, p. 179). Multiple strategies are more likely to keep the health message in the public eye, reach the priority population, appeal to a variety of learning styles, and increase the likelihood that the combined strategies will achieve program goals and objectives (McKenzie, Neiger, and Smeltzer, 2005, p. 205).

Coalition and community members, especially members of the priority population, should be involved in Implementing risk reduction strategies in order to:

- Change community norms and values, which are often tied to risk and protective factors
- Increase trust and credibility for the coalition.
- Create a wider base of support for changing behavior.
- Identify available strengths and resources in the community.
- Galvanize public support for the initiative.
- Integrate chosen strategies in other community activities to create long-term change.

Levels of Intervention

Coalitions must also decide whether they are going to intervene at the individual (intra- and interpersonal), institutional, or organizational level; the community level; or both. Coalitions are especially suited to making change at the organizational or community levels, but at times, they may work with partner organizations to enhance health services or programs that focus on the individual. Strategies that may be used to change *individual behavior* include these: using incentives to reward or encourage protective behavior (such as lower insurance rates for nonsmokers) and disincentives to penalize or discourage risky behavior (such as high taxes on cigarettes); providing support through peer counselors; creating mentor programs in which more experienced people work to help others change their behavior; enhancing resources by raising money, improving materials, linking with other programs and services, or increasing awareness of available resources; removing barriers to make the program more accessible (for example, school breakfast and lunch programs); creating, modifying, or terminating policy; providing information via informational campaigns and community outreach; providing skills training and modeling using peer education; and providing feedback on progress via risk reduction counseling (Community Tool Box, 2003a).

The strategies that are used to change *organizational and community knowledge, policies, and practices* include conducting public awareness and media campaigns (for example, street and community outreach), assessing communities, building coalitions and partnerships, changing access to products and services, developing resources to enhance family and peer support, enforcing existing policies and laws, conducting advocacy actions and nonviolent protests, and changing policies and laws (for example, information campaigns and direct action) (Community Tool Box, 2005a).

Replicating Community-Based Strategies

Programs that have demonstrated success in diverse settings (for example, urban, suburban, and rural areas) and with diverse populations (for example, different socioeconomic, racial, and cultural groups) create greater confidence that such programs can be transferred to new settings. As communities prepare to tackle complex health problems, such as substance abuse and obesity, knowledge that a specific program has had success in other settings with similar populations adds to its credibility. Coalitions must realize that to replicate promising practices effectively, members should be involved in identifying, selecting, and implementing the intervention, and adequate resources must be available. The intervention must be adapted to the new community or setting and its priority population. Furthermore, it will work best when implemented within systems and institutions that are open to and committed to its success (Rabinowitz, 2003a). Participants also must value the intervention and be committed to its success.

Interventions are more likely to be replicated when they are solid and based on proven and well-tried concepts; are practical, easy to understand, and can inspire local people to take ownership; transcend local issues; and connect people to focus on changing the world for the better. Programs are also easier to enact if the coalition staff and implementation team have access to people who have successfully implemented the program and if they obtain technical assistance and consultation from similar organizations, members of the priority population, or from a hired consultant with field experience (Schorr, 1997). The local coalition may offer its expertise, mobilize support, lend credibility and clout, and connect the intervention with local networks to make it more effective. Finally, funders must become aware of the fact that trying to replicate a successful program is a long-term commitment that does not necessarily guarantee success (Community Tool Box, 2005a). Resources, as well as practices, must be replicated (Schorr, 1997).

Sometimes, practices or interventions are difficult or impossible to replicate. According to Schorr (1997), even when an intervention is very successful, practitioners may not be able to explain exactly what they did, either because records were not kept or because the program developed intuitively over time. Likewise, an intervention also may depend on the dedication, skills, or sensitivity of a single individual or small group. Replicating a successful program may be very complicated, no matter how well-documented the program and its practices (Schorr, 1997).

Types of Intervention Strategies

Many types of strategies are commonly used by coalitions to change the attitudes, beliefs, and behaviors of individuals, as well as the broader practices and policies of organizations and communities. Most of these strategies involve modifying behavior either by changing the organizational culture (for example, offering healthy foods in school vending machines or adding time to the lunch hour for employee exercise); by providing incentives to increase desirable behaviors and disincentives to decrease undesirable ones (for example, offering monetary rewards for weight loss, increasing excise taxes for cigarettes, fining merchants for selling tobacco to minors); or by both. The Centers for Disease Control and Prevention (2003) uses the following categories of strategies, useful for coalitions to consider for a community-level intervention: health communication, health education, health policy and enforcement, health engineering, health-related community service, and community mobilization. Each of these is described here.

Health communication strategies. Almost all interventions implemented by coalitions include some form of communication (for example, speaking, reading, writing, mass media) that is designed to accomplish its goals and objectives. These objectives may include changing knowledge, attitudes, and behaviors; providing cues and motivation for action; increasing self-efficacy to accomplish skills; reinforcing positive behaviors; increasing demand and support for health services; and building social norms and capacity. Communication strategies also have the potential to reach the most individuals in the priority population and are more cost-effective and less threatening than most other strategies (McKenzie, Neiger, and Smeltzer, 2005, p. 180). Costs to implement these strategies range from minimal to very expensive, so they should be carefully planned with a coalition's resources in mind.

Communication strategies are usually divided by *communication channels,* or the routes through which messages are disseminated to the priority population. Arranged in ascending order by the number of people reached, the main communication channels are *intrapersonal, interpersonal, organizational and community,* and *mass media.*

Intrapersonal, or one-on-one, communication is the channel most often used, but also the most time- and resource-intensive. Computer technology enhances this process by delivering tailored electronic mail messages and health-promotion curricula. Telephones are used to deliver messages via hotlines, appointment reminders, and interactive professional health counseling (Soet and Basch, 1997).

Interpersonal channels usually use support groups and small classes to reach more people with fewer resources than intrapersonal communication can.

Organizational and community communication typically use existing channels such as posters, church bulletins, neighborhood and business newsletters, community bulletin boards, and activities (health fairs and walks) to disseminate health messages.

Mass media channels include print and electronic formats, such as billboards, direct mail, newspapers, magazines, television, and radio.

Information campaigns educate the public about how to reduce their risks for certain health problems through press conferences and media releases, news coverage, talk shows, public service announcements (PSAs), paid advertisements, letters to the editor, posters, brochures, speakers, hotlines, comic strips, and commentaries (Arkin, 1990).

Health education strategies. These strategies are usually associated with formal courses, seminars, and workshops, and may use methods such as lectures, discussions, small work groups, brainstorming, role plays, simulation, values clarification, debates, panel discussions, audiovisual and computerized instruction, demonstrations, case studies and problem solving, laboratory exercises, written material, and field trips (Gilbert and Sawyer, 2000). Health education often uses health communication messages (as described above) to inform or persuade an individual or group to voluntarily change behavior. However, these messages—for example, *Eat five fruits and vegetables per day*—do not provide direct or immediate reward or punishment. Education can create awareness about existing benefits but cannot deliver them, even though the resulting knowledge may have value or benefit in the long run, if the desired behavior change occurs (Rothschild, 1999). The learner is expected to voluntarily sacrifice to accrue promised benefits that often lie in the distant future, as exemplified by the message, *Stop smoking and reduce the chances of heart disease.* Educational strategies are more successful when combined with social marketing, media advocacy, and health policy strategies.

Health-policy and enforcement strategies. These types of strategies include executive orders, laws, ordinances, policies, position statements, regulations, and formal or informal rules, and are required by an administrative or legislative body to guide individual or collective behavior (McKenzie, Neiger, and Smeltzer, 2005, pp. 183–187). Coalitions have worked in this arena to promote state seat belt and helmet laws and no-smoking policies, and to create position statements to improve the food in school cafeterias. These strategies are sometimes controversial because they are not voluntary and restrict individual freedoms, even though they are implemented to protect the public's health (McKenzie, Neiger, and Smeltzer, 2005). However, coalitions find them effective when other health education strategies fail to change individual and collective behavior. When engaging in policy activities, coalitions should follow these guidelines to reduce controversy (McKenzie, Neiger, and Smeltzer, pp. 188–189):

- Obtain expert content and legal advice.
- Procure top-level support from public and private agencies involved.
- Have the priority population help identify the need for and create policy.
- Ensure that the health policy and enforcement strategies are based on solid research and sound principles; learn from the experience of others.
- Phase in the new regulation slowly, and provide education and behavior change programs to assist the priority population to implement these policy changes.
- Ensure that the regulations are enforceable, consistently and fairly enforced, and evaluated and revised, if necessary.

Health engineering strategies. These strategies are designed to change the structure or type of services or systems of care to improve the delivery of health care services (Centers for Disease Control, 2003). These environmental changes do not require that the priority population change their behavior, but that institutions and systems change. Equipping vehicles with safety belts and air bags, installing smoke alarms and fire doors in buildings, supplying school vending machines with healthy food and beverage choices, and installing foam padding under playground equipment are examples of such strategies. Health engineering strategies are most effective when they are combined with regulatory activities and health education strategies, such as providing after-prom shuttle services or posting no-smoking signs and point-of-purchase messages (McKenzie, Neiger, and Smeltzer, 2005).

Health-related community service strategies. These strategies include services, tests, and treatments to improve the health of the priority population. Such strategies are most effective when they are affordable and offered in easily accessible community settings. Risk reduction counseling involves intensive interactive work and straight talk about risky behavior in order to build skills (individually or in small groups) to change that behavior among high-risk participants. Other examples of these strategies include health risk appraisals, screenings, immunizations, examinations, and assisting with applications for low-cost insurance programs.

Community mobilization strategies. Participatory decision making and empowerment are at the heart of community organizing, building, and advocacy strategies. *Community organizing* is a process in which community groups are formed (usually by an outside person or professional organizer) to identify common problems, mobilize resources, and implement strategies for reaching collectively determined goals (McKenzie, Neiger, and Smeltzer, 2005, p. 221). *Community building* is similar, although the community assessment phase focuses on identifying community assets and capabilities. Minkler and

Wallerstein note that both community building and organizing are "fluid endeavors" that may start from a specific need or crisis and move to a "strengths-based community capacity approach" (2003a, p. 33). Different organizing strategies may incorporate needs- or strength-based approaches at different times and under different circumstances (Minkler and Wallerstein, 2003a).

Developing a community coalition or partnership is one example of a community organizing or building strategy. *Street outreach* is a strategy in which a specialist is sent to a given area to make regular, face-to-face contact with the priority population through canvassing, setting up information tables, or distributing information or supplies, whereas *community outreach* is done in a group setting, for example, by offering workshops and presentations. Community outreach strategies are usually one-time occurrences and must be combined with other strategies to be effective. Peer education programs usually employ members of the priority population, such as lay health workers, and send them into the community to act as positive role models for behavior and to distribute information. Peers can do one-on-one counseling, speaker's bureaus, or other activities.

Direct action strategies refer to a range of grassroots organizing strategies taken to directly confront or highlight an issue, institution, or authority through demonstrations, symbolic actions, street theatre, trespass actions, occupations and sit-ins, and blockades. Direct actions are often disruptive and more confrontational than other methods, and the people involved may end up being arrested. The confrontational nature of these tactics can alienate and polarize the public, especially if other methods of changing behavior have not been attempted.

Community advocacy is generally described as a process by which community members "become involved in the institutions and decisions that will have an impact on their lives" (McKenzie, Neiger, and Smeltzer, 2005, p. 191), but more specifically, it is a set of strategies and skills "used to create a shift in public opinion and mobilize the necessary resources and forces to support an issue, policy, or constituency" (Wallack, Dorfman, Jernigan, and Themba, 1993, p. 27). These strategies include personal visits to educate or lobby key decision makers and elected officials, rallies, telephone call campaigns to decision makers, letters to editors and legislators to campaign for a particular issue, and radio and television appearances to express views.

Advocacy assumes people have rights that they are entitled to and which are enforceable. Concerned with ensuring that institutions work the way they should, advocacy works best when it is focused on something specific (Wallack, Dorfman, Jernigan, and Themba, 1993, p. 28). Often, advocacy strategies challenge powerful institutions and the *status quo*. Advocacy efforts must be based on data, have clear goals and objectives, and be supported by the community. Broad-based coalitions are critical to meeting advocacy goals and building community. Advocacy strategies can build team spirit, increase membership, expand the leadership and its experience, and build community power (Wallack, Dorfman, Jernigan, and Themba, 1993, p. 40). However, before engaging in advocacy strategies, coalitions should ask whether they have the person power and financial resources to achieve advocacy goals.

In summary, a wide range of innovative interventions is available and should be used by coalitions when intervening at the community level. Two special kinds of interventions blend aspects of health communication with community mobilization or advocacy and are very often used by coalitions and partnerships. These interventions will be covered next in a bit more depth.

SOCIAL MARKETING

Social marketing is the use of marketing principles to influence human behavior for the purpose of improving health or benefiting society. While commercial marketing tries to change people's behavior for the benefit of the marketer, social marketing tries to change people's behavior for the benefit of the consumer or society as a whole (Community Tool Box, 2005b; Andreason, 2000).

Social marketing is a powerful persuasive tool, for instance, to convince people to stop polluting, adopt healthier diets, or use condoms. It emphasizes the need to listen to the priority population, learn what may motivate them to change, and confront the obstacles that block the path to positive behaviors. In the effort to stop the spread of AIDS, for example, social marketing promotes the concept of safe sex along with subsidized and readily available condoms (Andreasen, 2000).

Essential Elements of Social Marketing

All definitions of social marketing share at least four essential elements (Turning Point, 2005). First, the priority audience must be at the center of every decision made. Second, the focus of the endeavor is on voluntary behavior change. Third, that behavior change must be for the benefit of an individual, group, or population, not for profit or commercial gain. Fourth, if people are expected to give up or modify an old behavior, or accept a new one, they must be offered something very appealing in return.

To conduct an effective social marketing effort, the coalition must assess the community to identify what behavior(s) it intends to change and determine the intended audience (separated, or *segmented,* by age, gender, level of education, or race, for example) as well as the barriers to change. Once these factors are known, the coalition can plan how it intends to reduce the barriers and make the desired behavior easier, more accessible, and more attractive. It can then pre-test its ideas on a small number of people and modify the plan according to the results. Finally, the coalition should publicize both the benefits of change and its efforts to make change easier, and should evaluate the results of the campaign to see whether the desired change was achieved. Ultimately, the role of the coalition and its marketing team are to know where people stand along the continuum from attention to action, then design messages to move them along in the direction of the desired action or behavior (Community Tool Box, 2005b).

Features of Social Marketing

Some features of social marketing, such as identifying a priority audience, are not unique to social marketing, but have previously been identified by other planning models, such as PRECEDE-PROCEED (Green and Kreuter, 1999).

Audience segmentation. This involves identifying and selecting small groups of individuals for whom appropriate programs and interventions can be designed. The audience segments are grouped together based on shared characteristics and attributes that are linked to the behavior, such as values, knowledge, culture, behavioral determinants, opinions, beliefs, personality, and the channels that can be used to communicate with them effectively (Turning Point, 2003, p. 7).

Channels. Appropriate *channels* should be used to communicate social marketing messages and promote coalition programs. Interpersonal, small group, organizational, community, or mass media channels may be used, depending on the tendencies and preferences of the priority audience identified in formative market research. To determine the best channels to use, coalitions should consider the media habits of the priority population (electronic, print, radio, television), the costs of each medium, whether multiple channels may be used, how many will be reached, cultural appropriateness of the message, and frequency of contact (Kline and Huff, 1999).

The "4 P's" of Marketing. Social marketing helps a coalition reach its priority audience, customize its message, and create lasting behavior change in the priority population. Messages are communicated by using marketing principles known as the "4 P's": *product, price, place,* and *promotion* (Turning Point, 2005, pp. 7–8):

Product refers to the desired behavior asked of the audience and the associated promised benefits or services that support or facilitate behavior change. The product being marketed may range from a tangible, physical product (for example, food stamps), to a service (for example, transportation), to a practice (for example, participating in education), to an intangible, such as an idea, attitude, or belief. To have a viable product, people must first perceive that they have a need and that the product offered is a good answer for that need. For social marketing, the "product" may be a certain behavior that should be changed.

Price refers to the financial, emotional, psychological, and time costs or barriers that audience members face in making the desired behavior change. How much will it cost a person to stop (or adopt) a certain behavior (actual cost as well as time and effort costs)? If the customer believes the benefits will be greater than the costs, the likelihood of trial and adoption of the product is greater. To reduce costs, for example, an anti-litter campaign will try to place more trash cans around the city; a smoking cessation campaign might offer support groups to help with the effort, nutrition counseling to counteract weight gain, and nicotine patches to reduce withdrawal symptoms.

Place is the way in which the product reaches the consumer. Place is where and when the priority audience will perform the desired behavior, access program products or services, or think about the proposed health or safety issue. For an intangible product, place is less specific and may refer to the channels through which consumers are contacted with information or training, such as clinics, shopping malls, television, or in-home demonstrations. Another element of place is deciding how to ensure accessibility to the product and quality of the service delivery. Social marketing efforts make it easier to change behavior by ensuring the necessary supports are not only available but also easily accessible to the greatest possible number of people.

Promotion consists of the use of advertising, public relations, and media advocacy. The focus of promotion activities is on creating and sustaining demand for the product. Promotion includes the communication messages, materials, channels, and activities that will effectively reach the coalition's audience to publicize the benefits of the behavior change, as well as the product, price, and place features of its program. Messages may be delivered through public service announcements, paid ads, media events, print materials, small-group or one-on-one activities, editorials, in-store displays, and word-of-mouth communication. Promotion should consider the type of media the priority audience accesses, when and where they will receive messages, and characteristics of the communication.

Social Marketing's Four Additional "P's". The Appalachian Partnership for Welfare Reform (2005) identified four additional "Ps" that apply specifically to social marketing: *participation, partnership, politics,* and *policy.*

Participation incorporates the consumer's, or priority population's, input in planning, developing, and implementing a product it needs.

Partnership, or collaboration, is an effective strategy when other organizations in the community have similar goals.

Politics is part of the matrix because issues addressed by social marketing programs, such as health or poverty, are often controversial or complex; political diplomacy with community organizations may be needed to gain support and access to the priority audience or to deflect turf issues.

Policy refers to the use of laws or regulations to further encourage the desired behavior, as well as to understanding or changing those policies or laws that may act as barriers to the behavior.

Creating a Social Marketing Plan

Ten strategic questions can help the coalition work toward an initial marketing plan (Turning Point, 2005, p. 9):

- What is the social (or health) problem the coalition wants to address?
- What actions will best address that problem?
- Who is being asked to take that action? (audience)
- What does the audience want in exchange for adopting this new behavior?
- Why will the audience believe that anything offered is real and true?
- What is the competition offering? Is the coalition offering things the audience wants more than what the competition offers?

- What is the best time and place to reach members of the priority audience so that they are the most disposed to receiving the intervention?
- How often, and from whom, should the intervention be received if it is to work?
- How can a variety of interventions be integrated to act over time, in a coordinated way, to influence the behavior?
- Does the coalition have the resources to carry out this strategy alone; and if not, where can other useful partners be found?

Six-step social marketing process. A six-step social marketing process has been used in the CDCynergy program and is summarized here.

Step 1. Describe the problem. Use the coalition's local community assessment to help understand its specific health issues. For example, a SWOT analysis can identify the strengths, weaknesses, opportunities, and threats that might affect the social marketing program. Then, form a team of coalition members and community partners to create and implement the program plan (a subgroup of a work group or a separate task force).

Step 2. Conduct the market research. Once the issue to be addressed is decided, focus on the priority audience of the plan. The focus of research here is on consumer analysis (wants, needs, and preferences of the priority population), market analysis (the 4 "P's" and the competing behaviors, messages, and programs), and channel analysis (communication and promotion strategies) (McKenzie, Neiger, and Smeltzer, 2005, p. 257).

The coalition can conduct formative research as part of its community assessment (using interviews and focus groups) to help segment the market and position the program for a certain audience.

McKenzie and colleagues offer the following set of questions to guide the coalition's formative market research (2005, pp. 257–258):

- What type of programs would the priority population participate in, if offered?
- Where would they like the program offered?
- On what days and times would they like the program offered?
- Would individual or small group participation be preferred?
- How much (if anything) would the priority population be willing to pay for the program?
- What is the best way to communicate information about the program?

Step 3. Create the marketing strategy. Once the research is complete, and the issue, audience, and proposed behavior change have been identified, map out what the coalition is going to do and how it is going to be done. Pay attention to communication channels and the four P's. Describe the incentives that will be offered to the priority audience to adopt the desired behavior and the interventions the coalition will utilize.

Table 13.1. Marketing Campaign Development Tool.

Priority Audience	In order to help this priority audience . . .
Behavioral Change	Do this specific behavior . . .
Exchange or Benefits	The coalition will offer these benefits that the audience wants . . .
Strategy	And reduce these barriers, that is, address these "Ps" (price, product, place, and promotion) . . .

Through these strategies and tactics:

Strategies and Tactics	Behavior Change Goals	Program Delivery or Process (Reach) Objectives	Outcomes Objectives	Resource Needs

Source: Turning Point Social Marketing National Excellence Collaborative, 2003b. Turning Point Social Marketing National Excellence Collaborative, 2005. *The Basics of Social Marketing.* Reprinted by permission of Turning Point Social Marketing National Excellence Collaborative and The Robert Wood Johnson Foundation. For further information, please see www.turningpointprogram.org and www.socialmarketingcollaborative.org

Step 4. Plan the intervention. Develop interventions (such as new or improved products or services, staff training, policy change, or communication) that stick to the message and address a behavior benefit or cost. Create a plan, timeline, and budget for each intervention, noting where community partners are needed.

Step 5. Plan program monitoring and evaluation. Develop an evaluation plan to determine whether a change in attitude or another indicator(s) was linked to the targeted behavior and whether that change is at least partly due to the coalition's program. The plan should also measure the audience's exposure to and awareness or opinion of the social marketing message. These findings can help the coalition refine the intervention to be more effective.

Step 6. Implement the intervention and evaluation. Establish a schedule and stick to it.

Table 13.1 can be used to help coalitions develop their social marketing campaign by identifying the priority audience, expected behavioral change, benefits, strategies, and tactics.

MEDIA ADVOCACY

Advocacy is the act of speaking, writing, or acting in support of something or someone. Many of the partner organizations that work together in coalitions engage in advocacy when they help consumers obtain services, understand their rights, or work through their problems with the system by accompanying them to support groups and meetings with service providers or law enforcement personnel. They may even speak out publicly in support of a disenfranchised group or write opinion articles and letters to editors. However, media, or legislative, advocacy, which works to influence legislation to provide more funds or to create or improve services, is what most public health practitioners think of as advocacy.

Media advocacy strives to focus on the social and economic causes of health problems, not the individual behavioral ones. In essence, media advocacy creatively uses the mass media to pressure decision makers to support changes for healthy public policy (Wallack, 2005, p. 420).

The current concepts of media advocacy are best exemplified in the well-known American Stop Smoking Intervention Study (ASSIST) project (National Cancer Institute, 2005). Other public health programs, including the National Cancer Institute's Community Intervention Trial for Smoking Cessation (COMMIT) project, used a media advocacy approach prior to ASSIST. However, ASSIST advanced the use of media advocacy to bring about policy change within organizations, communities, and society. It capitalized on the tobacco industry's strategic use of the media to influence behavior and to change social norms. Although ASSIST did not accomplish all of its policy goals, it stimulated a number of policies that continue today. Smoke-free environments in public places are becoming the norm; excise taxes are recognized as effective in reducing tobacco use; states continue to raise taxes on tobacco products; and other coalitions have been inspired to use similar media advocacy tactics.

How Does Media Advocacy Work?

The coalition must take several steps to developing its advocacy initiative:

1. Identify its policy goal(s).
2. Decide with whom it wants to communicate and whether this group or organization has the power to make the policy changes that the coalition desires.
3. Frame the issue and develop a message.
4. Construct an overall media advocacy plan to deliver the message and create pressure for change.
5. Evaluate whether the policy has been accomplished.

Media advocacy uses the media first to *set the agenda* or bring attention to an issue. Second, it *frames the issue* by highlighting it and focusing on upstream or preventable causes. Third, it *advances a social or public policy initiative* to solve the issue or problem (Wallack, Dorfman, Jernigan, and Themba, 1993).

Setting the agenda and gaining access to the media. A local issue is more apt to be covered by the media or considered newsworthy if it is "timely, relevant, and defined to be in the public's interest" (Wallack, 2005, p. 425). The story is also considered newsworthy if it is sensational, tragic, unusual, or a human-interest story that shows people helping others or overcoming great challenges (Wallack, 2005, p. 425). Getting media access is also determined by where the issue falls in the media's "issue-attention cycle" (Downs, 1972). Keeping attention on the coalition's issue is complicated by the sheer number of other pressing and competing issues. Coalitions constantly have to keep their activities fresh, focused, and results-oriented to retain the involvement of the media and, consequently, the public.

Framing the debate. After gaining access to the media and setting the agenda, the next step that media advocacy must take is to frame the debate, or determine how health issues are defined. Environmental solutions that are prevention-oriented, population-based, and focused on social determinants are more likely to move people to action that will lead to sustained community change.

Developing the message. The message should be framed in a way that tells an audience how to interpret what they hear. "A campaign message must speak at one and the same time to the brain and to the heart" (The Advocacy Institute, 2005b). Clear, focused messages draw attention to social justice issues and help coalition partners to speak with a unified voice about their issues.

A good message is a brief, straightforward statement based on an analysis of what will persuade a particular audience. Using the same message repeatedly promotes retention and builds comfort and familiarity with ideas and issues over time. Examples of key messages that were used repeatedly in the tobacco control movement include these: *Passive smoking is a serious health hazard; Smoking kills more people than heroin, cocaine, alcohol, AIDS, fires, homicide, suicide, and automobile accidents combined;* and *Women are just as much at risk as men are for diseases caused by tobacco* (Advocacy Institute, 2005c). Advocates often develop a media campaign around the key message, which typically includes analysis of the problem, its cause, who is responsible for solving the problem, the proposed solution, and the action they ask others to take in support of the solution (Advocacy Institute, 2005d).

Advancing the policy initiative. The last stage of media advocacy is to support policies that improve the community's health. Media advocacy uses the mass media to pressure key leaders and policymakers. The real work of media advocacy is to get broad support for an issue and carefully plan a political approach.

Media Advocacy Strategies

In *Media Advocacy and Public Health*, Wallack and his colleagues offer these basic advocacy strategies (1993, pp. 206–207):

Root media actions in community support. Keeping community values and issues in mind, cultivating local expertise, and encouraging local advocacy actions are the foundation of promoting social change through the media.

Always think upstream. Focus on the root causes of problems and find solutions
to address them that are equitable and promote social justice.

Emphasize public health values. Emphasize public health values in the advocacy
actions that the coalition takes to change systems and institutions for those
most in need.

Anticipate opposition. Know the facts, be aware of the broad issues that the
coalition's issue involves, and understand the coalition's core values in order.

Think long term, evaluate, and reflect. Have an overall plan for social change
that determines which policies the coalition supports. Assess each media
activity to determine how well it fits into the coalition's goals.

Build strong relationships with the media. Building strong relationships with
reporters at each media outlet is the foundation of a good media relations program and ensures that newsworthy events important to the coalition's work
get news coverage. Tips to build a strong media relations program follow
(Brubach, 2005):

Tip 1: **Create a media contact list.** Create and maintain an accurate list of
community and statewide media contacts and outlets. Utilize the knowledge of partners to build an initial list, and then research additional
sources. Call, e-mail, or stop by each outlet to identify and meet the media
professionals that work on topics of interest to the coalition. The media
should be viewed as a partner in the coalition's work: The coalition needs
the media to tell its story and highlight solutions, and the media needs the
coalition to provide them with facts, access to local people and programs,
and ideas for stories (Wallack, Dorfman, Jernigan, and Themba, 1993).
This relationship must be nurtured over time to build rapport, trust, and
clear channels of communication.

Tip 2: **Decide how media contacts will be handled.** The media has a need to
attract audiences, provide entertainment, and sell newspapers or increase
audience ratings of news programming. Identifying an individual within or
close to the coalition, who has marketing or media background and can
serve as the primary contact with the media, is a good approach. He or she
can write press releases, assemble media packets, orchestrate media events
(such as interviews and news conferences), and run interference when
publicity is potentially negative. Many lead agencies have policies to protect
coalition staff and members from the media, such as fielding questions,
setting up interviews, and accompanying coalition members to them.

Tip 3: **Make the coalition a media resource.** Delivering regular updates on
key events, issues, and accomplishments of the coalition provides content
and ideas for slow news days and endears the coalition to the media.
Responding with research and community data when asked to do so by
reporters or offering to do interviews on those Sunday or early morning
health panels is often appreciated. These actions may be reciprocated
when the coalition contacts a health reporter to cover a community or
coalition event, or asks the news anchor to emcee a community forum.

Tip 4: Know the topic. Before getting started, be sure coalition contacts and spokespersons know the issue, the desired action, and who has the power to make change happen. Being confident about the topic and honest in presenting facts helps bolster the coalition's credibility.

Tip 5: Prepare press materials. Before contacting local media representatives about a particular issue, develop a press kit to respond to reporters' requests for information about the coalition's history, the area it serves, and its key initiatives. The press kit should include the following (Brubach, 2005; Community Catalyst, 2003, p. 22):

- Mission statement, brief history, and purpose of the coalition (or brochure covering these)
- Contact information for media people who want more information and for others interested in joining or supporting the coalition
- Coalition organizational roster that shows its diversity and representation
- Short biographies of influential members (one page)
- Relevant data on coalition issues
- Accomplishments and a few newspaper articles about the coalition and its achievements, to show that it is successful, acknowledged elsewhere, and actively works on the issue of interest
- Recent copy of the coalition newsletter

Tip 6: Utilize media outreach channels. Though innovation and creativity can help attract media attention, coalitions should consider using standard channels on a regular basis. Typical media outlets are described here and summarized in Table 13.2 on page 416 (Brubach, 2005):

- *News Releases.* A standard one- or two-page news release tells the reader the who, what, when, where, and why of the coalition's issue. It should get the attention of the reporter and convince him or her of the issue's newsworthiness. Samples of news releases are readily available (for example, CADCA's online news releases). The release should be followed by a call to the reporter, describing potential story angles and spokespersons.
- *Letter to the editor.* This is a brief letter (no more than 300 words) to a newspaper publisher, relating activities and opinions of the coalition concerning recently published stories.
- *Op-eds.* Short for "opposing editorials" because they traditionally were located opposite the editorial page, op-eds are actually letters to the editor. They provide an opportunity to discuss the coalition's opinion about current events or present an opinion that differs from those expressed by the newspaper.

Table 13.2. Media Outlets.

Medium	Access Points
Television	News, public affairs, entertainment, paid advertising, editorials, public service advertising (PSAs)
Newspapers	Front page, sports, lifestyle, paid advertising, arts, comics, financial letters to the editor, editorials, op-ed page
Radio	News, paid advertising, talk shows, editorials, public service
Billboards	Paid placement: in-kind supplements of more billboards or extended time of display

Source: Wallack, Dorfman, Jernigan, and Themba, 1993. From *Media Advocacy and Public Health* by L. Wallack, L. Dorfman, D. Jernigan & M. Themba, p. 87. Copyright © 1993 Sage Publications, Inc. Reproduced with permission of Sage Publications, Inc.

- *Editorial board meetings.* Presenting the coalition's view on an issue to the newspaper's editorial board may influence how the newspaper reports on a particular issue. The coalition should be well prepared and versed on the issue before the meeting and should follow up afterward.

- *Interviews.* Coalition spokespeople who are familiar with the coalition's work and with community-level data, and comfortable doing interviews, should be available to the media.

- *Press conferences.* A press conference may be held if the coalition has something it believes will attract media and community attention, such as launching an awareness campaign, recruiting a high-profile partner to the coalition, or reporting the results of a successful coalition program. These events require planning (including a guest list, speaker selection, and meeting logistics), and press conference-specific media kits. Community briefings that bring together key stakeholders in the community to discuss a community-wide issue and raise awareness can also produce media coverage.

Tip 7: Document media coverage. The coalition should keep track of the earned media it receives; use press clippings for its media kit; and evaluate media relations efforts to determine what works best.

Interview Basics

If a coalition spokesperson or representative is asked for an interview by the media, this is an ideal time to communicate the coalition's key messages. Interviewees should concentrate on two or three major points and develop memorable short phrases, or *sound bites,* to highlight the message (Goldman and Schmalz, 2005). They should prepare by anticipating difficult questions that might be asked and rehearsing answers to them that segue back to key messages. The dress for any interview should be conservative.

During the interview, the interviewee should be brief, non-defensive, and consider that everything that is said is "on the record" and could appear in the local newspaper. He or she should cite easily understood facts and admit to not knowing the answer to a question when such is the case. Goldman and Schmalz offer a set of interviewee rights that include the right to set the time and place for the interview and time limits, ask for time to prepare, know the general questions to be asked, refuse to answer personal or hypothetical questions, ask for time to think, and end the interview, if needed (2005, p. 17).

A good interview is one where the interviewee stays on track and ties everything to the key message(s); is quoted; presents complex or technical information in an understandable way; corrects any misinformation; appears to be in control; and resists becoming distracted, baited, or defensive (Goldman and Schmalz, 2005, p. 19). Afterward, interviewees should make corrections if facts are incorrect, follow up with a call thanking the reporter for the interview, and provide updates on the topic.

Developing an Advocacy Strategy

An advocacy strategy is generally one that uses education and persuasive communication to enact change. It may on occasion use lobbying, although nonprofits should be careful about how often, or even whether, this strategy is allowed under their articles of incorporation. Lobbying is used to urge decision makers to take a specific action, such as casting a vote, adopting a regulation, or writing an editorial (Advocacy Institute, 2005c). Coalitions should strive to build relationships that provide access to decision makers, serve as an information resource to them, and should be able to translate legislative practices and procedures to their own members. To be effective, coalitions must appreciate their limits in actually influencing votes; stay true to their principles while being flexible about timing and scope; understand the opposition; and share credit for victory with their members (Advocacy Institute, 2005c).

The Advocacy Center offers these key questions to guide coalitions in pursuing advocacy goals (Schultz, 2002):

- What is the coalition's objective? What change will actually solve the problem the coalition is concerned about? An advocacy objective must be defined at the start and be compelling enough to get people interested in working for it. It should also be modest enough that at least part of it can be achieved within a year or two, to keep people interested.
- Who must the coalition move? Who actually has the formal authority to give the coalition what it wants (city council, state legislature, the President)? Who else has the capacity to influence those with authority (the media, other citizen groups)? An effective advocacy effort requires a clear sense of who these audiences are and what access or pressure points are available to move them.
- What must the audience hear? What advocacy message will move these people toward the coalition's direction? Messages must be tailored or framed

differently for different audiences and usually appeal to the audience's sense of what is right and in their self-interest.

- Who should deliver the message to the audience? Which "messengers" can be recruited who will be the most persuasive? An advocacy campaign needs a mix of messengers: people who can speak from personal experience, or "authentic voices"; people with recognized authority or technical expertise; and others who might have some special pull with the audience. How can these messengers be equipped with the appropriate information and comfort level?

- What actions will the coalition take to make its point? What will the coalition mobilize people to do to deliver the message? Advocacy messages can be delivered in ways that range from non-confrontational (for example, lobbying) to educational (for example, a letter to the editor or town meeting), to direct action (for example, protest on the capitol steps). Generally, the best actions are those that require the least effort and confrontation, but which still "get the job done" (The Democracy Center, 2002).

- What resources does the coalition have? An effective advocacy effort assesses its strengths and builds on current resources, including past advocacy work, partnerships and relationships, staff and member capacity, information, and political intelligence.

- What should the coalition develop? After assessing advocacy resources, the next step is to identify needed resources. What partnerships and capacities related to outreach, research, and media efforts should be built?

- How should the coalition begin? What are some potential short-term goals or projects that would bring the right people together and create something achievable that lays the groundwork for the next step?

- How does the coalition know whether its advocacy strategy is working? Each of the above questions must be revisited, for example, *Are we focusing on the right audiences and reaching them?* Corrections can be made and unsuccessful activities discarded.

The Advocacy Team

Before focusing on strategy planning or message development and delivery, coalitions should examine the team that is responsible for the advocacy campaign. According to the Advocacy Institute (2005d), "The right combination of leadership roles can result in a coalition that responds faster, more flexibly, more strategically to its challenges, increasing its chances of success." An individual may fill more than one role, but if roles are missing, the coalition should develop its existing leaders or recruit new ones. The roles include

- *Visionaries,* who challenge conventional wisdom, take risks, and rethink priorities.

- *Strategists,* who decide what part of the vision is attainable, anticipate obstacles, and provide guidance to keep advocacy on track.

- *Statespersons,* the public figures who represent authority and trust, and raise the cause in the minds of both the public and decision makers.
- *Experts,* who have the knowledge and facts that lend credibility to the coalition's positions.
- *Outside "sparkplugs,"* agitators who energize the campaign and hold those in power accountable.
- *Inside advocates,* politically savvy and skilled negotiators, who are positioned to influence key policymakers.
- *Strategic communicators,* public teachers who translate complex data and policy into powerful messages that are easily understood by the general public.
- *Movement builders,* who quietly recruit new members, make everyone feel valued and needed, and promote inclusiveness and conflict resolution.
- *Generalists,* who have many talents and skills based on years of advocacy experience.
- *Historians,* who uphold the coalition's memory, build on past lessons, and convey its advocacy stories.
- *Cultural activists,* trusted public opinion leaders who use cultural preservation, history, and activism to sustain the coalition's advocacy efforts.

COALITION SPOTLIGHT: MEDIA ADVOCACY WITH LOS ANGELES COUNTY ALCOHOL, TOBACCO, AND DRUG POLICY COALITION

In 1997, a media advocacy campaign to restrict alcohol and tobacco billboards and storefront advertising was initiated by the Los Angeles County Alcohol, Tobacco, and Drug Policy Coalition. Residents were concerned about the number of alcohol and tobacco billboards, the number of community events that were sponsored by alcohol and tobacco companies, and the endorsements of alcohol and tobacco use by entertainers and sports figures. Cultural symbols, kid-friendly images, ethnic minority entertainers, and advertisements in Spanish, Korean, and hip-hop slang were also being used to target children of many cultural and ethnic groups. The Los Angeles City Council was the focal point of the coalition's effort because they had the power to enact an ordinance to restrict billboard and storefront advertising. The sixty-member coalition wanted not only to pass the ordinance but also to establish a county-wide, multiracial, multisector movement to protect youth from the impact of alcohol and tobacco advertising and to create a healthier environment.

The coalition identified its constituency, recruited members, and developed a vision, goals, and objectives. They created a winning message, assessed the opposition, and used creative tactics. Members knew that the key was to develop "a consistent message through consensus" (Gallegos, 1999, p. 4). The campaign focused on the issue of the concentration of alcohol and tobacco billboards in low-income minority communities and on protecting youth from these images. The opposition was expected to focus on the First Amendment issue of free speech, blaming parents for underage drinking and arguing that advertising had no impact on youth behavior.

The coalition mobilized youth to tell council members about the multitude of advertisements that encouraged them to smoke and drink. Parents spoke to council members about the difficulty of competing with messages that children received outside of the home and stressed their commitment to counseling their children not to smoke and drink. Coalition experts educated the council members about the legality of restricting alcohol and tobacco advertising.

The coalition gathered data about the community and provided fact sheets to council members and the media. Extant data included leading causes of death and injury among youth aged fifteen to twenty-four (the average age that children initiate smoking), the effect of alcohol advertising on youth attitudes toward alcohol, and the percentage of underage violent offenders who were under the influence of alcohol when committing crimes. Community surveys documenting the problems associated with alcohol and tobacco billboard advertising were used to help the city planning team draft the ordinance. Parents and youth surveyed the number of alcohol and tobacco billboards in their neighborhoods and near schools and found a disproportionate number of billboards and storefront advertisements in communities of color. A petition circulated by the coalition in support of the ordinance generated several thousand signatures. Together, these data proved to the city council that a problem existed and support for the ordinance was strong, and community members were mobilized to resolve the problem.

Just as the alcohol and tobacco industries had sponsored cultural events to promote their product, coalition member organizations planned a march on "El Día de Los Muertos," a Mexican holiday to honor the dead. They sent press releases to the media, who interviewed youth about the importance of honoring the dead and the role that the alcohol and tobacco industries played in contributing to high death rates. The coalition organized press conferences on the steps of city hall on council committee meeting days. Youth and parents addressed the media about the necessity of passing the ordinance. "The powerful images of youth, parents, and community members of many ethnic groups speaking with one voice to make a political change" led to further support from community members and, eventually, from the city council (Gallegos, 1999, p. 5).

The Los Angeles City Council passed the ordinance to restrict alcohol and tobacco billboard and storefront advertising in September 1998 (effective October 1999). The coalition continues to work with the Los Angeles City Department of Building and Safety and the Unified School District to enforce the ordinance, address "race and class inequalities" behind substance abuse problems, and "create an empowered citizenry that develops its own safe and healthy neighborhoods" (Gallegos, 1999, p. 15). The victory by grassroots members in this coalition reminds us of the positive social changes that can occur when community members work together as advocates.

LEGAL AND ETHICAL ISSUES IN COMMUNITY INTERVENTIONS

Ethics is a code of thinking and behavior governed by personal, moral, legal, and social standards of what is right (Community Tool Box, 2006). Although the definition of "right" varies with situations and cultures, its meaning in the context of a community intervention involves a number of guiding principles and responsibilities (see Exhibit 13.3). Acting ethically is advantageous for coalitions. It makes their programs

Exhibit 13.3. Ethical Guidelines for Community Interventions.

The following suggestions can guide coalitions in developing ethical community interventions.

- **Do no harm.** Sometimes, doing no harm can mean not starting a community intervention at all. Community interventions may sometimes harm participants by substituting for what they really need, that is, to be part of a real community, to be regarded in terms of their capacities rather than their deficiencies, and to have access to a steady source of income (McKnight, 1995).

- **Respect people as ends, not means.** Consider and treat everyone as a unique individual who matters, not as a number in a research study.

- **Respect participants' ability to play a role in determining what they need.** Do not assume that program staff or planners necessarily know what is best for a community or individual.

- **Respect everyone's human, civil, and legal rights.** This encompasses issues such as nondiscrimination and cultural sensitivity.

- **Do what is best for everyone under the circumstances.** Even if everyone cannot be helped all the time, try to do so as much as possible.

- **Do not exploit a participant to gain a personal advantage or to exercise power over another person.** This refers to taking advantage of participants or others for political, social, sexual, or financial gain.

- **Do not attempt an intervention in areas in which staff or volunteers are not trained and competent.** Sometimes any intervention is better than none at all; however, coalitions must distinguish between doing what they can and doing what is unethical and harmful.

- **Actively strive to improve the situations of program participants and the community.** Create the most effective program possible to meet the needs of participants, and address underlying conditions in ways that will benefit the community as a whole.

Source: Promotion and Community Development. (2006). Excerpt from "What do we mean by ethics?" from *Ethical Issues in Community Interventions* contributed by Phil Rabinowitz, edited by Bill Berkowitz and Tim Brownlee. Lawrence, KS: University of Kansas. Retrieved July 17, 2006 from the World Wide Web: http://ctb.ku.edu/tools/en/sub_section_main_1165.htm

more effective, builds credibility and moral leadership in the community, helps the coalition occupy the moral high ground when arguing the merits of their programs, and assures that the coalition remains in sound legal and professional standing (Community Tool Box, 2006). Everyone who works in a community program of any kind, or who deals with other people in a professional or paraprofessional capacity, is subject to a code of ethics in community interventions. A number of formal ethical codes apply to people in particular professional or other positions as well. Ethical behavior in community interventions relates to the treatment of people, information, and money, and to the general actions of the organization's or initiative's workers, even when they are not dealing directly with the community. The following list of ethical responsibilities is adapted from the Community Tool Box (2006):

Responsibility to funders. The coalition should be fiscally accountable for using funds properly and for trying to do what was promised. If a funder asks for something that the coalition is not willing to provide, it should not take (or apply for) the money just to get funding.

Responsibility to staff members. All persons in the program should be treated fairly, paid for the work they do, and have reasonable control over their jobs as well as opportunities to develop their skills and effectiveness through staff development, supervision, or both. Staff should be protected from harm, and warned and trained if physical or other dangers are part of their jobs.

Responsibility to participants. The coalition should provide the best and most effective services possible by searching for better methods and ideas; heeding participant feedback; building on program successes; and acknowledging, learning from, and correcting weaknesses. Participants' rights should be respected and everyone treated with respect.

Responsibility to community. The coalition should try to understand and meet the needs of the community, respond to their attitudes and opinions, and improve the quality of life for program participants and the community as a whole.

Liability

Because of concern over lawsuits, all coalition staff and volunteers involved with a community-based intervention should be covered by liability insurance, no matter how small the risk of physical or mental injury for participants. Providing a safe environment includes finding a safe location, free of hazards, and providing qualified staff, first-aid equipment, and an emergency care plan. Staff should also be aware of issues such as confidentiality, informed consent, disclosure, conflict of interest, and unethical behavior.

Confidentiality

Communications and information from participants in the course of a community intervention or program (including conversations, written or taped records, notes, test results, and so on) should be kept confidential. Confidentiality protects both participants and the coalition from invasion of privacy and establishes a bond of trust between participant and program. In all circumstances, ethical treatment of participants demands that they be informed about the program's confidentiality policies.

In most cases, they then have the choice of not participating if they are unhappy with those policies. In the case of court-mandated participation, at least they will know what to expect.

However, confidentiality may encompass a range of possibilities, including these:

- No one but the individual working with a participant has access to records or information about that participant without permission. Records and notes are usually kept under lock and key, and computer records are protected by electronic coding or passwords.

- Information is confidential within a program but shared among staff members for purposes of consultation and delivering better services to the participant.

- Information is confidential within a program or to a particular staff member but may be shared with staff members of other programs in which the participant is involved, either to improve services for the participant or to contribute to the other organization's reporting data. This usually requires participants to sign release forms giving the program permission to share records and information under appropriate circumstances.

- Information is confidential within a program but is submitted to funding sources as documentation of services provided. Some organizations provide the requested documentation without informing participants, on the assumption that funders are not likely either to have actual contact with participants or to misuse an individual record; others honor their promises and do not release anything without participants' permission.

- Information is not confidential or is only confidential under certain circumstances. Participation in a program may be court-mandated or mandated by an agency as a condition of receiving benefits or services. In these cases, participation often implies an agreement to share records and information, and may even be a matter of public record.

Informed Consent

Consent involves program participants giving program staff consent to share their records or information with others for purposes of service provision; participants giving informed consent to submit to particular medical or other services, treatment, research, or program conditions; or community members consenting to the location or operation of an intervention in their neighborhood. In some programs, a participant might sign a blanket form on entrance, but a separate form might be needed for each separate instance of information sharing outside the program itself. Ethical practice demands that participants be fully informed and that they be allowed to ask and have answered any questions about the program. In the case of research, participants have a right to know what the research is about, who will see and tabulate the results, what the results will be used for and how, what will happen to their personal records, and how their anonymity will be protected. They also have a right to refuse to be part of the study and cannot be denied services on that account.

In general, the best course is to be honest about intentions and attend to people's objections or concerns by keeping communication channels open.

Disclosure

Three types of disclosure are most often found in community interventions:

1. *Disclosure to participants of the conditions of the program,* in other words, confidentiality policies, the kinds of services that are available, time limits on the program, and whether it will cost anything. Participants have a right to know whether they will be part of a research study if they enter the program, and to understand the purpose of that study. Some coalitions put these disclosures in writing and make sure that every participant has a copy and understands it. It is ethically important both that participants know exactly what they are getting into and that they be treated as adults who can decide what makes sense for them.

2. *Disclosure of participant information to other individuals and agencies.* Information can only be disclosed with the participant's permission except in cases of mandated reporting, potential harm to self or others, or court testimony. Exceptions to this rule have to be spelled out to participants as they enter the program, so they can decide whether the services are worth any loss of privacy or anonymity.

3. *Disclosure by the program of any conflict of interest that the program represents to any staff or coalition members.* This includes individuals disclosing potential conflicts to the program or coalition, as well as the program disclosing potential conflicts to funders and other interested parties.

Competence

By offering services of any kind, a coalition essentially makes a contract with participants to do the job it says it will do. Implied in that contract is that the coalition and those doing the work are competent to accomplish their goals under reasonable circumstances. Competence means more than simply having the appropriate training and experience. A competent organization hires qualified staff members, provides supervision and staff development, and does everything it can to assure that the services it offers are the best available. If service appears to be ineffective or harmful, the program has the ethical responsibility to seek out or develop and then try methods that are more effective. If a staff member is not able to do the job, even with help from supervisors and others, that should be documented, and he or she should be dismissed. In some cases, service providers can lose their licenses or be sued for malpractice if they are found to be incompetent.

Conflict of Interest

A conflict of interest is a situation in which someone's personal (financial, political, professional, social, sexual, or family) interests could influence his or her judgment or actions in a financial or other decision, in carrying out a job, or in the person's relationships with participants. In community interventions, conflicts of interest may change how a program is run or how money is spent. Even if decisions or actions are not actually influenced by personal interest, in situations where people have a conflict of interest in either their public or professional lives, they must do everything possible to resolve it. The ethical remedy involves pointing it out to those who should know (the employer, funder, community, and program participant) and discussing possible solutions. Additionally, the solution might involve abstaining from participating in a particular decision, refusing funding from a particular source, ceasing to work with a particular participant, or even changing jobs.

COALITION SPOTLIGHT: COMPREHENSIVE COMMUNITY INTERVENTIONS—INJURY FREE COALITION FOR KIDS OF PHILADELPHIA

In 1998, the Injury Free Coalition for Kids (IFCK) of Philadelphia received a five-year grant from the Robert Wood Johnson Foundation to continue and expand injury-prevention efforts for children in West Philadelphia. For three years, IFCK laid the groundwork to build a strong and sustainable coalition of over fifty organizations focusing on the needs of children in West Philadelphia. The Hospital of the University of Pennsylvania and Mercy Hospital of Philadelphia are key partners in these injury-prevention initiatives, research, and activities.

Concern about pediatric pedestrian injuries led the coalition to explore where and how children were injured. Focus groups were held with parents and children, and a community-wide survey helped to identify the play spaces and activities that were most appreciated, least utilized, and most in need. The recreation department identified space and activity opportunities, and developed common goals and resources for making needed changes in the playgrounds. Pediatricians were enlisted to help develop a strategic plan to reduce injuries.

IFCK worked with fifth- through eighth-grade gifted students from two elementary schools to teach them about pedestrian safety and brainstorm ideas for teaching it. They studied pedestrian accidents, interviewed pedestrians and drivers for walking and driving skills, completed a behavior observation survey, and learned about collision-related injuries. A fun and memorable pedestrian safety video was created for first- through third-graders.

IFCK also developed an informational brochure on the dangers of walkers and used its partner neighborhood organizations to disseminate it. The walker exchange program (funded by the state American Trauma Society) provided safe exersaucers free to caregivers who either had a child requiring medical attention for a walker-related injury or who could not afford to replace their walkers. The aim was to reduce the number of injuries requiring emergency department treatment or hospital admission.

The BikeWise in West Philadelphia project, supported by IFCK and the Ronald McDonald House Charities, was formed to teach children how to bicycle safely and to create an atmosphere where safe riding becomes socially acceptable. BikeWise clinics were organized and promoted through recreation, summer, and after-school programs; Family Resource Center; and the Home Safety Project. Community and hospital volunteers were trained to teach safe riding strategies and the importance of wearing bike helmets, and to provide bike safety materials and free helmets to children who attended the clinic or who were treated for bike-related injuries in emergency rooms. Bike safety materials and education were provided at community events, such as bike rodeos, health fairs, and picnics. Positive reinforcement came from the *Catch a Kid Doing the Right Thing* campaign, which included rewards from local law enforcement, community-wide acknowledgment of safety behaviors, and local media coverage of children and parents who made the choice to be safe.

The Camera Club project was a partnership with IFCK Philadelphia and an elementary school in west Philadelphia to empower youth and encourage them to expand their strengths by serving their community rather than turning to violence. The program built skills in photography, anger management, and conflict resolution, while focusing on self-esteem. Children took pictures of their role models and things that made them proud or afraid, and a photo exhibit was held.

Home Safety Workshops were organized with community and faith-based organizations made up of parents who have young children in their homes, especially teen parents and grandparents. The groups provided child safety education and instruction, coupled with the distribution of free, easy-to-use safety devices to help teen parents provide safe home environments. The goal was to reduce the risk of injury to young children from falls, poisonings, cuts, burns, drowning, suffocation, and choking. A network of block captains in west and southwest Philadelphia neighborhoods were supportive of IFCK and hosted educational meetings, organizing families for the workshop and distributing literature and newsletters. Teen Parent Home Safety Discussion Groups, funded by the American Trauma Society, were offered in west and southwest Philadelphia to teen parents attending high schools or participating in specific teen programs.

To decrease injuries to children caused by motor vehicle collisions, IKFC (funded by the Allstate Foundation) partnered with the department of public health's HealthySTART program and one elementary school to create the Urban Car Seat Initiative. They conducted a workshop to teach parents how to use and install child safety seats properly, and distributed car seats to people who needed them. The children had previously learned about safe street crossing and the importance of car seats and booster seats. The workshop, entitled *Show Your Love, Put Your Child in a Car Seat,* was conducted on Valentine's Day after parents brought their children to school.

SUMMARY

Coalitions must constantly assess community needs, recognize community assets, and build on those strengths to develop new successful programs. They also must learn how to describe and present these programs to their members, community, and potential funders so that they receive the commitment and financial support needed for implementation. Choosing a promising practice or intervention is not simple. What works in one community may not work in another, and it may be difficult to determine how a successful intervention operates. Good programs have some elements in common, namely, that they are responsive, flexible, competent, committed to a clear mission for the long term, collaborative, managed well, and sensitive to the issue and the priority population. In addition to these general characteristics, programs are more likely to be effectively implemented if they adapt to local needs and cultures; are backed by an intermediary organization; understand the importance of the community and human context of the work; and focus on root causes as well as individual and community outcomes. Coalitions often work at different levels of the social ecology: individual (intrapersonal and interpersonal), institutional or organizational, and community levels. Likewise, coalitions have a whole range of strategies at their disposal: health communication, health education, health policy and enforcement, health engineering, health-related community service, and community mobilization strategies.

In marketing the services and products that coalitions use to promote behavior change at all levels of the social ecology, coalitions often rely on social marketing and media advocacy strategies. In social marketing, the priority audience must be at the center of every decision made. The focus is on voluntary behavior change that will benefit an individual, group, or population, not on profit or commercial gain. Finally, if people are expected to give up or modify an old behavior, or accept a new one, they must be offered some appealing benefit (or exchange) in return. Media advocacy initiatives create pressure to change the environment that determines much of those behaviors.

Ideally, the coalition and its partners should use both social marketing and media advocacy strategies to realize individual, family, organizational, and institutional change in the community. Social marketing strategies can be used to promote coalition programs focusing on education (improving knowledge, attitudes, and practices); better the quality of services; and link the priority population to needed services. Media advocacy strategies can be used to promote access to care, delivery of equitable services, and environmental changes (improved transportation, air quality, safety). Some coalition partners, such as traditional health agencies and health care providers, may be more comfortable with the social marketing approach, whereas other groups may embrace a more confrontational advocacy role.

Finally, ethical considerations are extremely important in community interventions. A program that is unethical ignores its mission and risks its credibility and effectiveness in the community. Because ethical issues are not always clear, community programs should develop their own ethical guidelines and policies before problems occur. Agreeing on standards for ethical issues, such as confidentiality and informed consent, and creating policies that help uphold those standards help ensure community respect and quality service delivery.

QUESTIONS FOR REVIEW

1. What are the advantages of phasing in or piloting a program before full implementation?
2. Discuss several criteria that a coalition can use to select interventions for implementation.

3. What factors make an intervention more likely to be successful?

4. Discuss some examples of community building interventions that coalitions are likely to use.

5. Under what circumstances should a coalition use social marketing versus media advocacy or other advocacy actions to effect broad community change?

6. How does ethical behavior benefit coalitions?

RESOURCES

Examples of Social Marketing Campaigns

American Legacy Foundation, anti-tobacco campaigns. www.americanlegacy.org

Centers for Disease Control and Prevention: Choose Your Cover, to promote sun protection. www.cdc.gov/ChooseYourCover/

Centers for Disease Control and Prevention: CDC and other agencies' Youth Media Campaign, to help youth develop exercise and eating habits that will foster a healthy life. www.VERBnow.com and www.bam.gov

Health Resource Service Administration (HRSA): Insure Kids Now!, to increase enrollment in children's health insurance. www.insurekidsnow.gov

National Cancer Institute: 5-a-Day campaign: www.5aday.gov

National Highway Traffic Safety Administration's Buckle Up America!, to increase seat belt and safety seat use. www.buckleupamerica.org

Robert Wood Johnson Foundation: Covering Kids and Families, to increase enrollment in children's health insurance. www.coveringkids.org

White House Office of National Drug Control Policy's National Youth Anti-Drug Media Campaign. www.mediacampaign.org

Other Social Marketing and Media Advocacy Resources

Advocacy Project, a nonprofit organization formed in 1998, serves the needs of civil society, particularly community-based advocates for peace and human rights. Special attention is given to helping NGOs and networks become self-sufficient in the use of information and communications technologies. The site offers the *AdvocacyNet* newsletter and other publications, as well as the opportunity to join the mailing list. www.advocacynet.org

Alliance for Justice is a national association of environmental, civil rights, mental health, women's, children's, and consumer advocacy organizations. Since its inception in 1979, the Alliance has worked to advance the cause of justice for all Americans, strengthen public interest in the community's ability to influence public policy, and foster the next generation of advocates. The site seeks to strengthen the capacity of the public-interest community to influence public policy. The Nonprofit Advocacy Project assists nonprofit organizations in this area through technical assistance, workshops, and a wealth of tools and information. www.afj.org

American Public Health Association (APHA) is a professional association dedicated to improving the public's health through education and advocacy. www.apha.org

American Psychological Association has a website featuring a number of areas relevant to ethics, including the APA Ethics Code (http://www.apa.org/ethics/code.html) and the Mental Health Patient's Bill of Rights (http://www.apa.org/pubinfo/rights/rights.html).

AtHealth is a large website with mental health information for both practitioners and consumers, and items relating to mental health patients' rights. http://www.athealth.com/Consumer/newsletter/FPN_3_11.html

Centers for Disease Control offers CDCynergy (2003, beta version), CD-ROMS with case examples of social marketing campaigns, planning models, and a wealth of reference resources and materials. www.cdc.gov/communication/cdcynergy_eds.htm.

Democracy Center Advocacy Training and Resources offers workshops, training, and counseling across the full range of advocacy activities: strategy development, policy and budget analysis, media advocacy, organizing and coalition building, and lobbying and influencing public officials. This site offers free advocacy support materials for use in trainings and as newsletter inserts, and other educational activities. http://www.democracyctr.org/advocacy/index.htm

Department of Transportation, National Highway Traffic Safety Administration has useful, downloadable *Community How-To Guides* on Coalition Building, Needs Assessments and Strategic Planning, Evaluation, Prevention and Education, Media Relations, Public Policy, Self-Sufficiency, and resources. http://www.nhtsa.dot.gov/people/injury/alcohol/community%20guides%20html/Guides_index.html

Quirks.Com has archived articles about all aspects of market research, including many from the nonprofit sector, in the magazine *Quirks*'s Marketing Research Review. http://www.quirks.com

ResearchInfo.com is a website of helpful links and free resources to assist coalitions in doing market research. Resources include the Market Research Roundtable, Research Conferences Calendar, Research Company Directory, Employment Board, Research Software Archive (trials and demos of over 50 MB of software specifically designed for the industry), Market Research Calculators (tools to assist in determining incidence, response rates, and confidence levels), Market Research Library, Legislative Watch, and Web-Survey Tutorial (how to create online survey content). http://www.researchinfo.com/

Social Marketing in Public Health Conference, held annually in June at Clearwater Beach, Florida, is sponsored by the University of South Florida. The preconference gives participants an overview of the social marketing approach along with basic principles and practices. www.publichealth.usf.edu/conted

Social Marketing Institute provides on-site team-based strategic guidance on social marketing approaches to programs, organizations, businesses, and foundations; conducts and disseminates research on social marketing best practices; trains and educates practitioners; sponsors academic research; and links with social change professionals, commercial marketers, academics, and funders eager to exchange ideas about social marketing. Their website provides a great list of publications and links. To join the Social Marketing Institute listserv, subscribe to listproc@listproc.georgetown.edu through e-mail, and type "subscribe soc-mktg < your name >" in the message body. http://www.social-marketing.org/papers.html. Accessed January 26, 2005.

Social Marketing Place is a communications firm that assists public, private, and nonprofit organizations to develop effective social marketing programs aimed at improving the health and well-being of the populations they serve. They also provide training through onsite workshops and conference presentations. http://www.social-marketing.com/

Tools of Change is a website founded on the principles of community-based social marketing. It offers specific tools, case studies, and a planning guide for helping people take actions and adopt habits that promote health or environmental issues. Several online courses are also offered for minimal fees. Address: Cullbridge Marketing and Communications; 61 Forest Hill Avenue, Ottawa ON, Canada K2C 1P7. Tel: (613) 224-3800; fax: (613) 224-3377; e-mail: toolsofchange@cullbridge.com; www.toolsofchange.com

Turning Point Social Marketing National Excellence Collaborative is a comprehensive site that offers web series for training, case studies, and print products, such as *CDCynergy-Social Marketing Edition—Media on Demand, The Basics of Social Marketing, The Manager's Guide to Social Marketing, Social Marketing and Public Health: Lessons from the Field, Social Marketing Resource Guide,* and the *CDCynergy One-Day Training Manual.* http://www.turningpointprogram.org/Pages/socialmkt.html. Accessed January 25, 2005.

Wisconsin Council on Developmental Disabilities funds DAWN as part of the State Plan on Developmental Disabilities. Disability Advocates/Wisconsin Network (DAWN) is a statewide grassroots cross-disability network of people who care about disability issues. DAWN supports legislative change in the programs and systems affecting people with all disabilities. The site includes a number of tools for media advocates. Address: 201 West Washington Avenue, Suite 110, Madison, Wisc. 53703. Tel: (888) 332-1677 or (608) 266-6660; fax: 608/267-3906; http://www.dawninfo.org/index.cfm

Publications

"Core Elements of Health Education and Risk Reduction Activities" in *Guidelines for Health Education and Risk Reduction Activities,* Centers for Disease Control and Prevention, 1995. Available online: http://wonder.cdc.gov/wonder/STD/RHER3704.PCW.html

"General Considerations Regarding Health Education and Risk Reduction Activities" in *Guidelines for Health Education and Risk Reduction Activities,* Centers for Disease Control and Prevention, 1995. Available online: http://wonder.cdc.gov/wonder/STD/RHER3702.PCW.html

Fawcett, S. B., and others, in collaboration with Johnston, J. *Reducing Risk for Chronic Disease: An Action Planning Guide for Community-Based Initiatives.* Lawrence, KS: University of Kansas, 1995.

Goldberg, M. E., Fishbein, M., Middlestat, S. E. (eds.). *Social Marketing: Theoretical and Practical Perspectives.* Washington, D.C.: The Academy for Educational Development, 1997.

Hawkins, J. D., Miller, J. Y., and Catalano, R. F., Jr.. *Communities That Care.* San Francisco, Calif.: Jossey Bass, 1992.

Making Health Communications Work. National Cancer Institute, 2002. http://www.cancer.gov or the Cancer Information Service at 1-800-4-CANCER

Ogden, L., Shepherd, M., Smith, W. A. *Applying Prevention Marketing.* Atlanta, Ga.: Centers for Disease Control and Prevention, Public Health Service, 1996. A free copy is available by calling the National AIDS Clearinghouse at (800) 458-5231 and requesting publication D905.

Valdiserri, R. O., Lyter, D. W., Leviton, L. C., Stoner, K., and Silvestre, A. "Applying the Criteria for the Development of Health Promotion and Education Programs to AIDS Risk Reduction Programs for Gay Men." *Journal of Community Health,* 1987, (12)4.

Wallack L., Woodruff, K., Dorfman, L., and Diaz, I. *News for a Change: An Advocate's Guide to Working with the Media.* Thousand Oaks, Calif: Sage Publications, 1999.

Weinrich, N. K. *Hands-On Social Marketing.* Thousand Oaks, Calif.: Sage Publications, 1999.

Ethics Websites

http://aspe.hhs.gov/search/admnsimp/pvcrec.htm
Recommendations of the Secretary of Health and Human Services to Congress on health privacy legislation.

http://www.ethicsweb.ca/resources/
This site features links to codes of professional ethics online.

http://www.bestpractices.org
United Nations Center for Human Settlements (Habitat) (UNCHS) and the Together Foundation. A catalog of good and best practices in a number of health, human service, and development areas.

http://www.cdc.gov/ncipc/dvp/bestpractices.htm
A downloadable 216-page sourcebook on youth violence prevention from the Centers for Disease Control.

http://www.cdc.gov/tobacco/bestprac.htm
A paper entitled "Best Practices for Comprehensive Tobacco Control Programs" from the Centers for Disease Control.

http://www.ed.gov/
Best practices in state and local education from the U.S. Department of Education.

http://www.health.gov/statelocal/best_prac.html
Best practices in community health from the U.S. Department of Health and Human Services.

http://hhs.gov/children/index.shtml
Reports on best practices in various areas of service for children and families from the U.S. Department of Health and Human Services. Rather than only referencing programs, it gives a detailed evaluation of best practices in each of several areas of child and family services.

http://www.ncjrs.org/html/ojjdp/jjbul9910-1/comm.html
"School and Community Intervention to Prevent Serious and Violent Offending," an article from the *Juvenile Justice Bulletin,* Sept. 1999. An evaluation of the effectiveness of eight different types of community youth violence prevention interventions from the National Criminal Justice Reference Service.

http://www.ncl.org/
National Civic League's Alliance for National Renewal. Providing resources to communities, including best practices.

http://www.reeusda.gov/1700/programs/programs.htm
About Promising Programs: a compendium of violence prevention programs that could be replicated elsewhere.

http://www.stedwards.edu/educ/eanes/ganghome.html
Best practices in gang prevention and intervention.

http://www.successlink.org/best/
Best practices awards in education from SuccessLink, a Missouri-based educational organization.

http://www.unesco.org/most/bpikreg.htm
UNESCO database on indigenous knowledge.

http://www.usmayors.org/uscm/best_practices/search.asp
The U.S. Council of Mayors' best practices database.

CHAPTER FOURTEEN

Evaluating Coalitions and Partnerships

Not everything that can be counted counts,
and not everything that counts can be counted.
—Albert Einstein (1879–1955)

E valuation is an essential organizational practice in public health; however, it is not practiced consistently across health issues, nor is it well integrated into program management (Breckon, Harvey, and Lancaster, 1998). Additionally, the evaluation process is often misunderstood by public health professionals, who may then use it in a limited or inconsistent way. Effective evaluation is a systematic way to improve and account for public health actions by using procedures that are useful, feasible, ethical, and accurate (Centers for Disease Control, 1999). Evaluation is, therefore, a central task for all coalitions and often determines whether the organization and its activities are sustained over time. Ten principles to guide coalition evaluation are presented here (Association for the Study and Development of Community [ASCD], 2001; Gabriel, 2000):

1. The evaluation should be designed, implemented, and interpreted in partnership between the coalition and the evaluator.

2. The evaluation design should be informed by existing research, prior evaluations, and the wisdom of people in the community.

3. The evaluation should be participatory and inclusive of all stakeholders.

4. The evaluation process should be used to assess, reflect, improve, and inform.

5. Expectations for the evaluation (including those related to goals, desired outcomes, processes, and roles) should be made explicit and clear for all stakeholders.

6. Issues of power and privilege, and of race and class, should be explicitly identified and addressed up front.

7. Trust and positive relationships among practitioners, community participants, funders, and evaluators should be constantly fostered and developed.

8. The evaluation process should be integrated into ongoing activities and functions.

9. Periodically, the evaluation process and design should be systematically re-evaluated to assure that it continues to meet the coalition's needs and to identify opportunities for using the findings to help decision making and learning.

10. The findings of the evaluation should be shared frequently with stakeholders (including members of the community) in a format that is useful and meaningful to them.

Evaluation, then, can help coalitions in the following ways and answer these critical questions (Goodman, 1998; Butterfoss and Francisco, 2004):

- Provides accountability to the community, stakeholders, and funding agencies. *(Are members satisfied and making a contribution? Did the coalition use resources wisely?)*

- Determines whether objectives are met. *(Did the program achieve its goals?)*

- Improves program implementation or develop better approaches. *(Were programs effective?)*

- Increases community awareness and support. *(Is the community aware of coalition efforts? Are they behind the coalition efforts?)*

- Informs policy decisions. *(Did elected officials support legislation proposed by the coalition?)*

- Contributes to the scientific understanding of what works. *(Does a coalition approach work?)*

This chapter opens by presenting various evaluation paradigms, focusing on the participatory types of evaluation that coalitions and partnerships use. Then key evaluation concepts, levels of coalition evaluation, and practical models that are used for accomplishing exemplary evaluations will be presented, and a step-by-step summary model will provide guidance on partnership program evaluation. Within these steps (and in the exhibits), the tools and measures that are most commonly used to evaluate coalitions and their programs are described. The chapter concludes with the challenges associated with evaluating community-based initiatives and recommended solutions to these dilemmas.

EVALUATION PARADIGMS

Fortunately, evaluation of public health organizations and programs is based on a rich tradition of paradigms that have been borrowed from other disciplines, such as psychology, sociology, and anthropology. To appreciate the roots of current evaluation trends, a summary of the most applicable ones is presented here.

Interpretivist, or constructivist, evaluation uses an anthropological approach instead of an explanatory one, to focus on understanding the phenomenon being studied through ongoing, in-depth contact and relationships with those involved (for example, observations and interviews). The resulting rich qualitative data describe the process and implementation of the program and its effects on participants (Maxwell and Lincoln, 1990). The main objective of the evaluation is to understand the program and its context from different perspectives in order to improve it (p. 11).

Theory-based evaluation attempts to address the problems associated with evaluating comprehensive, community-based initiatives and others not well suited to statistical analysis of outcomes (Chen, 1990; Weiss, 1995). Combining outcome data with an understanding of the process that leads to the outcomes informs one about the program's impact and its most influential factors (Connell and Kubisch, 1998). Theory-based evaluation starts with developing a program logic model that describes how the program works. Evaluators and staff use this theory of how the initiative effects change to develop key intermediate outcomes that ultimately lead to long-term outcomes. Documenting these intermediate outcomes demonstrates whether an initiative is on track and encourages modification of the logic model to increase the potential for achieving long-term impacts.

Participatory evaluation uses an egalitarian process, where the evaluator's perspective is given no more weight than any other stakeholder's or program participant's, to make the evaluation process and its results relevant and useful for future actions. Participatory approaches try to be practical and empowering to multiple stakeholders, and to improve program implementation and outcomes by actively engaging all stakeholders in evaluation. Participatory types of evaluation are well suited to community-based programs initiated by coalitions, because they articulate a strong belief in empowerment, recognize the power of participation, and work to enhance or sustain it through group dialogue and action (Coombe, 1997).

Collaborative or participatory types of evaluation are often characterized according to three features: (1) control of the evaluation process, which can range from decision making being completely in the hands of the evaluator or researcher, to control being exerted entirely by practitioners; (2) stakeholder selection for participation, ranging from restriction to primary users, to inclusion of all legitimate groups; and (3) depth of participation, from consultation with no decision making control or responsibility, to deep participation with involvement in all aspects of an evaluation, including design, data collection, analysis, reporting, and decisions about dissemination of results and use (Cousins and Whitmore, 1998). The different schools of evaluation are located on this continuum according to who controls the process, who participates, and how much.

Specific types include participatory evaluation, stakeholder-based evaluation, democratic evaluation, empowerment evaluation, participatory action research, and community-based participatory research (Butterfoss and others, 2001). Two types of participatory evaluation have been used most often by coalitions: empowerment evaluation and community-based participatory action research.

> **Empowerment evaluation** uses evaluation concepts and techniques to foster self-determination. This type of evaluation is flexible, collaborative, and focuses on program improvement. Its key objectives are training, facilitation, empowerment of individuals and groups, advocacy, and illumination of issues of concern (Fetterman, Kafterian, and Wandersman, 1996; Fetterman and Wandersman, 2005).
>
> **Community-Based Participatory Research (CBPR)** is similar to participatory action research, which is a "systematic investigation" that involves the collaboration of those affected by the matter being studied, for the purposes of educating, taking action, or effecting social change (Green and others, 1995). CBPR has a partnership approach to research and evaluation, whereby diverse partners are engaged in strategies aimed at obtaining multiple perspectives in order to address community-identified concerns (Israel and others, 2003).

To use these types of empowering research and evaluation approaches for transforming society to support health promotion, a more democratic and ecological approach is needed in which scientists, evaluators, and communities work together to learn from each other (Wing, 1998). However, this idealized approach is challenging and lengthy, as local communities, researchers, and collaborators must deal with issues of power, trust, research rigor, and conflicting agendas (Minkler, 2000).

COALITION EVALUATION: PROMOTING SELF-REFLECTION AND IMPROVEMENT

Effective evaluation is an ongoing process that can help coalition decision makers to better understand their organization and their projects, and how they impact participants, partner agencies, and the community. Effective evaluation provides ongoing, systematic information to strengthen coalition programs during their implementation and outcome data to assess the extent of change among participants or within the community. The type of evaluation that should be promoted for a community-based organization, such as a coalition, is collaborative and encompasses the following attributes (Cousins and Whitmore, 1998; W. K. Kellogg Foundation, 1998, p. 4):

- Uses multidisciplinary approaches to problem solving
- Is based on local community circumstances and issues
- Is participatory and values multiple perspectives
- Adapts and adjusts to the needs of an organization and its projects as they evolve
- Is concerned with the skills, knowledge, and perspectives acquired by the individuals who are involved with planning, implementing, and evaluating the initiative

People often benefit more from skills learned by participating in an evaluation *process* than from the *results* of an evaluation (Patton, 1997a); this has great potential for organizational learning and development within coalitions.

Participatory and collaborative approaches that maximize stakeholder involvement are advantageous because they increase local talent and capacity for evaluation, as well as the quality and breadth of evaluation feedback, which, in turn, increases the likelihood that evaluation results will be used. These approaches also provide a systematic, flexible process; improve communication with community audiences, because reports are written in usable formats; emphasize improving local practices rather than funder-based expectations; and produce practical, usable program materials (Dugan, 1996). Collaborative approaches have disadvantages as well, namely, that extra time and money are needed to train and build relationships; participants' motivation, commitment, and skills vary; highly technical reports are not usually produced; and some rigor may be lost (Dugan, 1996). However, rigor may be improved as participants' skills and commitment increase and by using systematic approaches and multiple methods.

The issues encountered in evaluating community-based initiatives and coalitions have been debated frequently, and the essence of these issues will be presented at the end of this chapter. First, the basics of evaluating coalitions will be examined, beginning with key evaluation concepts.

KEY CONCEPTS AND LEVELS OF COALITION EVALUATION

Studies suggest that members of coalitions may hold diverse views about how to measure success (Provan and Milward, 2001). Coalition leaders have defined successful coalitions in multiple ways, from achieving the goal to creating lasting networks and attaining longevity, to gaining or acquiring such resources as recognition from the target, community support, and new consciousness of issues or new skills (Mizrahi and Rosenthal, 1993).

Key Terms of Coalition Evaluation

Before delving into the fundamentals of effective evaluation, some key terms, such as *process, impact, and outcome evaluations,* and *formative and summative evaluations,* should be clarified.

Process evaluation is defined as the measurements obtained during the implementation of program activities "to control, assure or improve the quality of performance or delivery" (Greene, 1994, p. 364). Process evaluation documents the daily activities that take place within and outside the coalition and that determine how well things are going. These short-term indicators document the coalition's structure and procedures, budget allocations, staff hired, meetings, critical events, and media coverage. Process indicators also describe how the coalition's programs are responsive to, adapted for, delivered to, and received by the priority population for which they were intended. Linnan and Steckler identify seven components of any process evaluation (2002, p. 12):

1. *Context*—aspects of the social, political, and economic environment that may influence intervention implementation.
2. *Reach*—proportion of the priority population that participates in each intervention or component.
3. *Dose delivered*—number or amount of intended units of each intervention or component delivered or provided.
4. *Dose received*—extent to which participants actively engage with, interact with, are receptive to, or use materials or recommended resources.
5. *Fidelity*—extent to which the intervention was delivered as planned, in other words, the intervention's quality and integrity.
6. *Implementation*—composite score that indicates the extent to which the intervention has been implemented and received by the intended audience.
7. *Recruitment*—procedures used to approach and attract participants.

Impact evaluation is defined as the "immediate observable effects leading to the intended outcomes of a program" (Greene, 1994, p. 363). These intermediate outcomes measure the changes in knowledge, attitude, beliefs, behaviors, practices, and policies that should be linked to long-term outcomes.

Outcome evaluation is defined as the "ultimate goal of a program or treatment, generally measured in the health field by morbidity or mortality statistics in a population, vital measures, symptoms, and signs or physiological indicators on individuals" (Green, 1994, p. 364). For coalition evaluation, these *long-term outcomes* also include significant community changes, such as increased capacity and competence, institutionalization of coalition programs, and organizational empowerment.

To summarize, process evaluation documents the *short-term* specific activities that the coalition uses to create change. Impact evaluation documents the *intermediate* accomplishments of the coalition, such as the creation or modification of programs, services, or policies, and the changes in knowledge, attitudes, and practices of the priority population. And outcome evaluation documents the ultimate, *long-term* changes that result from the short-term and intermediate outcomes.

One other critical issue arises because coalitions often work with multiple partners from different professional backgrounds and, therefore, must use evaluation terms that are easily understood by all. The fields of organizational and community psychology, for example, use the same definition for process evaluation as the one described above, but they reverse the order for the other levels of evaluation; in other words, the levels of impact and outcome evaluations in public health are reversed in psychology. Using the terms *short-term, intermediate, and long-term evaluations* instead of *process, impact, and outcome evaluations* is more descriptive and may avoid confusion.

Formative evaluation is defined as the "measurements obtained and judgments made before or during the implementation of materials, methods, activities, or programs to control, assure, or improve the quality of performance or delivery" (Greene, 1994, p. 362). For coalition evaluation, this means the evaluation activities that occur during the formation, implementation, and maintenance of the coalition and its programs. Formative evaluation also covers the community assessment, or pre-planning, phase of the coalition and its work. Thus process evaluation is a type of formative evaluation that focuses on process, or short-term, outcomes.

Summative evaluation is defined as the "measurements and judgments that permit conclusions to be drawn about impact, outcome, or benefits of a program or method" (Greene, 1994, p. 366). For coalition evaluation, this refers to the evaluation of the impacts and outcomes of the coalition, or intermediate and long-term outcomes. In a practical sense, both formative and summative evaluation allow for the need to evaluate before, while, and after the coalition initiates any internal changes or any community program (McKenzie, Neiger, and Smeltzer, 2005, p. 295).

Ecological Levels of Outcomes

Outcomes can be further classified according to the ecological levels of change— that is, the changes in individuals and organizations, and across organizations, communities, or systems. For the most part, coalitions are more likely to measure change at the community, organizational, or systems levels.

Individual outcomes include changes in circumstances, status, quality of life or functioning, attitude or behavior, knowledge, skills, and transfer of skills.

Organizational outcomes include the adoption and enforcement of new policies or practices, the availability of new programs or services, and increased or new in-kind and financial resources. They can also include changes in the lives and career options, enhanced perceptions, or improved skills of staff, and changes in the mission, direction, or partners of the organization.

Inter-organizational outcomes focus on the linkages between public, private, nonprofit, and community-based organizations. Specific outcomes include these: the number of newly established relationships between organizations within the community and the extent to which these partnerships have progressed along a continuum of collaboration; bridging of community sectors that have not worked together in the past; and new relationships formed between the coalition and organizations outside of the community. They can also include improved communication, increased parent-child-school interactions, increased civic engagement and participation, decreased violence, shifts in authority and responsibility from traditional institutions to community-based agencies and resident groups, or more intensive collaboration among community agencies and institutions. These types of outcomes allow for pooling of resources and expertise, sharing of responsibility for an issue, and coordinating action.

Community, or systems, outcomes include broad outcomes in the population's health or social and physical environments due to changes in regulations, policies, and practices. The focus is on changes that result in healthier social and physical environments. Public policies (such as new bus routes or restrictions on alcohol sales), norms around community problem solving, and an increased sense of community are other community-level outcomes. Physical environments can also be transformed through coalition efforts such as improving the safety of playgrounds or developing walking trails.

Levels of Coalition Evaluation

Finally, in working with broad, community-based coalitions, coalition evaluation usually occurs at three levels: (1) processes that sustain and renew coalition infrastructure and function; (2) programs intended to accomplish targeted activities, or those that work directly toward the partnership's goals; and (3) changes in health status or the community. Every coalition should aim to evaluate *something* at each level. Complex evaluations can seem overwhelming, but every coalition has the ability to implement at least these three: conducting a member survey to assess satisfaction with how the organization functions (Level 1), evaluating one program or activity that the coalition conducts (Level 2), and collecting extant data on a set of health indicators of interest (Level 3). Together, these present a reasonable expectation for an annual evaluation plan. Each level is detailed below.

Level 1. Coalition infrastructure, function, and processes. In the early stages, coalitions create mission statements, set up work groups, conduct assessments, and develop action plans. To sustain momentum, a coalition has to recruit and orient new members, train leaders, prepare leaders-in-waiting to take over when there is turnover, address and resolve conflict, engage in public relations, celebrate its accomplishments, and raise funds. This process evaluation documents what was done, how people were recruited and engaged in coalition efforts, and whether organizations are functioning optimally and as originally intended. These are often *short-term* outcomes of the coalition's development as an organization.

This type of evaluation essentially assesses how well the coalition is functioning, including its management and organizational structure and operations. Process evaluation helps the coalition demonstrate that its efforts contributed to positive changes within the community. In conjunction with community assessment data, process evaluation can help coalitions improve and adjust efforts over time, resulting in improved functioning and a greater likelihood of reaching desired goals. Good record keeping is essential here; collecting and analyzing annual reports, attendance records, contribution records, meeting minutes, activity logs, and surveys that measure members' levels of satisfaction, commitment, and participation are methods and measures that may be used to document coalition structure and function.

Level 2. Coalition programs and interventions. To thrive, a coalition must engage in the tasks and produce the products for which it was created. In the implementation phase, coalition activities (for example, training, advocacy, education programs) are carried out. For instance, a community partnership to prevent asthma might develop after-school activities, parent training, and public awareness campaigns, or it might advocate for changes in clean indoor air policies. Successful implementation depends on available resources, a time-phased action plan, and a supportive environment. The likelihood of achieving program outcomes depends on the extent to which strategies are implemented and reach the priority populations. The purpose of program evaluation is not only to prove that programs work but also to improve them.

Intermediate outcomes, associated with changes in the priority population and the capacity of the coalition, the community, or both to achieve long-term outcomes, must be measured (Schorr and Kubisch, 1995). Evaluation should be ongoing and occur at every phase of a program's development, from planning to implementation, to expansion, to replication. This level of the evaluation focuses on the process outcomes, or how the program functions within its community and program setting, and the intermediate outcomes of the program, namely the changes in the community's knowledge, attitudes, practices, and policies. As described in Chapter Twelve, adaptations of interventions that have been previously evaluated or accepted as promising practices increase the likelihood that interventions will result in community change and, ultimately, in desired health and social outcomes.

Evaluating the extent to which specific program objectives have been met will also help planners assess coalition effectiveness. Observations of clinic functioning, home-visit logs and diaries, media-reach reports, and event participation logs provide short-term evidence of whether programs are implemented effectively and with fidelity. Reviewing patient records helps determine whether medical personnel adopt practice guidelines. Legislative records provide evidence of when and how proposed policies were introduced or passed. Finally, key informants can report whether school policies or curricula have changed because of coalition efforts.

Level 3. Health status and community change outcomes. For coalition members, communities, and funders, the bottom line for success depends on whether the coalition achieves its ultimate, long-term goals. Systems and community change do not happen quickly. Many outcomes are difficult to measure using traditional quantitative methods. Participatory and empowerment evaluation methods increase understanding about how and why community-based initiatives work. Epidemiological data will inform coalitions as to whether health status indicators have changed (for example, whether the prevalence of diabetes is reduced). Key informants can help identify the coalition programs that are institutionalized within their organizations.

In addition to key evaluation concepts, future evaluators should be familiar with the basic evaluation frameworks and models that have evolved for use in public health initiatives. Readers will recall that we followed a similar process in presenting planning models in Chapter Twelve.

EVALUATION FRAMEWORKS AND MODELS

Certain theoretical assumptions form the framework upon which most community coalitions are, or should be, built. The Community Coalition Action Theory, or CCAT (Butterfoss and Kegler, 2002), described in Chapter Three, suggests propositions for developing and maintaining coalitions and supporting successful actions and health outcomes. CCAT also may be used as the basis for developing a coalition evaluation plan. Many large-scale coalition efforts also develop their own logic models and evaluation plans, which can be readily obtained. Similarly, other practical frameworks and models can help a coalition choose effective evaluation methods and measures. Some examples are the Kansas University Work Group Framework for Participatory Evaluation of Community Initiatives (Fawcett and others, 1993; Francisco, Fawcett, Schultz, and Paine-Andrews, 2000; Fawcett and others, 2003); CDC's *Framework Featuring Steps and Standards for Program Evaluation* (Millstein, Wetterhall, and the CDC Evaluation Working Group, 2000); and the W. K. Kellogg Foundation's Steps to Program Evaluation (1998).

A description of each of these frameworks follows, and each will contribute to a composite model of evaluation that is the basis of this chapter. Note that the Center for Substance Abuse Prevention's *Getting to Outcomes* model (Chinman and others, 2001), presented in Chapter Eleven as a planning model, can also be used as an evaluation framework. The three frameworks that are discussed below are compared in Table 14.1.

Table 14.1. Summary of Public Health Planning Models.

Fawcett, and others, 1993	Millstein and others, 2000	W. K. Kellogg Foundation, 1998
1 Naming and framing the problem to be addressed	Engaging the stakeholders	Engaging the stakeholders
2 Developing a logic model or theory of action for how to achieve success	Describing the program	Focusing the evaluation
3 Identifying evaluation questions and appropriate methods	Focusing the evaluation design	Gathering credible evidence
4 Documenting the intervention and its effects	Gathering credible evidence	Developing and justifying conclusions
5 Making sense of the data	Justifying conclusions	Providing feedback of data and lessons learned to the community
6 Using the information to celebrate, make adjustments, and share data	Ensuring use and sharing lessons learned	Ensuring use of evaluation results

Kansas University Work Group's Framework for Participatory Evaluation of Community Initiatives

Kansas University Work Group's Framework for Participatory Evaluation of Community Initiatives (Fawcett and others, 2003; Fawcett and others, 1995; Francisco, Fawcett, Schultz, and Paine-Andrews, 2000) is as helpful for evaluation as it is for planning (as seen in Chapter Eleven). The six components are as follows:

1. *Naming and framing the problem or goal to be addressed.* Community representatives and stakeholders work together to develop a shared vision and mission. *(Where are we going? What issue are we trying to address?)*
2. *Developing a logic model or theory of action for how to achieve success.* Together, community representatives and stakeholders develop a road map that identifies the sequence of events needed to bring about the changes required to meet their goal. *(How will we get there?)*
3. *Identifying evaluation questions and appropriate methods.* Community representatives and stakeholders work to clarify the evaluation's purpose, which is what key stakeholders want to understand, and to identify the most appropriate and feasible evaluation methods to answer the research questions in their community. *(What do we want to know and how will we know it?)*
4. *Documenting the intervention and its effects.* Community representatives and stakeholders share responsibilities for the intervention and the evaluation.

Sometimes, it might be appropriate for them to help gather and record information; other times, it might not. Whichever is the case for the coalition, enabling these people to play an active role in examining the progress of the intervention is critical. *(What are we doing? Is it making a difference?)*

5. ***Making sense of the data.*** Community representatives and stakeholders bring their experience and knowledge to bear in interpreting the meaning of the information collected and what it says about the impact of the intervention. *(What are we seeing? What does it mean?)*

6. ***Using the information to celebrate, make adjustments, and share data.*** Community stakeholders collaborate to use the evaluation results to communicate successes and progress, celebrate accomplishments, and support next steps. Celebration and adjustment should occur not only at the end of a fiscal year, but all year long. *(Did we do what we said we would do? What course adjustments do we need to make based on the information we collected? What do we do now and how? With whom do we share the results?)*

CDC's Framework for Program Evaluation in Public Health

CDC's Framework for Program Evaluation in Public Health (Millstein and Wetterhall, 2000) helps answer these questions:

- What is the best way to evaluate?
- What is being learned from the evaluation?
- How will lessons learned from evaluations be used to make public health efforts more effective and accountable?

The framework guides its users in selecting evaluation strategies that are useful, feasible, ethical, and accurate. The challenge is to devise an optimal, as opposed to an ideal, evaluation that is attentive to program context and meets or exceeds relevant standards. The framework illustrated in Figure 14.1, was developed as a practical tool designed to summarize and organize the essential elements of program evaluation. Its six interdependent steps might be taken in any evaluation in order to increase understanding of a program's context (for example, the program's history, setting, and organization).

1. Engage the stakeholders (those involved in or affected by the program and the primary users of the evaluation).

2. Describe the program (need, expected effects, activities, resources, stage, context, logic model).

3. Focus the evaluation design (purpose, users, uses, questions, methods, agreements).

4. Gather credible evidence (indicators, sources, quality, quantity, logistics).

5. Justify conclusions (standards, analysis or synthesis, interpretation, judgment, recommendations).

6. Ensure use and share lessons learned (design, preparation, feedback, follow-up, and dissemination.

CDC's *Standards for Effective Evaluation* were adopted from the Joint Committee on Standards for Educational Evaluation (1994) and are recommended as criteria for judging the quality of program evaluation efforts in public health.

Standard 1: Utility. Utility standards ensure that information needs of evaluation users are satisfied. They address such items as identifying those who will be impacted by the evaluation, the amount and type of information collected, the values used in interpreting evaluation findings, and the clarity and timeliness of evaluation reports.

Standard 2: Feasibility. Feasibility standards ensure that the evaluation is viable and pragmatic. They emphasize that the evaluation should employ practical, nonobtrusive procedures; the varied political interests of those involved should be anticipated and acknowledged; and the use of resources in conducting the evaluation should be prudent and produce valuable findings.

Standard 3: Propriety. These standards ensure that the evaluation is ethical and address such items as developing protocols and agreements for guiding the evaluation; protecting the welfare of human subjects; weighing and disclosing findings in a complete and balanced fashion; and addressing conflicts of interest openly and fairly.

Standard 4: Accuracy. These standards ensure that the evaluation produces findings that are considered correct and include such items as describing the program and its context; clearly articulating the purpose and methods of the evaluation; using systematic methods to gather valid and reliable information; using appropriate qualitative or quantitative methods during analysis and synthesis; and producing balanced reports with justified conclusions.

A graphic representation of the framework follows:

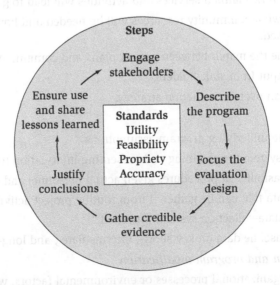

Figure 14.1. Recommended Framework for Program Evaluation.

The Kellogg Foundation's Steps to Program Evaluation

The Kellogg Foundation's Steps to Program Evaluation was developed to improve programs rather than to prove whether programs work (W. K. Kellogg Foundation, 1998). Like CDC's Framework for Evaluation, it follows six steps:

1. Engaging members and community stakeholders in evaluation
2. Focusing the evaluation
3. Gathering credible evidence
4. Developing and justifying conclusions
5. Providing feedback of data and lessons learned to the community
6. Ensuring use of evaluation results

Every step has political implications, which affect the issues of focus, decision making, how the outside world perceives the project, and whose interests are considered. Evaluators must understand the implications of their actions; be sensitive to the concerns of all stakeholders; and talk openly about how conflicting agendas, limited funds, diverse perspectives, and lack of a common knowledge affect the evaluation process, to improve relationships between these players (W. K. Kellogg Foundation, 1998, p. 9). This framework also lists certain *evaluation activities* that should be accomplished, from pre-evaluation to start-up, to implementation and sustainability:

Pre-Evaluation

- Assess needs and assets of priority population or community.
- Specify goals and objectives of planned services and activities.
- Describe how planned services and activities will lead to goals.
- Identify what community resources will be needed and how they can be obtained.
- Determine the match between project plans and community priorities.
- Obtain input from stakeholders.
- Develop an overall evaluation strategy.

Start-Up

- Determine underlying program assumptions.
- Develop system for obtaining and presenting information to stakeholders.
- Assess feasibility of procedures given actual personnel and funds.
- Assess data that can be gathered from routine project activities.
- Develop data-collection system, if needed.
- Collect baseline data on key short-, intermediate-, and long-term outcomes.

Implementation and program modification

- Assess organizational processes or environmental factors, which may inhibit or promote success.

- Describe project and assess reasons for changes from original implementation plan.
- Analyze feedback from staff and participants about successes and failures; use it to modify the program.
- Provide information on short-term outcomes for stakeholders and decision makers.
- Use short-term outcome data to improve the project.
- Describe how short-term and intermediate outcomes are expected to affect long-term outcomes.
- Continue to collect data on all outcomes.
- Assess assumptions about how and why program works; modify as needed.

Maintenance and sustainability

- Share findings with community and other projects.
- Inform various funding sources about accomplishments.
- Continue to use evaluation to improve project and monitor outcomes.
- Continue to share information with multiple stakeholders.
- Assess long-term impact and implementation lessons; describe how and why program works.

Replication and policy

- Assess project fit with other communities.
- Determine critical elements of project that are necessary for success.
- Highlight specific contextual factors that inhibited or facilitated success.
- Develop strategies for sharing information with policy makers to make relevant policy changes.

EVALUATION STEPS

Using the above models as a jumping off point, the following model utilizes the best approaches from each in a new model that is especially geared to evaluating the coalition and its programs. The main difference is an added planning stage that includes mobilizing the stakeholders. The six steps are (1) plan the evaluation and engage stakeholders; (2) describe the program and develop evaluation questions; (3) focus the evaluation design; (4) decide on data-collection methods and collect the data; (5) analyze and interpret the data; and (6) communicate and ensure use of evaluation findings. The steps are described next and frame the rest of this chapter.

1. *Plan the evaluation: Engage stakeholders and establish an evaluation team and evaluation resources.* Engaging stakeholders means fostering input, participation, and power sharing among those persons who have an investment in the evaluation and the findings. Stakeholders include those involved in program operations (for example, sponsors, collaborators, coalition partners,

funders, administrators, managers, staff); those served or affected by the program (for example, clients, family members, neighborhood organizations, academic institutions, elected officials, advocacy groups, professional associations, skeptics, opponents, staff of related or competing organizations); and primary users of the evaluation (W. K. Kellogg Foundation, 1998, p. 49). A special effort should be made to include less powerful groups or individuals. Stakeholders might have varying levels of involvement in the evaluation that correspond to their own perspectives, skills, and concerns. For example, stakeholders can help design and conduct the evaluation as part of a team that makes decisions throughout the evaluation (Poreteous, Sheldrick, and Stewart, 1997; Taylor-Powell, Rossing, and Geran, 1998).

Besides strengthening partnerships and building evaluation capacity in the community, a collaborative approach helps reduce suspicion of research; increases knowledge, awareness, and commitment of diverse partners; and increases the likelihood of achieving objectives and using findings (Centers for Disease Control, 1998; Taylor-Powell, Rossing, and Geran, 1998; Greene and others, 1998). A diverse team is more likely to conduct a culturally competent evaluation that is sensitive to the program's participants, contexts, and conditions (Bonnet, 1999; Smith, 1991). Other stakeholders can be kept informed of evaluation progress through meetings, reports, and other communication channels. Sharing power helps avoid overemphasizing values by any one stakeholder (Connell and Kubisch, 1998).

The evaluation team must understand the roles, responsibilities, organizational structure, history, and goals of the coalition, and how politics and values affect the implementation and impact of its programs. These objectives can be attained by creating an environment where stakeholders are expected to discuss their values, philosophies, and assumptions. The team should be open to findings and willing to learn. Finally, team members must be clear about how policies and decision making can lead to community change, and must develop specific policy goals for the evaluation. Asking the following questions is a good way to begin: *What levels and types of policies are we hoping to change? Who are we trying to influence? What do they need to hear?* Educating community members about relevant issues creates future advocates to help shape policy. Program participants are often the strongest advocates for policy change because they speak from lived experiences about how the coalition's programs affected their quality of life.

Hiring a professional evaluator. The coalition may decide to hire a professional evaluator from outside the coalition and its lead agency, to lead the evaluation team. This person may have broader experience than an insider and be more neutral but may have limited knowledge of the project's needs and goals and limited access to project activities. An internal evaluator may be more familiar with the project and its staff and community members, have access to organizational resources, and have more opportunities for informal feedback with project stakeholders. However, he or she may lack the outside perspective and technical skills of an external evaluator. A good compromise is to have local stakeholders to identify and direct the program content of the evaluation, and an outside evaluator to facilitate its technical aspects. The outside evaluator assumes a facilitative role to bring a different and helpful perspective, raise difficult questions or issues that have not been considered, create methods of data collection and analysis, and be a positive supporter (Butterfoss, Francisco, and Capwell, 2001). He or she must ensure that the coalition and key stakeholders own the evaluation process. Whichever option is chosen, the evaluator's role and qualifications must be carefully considered. Some coalitions require someone with knowledge of the community or experience working with the priority population; others may desire an evaluator who is experienced in a specific subject or certain kinds of evaluations.

Evaluator skills. The critical skills of an effective evaluator include the ability to listen, negotiate, bring together multiple perspectives, analyze the specific situation, and assist the evaluation team in developing a design that will lead to the most useful and important information and final products. The evaluator should have formal training in evaluation, evaluation experience, and a personal style that meshes with that of the coalition (Worthen, Sanders, and Fitzpatrick, 1996). He or she should be expected to assist in building and using the skills, knowledge, and abilities of other staff and stakeholders. Evaluators must have integrity and uphold standards; be ethical and honest; stay focused on evidence while adapting to rapid changes in context, issues, and focus; include and facilitate different perspectives and values; resolve conflict; and deal well with the media and publicity in presenting findings (Patton, 1997a, p. 131).

The best evaluators of community-based programs also are culturally competent, that is, they invest time in learning about the history and culture of the priority population(s), find out what questions should be asked and what methods are culturally appropriate, use multiple data sources, and identify appropriate channels in the community to disseminate evaluation results (Butterfoss and Francisco, 2000). The American Evaluation Association Task Force's *Guiding Principles for Evaluators* (2004) maintains that evaluators should "respect the security, dignity, and self-worth of the respondents, program participants, and other stakeholders with whom they interact" and "articulate and take into account the diversity of interests and values that may be related to the general and public welfare" (the guidelines are included in Exhibit 14.1). Bishop, Earp, Eng, and Lynch (2002) describe a culturally competent evaluation of a lay health advisor program to increase mammography screening for African-American women in rural North Carolina. By working with a local advisory committee, the evaluators were actively involved in the community, asking the right questions and learning what worked and how to improve the program to focus on true community needs. See Exhibit 14.2 on page 452 for a checklist for selecting a competent evaluator.

Exhibit 14.1. Guiding Principles for Evaluators.

A. Systematic Inquiry: Evaluators conduct systematic, data-based inquiries, and thus should
1. Adhere to the highest technical standards appropriate to the methods they use.
2. Explore with the client the shortcomings and strengths of evaluation questions and approaches.
3. Communicate the approaches, methods, and limitations of the evaluation accurately and in sufficient detail to allow others to understand, interpret, and critique their work.

B. Competence: Evaluators provide competent performance to stakeholders, and thus should
1. Ensure that the evaluation team collectively possesses the education, abilities, skills, and experience appropriate to the evaluation.
2. Ensure that the evaluation team collectively demonstrates cultural competence and uses appropriate evaluation strategies and skills to work with culturally different groups.
3. Practice within the limits of their competence, decline to conduct evaluations that fall substantially outside those limits, and make clear any limitations on the evaluation that might result if declining is not feasible.
4. Seek to maintain and improve their competencies in order to provide the highest level of performance in their evaluations.

C. Integrity and Honesty: Evaluators display honesty and integrity in their own behavior and attempt to ensure the honesty and integrity of the entire evaluation process, and thus should
1. Negotiate honestly with clients and relevant stakeholders concerning the costs, tasks, limitations of methodology, scope of results, and uses of data.
2. Disclose any roles or relationships that might pose a real or apparent conflict of interest before accepting an assignment.
3. Record and report all changes to the original negotiated project plans and the reasons for them, including any possible impacts that could result.
4. Be explicit about their own, their clients', and other stakeholders' interests and values related to the evaluation.
5. Represent accurately their procedures, data, and findings, and attempt to prevent or correct misuse of their work by others.
6. Work to resolve any concerns related to procedures or activities likely to produce misleading evaluative information; decline to conduct the evaluation if concerns cannot be resolved; and consult colleagues or relevant stakeholders about other ways to proceed if declining is not feasible.
7. Disclose all sources of financial support for an evaluation and the source of the request for the evaluation.

Exhibit 14.1. (*Continued*)

D. Respect for People: Evaluators respect the security, dignity, and self-worth of respondents, program participants, clients, and other evaluation stakeholders, and thus should

1. Seek a comprehensive understanding of the contextual elements of the evaluation.

2. Abide by current professional ethics, standards, and regulations regarding confidentiality, informed consent, and potential risks or harms to participants.

3. Seek to maximize the benefits and reduce any unnecessary harm that might occur from an evaluation, and carefully judge when the benefits from the evaluation or procedure should be foregone because of potential risks.

4. Conduct the evaluation and communicate its results in a way that respects stakeholders' dignity and self-worth.

5. Foster social equity in evaluation when feasible so that those who give to the evaluation may benefit in return.

6. Understand, respect, and take into account differences among stakeholders such as culture, religion, disability, age, sexual orientation, and ethnicity.

E. Responsibilities for General and Public Welfare: Evaluators articulate and take into account the diversity of general and public interests and values, and thus should

1. Include relevant perspectives and interests of the full range of stakeholders.

2. Consider not only immediate operations and outcomes of the evaluation but also the broad assumptions, implications, and potential side effects.

3. Allow stakeholders' access to and actively disseminate evaluative information, and present evaluation results in understandable forms that respect people and honor promises of confidentiality.

4. Maintain a balance between client and other stakeholder needs and interests.

5. Take into account the public interest and good, going beyond analysis of particular stakeholder interests to consider the welfare of society as a whole.

Source: American Evaluation Association, 1994, revised 2004. *Guiding Principles for Evaluation.* Reprinted by permission of the American Evaluation Association.

Evaluation budget. Conducting an evaluation requires an organization to invest valuable resources, including time and money, usually between 5 and 7 percent of a project's total budget. A mechanism for reviewing and revising the evaluation budget based on what happens during the course of the evaluation is recommended. Evaluation budgets should also allow sufficient resources for the analysis and interpretation step. A useful

Exhibit 14.2. Checklist for Selecting an Evaluator.

	Evaluator appears to be: (Check one for each item)		
	Not Well Qualified	Cannot Determine Whether Qualified	Well Qualified
1. To what extent does formal training of evaluator qualify him or her to conduct evaluation (for example, major and minor degree specializations; courses in evaluation methodology; whether evaluator has conducted applied research in human service setting)?			
2. To what extent does previous evaluation experience qualify evaluator to conduct evaluation (for example, length and relevance of experience)?			
3. To what extent does previous performance of evaluator qualify him or her to conduct this evaluation? What prior experience does she or he have in similar settings? (Look at work samples; contact references.)			
4. To what extent is evaluator's professional orientation a good match for evaluation approach required (for example, philosophical and methodological orientations)?	Unacceptable match	Cannot determine match	Acceptable match
5. To what extent are evaluator's personal styles and characteristics acceptable (for example, honesty, character, communication skills, personal mannerisms, cultural competence, ability to resolve conflicts)?	Unacceptable	Cannot determine acceptability	Acceptable
Summary: Based on questions above, to what extent is evaluator qualified and acceptable to conduct the evaluation?	Not well qualified, unacceptable, or both	Cannot determine whether qualified or acceptable	Well qualified and acceptable

Source: W. K. Kellogg Foundation (1998). From *W. K. Foundation Evaluation Handbook.* Reprinted by permission of the W. K. Kellogg Foundation.

framework for developing an evaluation budget follows (Worthen, Sanders, and Fitzpatrick, 1996):

- *Evaluation staff salary and benefits.* The amount of time staff must spend on evaluation and the level of expertise needed to perform particular evaluation tasks will affect costs.
- *Consultants.* If staff need assistance in conducting the evaluation, contract with external consultants to provide special expertise, different perspectives, or both throughout the evaluation.
- *Travel.* Expenses for staff and evaluator travel vary from project to project.
- *Communications.* Costs such as postage and telephone calls are included here.
- *Printing and duplication.* These costs cover preparation of data-collection instruments, reports, and any other documents.
- *Printed materials.* Costs of acquiring data-collection instruments and library materials are included.
- *Supplies and equipment.* This category contains the costs of specific items such as computers or packaged software that must be purchased or rented.

2. *Describe the program and develop evaluation questions.* A program description should focus on the need(s) addressed by the program, its goals, objectives and criteria for success, and how activities are expected to lead to changes. It includes information about the way the program is intended to function and how it will be implemented. A good description provides a balanced assessment of strengths and weaknesses and helps stakeholders understand the relationship between program activities and expected changes (perhaps through a logic model). Finally, it should show how the program fits with the coalition and the community and how it links to other efforts.

Drafting an evaluation plan will usually require many meetings with the evaluation team and other stakeholders. One of the first steps the team should work through is setting the goals of the evaluation, or what questions must be answered, such as:

- What should the program accomplish and how will it be demonstrated?
- What activities will the project undertake to accomplish its goals?
- What factors might help or hinder the program in accomplishing its goals?

Mosaica (2005c) provides a seven-step evaluation planning worksheet that may be useful:

1. What are the overall project goals and objectives for this program?
2. What are the measurable objectives for the strategy you plan to evaluate? (If you do not have measurable objectives, describe the kinds of objectives identified for the program.)

3. What staff or other resources (internal or outside) are available for the evaluation? Indicate who can help, how much time they have, and whether they have experience.

4. What type(s) of evaluation do you want to conduct (for example, process, outcome, or both)?

5. What existing documentation is available as input to the evaluation (for example, contact information on participants, number and types of activities completed) and how will it be used?

6. What evaluation methods will be used (for example, surveys, key informant interviews, focus groups)?

7. Describe the evaluation plan, including major tasks (for example, develop survey, plan focus groups); for each task, indicate who will be responsible and a projected timeline.

Logic models. A logic model describes the sequence of events for bringing about change by arranging the main program elements into a flowchart, map, or table that displays how the program is supposed to work (Julian, 1997; McEwan and Bigelow, 1997). It serves as a road map of the program, highlighting priority activities and how desired outcomes will be achieved. A logic model summarizes the program's mechanism of change by linking processes to eventual outcomes and displays the infrastructure needed to support program operations (Centers for Disease Control, 1999). Elements that are connected within a logic model generally include inputs (for example, trained staff), activities (for example, identification of cases), outputs (for example, persons completing treatment), and results ranging from immediate (for example, curing persons with cancer), to intermediate (for example, reducing cancer rate), to long-term effects (for example, improvement of population health status) (Centers for Disease Control, 1999).

Developing a logic model requires stakeholders to work together to clarify the program rationale, its strategies, and the conditions that will make success more likely. In fact, most of a logic model's value "lies in the process of creating, validating, and then modifying it" (W. K. Kellogg Foundation, 1998, p. 11). The logic model can be used to explain the program to others and to build ownership among stakeholders. It provides an effective way to chart the progress of complex initiatives and make continuous improvements in them. An effective logic model will be refined and changed many times throughout the evaluation process as more is learned about the program, how and why it works, and how it is operationalized.

Logic models can be created in different ways. The starting point is to identify the elements of an existing program and organize them into a logical flow. For a new program, the starting point could be the mission and long-term goals of the program, to which the short-term and intermediate objectives that lead to those long-term goals are added (McLaughlin and Jordan, 1999). An activity logic model can be built in the same way; long-range activities are linked to short-term and intermediate activities. Exhibit 14.3 provides a sample logic model for a comprehensive cancer coalition.

3. Focus the evaluation design. Focusing the evaluation design for its intended uses increases the likelihood that the evaluation will succeed by identifying procedures that are practical, politically viable, ethical, accurate, and cost-effective (Centers for Disease Control, 1998; W. K. Kellogg Foundation, 1998). The evaluation should address the issues of greatest concern to stakeholders and adapt itself to the needs of the priority population, while being efficient of time and resources. Explicit evaluation questions to be asked must be decided upon and practical methods developed for sampling, data collection, data analysis, and interpretation. See Exhibit 14.4 for a sample grid of evaluation questions, design, and methods, and Exhibit 14.5 for an evaluation timeline.

(*Text resumes on page 458.*)

Exhibit 14.3. Narrative: Smokefree (SF) Environments Logic Model

This logic model shows the interconnections of inputs, outputs (activities and reach) and outcomes in public policy to achieve smoke-free environments (goal). Smoke-free environments refer to municipal buildings, grounds and vehicles, public areas/events, worksites (including restaurants) and residences. A coalition may be working on any one or several of these SF environments.

Starting at the left side, this logic model shows that a variety of human and materials resources (INPUTS) are invested. These include coalition members, funding, partners, the media, existing research and best practices, and supportive policy makers. These INPUTS link to three interconnected chains of events.

1. Campaign. A whole series of activities make up the smoke-free campaign directed to many individuals and groups (REACH). As a result, certain changes occur in the short term. These immediate (short-term) changes include increased awareness of the importance of public policies, increased knowledge of SF benefits and options; increased commitment, support and demand for SF environments; and for the community activists, increased knowledge and skills in participating in public policy change and increased understanding of the need for cessation services and support. These short-term outcomes link to a number of medium term outcomes that include demonstrations of public support for SF public policies; SF policies drafted; SF policies implemented; SF policies enforced and increased availability of cessation services and support. It is expected that initial demonstrations of public support create additional commitments that in turn lead to further public support (illustrated by two-headed arrow) necessary for public policy change.

2. Youth involvement. Another area of emphasis in SF policy change is youth advocacy (also see Youth Logic Model). Youth are identified as a specific target group and are linked to the chain of outcomes as depicted in the overarching logic model.

3. Integrating cessation. The third main activity area for achieving the long-term outcomes is the integration of cessation resources into policy change efforts. This activity area is directed primarily to worksites and community groups in order to increase their understanding of the need for cessation services/support (Short-term outcome). This, in turn, is expected to lead to the increased availability of such services and support (Medium-term outcome).

(*continued*)

Exhibit 14.3. Narrative: Smokefree (SF) Environments Logic Model. (*Continued*)

Overarching Logic Model: Smoke-Free (SF) Environments

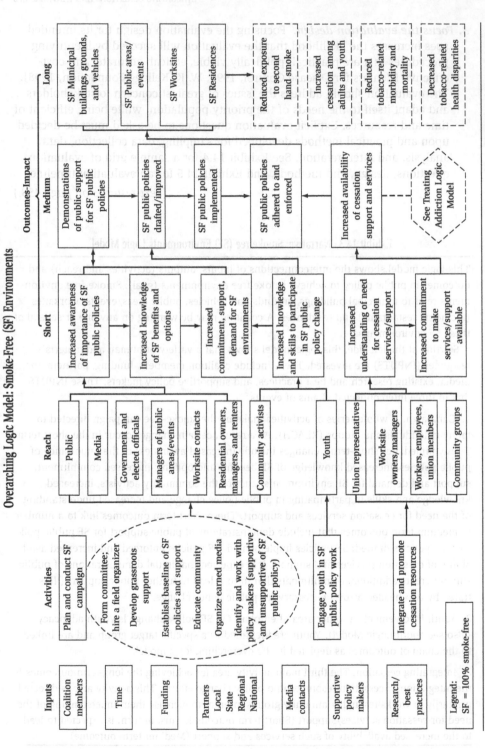

Source: UW-Extension-Cooperative Extension, Local evaluation project. 2003 http://www.uwex.edu.ces/pdande/evaluation/pdf Accessed Jan. 18, 2007

Exhibit 14.4. Evaluation Questions and Methods.

Key Evaluation Question(s)	Type of Management Information and Evaluation Measure(s)	Type of Data Collection					Experimental Design		
		Survey/Scale	Structured Interview	Self Report/Log	Direct Observation	Archival Records	Case Study	Pre-Post-Test Control Group	Time Series
A. Planning and Implementation Issues	**A. Descriptive and Process Measures**								
1. Who participates?	1. Demographic data	X	X				X		
2. Why do participants drop out?	2. Participants' reasons for dropping out	X	X				X		
3. Are different activities generated?	3. Type and frequency of activities				X	X	X		
B. Assessing Attainment of Objectives	**B. Outcome Measures**								
1. How many participate?	Number of participants			X	X	X	X		X
2. How many hours are participants involved?	Number of hours by activity			X	X	X	X		X
3. How many people are trained?	Number of participants per workshop			X	X	X	X		X
C. Impact on Participants									
1. How do attitudes and behavior change by participating in program?	Changes in attitudes and behavior	X	X	X	X	X		X	X
2. Does participation affect the incidence of problems?	Incidence of problems (for example, substance abuse, gang involvement)		X			X		X	
3. Are participants satisfied with the experience?	Participants' satisfaction ratings	X					X		
D. Impact on Community									
1. What resulted from program?	Changes in programs, policies, and practices of partner organizations	X	X	X	X	X			X
2. Do program benefits outweigh costs?	Cost-benefit data			X	X		X	X	
3. Are community members satisfied with participants and service they provide?	Beneficiaries and community members/satisfaction ratings	X					X		

Source: From "Getting off to a good start with your evaluation," by V. T. Francisco, E. M. Capwell and F. D. Butterfoss in *Health Promotion Practice*, 1(2), p. 130. Copyright © 2000 Sage Publications, Inc. Reproduced with permission of Sage Publications, Inc. via Copyright Clearance Center.

Exhibit 14.5. Evaluation Timeline.

Documentation System	Year 1 JFMAMJJASOND	Year 2 JFMAMJJASOND	Year 3 JFMAMJJASOND	Year 4 JFMAMJJASOND
Establish system	xxxxxx			
Train participants and staff in data entry	xxx			
Maintain system (data collection and reporting)	xxxxxxxxxxxxxxxxxxxxxxxxxxxxxxxxxxxxxxxxxxxxxxxxxxxxxxxxx			
Critical Events				
Identify key people	xxxx	xxxx	xxxx	
Conduct interviews	xxx	xxx	xxx	
Report results	xxxx	xxxx	xxxx	
Community-Level Indicators				
Identify local indicators	xxxx			
Identify comparison site	xxxx			
Secure data	xxxxxxxxxxxxxxxxxxxxxxxxxxxxxxxxxxxxxxxx			
Report results	xxxx	xxx	xxxx	
Other Indicators (for example, behavioral surveys, data observations)				
Identify indicators	xxxxxxxxx			
Secure data	xxxxxxxxxxxxxxxxxxxxxxxxxxxxxxxxxxxxxxxxxx			
Report results	xxxx	xxxx	xxxx	

Source: From "Getting off to a good start with your evaluation," by V. T. Francisco, E. M. Capwell and F. D. Butterfoss in *Health Promotion Practice*, *1*(2), p. 130. Copyright © 2000 Sage Publications, Inc. Reproduced with permission of Sage Publications, Inc. via Copyright Clearance Center.

A written protocol or agreement that summarizes the evaluation procedures, with clear roles and responsibilities for all stakeholders, is often helpful. The evaluation plan should be revised when critical circumstances change. The evaluation team must be sensitive to cultural issues in the community; know what resources are available for evaluation and request additional resources if necessary; understand the existing capacity and limitations of the program; and take time to deal with unexpected problems (Centers for Disease Control, 1999; W. K. Kellogg Foundation, 1998, p. 71).

Evaluation designs. Evaluation methods should be selected to provide the appropriate information to address stakeholders' questions. The more closely the evaluation design is linked to the priority questions, the more likely the questions will be effectively addressed. The choice of design has implications for what data will be collected and how it will be collected.

- An *experimental design* involves using random assignment to experimental and control groups, measuring both, and provides the greatest control over variables that can influence the results.

- The *quasi experimental pre-post-test design*, which uses a comparison group that is measured before and after the program, is a more common and feasible design used in most programs that coalitions initiate or to compare one coalition to another.

- A *time series design* (used with either experimental or quasi-experimental designs) occurs when several measurements are taken over time, before and after a program is implemented. This design helps identify other factors that may account for a change in pre- and post-test measurements, and measures delayed program effects (such as weight loss).

- A *case studies design* is the design most often used to study the structure and function of a partnership or group of partnerships. Cresswell defines this method as the "exploration of a bounded system (case or multiple cases) over time through detailed, in-depth data collection involving multiple sources of information rich in context, which include observations, interviews, audiovisual material, documents, and reports" (1998, p. 61). The case can be a community (based on geography, locality, or identity) in which members share common culture or characteristics (Quinn, 1999). Similarly, one can see the case study design is ideal for evaluating a coalition or group of coalitions, because controls or comparison groups would be difficult or impossible to locate.

    Methodological decisions clarify how the evaluation will proceed (for example, to what extent program participants will be involved; how information sources will be selected; what data-collection instruments will be used; who will collect the data; what data management systems will be needed; and what methods of analysis, synthesis, interpretation, and presentation are appropriate).

4. *Decide on data-collection methods and collect data.* After deciding on the questions to address, the coalition must decide what data is needed to answer these questions, from whom and how it can best be obtained, and how it should be analyzed and used. Adequate data might be available and easily accessed, or new data may have to be collected. Having credible evidence strengthens evaluation judgments and the recommendations that follow from them. Whether evidence is credible to stakeholders depends on how the questions were posed, the sources of information, conditions of data collection, reliability of measurement, validity of interpretations, and quality control processes.

No simple formula exists to decide how evaluations should be conducted. When selecting methods for gathering evaluation data, the team must decide what type of information is feasible, desired by, and acceptable to the stakeholders. They should determine, for example, whether data should document effectiveness, answer specific questions, be generalizable to a larger population, or provide deeper understanding of an event, attitude, or relationship (Butterfoss, Francisco, and Capwell, 2000). Just as no single program design can solve complex social problems, one evaluation method cannot document and explain the complexity and richness of a project (W. K. Kellogg Foundation, 1998, p. 71; Reichardt and Rallis, 1994). An evaluation should collect data that provide a well-rounded picture of the coalition and its programs in order for stakeholders to perceive the results as believable and relevant. Such evidence can be experimental or observational, qualitative or quantitative, or it can include a mixture of methods.

Qualitative evaluation methods provide greater depth of understanding about a small number of people, help identify new variables for study and relationships among variables, and enhance the understanding of what evaluation findings mean or successes in applied programs (Francisco, Butterfoss, and Capwell, 2001, p. 21). However, generalizations to broader groups of people are limited, findings are not always replicable, and making inferences beyond the data is minimized.

Quantitative methods, on the other hand, provide data from large numbers of people that lead to a greater breadth of understanding (as opposed to the depth provided by qualitative methods) and strong inferences; are more systematic, making them easier to replicate; and focus on the strength of relationships among variables (Francisco, Butterfoss, and Capwell, 2001b, p. 21). These methods are limited because they can only confirm hypotheses about current variables and cannot be used to demonstrate the meaning of findings to people's lives.

Methods may also be classified as obtrusive (interactive) and unobtrusive (noninteractive) (Bernard, 1998; Shadish, Cook, and Leviton, 1991). *Obtrusive measures* are those that are completed in the open and with the direct knowledge of the participants, such as surveys and diaries. *Unobtrusive measures,* such as observation of public behaviors, are those that are done in the absence of direct awareness by participants, although they do not preclude participants' prior knowledge and permission.

The methods that are used in evaluation are often the same as those used in community or organizational assessments as covered in Chapter 11. The main difference concerns the intent of gathering information. In assessment, the data is used to draw a picture of the community in question—its residents, quality of life, strengths, and challenges. In evaluation, the purpose of using such methods is to determine whether a particular organization, institution, system, practice, policy, or program is working as it should (that is, achieving its intended short-term, intermediate, and long-term outcomes); how participants and other stakeholders view that organization or program and its outcomes; and how to make it more effective. Figure 14.2 illustrates that many options are available for gathering data obtrusively or unobtrusively, as well as quantitatively, qualitatively, or a combination of both methods. (Capwell, Butterfoss, and Francisco, 2000, p. 312).

Mixed methods seem to yield stronger data or at least the ability to make stronger inferences or conclusions from those data (Yin, 1994). Integrating qualitative and quantitative data also increases the likelihood that the data will be balanced and accepted by all stakeholders (Greene, 1994; Greene and Caracelli, 1997; Steckler and others, 1992). See Exhibit 14.6 for a sample evaluation plan that use mixed methods.

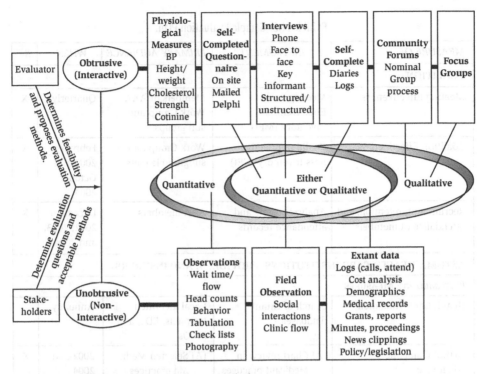

*Note the following steps in selecting evaluation methods:
1-Evaluator and stakeholders reach agreement on evaluation question to be answered
2-Consider feasibility and acceptability of obtrusive and/or unobtrusive measures
3-Consider preference for quantitative and/or qualitative methods
4-Select specific evaluation method(s) that meet(s) need

Figure 14.2. Options for Selecting Evaluation Methods.

From "Choosing Effective Evaluation Methods," by F. D. Butterfoss, V. T. Francisco, & E. M. Capwell in *Health Promotion Practice, 1*(4), 307–313. Copyright © 2000 by Sage Publications, Inc. Reproduced with permission of Sage Publications Inc. via Copyright Clearance Center.

Before data are collected or analyzed, the coalition must determine whether the data will be relevant to the problems the coalition is trying to solve. Several questions may help the coalition decide (U.S. Department of Health and Human Services, 2000):

- Will data match the perceived problems? People may not be aware of the problems evidenced by the data, but they know about the problems they face.
- Will data match the community's values and beliefs about what is right? Do they elevate important shared community values and beliefs?
- Will data consider the different cultural perspectives of respondents, such as language and literacy needs?

Exhibit 14.6. Sample Evaluation Plan.

MEASURE OF	INSTRUMENT	PRIMARY AUDIENCE	WHEN	X
COALITION				
Meeting Effectiveness	Meeting Effectiveness Inventory (MEI)	Members of AAA Work Group and sub groups	Quarterly	X
Coalition Effectiveness	Coalition Effectiveness Inventory (CEI)	Work Group and subgroup leaders	February 2002 and October 2004	X
Recruitment, retention, and attendance of members	Analyze rosters and attendance records	AAA members	December 2002, 2003, and 2004	X
ASTHMA HEALTH CARE INSTITUTIONS, PROVIDERS, AND INSURERS				
INTERMEDIATE MEASURES				
Health Care Utilization	Search of extant databases	Local identified hospitals, EDs, and MCOs	Annually	
NHLBI Guideline adherence	(A) Chart review in Medicaid practices (B) Chart review in EDs	(A) Selected Medicaid practices (B) Selected EDs	2002 and 2004	X
Knowledge of asthma management	Surveys	Physicians attending training	2002 and 2003	X
Satisfaction with care of asthmatics	Physician focus groups	Physicians (P, FM, and ED)	2004	X
Health care utilization and self-management	ED survey	Selected EDs	2001 and 2004	
Asthma knowledge and management skills	Parent focus groups	Parents	2004	X
Communication among nurses and providers	School nurse focus groups	School nurses	2004	X

PROCESS MEASURES:

1. number of algorithms displayed
2. number of appropriate educational brochures and materials distributed
3. number of records reviewed
4. number attending educational sessions (December 2002, 2003, 2004)
5. number of Action Plans available in health records in schools and practices
6. number of pieces of equipment distributed
7. satisfaction with communications form
8. number of physician practices enrolled in hotline
9. number of Asthma Management Kits distributed

Exhibit 14.6. (*Continued*)

MEASURE OF	INSTRUMENT	PRIMARY AUDIENCE	WHEN	X
GENERAL COMMUNITY AND PARENTS OF ASTHMATIC CHILDREN				
INTERMEDIATE MEASURES				
Asthma knowledge and management skills	Post training survey	Parents and community members	2002, 2003, and 2004	X
Asthma knowledge and management skills	Survey	Ambassador program	2004	X
Asthma knowledge and management skills	Parents of Head Start children	EZ Breathers program	2002, 2003, and 2004	

PROCESS MEASURES:

1. number of public service announcements aired and when
2. number of inches of print media devoted to asthma
3. number of posters and brochures distributed
4. number of educational sessions and workshops held
5. number of parents attending training and health fairs
6. number of Asthma Management Kits distributed
7. number of hits to asthma website
8. number of families reached by EZ Breathers
9. number of families reached by Ambassadors
10. number attending Legislative Breakfast
11. number of bills introduced
12. number of letters to the editor
13. number of reports distributed
14. number of decals distributed
15. number attending Summit
16. number of homes taking smoke-free pledge
17. number of Asthma-Proof Your House Kits distributed

Source: Kelly, Butterfoss, and Taylor-Fishwick, 2004.

- Will data lead to the empowerment of marginalized groups, especially if these groups are most at risk for the problems that the coalition is attempting to solve?
- Will data inform decision making about community goals and objectives?
- Will data show how the community changed over time?

Sources of data are the persons, documents, or observations that provide information for the evaluation. More than one source might be used to gather data for each indicator to be measured. Selecting multiple sources (for example, from internal documents, staff interviews, and participant observations) provides different perspectives of the program and enhances the comprehensiveness and credibility of the evaluation (McQueen and Anderson, 1999). For instance, data in community report cards are used to promote awareness of problems and advocacy goals. Some large data sets, like census data (including economic data and demographics), health status indicators (such as immunization rates), and health survey data (such as the Behavior Risk Factor Surveillance Survey) represent likely data sets used by health departments and initiatives working on public health problems. More targeted data sets, such as self-reported drug- and alcohol-use survey data, are used by communities and required by state agencies working on drug and alcohol prevention issues. Finally, some community and state data sets include behavioral outcome data, such as vehicle accidents and alcohol-related emergency medical transports. Community-level indicators can also be found in the various health objectives in Healthy People and Healthy Communities documents.

Indicators that can be defined and tracked include (1) measures of coalition effectiveness (for example, participation in meetings and activities, usefulness of coalition structures, and satisfaction with coalition procedures) and measures of program activities (for example, the program's capacity to deliver services, the participation rate, levels of patient satisfaction, the efficiency of resource use, and the amount and duration of exposure to the intervention); and (2) measures of program effects (for example, changes in participant behavior, community norms, policies or practices, health status, quality of life, and the settings or environment around the program). The logic model can be used as a template to define the indicators that lead from coalition activities to expected effects.

The main issues to be aware of when considering community-level indicators as markers of success for any community initiative are accuracy, sensitivity, and feasibility. If coalitions use data that supposedly reflects the population in its geographic area, yet was actually drawn from only one small sample, the data do not accurately reflect the entire population. For example, if a coalition (that represents two counties) develops a pregnancy prevention initiative based on survey responses from only one county, the data may not accurately reflect the entire population of teens.

If a coalition focuses on a public health issue, such as cardiovascular disease prevention, and its interventions include social marketing of low-fat purchases and public walking trails, then it must track indicators closer to these interventions. Examining statewide indicators such as serum triglycerides and hypertension levels will not be sensitive enough to detect the results of a local prevention initiative.

Finally, data collection must be feasible, or reliable data sets cannot be created, no matter how good the ideas behind them.

Data-collection methods. When deciding on which methods to use, several questions should be considered (W. K. Kellogg Foundation, 1998, p. 72):

- How credible will the evaluation be with the methods chosen? Would other methods be more credible or reliable and still be cost-effective?

- Are the instruments used in these methods valid—in other words, do they measure what they claim to measure? Are the instruments reliable—that is, will they provide similar answers with the same population even if they are administered at different times or in varied places?

- Are the methods and instruments suitable for the population and problem being assessed?
- Can the methods and instruments detect critical program issues, meaningful changes, and outcomes?
- Is the expertise needed to carry out these methods available from staff or consultants?

Although all types of data have limitations, if stakeholders develop clear procedures for gathering, analyzing, and interpreting data, and for training persons to collect high-quality data, an evaluation's credibility will be improved. When stakeholders help define and gather data that they find credible, they will be more likely to accept the evaluation's conclusions and to act on its recommendations. The quality of data obtained should be monitored periodically and improved as necessary.

> **Collecting data.** Once the evaluation questions and methods are determined, arrangements for data collection must be made. Training is essential, especially if the persons collecting the data are coalition or community members who do not have experience with community-based research. Staff, students, and coalition partners who collect data can then revise data-collection strategies based on initial analyses of what is working and what pieces of data are still missing. This step helps the team revise the design and methods based on available financial and human resources; examine how the evaluation process is received by participants from whom data is collected; and assess the usefulness of the collected data. The tracking and organizing of data is critical for keeping the evaluation in progress and protecting the confidentiality of the data. Coalitions are reminded to avoid "drowning in data," and to collect only data that will be used and use all data collected. The team should keep asking how each piece of data collected will be used, fit with other data, and help answer the evaluation questions.

Several questions might be asked concerning the rigor with which data are collected, to assure that it is accurate and sensitive (USDHHS, 2000):

- Are the data reflective of the people who live in the community? The demographics of respondents should match the demographics of the priority audience.
- Do these data reflect the behavior of the priority population, or are they logically connected to intermediate outcomes of behavior change? Sampling strategies should be able to detect the behaviors targeted by the initiative.
- Are the data plausible? Sometimes sampling strategies do not detect what is actually happening; more robust, statistically appropriate methods may be needed.

5. *Analyze and interpret the data.* After designing an evaluation and collecting data, the information must be described, analyzed, and synthesized to summarize findings, and then interpreted according to the context of the program, coalition, and community. Judgments should be made according to clearly stated values that classify a result as positive or negative, high or low. Sometimes this means considering alternative ways to compare results (for example, by using program objectives, a comparison group, national norms, or past performance) and indicating why these explanations are significant (Joint Committee on Standards for Educational Evaluation, 1994). Conclusions should be limited to the situations, time periods, persons, contexts, and purposes for which the findings are applicable, and linked to the recommended actions or decisions. The conclusions are justified when they are linked to the evidence gathered and consistent with the agreed-upon values of the stakeholders.

Quantitative data analysis requires interpreting the results and seeing whether they make sense given the project's contextual factors. Increasingly, most quantitative data are analyzed by sensitive computer programs. One should look for alternative explanations for unusual findings and make sure the data are complete and accurate. Again, a primary goal of evaluation is using these findings for program improvement.

Qualitative data collected from interviews and observations are often recorded in field notes or tape-recorded and transcribed. Frequently, qualitative data are seen as anecdotal information that illuminates the quantitative data, but they may be more helpful in explaining how a program works and why it faces barriers.

Qualitative data should be analyzed systematically. Examining interview transcripts, observation field notes, or open-ended surveys for patterns and themes involves categorizing notes into recurring topics that seem relevant to the evaluation questions (Miles and Huberman, 1994). The materials are first read to identify themes and patterns, then sorted into key categories by using paper-and-pencil techniques or computer-assisted qualitative data analysis software (CAQDAS), such as the traditional Ethnograph® software and the newer NUD*IST® or ATLAS/ti® programs. This type of organization makes it easier to find patterns, develop new hypotheses, or test hypotheses derived from other sources (W. K. Kellogg Foundation, 1998, p. 89). Contextualization techniques, such as case studies and narrative summaries, clarify the connections that are hidden when transcripts and qualitative data are sorted into categories.

Not only are new CAQDAS programs being constantly developed, but new versions of the same packages are also released regularly, offering substantial changes to previous versions. Different packages and different versions do have differential effects on the analysis process. The programs appear to differ along two dimensions: structure of the software and how this impacts the analysis and complexity of the research project (Barry, 1998). The structure of the software is a matter of evaluator preference, which might change over the researcher's career but is likely to remain static across different types of research. The degree of complexity of the project will, however, change according to the type of work a researcher does. In choosing software programs, evaluators must consider their preferred methods of working with computers, the types of projects they currently engage in, and the types of projects they may do in the future. Whichever software programs are used, they help to "automate and speed up some analysis tasks, allow more instant access to data once coded, facilitate more complex questioning of the data, and provide creative aids to stimulate theoretical development" (Barry, 1998).

Besides statistical analysis, many other forms of analysis exist to help explain what is happening with coalition programs and services. Investing enough time and resources in the analysis and interpretation step is critical, because this is when decisions are made and actions are taken. Once the data are collected, they are fed back to the participants for collective reflection and verification. The evaluation team initially synthesizes the data and presents them to the participants with questions, draft conclusions, and recommendations. In this way, the validity of the data is checked, and gaps in knowledge are acknowledged. The evaluation team must look beyond the raw data to ask questions about what the results mean, what led to the findings, and whether they are significant.

While analyzing and interpreting both quantitative and qualitative data, the team should be aware of several pitfalls (W. K. Kellogg Foundation, 1998, p. 95). They should not assume that the program is the only cause of documented changes; other factors that are unrelated to project activities may be responsible and should be acknowledged. They should also recognize that evaluation methods could be unreliable. The same method may give different results when used by different people, or respondents may tell an evaluator what they believe he or she wants to hear. Finally, the team should not claim that local results apply to a larger group or geographic area.

Ansari and Weiss (2006) suggest that when conducting quantitative research, coalitions must be vigilant in ensuring that quantitative items and scales within questionnaires adequately measure partnership-level phenomena rather than an aggregate of individual-level phenomena; that they measure partnership changes over time, because some measures of coalition function are time-sensitive and not durable; that they are broad enough to capture group characteristics, process, and short- and long-term effects; that they are reliable and valid in relation to each other; and that they take positive response bias of partners into account (pp. 177–178). For qualitative research, Ansari and Weiss caution coalitions to ensure that the process and conclusions respect and capture the subtle differences among participants by having partners help refine and verify interpretations and that they accurately portray the contextual settings of the coalitions and original questions that were asked. Furthermore, they should be backed by an "audit trail" of raw data and descriptions of the processes used to develop instruments and analyze data (2006, p. 177).

6. *Communicate and ensure use of evaluation findings.* Lessons learned through an evaluation do not always lead to decision making and appropriate action. The evaluation team should provide continuous feedback to stakeholders regarding interim findings and interpretations to ensure that evaluation conclusions lead to appropriate program actions or decisions. During each step, relevant stakeholders and the evaluation team should discuss the most useful ways to communicate evaluation findings and use them. Frequent communication will increase ownership and commitment to act on the results, as well as to refine the evaluation design, questions, methods, and interpretations (Torres, Preskill, and Piontek, 1996).

Generally, having a positive experience with evaluation changes participants' attitudes and behaviors. For example, they begin to base decisions on sound judgments instead of on their assumptions (Patton, 1997b). Staff and stakeholders are more likely to use evaluation findings if they have ownership of the evaluation process and function cohesively as a team (Fawcett, Paine-Andrews, Francisco, and others, 2001). When more people are aware of and actively involved in evaluation, using evaluation findings to accomplish the following objectives becomes easier (W. K. Kellogg Foundation, 1998, p. 102):

- Improve the coalition and its programs by identifying strengths and weaknesses or continuous quality improvement (CQI) strategies that focus on management, organizational systems, or relationships with program participants.

- Support decisions related to program effectiveness and accountability, such as whether to continue funding or expand a program.

- Generate new knowledge about effective practice, crosscutting themes, or connections between existing or new theories and practice to inform policy-making decisions.

- Build shared understanding and communication between the stakeholders, community, and priority population.

- Integrate data collection and analysis into programs to enhance design and implementation.

- Build evaluation capacity and skills among staff, participants, and stakeholders to identify problems; collect, analyze, and interpret data; and develop alternative solutions.

Communicate findings. In addition to ongoing internal communication mechanisms, more formal products and presentations about the program and its evaluation findings should be developed and disseminated by the coalition to outside audiences. This information can improve how coalitions, their partner organizations, and related programs function; provide evidence to funding and regulatory bodies; convince diverse audiences of the program's importance; and generate further support and involvement in local coalitions and their programs (Capwell, Butterfoss, and Francisco, 2000).

Key findings and lessons learned could be disseminated by networking with coalitions and communities working on similar issues, and by replicating programs in other communities. When communicating findings, the coalition must recognize that decision makers want useful information that will help them understand the problem and how policies will improve people's lives. Real-life stories about the coalition's programs and people served may be used to showcase findings and lessons in compelling ways. Examples of communication products that can also be counted as project outcomes include these:

- Published articles about findings in local newspapers, newsletters, or professional journals; press releases and press conferences
- Evaluation report with executive summary and appendices
- Presentations to community, government, and media outlets with graphics, charts, and displays
- Video presentation or webcast
- Debate or panel about findings at a town meeting or conference

Evaluation reports. Interim and final evaluation reports should be provided as early as possible to assure that they will be used for decision making. The content, format, and style should be appropriately tailored for the intended audiences. Coalition partners and community members can preview the reports to make sure they are understandable and will have the intended impact. The following checklist can help assure readability and effectiveness in written reports (Joly, 2003; Worthen, Sanders, and Fitzpatrick, 1996):

- Start with an executive summary; organize sections logically, and include illustrations and graphics.
- Describe the stakeholders and how they were engaged; include stories from the participants.
- Describe essential features of the program, and include a simple logic model.
- Explain the evaluation's focus and its limitations.
- Summarize the evaluation plan and procedures.
- Remove technical jargon; provide all necessary technical information in appendices.
- Specify standards and criteria for evaluative judgments and how they are supported by data evidence.
- List both strengths and weaknesses of the evaluation.
- Provide recommendations with their advantages, disadvantages, and resource implications.

- Ensure protections for program clients and other stakeholders.
- Anticipate how people or organizations might be affected by findings.
- Present minority opinions or rejoinders where necessary.
- Verify that the report is accurate and unbiased.

COALITION MEASURES

Over the past two decades, coalition and community-based researchers have identified a number of measures to document changes in knowledge, attitudes, practices, community environment, policies, and health status. Most of the measures that follow are derived from process evaluation. Practitioners and researchers value process evaluation as a means of discovering the extent, fidelity, and quality of health-promotion and disease-prevention interventions (Joffres and others, 2004). Process evaluation encourages refinement of constructs during implementation and focuses on program operations and *how* outcomes are achieved, as opposed to outcome evaluation, which studies the program's influence on health outcomes (Goodman and others, 1996; Joffres and others, 2004).

Documentation of process outcomes can help assess progress, recognize positive achievements, and refine programs (Berkowitz, 2001). When faced with project timelines of three to five years, process data is helpful in maintaining community interest before longer-term outcome data is available (Butterfoss and Kegler, 2002; Cheadle and others, 1997; Fawcett and others, 1997; Florin, Mitchell, and Stevenson, 1993; Francisco, Paine, and Fawcett, 1993; Goodman and Wandersman, 1994; Mittlemark, Hunt, Heath, and Schmidt, 1993). Assessment and feedback of process evaluation results can strengthen programs and reassure community participants that their efforts are worth the time and effort that they invest.

Measurement of process indicators alone, however, is insufficient (Berkowitz, 2001; Chavis, 2001; Schooler, Farquahr, Fortmann, and Flora, 1997). Researchers and evaluators must learn innovative ways to link process evaluation to intermediate and long-term goal attainment (Butterfoss, 2006). Measures that have been used by a number of researchers for Level 1 evaluation, or evaluation of coalition infrastructure, function, and processes, are presented here. Granner and Sharpe (2004) summarized very well these short-term, or process, measures as well as some of the intermediate and long-term outcome measures found in Level 2 and 3 evaluations. The authors note that very little attention has been paid to validating measures of partnership functioning and that many measures overlap or may not be measuring distinct constructs. Complete tables including correlations and associations for these measures can be found at http://prevention.sph.sc.edu/tools/CoalitionEvalInvent.pdf.

Level 1. Measures of Coalition Infrastructure, Function, and Processes

Again, these are often *short-term* outcomes of the coalition's development as an organization that indicate how well the coalition is functioning, including its management and organizational structure and operations. They are used to document changes in the number and type of partners, the perceptions or skills of staff and members, and the mission or direction of the coalition.

Member representation—the representation of organizational partners by community sector, diverse racial and ethnic groups, and members' perceptions of representativeness (Hays, Hays, DeVille, and Mulhall, 2000; Rogers and others, 1993).

Member skills and experience—the number of years worked on the issue, skills and expertise related to the issue, collaboration, coalition management, and other strengths (Kegler, Steckler, McLeroy, and Malek, 1998b; McMillan and others, 1995; Rogers and others, 1993).

Recruitment—the number of community sectors represented and the average length of membership, as well as success in recruiting new members and steps taken to ensure representativeness (Cook, Roehl, Oros, and Trudeau, 1994; Kegler, Steckler, McLeroy, and Malek, 1998b).

Participation—the length of service; the level of participation (high or low, active or inactive); average meeting attendance; number of meetings or coalition activities attended; drop-out and retention rates; number of hours spent per month on coalition work; whether involvement has increased, decreased, or stayed the same over time; service on committees; service in leadership role; voluntary, paid, or consultant role; types of activities engaged in; the extent of personal and organizational contributions; and the effective use of member abilities (Butterfoss and others, 1996; Chinman and others, 1996; Fawcett and others, 1993; Florin, Mitchell, Stevenson, and Klein, 2000; Giamartino and Wandersman, 1983; Hays, Hays, DeVille, and Mulhall, 2000; Kegler, Steckler, McLeroy, and Malek, 1998b; McMillan and others, 1995; Prestby and others, 1990; Taylor-Powell, Rossing, and Geran, 1998).

Role clarity—the knowledge about coalition mission, structure, and operations; and whether role perception of members matches that of staff's concerning the coalition's involvement in developing the action plan, budget, plans, and objectives (Rogers and others, 1993).

Costs and benefits of participation—include personal, social and solidarity, purposive, and material benefits as well as the extent to which participation has changed members' knowledge, beliefs, and skills (Butterfoss and others, 1996; Chinman and others, 1996; McMillan and others, 1995; Rogers and others, 1993; Taylor-Powell, Rossing, and Geran, 1998). Costs include personal or coalition difficulties such as personal, social, material, and purposive costs (Butterfoss and others, 1996; Chinman and others, 1996; McMillan and others, 1995; Prestby and others, 1990; Rogers and others, 1993). An overall assessment of benefits versus costs of participation can also be made (Kegler, Steckler, McLeroy, and Malek,1998b; Rogers and others, 1993).

Satisfaction—the global satisfaction with the work of the coalition, personal involvement, the committee's or team's work and plan, or specific aspects of group function and achievement, as well as the progress and strength of the organization (Butterfoss and others, 1996; Cook and others, 1994; Giamartino and Wanderman, 1983; Kegler and others, 1998; Kumpher, Turner, Hopkins, and Librett, 1993; McMillan and others, 1995; Rogers and others, 1993).

Commitment—the strength of member commitment to the coalition, sense of pride, endorsement of mission and efforts, and caring about its future (Kumpher, Turner, Hopkins, and Librett, 1993; McMillan and others, 1995; Rogers and others, 1993).

Collaboration—the degree to which the partnership increases cooperation, joint planning of activities, networking, and information exchange. Factors that determine collaboration include shared vision, political climate, community history, understanding of goals and objectives, clear roles and responsibilities, decision-making procedures, connectedness, conflict management, changing membership, leadership, plans, policies, relationships, trust, internal and external communication, community development, resources, and evaluation (Borden and Perkins, 1999; Cook, Roehl, Oros, and Trudeau, 1994; Hays, Hays, DeVille, and Mulhall, 2000; Taylor-Powell, Rossing, and Geran, 1998).

Sense of ownership—the staff and members' commitment, sense of pride, and concern for the coalition's future; individual perception of influence on organizational processes; and perceived influence that partners have on program or group goals, processes, and structure (Flynn, 1995; Israel and others, 1994; Rogers and others, 1993).

Sense of community—the feelings of connection, support, and collective problem solving; and perceived severity of community problems (McMillan and others, 1995).

Expectations—the expectation or likelihood that the coalition will have an effect on the health issue, that members will engage in activities, that planned activities will be fully implemented, and that the group will accomplish its planned outcomes (Kumpher, Turner, Hopkins, and Librett, 1993; McMillan and others, 1995; Rogers and others, 1993).

Perceived effectiveness—the perception that the coalition is effective in its activities, fund raising, coordination, training, goal setting, communication, public relations, and evaluation (Gottlieb, Brink, and Gingiss, 1993).

Leadership—the leader support style (egalitarian, empowering, encouraging); decision-making style and control (democratic or authoritarian); competence; effectiveness in articulating vision, decision making, incentive management, conflict management; also, defining roles, facilitating meetings, nurturing collaborative group commitment and achievement, and providing guidance, support, and feedback (Butterfoss and others, 1996; Goldstein, 1997; Hays, Hays, DeVille, and Mulhall, 2000; Kegler, Steckler, Malek, and McLeroy, 1998a; Kumpher, Turner, Hopkins, and Librett, 1993; Rogers and others, 1993; Prestby and others, 1990; Taylor-Powell, Rossing, and Geran, 1998).

Staff performance—the staff time devoted to the coalition; expertise, priorities, interest, availability, and turnover; transfer of knowledge and skills from staff to members; relationship with members; efficiency in managing coalition process and operating procedures; ability to guide and support coalition; share responsibility with members; and the costs and benefits of maintaining the coalition (Butterfoss and others, 1996; Gottlieb, Brink, and Gingiss, 1993; Kegler, Steckler, Malek, and McLeroy, 1998a; Rogers and others, 1993).

Formal organizational structure and planning products—the level of formality and complexity of the coalition's structure and operation. It is usually measured by assessing the presence and adequacy of bylaws, written agendas, minutes and action plans, functioning steering committee and work groups, planning mechanisms, memoranda of agreement, procedures for leadership stability and renewal, member orientation and training, communication, decision making, and conflict resolution (Butterfoss and others, 1996; Fawcett and others, 1994; Florin, Mitchell, Stevenson, and Klein, 2000; Goldstein, 1997; Kegler, Steckler, Malek, and McLeroy, 1998a; Rogers and others, 1993; Taylor-Powell, Rossing, and Geran, 1998).

Task focus and meeting effectiveness—the task focus of meetings, order and organization of the group, meeting effectiveness and efficiency, formal structures, and accomplishment of tasks by stage of development (Butterfoss and others, 1996; Florin, Mitchell, Stevenson, and Klein, 2000; Goldstein, 1997; Kegler, Steckler, Malek, and McLeroy, 1998a; McMillan and others, 1995).

Organizational climate—the involvement, inclusion and task focus, organizational barriers, satisfaction level and commitment, cohesion, leader support and control, task orientation, expression, independence, self-discovery, anger and aggression, innovation, and organization and order within the coalition (Butterfoss and others, 1996; Giamartino and Wandersman, 1983; Gottlieb, Brink, and Gingiss, 1993; McMillan and others, 1995; Moos, Insel, and Humphrey, 1974).

Group relationships—partnership relations, that is, the nature, quality, and frequency of interactions; trust, conflict management, team work, use of talents, recognition; and the comfort and satisfaction that one is heard and valued by the group (Cook, Roehl, Oros, and Trudeau, 1994; Kegler, Steckler, Malek, and McLeroy, 1998a; Taylor-Powell, Rossing, and Geran, 1998).

Communication—the quality, frequency, and productivity of member-staff and member-member communications, as well as the use of various methods of communication (Butterfoss and others, 1996; Kegler, Steckler, Malek, and McLeroy, 1998a; Rogers and others, 1993).

Conflict—the amount of tension that is caused by opinion differences, personality clashes, hidden agendas, and power struggles (Kegler, Steckler, Malek, and McLeroy, 1998a).

Decision making—the extent of influence that individuals, group, staff, and leaders have in determining a coalition's policies and actions, as well as member inclusion or involvement in the group (Butterfoss and others, 1996; Kegler, Steckler, Malek, and McLeroy, 1998a; McMillan and others, 1995).

Resources—the personnel, sponsorships, contracts, grants, funds, and in-kind donations mobilized by the coalition, whether they are sufficient and effectively used, and whether members are satisfied with the use of funds in the community (Fawcett and others, 1993; Kegler, Steckler, Malek, and McLeroy, 1998a; Rogers and others, 1993; Taylor-Powell, Rossing, and Geran, 1998).

Action plan quality—evaluation of the coalition's action plan and planning process to include the scope, comprehensiveness, clarity, effectiveness, and quality of plans. Specifically, these measures look for clear and achievable mission, goals, objectives, tasks, defined responsibilities, and good use of community resources (Butterfoss and others, 1996; Florin, Mitchell, Stevenson, and Klein, 2000; Hays and others, 2000; Kegler, Steckler, Malek, and McLeroy, 1998a; Taylor-Powell, Rossing, and Geran, 1998).

General functioning—the coalition's capacity for group functioning and effective action related to community ownership; organizational effectiveness; comprehensive prevention approach; commitment to results orientation; group and organizational accomplishments; and relationships among the coalition, other organizations, and the community. It includes activities or factors involved in recruitment, member benefits, goals, commitment, leadership, role responsibilities, decision making, building trust, fund-raising, making linkages and referrals, securing resources, strengthening policy or regulations, managing negotiations, cultural competence, planning, recruitment, training, evaluating, and building capacity (Brown, 1984; Butterfoss and others, 1996; Cook and others, 1994; Florin, Mitchell, Stevenson, and Klein, 2000; Hays, Hays, DeVille, and Mulhall, 2000; Kumpher, Turner, Hopkins, and Librett, 1993; McMillan and others, 1995; National Network for Health, 2001; Taylor-Powell, Rossing, and Geran, 1998; Center for Prevention Research and Development, 1999).

Level 2. Measures of Coalition Programs and Interventions

These are the short-term and intermediate outcomes that focus on the activities and programs that the coalition accomplishes; the people, organizations, and groups it has served or impacted; and the scope of its various efforts. These include accomplishment of specific program outcomes, such as changes in knowledge, attitudes, beliefs, and behaviors.

Implementation—an overall assessment of the extent of implementation of the action plan, type and number of completed activities, resources generated, and capitalization of opportunities outside of the plan (Gottlieb, Brink, and Gingiss, 1993; Kegler, Steckler, Malek, and McLeroy, 1998a).

Media coverage—the coverage of coalition events or issues by radio, television, and print media (for example, the number of radio spots, number of news outlets featuring the ads, amount of time recorded, or inches of print) (Fawcett and others, 1993).

New or modified services or programs—the classes, programs, workshops, publications, or other communications or services provided for the community by the coalition and its partners, such as a required well baby course for parents that is established for all women who deliver infants in community hospitals (Fawcett and others, 1993).

Community actions taken—the actions taken to encourage change in the community, such as promoting multiple administration of vaccines at health department clinics or creating a safety checklist that parks and recreation department staff use to regularly monitor the condition of playground equipment (Fawcett and others, 1993).

New or modified policies—policies that have been promoted by the coalition and its partners, such as restricting sales of cigarettes to minors or enacting a smoke-free restaurant ordinance.

New or modified practices—practices promoted by the coalition and its partners, such as following a standard pediatric asthma pathway to improve treatment of childhood asthma in the hospital emergency department.

Level 3. Measures of Health Status and Community Change Outcomes

This phase of evaluation focuses on attainment of the coalition's long-term goals and objectives and whether its strategies have affected, the ultimate impacts that the coalition has beyond specific program outcomes. These are mostly the long-term outcomes, such as changes in health status, quality of care, stability and effectiveness of community institutions, and overall changes in the community's capacity and competence to deal with emerging problems.

Community capacity—the community's ability to plan, problem solve, implement programs, network, collaborate, conduct research and evaluate its work (Kegler, Steckler, Malek, and McLeroy, 1998a).

Organizational viability—an assessment that includes noting whether groups continue to meet and function, the level of institutionalization of coalition programs, organizational empowerment (coalition's impact on organizational policies and resources generated and used), and community competence (Eng and Parker, 1994; Giamartino and Wandersman, 1983; Goeppinger and Baglioni, 1985; Goodman, McLeroy, Steckler, and Hoyle, 1993; Israel, Checkoway, Schultz, and Zimmerman, 1994; McMillan and others, 1995).

Health status indicators—include the sought-after ultimate changes that relate to the coalition's mission. For example, alcohol, tobacco, and other substance abuse prevention coalitions would look for reduced DUI-related accidents and arrest rates; teen pregnancy prevention coalitions would expect reduced rates of teen pregnancy; chronic disease prevention coalitions would expect reduced rates of cardiovascular disease and cancer; and coalitions focused on asthma management would expect reduced levels of asthma exacerbations, evidenced by reduced hospitalization and emergency department admissions due to asthma.

Citing all the possible examples of measures that coalitions can use to document their intermediate and long-term outcomes is beyond the scope of this text. However, these indicators are available for each health and social issue of concern to national, state, and local organizations. An example is provided in the following menu of intermediate and long-term alcohol, tobacco, and other drug indicators by Join Together (2005):

Availability—the number of sites or locations with licenses to sell alcoholic beverages; existence of smoke-free workplace and secondhand smoke regulations; number of cigarette sales outlets; prevalence, location, and restrictions on alcohol advertising; and amount of taxes levied on alcohol or tobacco substances.

Use—the percent of youth and adults who report substance use; volume of alcohol sold or distributed per person in a geographic area; and percentages of arrestees who test positive for drug or alcohol use at time of arrest.

Prevention—the presence or absence of environmental policies to prevent or reduce substance use in the community; and presence of evidence-based educational programs and policies on alcohol, tobacco, and other drugs in public and private primary and secondary schools.

Community coalitions—the presence of coalitions working on substance use issues in the community.

Treatment—the number of people currently enrolled in public and private addiction treatment programs in the community; average length of stay in treatment, the percentage of clients completing treatment, and the use of aftercare plans; use of medically assisted treatment; policies and programs focused on screenings, brief interventions, and referrals in the community; number of weekly open self-help meetings held in the community; and use of hotlines to help people quit smoking and find drug and alcohol treatment.

Criminal justice—the arrests for drug- and alcohol-related violations; and sales of alcohol and tobacco to minors.

Harm—the number of hospital and emergency department admission with alcohol or drug use diagnoses; number of deaths resulting, directly or indirectly, from alcohol or substance use, such as alcohol-related crashes that result in a fatality; and number of new drug-related AIDS, hepatitis C, and STD cases.

COALITION EVALUATION INSTRUMENTS

In deciding which instruments to use for evaluating their partnership and its activities, coalitions have a wide range of opportunities. The team can develop its own survey instruments or interview frameworks, use validated and reliable tools that have already been created, or modify existing tools to meet its needs. The latter is often preferable, as the coalition may want to explore some issues that are not covered in existing instruments, or the team may prefer to use a tool that has been adapted to fit its priority population, community culture, and the way its issue(s) is framed. Researchers have developed a number of instruments in the field of collaboration and coalition building. Some of these are located at the end of each chapter in this book, according to the topic covered. A comprehensive list of general evaluation instruments is presented in the Resources section at the end of this chapter, and a few short tools are featured in Exhibits 14.7–14.10 on the following pages, although space will not permit printing all of the existing instruments.

(*Text resumes on page 486.*)

Exhibit 14.7. Checklist of Policy Indicators for Alcohol, Tobacco, and Other Drugs.

This checklist can help you to assess the number and types of policies within your community and where you might best extend your efforts.

ALCOHOL—*Public Policies*	Yes	No
1. Excise taxes (local)	___	___
2. Limits on hours or days of sale	___	___
3. Restrictions of density, location, or types of outlets	___	___
4. Mandatory server training and licensing	___	___
5. Dram shop and social host liability	___	___
6. Restrictions on advertising and promotion	___	___
7. Mandatory warning signs and labels	___	___
8. Restrictions on consumption in public places	___	___
9. Prevention of preemption of local control of alcohol regulation (home rule)	___	___
10. Minimum bar entry age	___	___
11. Keg registration or tagging ordinances	___	___
12. Compulsory compliance checks for minimum purchase age and administrative penalties for violations	___	___
13. Establishment of minimum age for sellers	___	___

ALCOHOL—*Organizational Policies*	Yes	No
1. Restrictions on alcohol advertisements (*media*)	___	___
2. Restrictions on alcohol use at work and work events (*businesses*)	___	___
3. Restrictions on sponsorship of special events (*communities, stadiums*)	___	___
4. Police walkthroughs at alcohol outlets	___	___
5. Undercover outlet compliance checks (*law enforcement agencies*)	___	___
6. Responsible beverage service policies (*outlets*)	___	___

(*continued*)

Exhibit 14.7. Checklist of Policy Indicators for Alcohol, Tobacco, and Other Drugs. (*Continued*)

ALCOHOL—*Organizational Policies*	Yes	No
7. Mandatory checks of age identification (*businesses*)	_____	_____
8. Server training (*businesses*)	_____	_____
9. Incentives for checking age identification (*businesses*)	_____	_____
10. Prohibition of alcohol on school grounds or at school events (*schools*)	_____	_____
11. Enforcement of school policies (*schools*)	_____	_____
12. Prohibition of beer kegs on campus (*colleges*)	_____	_____
13. Establishment of enforcement priorities against adults who illegally provide alcohol to youth	_____	_____
14. Sobriety checkpoints (*law enforcement agencies*)	_____	_____
15. Media campaigns about enforcement efforts (*media*)	_____	_____
16. Safe ride programs (*businesses*)	_____	_____
17. Identification of source of alcohol consumed prior to DUI arrests (*law enforcement agencies*)	_____	_____

TOBACCO—*Public Policies*	Yes	No
1. Excise taxes (*local*)	_____	_____
2. Tobacco sales licensing system	_____	_____
3. Prohibition of smoking in public places	_____	_____
4. Prevention of preemption of local control of tobacco sales	_____	_____
5. Restrictions on advertising and promotion	_____	_____
6. Ban on vending machines	_____	_____
7. Compulsory compliance checks for minimum purchase age and administrative penalties for violations	_____	_____
8. Minimum age for sales of age eighteen	_____	_____
9. Warning labels	_____	_____
10. Mandatory seller training	_____	_____
11. Ban on self-service sales (*all tobacco behind the counter*)	_____	_____
12. Minimum age for sellers	_____	_____
13. Penalty for underage use	_____	_____

Exhibit 14.7. *(Continued)*

TOBACCO—*Organizational Policies*	*Yes*	*No*
1. Establishment of smoke-free settings *(restaurants, workplaces, hospitals, stadiums, malls, day care facilities)*	____	____
2. Counter advertising *(media)*	____	____
3. Restrictions on sponsorship of special events *(communities, colleges, stadiums)*	____	____
4. Prohibition of tobacco use on school grounds, in buses, and at school events	____	____
5. Enforcement of school policies *(schools)*	____	____
6. Mandatory checks for age identification *(businesses)*	____	____
7. Seller training *(businesses)*	____	____
8. Incentives for checking age identification *(businesses)*	____	____
9. Undercover shopper or monitoring program *(businesses)*	____	____

OTHER DRUGS—*Public Policies*	*Yes*	*No*
1. Control of production and distribution	____	____
2. Zoning and building codes that discourage drug activity and penalties for property owners who fail to address known drug activity	____	____
3. Mandated school policies	____	____

OTHER DRUGS—*Organizational Policies*	*Yes*	*No*
1. Employer policies *(businesses)*	____	____
2. Surveillance of high-risk public areas *(law enforcement agencies, neighborhood watch groups)*	____	____
3. Enforcement of zoning and building codes *(law enforcement agencies, building authorities)*	____	____
4. Appropriate design and maintenance of parks, streets, and other public places (e.g., lighting, traffic flow) *(city agencies, housing authorities)*	____	____
5. Enforcement of school drug policies *(schools)*	____	____

Source: Center for Prevention Research and Development (CPRD) [http://www.coalitioninstitute.org/Evaluation-Research/CoalitionAssessmentTools/Checklist-of-PolicyIndicators.doc], accessed January 31, 2006. Reprinted by permission of the Center for Prevention Research and Development and Community Anti-Drug Coalitions of America.

**Exhibit 14.8. Community Anti-Drug Coalitions of America
Coalition Self-Assessment Instrument.**

1. What is the strategy you are using to mobilize your community or address your most pressing substance abuse problems? Why is this strategy effective? How will you be able to sustain the selected strategy over time, or make changes with shifts in your community?

2. What are the most important substance abuse problems(s) in your community that you are trying to address? Why have you chosen to address it (or them)? How do you know that those are the most serious substance abuse problems in your community? (What data and experience confirm your conclusions?)

3. What specific programs, policies, mobilization efforts, or additional actions must you and others take to address your priority issues? Why are these actions likely to be effective?

4. What other community institutions and leaders must be involved for your efforts to achieve greater success? How do you expect to get their collaboration and what roles do you want them to fulfill?

5. How do you know that your efforts are achieving the expected results? Who collects and analyzes the information necessary for you to make these conclusions? How is this data used to improve your prevention efforts?

6. What governance structure have you established to achieve your strategy and hold yourselves accountable and to ensure continuing community and financial support?

7. What mechanisms have you developed to ensure that your coalition reviews and publicly reports information about its efforts and about community changes that may affect your priorities, strategies and activities?

8. How does your coalition train, encourage and mobilize your current and future leaders, workers, and volunteers?

9. What are your resource development plans to ensure that you meet matching requirements and have long-term sustainability for your strategies?

10. What are your plans for strengthening your governance structure to achieve your strategies and policies for getting money, maintain focus on your highest priorities, and meet the needs of the project itself?

11. How do you relate to your host institution (where applicable)? What do you expect financially from the groups that you work with? What is the mix of public and private funding that you have to address the priority issue(s) identified in your planning process?

Source: Center for Prevention Research and Development [http://www.coalitioninstitute.org/Evaluation-Research/CoalitionAssessmentTools/CoalitionSelf-AssessmentInstrument.doc], accessed January 31, 2006. Reprinted by permission of Community Anti-Drug Coalitions of America (CADCA), National Coalition Institute.

Exhibit 14.9. Diagnosing the Health of Your Coalition Assessment Instrument.

Goal: To help you assess, individually, what you believe to be the current reality of your collaborative partnership. This tool is used most effectively when provided to multiple parties with varied perspectives on the initiative. Communicate results and facilitate conversation among members to generate ideas about how to move the group forward. Time: twenty-five minutes.

1. For about two minutes, scan the checklist to see whether it seems right for you and your partnership. Even if the entire piece may not seem relevant, consider that most initiatives benefit from reflection on these questions.

2. Respond to the checklist items thoughtfully, and tally up your scores.

3. Discuss with a partner how you might make use of this instrument in your home organization or community. Who else will you include? How will you collect and communicate the results? Can you imagine forming a task force or holding a retreat of all members to generate recommendations based upon the results? How might you seek consensus or otherwise implement recommendations? What would be required to ensure that adopted changes are implemented in actual practice? How often do you imagine using this process?

4. Return to the large group to discuss reactions to the assessment, what was learned, and how it might be used to improve the functioning of your organization.

Carrying It Forward: Reflect on the value of assessing the functioning of your group. What did you learn? How might it pay off for your collaborative partnership? How might you use this information to support maintenance or renewal of your organization?

Using the scale below, rate each component of your organization, then tally your score on the worksheet provided at the end.

Strong or Always				*Weak or Never*
5	4	3	2	1

1. The clarity of your coalition's vision, mission, and goals

   ___ A. Your coalition's vision (your dream) and mission (what you are going to do) take into account what is happening in the community.

   ___ B. Your vision, mission, and goals are written down.

   ___ C. Residents and institutions are aware of your coalition's vision, mission, and goals.

   ___ D. Your coalition periodically re-evaluates and updates its vision, mission, and goals.

   ___ E. Your coalition's activities are evaluated in relation to its vision, mission, and goals.

(continued)

Exhibit 14.9. Diagnosing the Health of Your Coalition Assessment Instrument. *(Continued)*

2. The effectiveness of your coalition structure

____ A. Your coalition has a regular meeting cycle that members can count on.

____ B. Your coalition has active committees.

____ C. All of your members have copies of the bylaws.

____ D. Your executive board and committees communicate regularly.

____ E. Your executive board meets on a regular basis with good attendance.

3. The effectiveness of your outreach and communication

____ A. Your coalition has a newsletter or another method of communication that keeps the community updated regularly and informed about your activities.

____ B. You use a survey or other method to collect information about members' interests, needs, and concerns.

____ C. You always publish survey results and use them to guide your coalition's projects.

____ D. The survey is conducted every year or so because the community and residents change.

____ E. Your coalition "goes to where members are" to do outreach, including where people live, shop, and work.

4. The effectiveness of coalition meetings

____ A. Members feel free to speak at a meeting without fear of being confronted for their views.

____ B. Your coalition advertises its meetings with sufficient notice by sending out agendas and fliers in advance.

____ C. You provide childcare and language assistance when needed.

____ D. You accomplish the meeting's agenda in meetings that start and end on time.

____ E. You hold meetings in centrally accessible, comfortable places and at convenient times for all members.

5. Opportunities for member responsibility and growth

____ A. Your coalition makes a conscious effort to develop new leaders.

____ B. You offer training and support to new and experienced leaders, either through your coalition or through outside agencies.

____ C. Your "buddy system" matches less experienced members with leaders to help the former learn jobs and make contacts.

____ D. You give committees serious work to do.

____ E. Leadership responsibilities are shared; for example, you rotate the chairing of a meeting between members.

6. The coalition's effectiveness at planning, implementing, and evaluating projects

____ A. At the beginning of each new year your coalition develops a plan that includes goals and activities to accomplish during the year.

Exhibit 14.9. (*Continued*)

____ B. These plans are based at least in part on information collected from member surveys.

____ C. After each activity or project, the leadership or the committee evaluates how it went in order to learn from the experience.

____ D. Your coalition always organizes visible projects that make a difference to members.

____ E. When you undertake projects, you develop action plans that identify tasks, who will do them, and by what target dates.

7. Your coalition's use of research, external resources, or both

____ A. Your coalition works with other coalitions in the community on common issues, and with citywide organizations that address critical community concerns.

____ B. Your coalition utilizes the resources and information of other organizations that can help the community, such as training workshops.

____ C. Your coalition keeps abreast of issues affecting communities across the city and state.

____ D. Outside speakers come to meetings to address topics of interest to members.

____ E. When your coalition wants to work on an issue, leaders know where to go to get necessary information such as statistics, forms, and so forth.

8. The coalition's sense of community

____ A. Your coalition builds social time into meetings so that people can talk informally and build a sense of community.

____ B. You plan social activities.

____ C. Everyone in your organization is treated equally.

____ D. You recognize and reward all member contributions, large or small.

____ E. You make all residents welcome in the coalition regardless of income, race, gender, age, or education level.

9. How well the coalition meets needs and provides benefits

____ A. You make resource lists and important contacts available to members on a regular basis.

____ B. You hold workshops with experts who can provide specific services to members.

____ C. Your coalition helps members with issues of individual need.

____ D. If a member survey indicates that personal issues (such as child care or landlord–tenant problems) are interfering with member involvement, your coalition responds to those issues.

____ E. Your coalition holds meetings and workshops in which residents can meet elected officials and city service personnel to voice their opinions and learn about resources and programs in the community.

(*continued*)

Exhibit 14.9. Diagnosing the Health of Your Coalition Assessment Instrument. (*Continued*)

10. Your coalition's relationship with elected officials, institutional leaders, and other power players

   ___ A. Coalition leaders know how to negotiate successfully with elected officials and institutional leaders about member concerns.

   ___ B. Your coalition has one or more regular representatives who attend important community meetings.

   ___ C. Coalition leaders and members understand the lines of authority, decision-making power, responsibility, and other aspects of the community power structure.

   ___ D. Your coalition meets with officials on a regular basis about the issues that concern members.

   ___ E. Your coalition participates in citywide activities and demonstrates focus on community issues.

Source: Kaye, 2001.

DIAGNOSING THE HEALTH OF YOUR COALITION SCORE SHEET

Fill out this score sheet using the total numbers from each section of the organizational diagnosis:

Section	Total Score:
1. Vision, mission, and goals	_____
2. Coalition structure	_____
3. Outreach and communication	_____
4. Coalition meetings	_____
5. Member responsibility and growth	_____
6. Projects	_____
7. Research and external resources	_____
8. Sense of community	_____
9. Needs and benefits	_____
10. Relationships with power players	_____

For each section, follow the guidelines below:

If you scored between:

5–15 Watch out! You may need an overhaul in this area.

15–20 Checkup time! It's time for tune-up to get everything in good working order.

20–25 Congratulations! You're running smoothly and all systems are go. Keep up the good work.

Source: Developed by Gillian Kaye, President, Community Development Consultants, Brooklyn, N.Y.

Exhibit 14.10. Tobacco-Free Youth Coalition Self-Evaluation Instrument.

Ongoing self-evaluation is an important part of the coalition development process. Evaluation can be used to assess accountability, program effectiveness, and program improvement. This evaluation questionnaire is especially useful when it is completed by active members after a major coalition activity.

Instructions: Rate each aspect of the coalition's capacity to take effective action, from 1 (low) to 5 (high). Make comments about factors that influenced your rating.

1. **Goals.** Common goals for coalition should be shared and understood by members. Rate members' understanding of coalition's goals.

    Low   1   2   3   4   5   High

    _____

    _____

2. **Outcomes.** Coalition members should identify benefits that can be achieved by working together and clearly understand coalition expectations. Rate members' awareness of benefits to them and their organizations.

    Low   1   2   3   4   5   High

    _____

    _____

3. **Leadership.** Leadership should help coalition move toward agreed upon goals in timely manner. Rate effectiveness of coalition's leadership.

    Low   1   2   3   4   5   High

4. **Commitment.** Each member should be committed to work together toward coalition's mission, goals, and priorities. Rate members' commitment to coalition.

    Low   1   2   3   4   5   High

5. **Communication.** Plans should be made to ensure clear and prompt communication within coalition as well as for media contacts and spokespersons on specific issues. Rate effectiveness of coalition's communication, both formal informal.

    Low   1   2   3   4   5   High

(continued)

Exhibit 14.10. Tobacco-Free Youth Coalition Self-Evaluation Instrument. (*Continued*)

6. **Turf.** Coalition should be aware of participant's commitments outside coalition and possible areas of conflict of interest. Rate positive resolution of turf issues within coalition.

  Low   1   2   3   4   5   High

_____

_____

7. **Diversity.** Coalition should strive for diversity in backgrounds of members. Coalition leadership should reflect gender, ethnic, and racial backgrounds of members. Rate diversity in coalition's membership and leadership.

  Low   1   2   3   4   5   High

_____

_____

Source: National Network for Health, 2004.

CHALLENGES OF EVALUATING COMMUNITY-BASED INITIATIVES

The inherent challenges in evaluating complex, community-wide prevention initiatives are considerable. The difficulties include unit of analyses issues, secular trends, and the synergistic effects of multiple strategies (Mittlemark, 1999). Limited resources, increasingly complex social problems, changing political climate, and a shift in public opinion about the extent to which government and other institutions should support disadvantaged populations also have influenced how these initiatives are evaluated. Major funders of such initiatives have been more concerned with the accountability of initiatives (proving they work) than their quality (working to improve) (W. K. Kellogg Foundation, 1998, p. 6). As a result, evaluations often do not address issues of process, implementation, and improvement well. They should question how and why programs work, for whom, and under what circumstances.

Moreover, quantitative evaluation designs have been overemphasized, while little attention has been given to naturalistic, qualitative designs aimed at program improvement (McQueen and Anderson, 1999). Complex, comprehensive community initiatives often are seen as incapable of being evaluated, or they are evaluated in traditional ways that do not capture the complex, "messy" ways in which these initiatives effect change (Connell, Kubisch, Schorr, and Weiss, 1995; Connell and Kubisch, 1998). Many of these initiatives are not evaluated at all, making it difficult for communities to provide effective evidence. Others are evaluated using traditional methods that narrow the project to fit the evaluation design. Still others use a traditional impact report that shows the initiative had limited impact (because impact may occur over a longer time or because intermediate outcomes that are difficult to quantify are overlooked). Valuable resources are then wasted, and little is learned about how these initiatives really work and what their true potential may be (Connell, Kubisch, Schorr, and Weiss, 1995).

THE CHALLENGES OF COALITION EVALUATION

As we have discussed in the previous chapters, implementing community coalitions has proved to be "far more complicated and different than most initially believed," partly because coalitions are different from most other health promoting institutions (Chavis, 2001, p. 310). Similarly, evaluating coalitions is often fraught with controversy and challenges. If coalitions expect to improve the health status of the community, then the impact they have on improving the social and health systems and long-term outcomes of the community must be evaluated (Sink and Stowers, 1989). As partnership interventions become more complex, they focus on changes in policies, practices, and systems. Measuring these community-level or system changes (for example, improving environmental quality or changing insurance coverage policies), however, is much more difficult than evaluating program outcomes (Kagan, 1991). These evaluations have to focus across multiple levels and take into account community readiness (Goodman, Wandersman, Chinman, Imm, and Morrisey, 1996).

Coalitions have been portrayed in the literature both as "expensive, insufficient, weak, and lacking sufficient data to support their continued use" and as "holistic, comprehensive, flexible, responsive, innovative," (Birkby, 2003, p. 2) and as creating significant impacts on health promotion. Whether coalitions actually achieve measurable outcomes, results are limited, mixed, and inconsistent. Berkowitz suggests that one obstacle to conducting solid evaluation studies with coalitions is not knowing how many coalitions exist because many have not published and are unknown beyond their local boundaries (Berkowitz, 2001, p. 215). Without a coalition registry, having a large enough sample within any one health-issue area remains difficult. Thus, most of the published coalition evaluation research consists of single or multiple case studies that do not support strong conclusions about the impact of partnerships on population-level outcomes, such as changes in health status (Morrow and others, 1998; Kegler, Steckler, McLeroy, and Malek, 1998b; Kreuter, Lezin and Young, 2000; Roussos and Fawcett, 2000; Zakocs and Edwards, 2006). Berkowitz (2001) suggests that most coalition evaluations have not used rigorous designs (experimental designs with random assignment and comparison groups) and methods that make measuring outcomes feasible.

Kreuter and colleagues (2000) reviewed sixty-eight published studies on health-promotion coalitions and reported "only marginal evidence" that their programs and other activities lead to changes in health status or systems, and expectations for success may be overly optimistic. Roussos and Fawcett reviewed thirty-four studies of 252 partnerships and found the results insufficient to make strong conclusions about the effects of these partnerships on population-level outcomes (2000, p. 375). Zakocs and Edwards (2006) reviewed partnership literature published between 1980 and 2004, to examine the relationships among coalition-building factors and indicators of coalition effectiveness. The twenty-six selected studies yielded nineteen indicators that measured coalition functioning and two indicators that measured changes in rates of community-wide health behaviors. Of the fifty-five coalition-building factors associated with indicators of coalition effectiveness, only six were common enough to compare results about coalition effectiveness (formalization of rules and procedures, leadership style, member participation, membership diversity, agency collaboration, and group cohesion). Others have criticized well-funded coalition initiatives, such as the Fighting Back substance abuse prevention program, as being too costly to maintain and challenged in its capacity to implement comprehensive, effective strategies (Green and Kreuter, 2003; Hallfors, Cho, Livert, and Kadushin, 2003; Klitzner, 1991; Merzel and D'Affliti, 2003).

On the other hand, some coalitions have reported achieving positive outcomes when addressing issues such as disability advocacy, education, access to prenatal care, housing for the mentally ill, and physical exercise (Berkowitz, 2001). Case studies and larger community-wide successes also have reported significant outcomes for the following issues: media advocacy (McKinlay, 2000); pregnancy prevention (Kegler, Wyatt, and Rodine, 2005); arson prevention and immunization rates (Morrow and others, 1998; Wandersman and Florin, 2003); alcohol and other drug abuse prevention (Hingson and others, 1996; Shaw and others, 1997; Yin, Kafterian, Yu, and Jansen, 1997); policy changes benefiting childhood asthma management, including quality of health care, outdoor air quality, and housing (Lara and others, 2006; Nicholas and others, 2006); and lead poisoning prevention (Klitzman, Kass, and Freudenberg, 2005). Although partnerships have modestly changed community-wide behavior, the strongest evidence shows that they most often contribute to changes in programs, services, and practices (Roussos and Fawcett, 2000).

Coalitions also hold promise as catalysts for policy change. For example, the SmokeLess States: National Tobacco Policy Initiative to support statewide efforts to reduce tobacco use, particularly among children and youth, was funded by the Robert Wood Johnson Foundation from 1993 to 2004 (Robert Wood Johnson Foundation, 2005b). SmokeLess States made grants to forty-eight statewide coalitions and two other coalitions (in the District of Columbia and Tucson, Arizona), who worked in partnership with community groups to develop and implement comprehensive tobacco-control programs that included education, treatment, and policy initiatives. Key results from the evaluation show that the coalition policy campaigns, underwritten by matching funds, led to

- Increased excise taxes by an average of 51.3 cents in thirty-five states; five states raised taxes by more than a dollar.
- Clean indoor air legislation in ten states, with nearly 30 percent of the U.S. population now covered by strong workplace smoking restrictions, a 50 percent increase from 2002.
- Ordinances to restrict youth access to tobacco products in thirteen states, involving hundreds of counties, towns, and municipalities.
- The defeat or blockage of preemption bills in ten states, and repealing or partially repealing them in seven states.

- Securing substantial commitments (at least $10 million) from sixteen states for comprehensive tobacco prevention and control programs from the 1988 Master Settlement Agreement with the tobacco industry.

Given the lack of agreement about whether coalitions are effective or not, researchers do agree on one thing—coalition effectiveness *is* difficult to evaluate due to some of the practical and methodological issues that are discussed here (Berkowitz, 2001; Birkby, 2003; Butterfoss and Francisco, 2004; Drug Strategies, 2001; Gabriel, 2000; Wandersman and Florin, 2003; Yin and Ware, 2000; Weiss, 1995; Zakocs and Edwards, 2006):

Evaluation is often not built into the coalition's planning process. Resources are more likely to be spent on interventions, which are visible to stakeholders. If funds are made available for evaluation, they are often inadequate. Because evaluation can be costly in terms of time and resources, the coalition's lead agency, staff, and members are not always committed to doing it. If it is supported, coalition coordinators and program managers are motivated to make programs "look" effective in order to maintain funding or their jobs. Evaluation may not be based on a solid logic model or theory, and often ends up being a do-it-yourself model. According to Wolff, coalitions often fail to evaluate their efforts because they lack "the motivation, interest, and intent" to carry out an evaluation, fail to find the right evaluators and establish "mutually effective and respectful relationships" with them, and lack access to usable tools for evaluating the process and outcome of their efforts (2002, p. 1). Often coalition representatives fail to find coalitions useful in improving their own organizations or those organizations' activities.

Each coalition is unique. Because coalitions are embedded within their communities and responsive to a variety of cultural contexts, they tend to be unique, difficult to replicate, and may not be representative of other coalitions, even those that address similar issues. Thus using experimental approaches that require control or comparison coalitions from similar communities is extremely difficult. Moreover, if comparison communities are found where no coalition exists (in order to test whether this approach makes a difference), it is unethical to withhold a treatment (in other words, the coalition and its services) from the priority population in the comparison city.

Design and methods issues make it difficult to generalize about coalitions. The difficulties inherent in establishing and measuring outcomes, specifying and controlling extraneous variables that interact with the outcomes, factoring in secular trends over the life stages of the coalition, and dealing with the political realities of satisfying funders make evaluating coalitions and detecting community-level change challenging (Berkowitz, 2001). First, extraneous variables (such as new government programs, funding streams, and changes in demographics) are difficult to control for and vary across communities. These variables may influence coalition outcomes by changing how programs are implemented or by interacting or influencing each other.

Second, coalitions sometimes choose unique outcomes that make comparisons across coalitions difficult (Zakocs and Edwards, 2006). Even when comparable long-term outcomes are used across sites, baseline data may not be available. For example, the Allies Against Asthma initiative funded by the Robert Wood Johnson initiative chose reduction in emergency room visits for asthma as a comparable outcome measure across sites; however, most sites had difficulty accessing baseline data from multiple hospitals or from inadequate state databases. Similar issues arise with obesity prevention coalitions, where baseline body mass index statistics are not easily available or reliably measured. Intermediate outcomes from surveys and interviews with parents of children with asthma may be problematic because social-desirability or self-selection biases are possible.

Third, coalitions do not always identify outcome measures. If they do, they have difficulty identifying and linking appropriate intermediate outcomes to these long-term outcomes. Distinguishing between cause and effect, or what percentage of the outcome can be attributed to which coalition program or activity, is difficult. Coalitions tend to focus on "quick wins" and awareness activities that do not, in and of themselves, lead to significant changes in systems or health status (Roussos and Fawcett, 2000; Mittelmark, 1999; Kreuter, Lezin, and Young, 2000; Berkowitz, 2001). These quick wins and short-term successes are needed to increase member commitment and build the coalition's credibility before it can focus on programs entailing greater complexity (Brown, 1984; Hord, 1986; Cohen, Baer, and Satterwhite, 2002). This short-term focus is unlikely to lead to significant outcomes and may explain why some programs are not able to achieve systems or health outcomes change (Kreuter, Lezin, and Young, 2000).

SOLVING THE COALITION EVALUATION DILEMMA

Coalitions may be the best answer at present to address the persistent health problems of our time (Berkowitz, 2001). Therefore, we must be patient with the trial-and-error phase of testing the effectiveness of this approach until research "catches up with practice" (Butterfoss, Cashman, Foster-Fishman, and Kegler, 2001, p. 239). Proposed solutions to coalition evaluation issues are complex and include the following:

Use more innovative, qualitative evaluation methods. Foster-Fishman notes that relying on qualitative methods that better represent the community and trying to figure out *how* coalitions make a difference are good starting points (Butterfoss, Cashman, Foster-Fishman, and Kegler, 2001, p. 230). Evaluators often resort to traditional evaluation methods and fail to use methods appropriate for measuring the impact of these coalitions. Innovative methods should be developed in order to respond to the dynamic nature of coalitions (Gabriel, 2000).

Focus efforts on evaluating practice-proven strategies. Kegler questions whether coalitions select the most effective strategies in building ownership and fostering meaningful participation, and suggests that coalitions may be best suited to assessment and priority setting rather than implementing specific projects (Butterfoss, Cashman, Foster-Fishman, and Kegler, 2001, p. 231).

Focus efforts on measurable outcomes. Evaluators must concern themselves with short-term or direct effects of the program, as well as with the long-term, ultimate effects desired by a community organizing effort or program. In addition to coalition outcomes associated with health or social issues, another set of outcomes is associated with increases in a community's capacity to solve problems (Goodman and others, 1998). Coalitions can impact a community's capacity by positively or negatively affecting participation, leadership, networks of individuals and organizations, skills, resources, and sense of community. Current evaluation research has begun to focus on outcomes associated with community capacity issues (Norton, Kegler, and Aronson, 2003).

Similarly, Reininger, and colleagues (1999–2000) identified early and late benchmarks (or indicators) for empowerment. The ten *early benchmarks* of a community partnership that is moving toward empowerment include a communication system; inclusive representation, participation, and action by diverse groups; community self-reliance that generates high levels of belonging and responsibility; capacity to engage in risk-taking, creative activities; building a long-term, proactive strategic plan; engaging in change by implementing the strategic plan; resource attainment from within and outside the community; developing new leadership over time; advocacy based on training, group demonstration, and dissemination of political information; and changing community norms. Although some processes, such as building a communication system, may take up to five years to develop, this early benchmarks system allows evaluators to visualize whether a coalition is on track to become empowered and sustained.

Late benchmarks may be viewed as outcomes of the earlier ones and include building social and physical community infrastructure; establishing capacity-building human services; increasing the sense of security within the community; increasing economic enhancements within the community; increasing educational opportunities; maintaining the surroundings; achieving desired policy changes; and the psychological realization that members are interconnected and interdependent.

Provide needed training and technical assistance in evaluation. Many researchers agree that we should not "throw the baby out with the bathwater," but rather should assure that the proper training, technical assistance, and community resources are available to make each coalition the best that it can be. Some evaluators have built their professional credibility on helping collaborations to succeed through evaluating their efforts. The plain truth is that evaluation should not be done if it has no utility (Wolff, 2002). Therefore, the key is to translate evaluation results into actionable tasks that can be accomplished by collaborative organizations and their members, funders, and the community.

Help coalitions and partnerships to "begin where they are." Most coalition coordinators, staff, members, and leaders see evaluation as a formidable task. They are overwhelmed by the endless range of evaluation tasks, the numerous potential methods, prerequisite time and financial costs, and the concern that they might not measure up. Add to this the fact that much of the evaluation literature is based on large, grant-funded projects with teams of contracted evaluators. The result is that many coalitions choose to evaluate nothing at all. A better strategy is to "evaluate something, not everything." In other words, at the outset, the coalition should choose to evaluate one thing about its activities from each of three levels—short-term (process), intermediate (impact), and long-term (outcome). As a starting point, chances are the coalition has existing data that can be used at practically no cost, such as evaluating the diversity of membership by assessing the partner roster or analyzing the content of coalition minutes to discern attendance numbers and patterns. As confidence and skills grow by so doing, coalitions may be encouraged to engage in new and more complex evaluation tasks.

COALITION SPOTLIGHT: THE CALIFORNIA COALITION FOR CHILDHOOD IMMUNIZATION

The following example shows how evaluation can help sustain a community program over time to promote public awareness of a health issue. With the goal of raising awareness of childhood immunization and launching a high-profile 1996 National Infant Immunization Week, the California Coalition for Childhood Immunization developed the mock measles outbreak. The outbreak capitalized on a winning combination—visuals of children at play juxtaposed with a serious public health message. The event involved the collaborative efforts of local immunization coordinators, county health departments, and local business and community partners to generate widespread media coverage promoting the importance of early immunizations. The events, featuring toddlers dressed in doctor's smocks attending to their "sick" peers adorned in red dots, were held at five sites the first year. The program was carefully evaluated, and based on its early success, the outbreak was again staged in 1997, with an increased number of participating counties (thirteen) and actual sites (seventeen). Two dozen daily newspapers gave the "outbreak" prominent space; twenty television stations and eight radio stations aired forty-five PSAs; three radio stations and numerous television stations held live broadcasts of the events; and several other newspapers printed op-ed and editorial pieces on immunizations (Every Child By Two, 1997). In 1998, the event realized its most dramatic success to date. Seventeen counties participated at nineteen separate sites—nearly four times as many as the inaugural year. The breakdown of counties represented all regions of the state, from southern California to the Central Valley, and north to the Bay Area and Sacramento regions. The events generated widespread media coverage in every major media market in the state. More than twenty-five individual television stations ran more than thirty news segments. By mid-May, twenty-four newspapers published more than thirty articles and editorials on immunizations and the mock measles outbreak. Media impressions totaled 1 million dollars for print, with more than

25 million Californians exposed to the story on television and radio. Immunization messages were communicated to more than 300 key health care and community media representatives through a comprehensive press kit and targeted follow-up.

Inherent in this public awareness campaign was a timely and important public health story that emphasized the need for parents to properly immunize their children. Calls to immunization hotlines increased significantly. Due to the high volume of calls and extensive media coverage, some state officials actually called to inquire if indeed a measles outbreak had occurred! More important, local partnerships were developed with businesses and community organizations that continue to support immunization activities statewide. From bridge calls before the event, to post-event evaluations, communication among organizers was critical to the success of the mock measles outbreaks (Capwell, Butterfoss, and Francisco, 2000; Every Child By Two, 1997).

SUMMARY

Coalitions can be time-consuming and difficult, especially when resources are limited (Cheadle and others, 1997). If a coalition is successful, evaluation must be performed that demonstrates a sustainable infrastructure and purpose, programs that accomplish their goals, and measurable community impacts. Evaluation is, therefore, a crucial coalition task and often determines whether the organization and its activities are sustained over time. However, evaluators face many challenges when trying to conduct effective evaluations of coalition initiatives. Evaluations that focus on measurable outcomes and use qualitative as well as quantitative approaches, multiple methods of data collection, and instruments that are adapted to the cultures and populations that coalitions serve are more likely to be effective.

QUESTIONS FOR REVIEW

1. What are the six main purposes of coalition evaluation, and what evaluation data should be collected to serve each purpose?
2. Identify and describe briefly the elements or steps that each of the four evaluation frameworks featured in this chapter have in common.
3. How can coalition evaluators best deal with the challenges that face them?
4. How are formative and summative evaluation; processes, impacts, and outcomes; and short-term, intermediate, and long-term outcomes related?
5. Why do participatory evaluation principles make sense for coalitions?
6. Are assessment and evaluation synonymous? If not, why not?
7. Provide examples of process and outcomes indicators. What is the purpose of collecting each?

RESOURCES

General Evaluation Instruments

The Coalition Institute's coalition assessment tools—twenty-nine instruments, most of which can be downloaded in pdf format; the agency can be contacted by e-mail. Accessed February 14, 2006 at http://www.coalitioninstitute.org/ Evaluation-Research/Coalition_Assessment_Tools.htm

Fighting Back: Current project director, board chair, and community leader surveys—nineteen pages, thirty-seven multiple-part items, closed and open-ended mail surveys that gather information from project directors and board chairs on resources, governance, administration and impact on the community, and the community leaders' perceptions of the local Fighting Back initiative, impact on leaders' organizations, and impact on the community. Address: Fighting Back National Program Office, Join Together, One Appleton Street, Boston, Mass. 02116. http://www.coalitioninstitute.org/ Evaluation-Research/CoalitionAssessmentTools/FightingBack-ProjectDirectorSurvey.doc

1996 Task Force Member Survey—twenty- to twenty-five-minute mail survey of members involved in substance abuse prevention task forces in Rhode Island. Assesses member participation in the community task force, perceptions of effects of member participation, information on the community served by the task force, and views of the community task force and its effects. Address: Communities United for Prevention, Communities Research and Services Team, Department of Psychology, University of Rhode Island.

Key Informant Interview—a ten-minute telephone survey of community key informants (chair of city or town council, superintendent of schools, police chief for city or town). Assesses substance abuse prevention task force impact in the community, their perceptions of substance abuse issues in the community, and supports and barriers in the community. Consortium for Community Initiatives, Communities Research and Services Team, Department of Psychology, University of Rhode Island. In Florin, P., Mitchell, R., and Stevenson, J. "Predicting Intermediate Outcomes for Prevention Coalitions: A Developmental Perspective." *Evaluation Program Planning,* 23, 341–346.

Checklist of Policy Indicators for Alcohol, Tobacco, and Other Drugs—a checklist to help coalitions assess the number and types of policies within the community and where they might best extend their efforts. Address: Center for Prevention Research and Development, Institute of Government and Public Affairs, University of Illinois at Champaign-Urbana, 510 Devonshire Drive Champaign, Ill. 61820. Tel: (217) 333-3231; fax: (217) 244-0214; http://www. coalitioninstitute.org/Evaluation-Research/CoalitionAssessmentTools/ Checklist-of-PolicyIndicators.doc

Coalition Member Survey—a tool to use on an annual basis to gauge coalition members' opinions about their involvement with the coalition. It covers topics such as the role members play in the coalition, interaction with other partners, perceived coalition impact on ATOD issues in the community, and an assessment

EVALUATING COALITIONS AND PARTNERSHIPS **495**

of the coalition leadership. Address: Center for Prevention Research and Development (CPRD), Institute of Government and Public Affairs, University of Illinois at Champaign-Urbana, 510 Devonshire Drive, Champaign, Ill. 61820. Tel: (217) 333-3231; fax: (217) 244-0214; http://www.coalitioninstitute.org/ Evaluation-Research/CoalitionAssessmentTools/CoalitionMember Survey.pdf

Coalition Self Assessment—eleven open-ended qualitative questions that coalitions can use to help articulate their strategic plan or logic model, developed as part of the Fighting Back project. Address: Community Anti-Drug Coalitions of America (CADCA), National Community Anti-Drug Coalition Institute. http://www.coalitioninstitute.org/Evaluation-Research/ CoalitionAssessmentTools/CoalitionSelf-AssessmentInstrument.doc

Collaboration Evaluation Worksheets—compilation of various assessment tools: Annual Satisfaction Survey for Community Coalitions; Diagnosing Your Coalition; Risk Factors for Participation; Assessing Your Collaboration's Commitment to Agency-Based and Community-Based Approaches; Climate Diagnostic Tool: The Six R's of Participation; Responsibility Charting; Inclusivity Checklist; Task Force Evaluation and Resource Allocation; Sustainability Benchmarks; and Coalition Annual Report. All can be obtained through Tom Wolff's website at http://www.tomwolff.com/and are contained in the following publication: Wolff, T. "A Practical Approach to Evaluating Coalitions. In T. Backer (ed.), *Evaluating Community Collaborations.* New York, N.Y.: Springer Publishing, 2002. Available at http://www. tomwolff.com/resources/backer.pdf.

Collaboration Progress Checklist—a checklist for members to rate the extent to which they feel certain factors are part of their collaboration (goals, communication, sustainability, research and evaluation, political climate, resources, and so forth). Thirteen factors are rated using a five-point scale (strongly agree to strongly disagree). The checklist is found at http://crs.uvm.edu/nnco/cd/ checklis.htm, and in *National Network for Collaboration Training Manual* at http://crs.uvm.edu/nnco/cd/.

Diagnosing the Health of Your Coalition—to help members assess, individually, what they believe to be the status of their collaborative partnership. This tool is used most effectively when it is provided to multiple parties with varied perspectives and the results are communicated to the group. It can facilitate conversation among members and generate ideas about how to move the group forward. Developed by Gillian Kaye, President, Community Development Consultants, Brooklyn, N.Y. http://www.coalitioninstitute.org/ Evaluation-Research/CoalitionAssessmentTools/Diagnosing-the-Health-of-your-Coalition.doc

DrugStrategies Instruments (2001)—tools used in assessment of twelve community antidrug coalitions in eleven Knight Foundation cities.

The Case Study Questionnaire is a questionnaire designed to explore coalitions' experiences in addressing key elements, including how they are established and funded; how they define their objectives and whether they can be translated into outcome indicators; what process data are collected; and how data are used to maintain public support, media interest, and financial backing. The questions evaluate how the coalition interacts with the community, develops a strategic plan, chooses programs, and identifies training needs. http://www.drugstrategies.org/acrobat/CommCoal.pdf

The Coalition Mail Survey is an eighteen-item survey mailed to coalition leaders regarding basic coalition structure and functioning, including early history, composition of membership, staffing, type of interventions, obstacles, and funding history.

The Coalition Telephone Survey is a forty-five-minute telephone survey with coalition leaders to further explore coalition structure and functioning, including decision-making structure, program goals and compliance with goals, purpose of coalitions' interventions, evaluation efforts, barriers, and community readiness.

Expert Advisory Panel Questions are nine questions for experts in the prevention field designed to identify various aspects of community coalitions. They include different coalition types, implementation methods, community influence, barriers to and key elements of success, need for training, and evaluation.

The Key Informant Survey is a twenty-minute phone survey of non-coalition community leaders in business, law enforcement, education, media, faith, social services, and government, to assess their perspectives on issues of substance abuse in their community and whether they know of coalition efforts.

Survey on Participation in Community-Based Substance Abuse Prevention— designed to capture information about involvement with a community coalition to prevent substance abuse, and members' prevention experiences. RAND—Survey Research Group. Contact: Dr. Abe Wandersman, University of South Carolina, at WanderAH@gwm.sc.edu.

The Coalition Self-Assessment Survey (CSAS)—a sixteen-page quantitative questionnaire for members and staff that looks at coalition leadership, membership, structure, function, and processes. Kenney, E., and Sofaer, S. *The Coalition Self-Assessment Survey: A Manual for Users.* New York: City University of New York, Baruch College, School of Public Affairs, 2000. Available at www.baruch.cuny.edu/spa/Faculty/ShoshannaSofaer.jsp or on CD-ROM from shoshanna_sofaer@baruch.cuny.edu.

Partnership Synergy Tools—instruments developed by the Center for the Advancement of Collaborative Strategies in Health (CACSH) to enhance the capacity of communities to implement health-promoting partnerships. http://www.cacsh.org

Coalition Effectiveness Inventory (CEI)—a self-assessment tool that identifies whether coalition elements related to participants, processes, and structures are present, and that determines the coalition's stage of development and how well tasks are accomplished within each stage: fully (score = 2), minimally (score = 1), or not at all (score = 0) (Butterfoss, 2004; Goldstein, 1997). The tool can be obtained from ButterFD@evms.edu.

Partnership Self-Assessment Tool—an easy-to-use instrument that previously was available online. Copies can now be accessed by contacting the Center for the Advancement of Collaborative Strategies in Health at The New York Academy of Medicine. This tool gives partnerships a way to assess how well their collaborative process works and to identify specific areas they can focus on to make the process work well. It measures the partnership's level of synergy and identifies its strengths and weaknesses in areas such as leadership, efficiency, administration and management, and sufficiency of resources. It measures partners' perspectives about the coalition's decision-making process, the benefits and drawbacks they experience by participating, and their overall satisfaction with the partnership. Findings from the National Study of Partnership Functioning are also available at http://www.cacsh.org/researchandinstruments.html#nspf.

Framework for Achieving Partnership Synergy: http://www.cacsh.org/synergypaper.html

Center for the Advancement of Collaborative Strategies in Health—research instruments to measure partnership synergy and potential predictors of synergy. http://www.cacsh.org/cresources.html#researchinstr

Other Resources

American Evaluation Association has a comprehensive site that includes several handbooks and texts available in their entirety online. Most are multi-chapter documents focusing on "how-to's" of evaluation-related subjects. http://www.eval.org/Resources/onlinehbtxt.htm

Annie E. Casey Foundation is a private charitable organization dedicated to helping build better futures for disadvantaged children in the United States. *Kids Count On-line Data Book* contains state-level data for over seventy-five measures of child well-being. This online database helps in generating custom reports for a geographic area (profiles) or comparing geographic areas on a topic. http://www.aecf.org/kidscount/sld/

Association for the Study and Development of Community. *Principles for Evaluating Comprehensive Community Initiatives.* Washington, D.C.: National Funding Collaborative on Violence Prevention. This document covers issues and approaches in a particular context and was developed for evaluators who have in-depth knowledge of the challenges of evaluating comprehensive community initiatives. Funders and practitioners also might find it useful. Address: National Funding Collaborative on Violence Prevention, 1522 K Street, N.W., Suite 1100, Washington, D.C. 20005-2201. Tel: (202) 393-7731; www.peacebeyondviolence.org

Basic Guide to Program Evaluation: http://www.mapnp.org/library/evaluatn/fnl_eval.htm

Center for the Advancement of Collaborative Strategies in Health at the New York Academy of Medicine helps partnerships, funders, and policy makers realize the full potential of collaboration to solve complex problems related to health or any other area. Working closely with people and organizations involved in collaboration, the Center conducts research studies, policy analyses, and joint learning activities to identify and explore key challenges associated with collaborative problem solving. The Center also develops practical tools and training programs based on the knowledge it obtains: The Center's Focus and Conceptual Models, *Pathways to Collaboration: A Knowledge-Building Workgroup,* and the web-based *Partnership Self-Assessment Tool.*

Centers for Disease Control and Prevention. *Framework for Program Evaluation in Public Health.* Morbidity and Mortality Weekly Report, 48(RR-11), 1999. The framework was produced to guide public health professionals in program evaluation and in integrating evaluation into program activities. It summarizes the essential elements of program evaluation, steps in program evaluation, and standards for effective program evaluation. Download at www.cdc.gov/eval/framework.htm#cbph.

Community Anti-Drug Coalitions of America (CADCA). *The Coalition Institute's Guiding Principles for Coalition Evaluation.* Washington, D.C.: Author, 2004. http://www.coalitioninstitute.org/Evaluation-Research/Strategizer48.pdf. Accessed February 17, 2006.

Collaborative Solutions. Tom Wolff and Associates provide tools and resources necessary to mobilize the power of collaborative processes in communities and organizations. They have services for those who want to create collaborative solutions, enhance healthy communities, and build community coalitions. Contact via the website http://www.tomwolff.com/ or call (413) 253-2646. Resources such as publications and the twenty-eight *Coalition Building Tip Sheets* that cover issues from start-up to sustainability can be ordered online or downloaded.

Community Toolbox. *Evaluating Community Programs and Initiatives.* A web-based resource created and maintained by the University of Kansas Work Group on Health Promotion and Community Development in Lawrence, Kans., and AHEC/Community Partners in Amherst, Mass. It contains user-friendly instructions for planning, implementing, and evaluating community health and development initiatives. The evaluation section includes step-by-step guidelines, examples, checklists of major points, and training materials for evaluating community health and development efforts. http://ctb.ukans.edu

Drug Strategies. *Assessing Community Coalitions.* Washington, D.C.: Author, 2001. This manual, funded by the Robert Wood Johnson and Knight Foundations, offers a history of drug abuse prevention coalition efforts in the United States and the history of their evaluations, and explores the elements felt to contribute to their effectiveness. Resources and survey instruments are referenced here. http://www.drugstrategies.org/acrobat/CommCoal.pdf

Empowerment Evaluation. The Collaborative, Participatory, and Empowerment Evaluation group is part of the American Evaluation Association. This site includes online survey software and self-help manuals. http://www. stanford.edu/~davidf/empowermentevaluation.html

Fawcett, S., and others. *Work Group Evaluation Handbook: Evaluating and Supporting Community Initiatives for Health and Development.* Lawrence, Kans.: Work Group on Health Promotion and Community Development, University of Kansas, 1995.

Healthy People 2010, Health Objectives for the Nation. http://www.healthypeople.gov/

Innovative Network (InnonNet). Helping Agencies Succeed. www.innonet.org. This web-based resource was developed to make evaluation tools and resources available to nonprofits and funders across program type, organization size, and geographic boundaries. An interactive "workstation" leads the user through steps to define program goals, identify activities needed to achieve those goals, design steps for evaluating the activities and outcomes, and budget expenses for conducting the program and evaluation. The user can also submit the plans for comments by InnoNet staff.

Join Together. How Do We Know We Are Making a Difference? A Community Alcohol, Tobacco, and Drug Indicators Handbook. Boston, Mass.: Author, 2005. http://indicatorshandbook.org/indicators/

Linney, J., and Wandersman, A. *Prevention Plus III: Assessing Alcohol and Other Drug Prevention Programs at the School and Community Level.* Rockville, Md.: U.S. Department of Health and Human Services, Centers for Substance Abuse Prevention (CSAP), 1991. School and community leaders involved in community partnerships and coalitions to prevent alcohol and drug use can use this resource to help them assess the effectiveness of their prevention efforts. It uses simple language to guide them through a series of steps to assess and document their individual activities. Address: National Clearinghouse for Alcohol and Drug Information, 11426 Rockville Pike, Suite 200, Rockville, Md. 20852. Tel: (800) 729-6686; www.ncadi.samhsa.gov

National Science Foundation. The 2002 User-Friendly Handbook for Project Evaluation. Arlington, Va.: National Science Foundation, 2002. This handbook was developed for managers of National Science Foundation (NSF)-funded education programs to increase program managers' understanding of the evaluation process and NSF's requirements for evaluation, as well as to build their capacity to communicate with evaluators and manage the evaluation. Download at www.nsf.gov/pubs/2002/nsf02057/start.htm.

National Neighborhood Indicators Project is a collaborative effort by the Urban Institute and local partners to further the development and use of neighborhood information systems in local policy making and community building. http://www.urban.org/nnip/

Rossi, P. H., Freeman, H. E., and Lipsey, M. W. *Evaluation: A Systematic Approach,* 6th ed. Thousand Oaks, Calif.: Sage Publications, 1999.

Self-help software for survey development:
- SurveyKey®–http://www.surveykey.com/
- Survey Suite®–http://intercom.virginia.edu/cgi-bin/cgiwrap/intercom/SurveySuite/ss_index.pl

- Formsite®—http://www.formsite.com
- Zoomerang®–http://www.zoomerang.com

Sierra Health Foundation. *We Did It Ourselves: An Evaluation Guide Book.* Sacramento, Calif.: Sierra Health Foundation, 2000. This reference guide helps community practitioners design and conduct an evaluation of their individual collaboratives. It contains step-by-step instructions, worksheets, and exercises for individuals who have never done an evaluation before. Address: Sierra Health Foundation, 1321 Garden Highway, Sacramento, Calif. 95833. Tel: (916) 922–4755; www.sierrahealth.org

Thompson, N. J., and McClintock, H. O. *Demonstrating Your Program's Worth: A Primer on Evaluation for Programs to Prevent Unintentional Injury.* Atlanta, Ga.: CDC, National Center for Injury Prevention and Control, 1998.

United Way of America Measuring Program Outcomes. Alexandria, Va.: United Way of America, 1996. This step-by-step guide is intended to help executive directors and program managers in a broad range of human services measure their program outcomes. These include not only direct services but also advocacy, public education, capacity building, and other related efforts. It leads the user through a series of steps for measuring program outcomes, from getting ready to do it, to actually using the findings. Address: The United Way of America, Effective Practices and Measuring Impact, 701 North Fairfax Street, Alexandria, Va. 22314. Tel: (703) 836-7100.

University of Wisconsin—Cooperative Extension. *Evaluating Collaboratives.* Madison, Wisc.: Cooperative Extension Publications, 1998. Individuals interested in evaluating the work of coalitions and collaborations will find this workbook useful. It provides a compendium of ideas and research for users to consider and choose from to increase their collaboratives' effectiveness. Address: Cooperative Extension Publications, Room 170, 630 W. Mifflin Street, Madison, Wis. 53703. Tel: (608) 262-3346.

W. K. Kellogg Foundation. *Evaluation Handbook.* Battle Creek, Mich.: W. K. Kellogg Foundation, 1998. Download at www.wkkf.org. This handbook was developed primarily for project directors who are responsible for evaluating projects funded by the W. K. Kellogg Foundation. It provides a framework for considering evaluation as a useful tool for program improvement as well as enough information for program staff to plan and conduct an evaluation with or without the assistance of an external evaluator.

CHAPTER FIFTEEN

Coalitions and Partnerships: Their Promise and Future

When you cease to make a contribution, you begin to die.
—Eleanor Roosevelt, 1884–1962

In this final chapter, asking once again why we *need* coalitions is a legitimate question. Opinions about the value of coalitions range from those who consider them a waste of time to those who cannot imagine working in community in any other way. The Advocacy Institute (2004) phrased the unique accomplishments of coalitions quite eloquently:

> Coalitions expand the numbers and expertise of those working on an issue; they
> can unite unlikely allies and bridge essential gaps. When effective, coalitions
> mass and focus the collective skills, resources, and energies of their constituents.
> When ineffective, they can drain energy and resources, exacerbate institutional
> and personal rivalries and conflicts, paralyze flexibility, and deaden initiative.

Coalitions may be seen as panaceas, as tools for accomplishing complex tasks, or as ways to build community capacity and self-determination. But can community coalitions and partnerships be powerful agents for social change? Can they help solve complex public health challenges?

REFLECTIONS ON THE POWER OF WORKING IN PARTNERSHIP

Without a doubt, community coalitions and partnerships are at the core of most modern health-promotion movements. However, as we have found, their underlying energy must be focused in a realistic and systematic approach. To reach their goals, coalitions must recruit competent leaders who can encourage members to invest significant resources and share in decision making; coordinate their strategies, messages, and action plans; and accept and work through differences in a trusting environment. Members agree to participate in coalitions because of the inherent benefits that can be accrued by working together. To recap, these benefits include (Community Catalyst, 2003, pp. 6–7; The Advocacy Institute, 2005f):

Strength in numbers. Working together creates pressure on decision makers and increases individuals' risk-taking abilities. This powerful community voice exerts collective influence to achieve desired outcomes.

Strength in diversity. Bringing together people who are not just the "usual suspects" provides strength, credibility, diverse perspectives, better problem solving, more effective outreach and, ultimately, the impacts and outcomes that the group sought in the first place. A coalition effort appears more legitimate and reliable, attracts more attention, and commands more respect from both allies and potential opponents than do individual efforts.

Strength in community relationships. Coalitions provide opportunities for groups and individuals who have never before worked together to collaborate across age, race, ethnic, and socioeconomic groups. These shared experiences can forge enduring bonds between organizations, build confidence, strengthen community loyalties, and enhance synergy among members, as well as a belief that change is possible.

Increased access to resources. By pooling valuable resources and talents, coalition members complement each other to maximize their effectiveness. Sharing the workload enables them to implement a comprehensive plan of action and reduces the burden on any one organization.

Participating in an organization that models a just society. Coalitions provide opportunities to develop the skills needed for a strong democracy and foster the belief that change is possible.

LESSONS LEARNED FROM COALITION EVALUATIONS

In trying to arrive at a set of lessons learned for coalitions, six multisite coalition initiatives covering diverse issues were reviewed: the six Community Partners for Health coalitions in Nigeria (Brieger and others, 2000–2001) and the 155 Catchment Area Planning and Action (CAPA) coalitions that focused on varied maternal-child health issues in three African countries (Brieger, Salami, and Ogunlade, 2004); seven Allies Against Asthma coalitions in the United States and Puerto Rico (Clark, Friedman, and Lachance, 2006); twenty California Healthy Cities and Communities partnerships in California (Kegler, Norton, and Aronson, 2003); SmokeLess States coalitions in forty-eight states, one city, and the District of Columbia (Robert Wood Johnson Foundation, 2005b); the Center for Substance Abuse Prevention (CSAP)/Substance Abuse and Mental Health Services Administration's (SAMHSA) 251 community partnerships for substance abuse prevention in forty-five states and Puerto Rico, in which forty-eight communities with and without partnerships were compared (Yin, Kafterian, Yu, and Jansen, 1997; Substance Abuse and Mental

Health Services Administration, 2000); and thirteen teen pregnancy coalitions in the urban United States (The National Campaign to Prevent Teen Pregnancy, 2003). This cross-section of coalitions, funded within the past decade, and many of which are still operating, is not an exhaustive list but serves to highlight common lessons learned from coalition evaluation.

Building a coalition is an incremental, long-term process. Evaluations from each of these projects agreed that this was the first and greatest lesson. Establishing trust among individuals and organizations with different views about prevention required leaders with consensus-building skills. As partners experienced success in defining a common agenda and carrying out discrete projects, such as needs and assets assessments, the coalition began to solidify, making it possible to attract new organizations and individuals to the effort.

Building truly diverse coalitions is even harder. Many of these initiatives agreed that they were not as successful as they hoped in building diverse coalitions (Brieger and others, 2000–2001; Clark, Friedman, and Lachance, 2006; Robert Wood Johnson Foundation, 2005b; The National Campaign to Prevent Teen Pregnancy, 2003; Substance Abuse and Mental Health Services Administration, 2000). Addressing diversity required substantial time and resources and an awareness that efforts would be unsustainable if a representative group did not embrace the issue and engage in the work. In most cases, coalitions expanded their base of support by casting a wider net to attract new partners.

One size does not fit all. Partnerships grew out of the unique characteristics that defined each community. The ways that most communities built coalitions, prepared needs and assets assessments, and developed action plans were as diverse as the communities themselves (Kegler, Norton, and Aronson, 2003; The National Campaign to Prevent Teen Pregnancy, 2003). For instance, in the California Healthy Cities and Communities initiative, each community selected a meaningful and feasible priority focus that addressed a pressing issue. Then they designed strategies and activities based upon available resources and capacities to leverage others as needed. The project provided great latitude for communities to conduct a community development process that they defined themselves. As a result, twenty unique projects were developed (each consisting of many health promotion programs, community and policy development strategies, and community-building and awareness activities), and twenty collaborative structures, shaped by local context, were created to support them (Kegler, Norton, and Aronson, 2003).

Every coalition faces challenges. Communities with considerable experience in their health issue and those with less experience both encountered barriers. Communities had many competing issues, and the coalition's issue was often a low priority for them. Real collaboration began when partners stopped thinking only of the funds they would receive and concentrated on how each could contribute to the well-being of the coalition (Substance Abuse and Mental Health Services Administration, 2000). When the health or social issue was controversial, recruiting partners from such sectors as the business and faith communities was more difficult. Sometimes adopting a youth- or family-development approach helped bridge strong differences of opinion, but the coalition had to make sure that its issue was not lost in the broader agenda (The National Campaign to Prevent Teen Pregnancy, 2003, p. 34).

Coalitions need to balance size and participation. More partners were needed in order to have social and political impact on the community and priority population. Participation, on the other hand, was inhibited when coalitions were too small. Membership growth was one piece of evidence that the coalition or its ideas had credibility in the community.

Coalitions need to be realistic in carrying out their work. Coalitions discovered that it was easy to take on too much. Before starting an initiative, the scope, budget, staff, and resources available for the effort must be carefully defined. Coalitions recognized that involving coalition partners, residents, and youth in research activities compromised some of the research goals but resulted in wider community buy-in (Butterfoss and others, 2006; The National Campaign to Prevent Teen Pregnancy, 2003). When prevention efforts were organized at the neighborhood level, residents were more likely to volunteer because they understood how and why it might help their own situation (Substance Abuse and Mental Health Services Administration, 2000).

The approach to developing the action plan and the appropriate roles for staff, coalition partners, and the larger community should be defined from the outset. Often roles and expectations were not clarified before the time-sensitive projects were initiated, and conflicts ensued (Robert Wood Johnson Foundation, 2005b; The National Campaign to Prevent Teen Pregnancy, 2003; Yin, Kafterian, Yu, and Jansen, 1997). By conducting strategic and timely reviews of programs and offering technical assistance and training, some of this confusion could have been avoided. One key to future success is how the partnership, its steering committee, and lead agency interpret and divide their responsibilities for critical functions, such as hiring and firing or deciding on strategic directions (Substance Abuse and Mental Health Services Administration, 2000; Yin, Kafterian, Yu, and Jansen, 1997). Moreover, coalitions needed to strike a balance between planning and action. For many busy community and business leaders, youth, and neighborhood residents, a little bit of planning was all they wanted. To stay engaged, partners needed concrete activities and tangible results from programs that encouraged them to build on that momentum (The National Campaign to Prevent Teen Pregnancy, 2003). Staff members often played important behind-the-scene roles in running coalitions. They had to be aware of and responsive to members' needs and the changes in their roles over time, from offering resources to conducting program activities, to providing official or unofficial leadership.

Effective community collaboration leads to institutionalization of coalition programs and services, but additional external funding makes this more likely. As examples, the tobacco tax and Master Settlement dollars propelled the SmokeLess States coalitions to encourage their partners to incorporate coalition programs into their operations, whereas for Allies Against Asthma coalitions, an infusion of new federal and foundation grant dollars for related chronic disease issues fueled the institutionalization of their programs (Robert Wood Johnson Foundation, 2005; Clark, Friedman, and Lachance, 2006). In the Nigerian coalitions, local investments such as cooperatives and businesses provided an important foundation, and payment of dues was used to show commitment, even though it did not yield much money. Guiding these coalitions in securing grants was the third strategy that was recommended to build capacity (Brieger and others, 2000–2001). Coordinating existing activities and programs, and identifying ways in which agencies and organizations could collaborate with the coalition, rather than compete for funds, helped secure new resources (Substance Abuse and Mental Health Services Administration, 2000).

Clear benchmarks and other measures of success should be identified and defined from the outset (Robert Wood Johnson Foundation, 2005b). Some common intermediate and long-term outcome measures were helpful in comparing coalitions across sites (Butterfoss and others, 2006; Kegler, Norton, and Aronson, 2003).

Training is an essential resource for coalition building and for developing new roles for members. Good training depends on developing standardized curricula and manuals, finding competent trainers, and securing funding to cover basic expenses (Brieger and others, 2000–2001).

A central coordinating body or program office for multisite coalitions is beneficial. Such a group ensured that coalitions did some or all of the following: used promising practices, were financially accountable, had access to technical assistance, communicated regularly and were mentored by other coalitions, and shared data and lessons learned across all coalitions (Brieger and others, 2000–2001; Butterfoss and others, 2006; Robert Wood Johnson Foundation, 2005b).

SUMMING UP: FACTORS THAT PROMOTE COALITION SUCCESS

In addition to lessons learned from formal evaluations, many coalition practitioners and researchers have recommended factors that lead to successful coalition implementation and attainment of valued outcomes, such as changes in behavior(s) and in more distal outcomes (Chavis, 2001; DrugStrategies, 2001; Fawcett, Francisco, Paine-Andrews, and Schultz, 2000; Roussos and Fawcett, 2000; The Advocacy Institute, 2004; Wolff, 2001c). Many of them mirror what was learned from large-scale evaluations as follows:

Community readiness. A coalition is more likely to work when the community itself originates it and has collaboration experience, and when competition among potential partners is minimal (Wolff, 2001c).

Structural and organizational capacity. Coalitions can be formal or informal, strictly or loosely organized—no single structural arrangement is mandated. Coalition members should be involved in choosing a functional structure for the coalition that fits its issue and the community's culture of working together. The structure should facilitate shared mission, careful community assessment, understandable and attainable goals, measurable objectives, and an overall strategic plan that is theory-based, community owned, and focused on change.

Broad, diverse coalition membership. Members should include professionals from service agencies and institutions and grassroots representatives from community-based organizations and neighborhoods. The most effective coalitions are composed of a core of fully committed organizations that have access to businesses, media, funds, and other resources. These members can then recruit other allies for campaigns or special projects. Over all, the coalition should be recognized as being open, inclusive, constantly recruiting, and committed to its members.

Strong, inspired leadership. A coalition should strive to develop leadership among its members with a process for leader succession. While recognizing members' self-interests, leaders can help find the common ground where trust and respect can be nurtured. Good leaders are visionaries who help sustain member commitment, manage conflict, and build consensus. The coalition's leaders must also have strong ties to the major organizations.

Paid, competent staff. Effective coalitions have staff who are fairly compensated and passionate about the coalition's issue(s) and committed to the members and taking care of the coalition itself. They manage the coalition's resources (budget and personnel), promote open and productive communication and decision making, and share power and tasks well with members. Having strong community ties and links to other major organizations is beneficial.

Relationships, relationships, relationships. Building a coalition is really about building relationships. Its success depends on developing an accepting climate that welcomes newcomers, celebrates differences, and resolves conflicts when they arise. Nurturing new relationships both in and outside of the coalition ushers in fresh ideas and perspectives. Providing incentive grants to other organizations and recognizing successful efforts reap later rewards. The coalition's mission must be communicated clearly so that potential partners will understand the nature of their commitment.

Planning and taking action. Coalitions must balance careful planning with strategic action. Members can then choose where best to put their energies; some members are natural planners, whereas others prefer to engage in direct action. Coalition tasks and responsibilities should be clearly defined and equitably shared. In being sensitive to the environment and responsive to the community, coalitions will be more likely to accomplish community change. Frequent communication and feedback and wide publicity about the coalition's activities help build support for the issue(s). Coalitions serve three main functions: coordinating and integrating services, policies, and activities; delivering model programs, services, or both (Krieger and others, 2006); and creating changes in community policies and practices (Lara and others, 2006).

Diversified funding sources. Having adequate resources and funding is necessary, but not sufficient for success. The level of coalition funding often determines what kinds of activities a coalition undertakes—one-time events or multi-component strategies. It also influences the reach and intensity of a coalition's interventions. If a coalition is working to sustain itself and institutionalize its programs, a broad spectrum of resources, including contracts, grants, donations, and in-kind resources, is preferable. When coalition members are involved in fund-raising or grant writing, they begin to emotionally invest in the coalition as well.

Training and technical assistance. To grow and mature, coalitions need consultation and mentorship, technical assistance, and general support. Effective training can lead to improvements in many areas of collaborative work—recruitment, strategic planning, developing and replicating promising practices, legislative and media advocacy, and leadership. Many community organizations offer training for nonprofit leaders at minimal cost, and web-based training is often available. Regular training retreats for coalition members and leaders are a tangible benefit and promote participation.

Research and evaluation. Ongoing, planned evaluation is essential. Evaluation provides evidence of coalition activity and positive outcomes, often required by the local government and institutions, the coalition's lead agency and key partners, funders, media outlets, and the broader community. A participatory evaluation process and evaluation plan help ensure that data will be reliably collected, analyzed, and reported.

Taking the long view. The complex issues that many coalitions address take concerted and long-range efforts. As interventions become more complex and focused on organizational and community change, the coalition must work across multiple levels and take into account community readiness (Goodman and others, 1996). Successful community organizing efforts and programs should be offered frequently, which may require institutionalizing them either in the coalition or in one of its member organizations. Sustaining the coalition itself or its functions should be a long-range goal and a milestone of coalition success.

IMPLICATIONS AND FUTURE RESEARCH

This text has presented what is currently known about coalitions and partnerships based on the research, evaluations, and experiences of practitioners, community organizers, researchers, and evaluators. What are the prospects for coalitions, given the current state of knowledge and state of the public's health? George Orwell predicted a dismal totalitarian government fueled by high technology in his book *1984*. In that year, Cheri Brown published her classic manual, *The Art of Coalition Building*. Brown's vision, however, clearly showed us the promise and possibilities that come from working together in democratic partnership. Coalitions took a while to catch on, but catch on they did. Coalitions and partnerships of all shapes and sizes have sprung up across the United States and in other parts of the world as well. Now, more than twenty years later, we still question whether this approach makes sense and is worth pursuing.

I am convinced that we have just begun to see what coalitions can accomplish. I have been accused of being an eternal optimist or a dreamer. I have been labeled a coalition guru, groupie, and cheerleader. But, in fact, I am a believer in the power that lies within each of us to hatch a new idea, dare to do things differently, and succeed despite challenges. I have witnessed what can happen when people and organizations celebrate their differences, ask the hard questions, reach into their pockets, and put their collective talents to work for change. Given the mere ten to fifteen years that we have harnessed the community's energy and commitment to work together to ensure a healthier future, abandoning the concept of coalitions is really quite premature. In fact, I think we have really been asking the wrong question all along. The question is not, *Do coalitions work?* but, *What do we still have to learn about how to make them work better?* To know for sure, coalitions must be seriously studied for five to seven years beyond their inception.

Some wisely advocate scaling back expectations of what can be accomplished through community participation and collaboration via a coalition approach (Kreuter, Lezin, and Young, 2000; Minkler and Wallerstein, 2003a). Instead of focusing only on whether coalitions achieve desired long-term outcomes in a given community, we should widen our focus to appreciate what works and what does not work in the steps along the way to those outcomes. Birkby states that coalitions may be "a necessary, but not sufficient, part of the solution" and "a means to an end" (2003, p. 5). The specific strategies that coalitions promote are variable; their real potential lies in the structures and processes they create for planning and intervention and in the community capacity they build.

Countless community-based interventions aim to improve health at the community level, especially those that are community-driven. Kegler, Norton, and Aronson advise that we should become even more committed to understand the influence of social, political, and environmental determinants on health and "develop communities' capacities for enhanced health, even as we try to figure out the best technical support and tools to facilitate this community-driven work" (2003, p. 98). Community readiness should also be considered before implementing a coalition; communities may not be ready, or competent, to engage in this process.

A coalition's developmental history also affects its potential for success, as demonstrated in the Allies Against Asthma initiative that traced the natural history or development of the coalitions through stages, and the internal and external factors that influence their development (Butterfoss and others, 2006). Even though the coalitions were very different initially (some were brand new and some very mature), they all progressed through the implementation stage; all but one reached maintenance; and five of seven coalitions began institutionalization.

The experiences of this multisite initiative and the insights gleaned about developmental stages of coalitions might encourage coalitions to track and pay attention to their development. The resulting awareness may alter their expectations for what can realistically be achieved in a given time period and encourage them to link with more experienced coalitions to learn from them. Similarly, funders may consider funding coalitions in varying amounts depending on their stage of development or readiness. Initial smaller grants could fund promising communities to build coalitions throughout a two- to three-year period, which could be followed by larger intervention grants, if coalitions proved worthy. Established, proven coalitions, on the other hand, could be given significant funding from the outset.

The type of issue a coalition focuses on may also affect its development. Much of our knowledge and experience with public health coalitions focus on preventing risky behaviors (for example, tobacco, drug, and alcohol abuse or unprotected sex) or promoting healthy behaviors and accessing care (for example, immunizations, seat belt use, physical activity, cancer screening). Chronic disease management (for example, asthma, diabetes, obesity) appears to be more complex than preventing disease or accessing primary care services. Managing asthma or diabetes, for example, is more costly and time-intensive than promoting immunizations. These diseases require many clinical visits, costly medications, and equipment, and demand intensive education and skills as well as adherence to daily regimens of exercise, diet, and treatment. Moreover, the educational, clinical, and public awareness strategies must be tailored to specific priority populations, unlike health-promoting messages that urge general audiences to be immunized or stay drug-free. Some coalitions have figured out how to navigate through these complex issues to demonstrate how services can be coordinated and integrated effectively. As coalitions mature, they often move from providing services (that potentially compete with their partners') to engaging in policy and advocacy work for which they are better suited. What can be done to ensure that the transition is smooth and well-timed?

Several characteristics of the California Healthy Cities and Communities Program make it stand out: its noncategorical approach to public health and health promotion; its flexible approach to community development; its commitment to technical assistance and supportive, competent staff; and its principles of building collaboration and cohesion while encouraging sensitivity to local context. The program strengthened the ability of local communities to strategically promote their goals for health improvement, which is evidenced by the diverse funding sources that eventually recognized the partnerships' potential to attain significant change (Kegler, Norton, and Aronson, 2003, p. 99).

In a like fashion, more coalition researchers and evaluators must learn innovative ways to link process outcomes to intermediate and long-term goals. Short-term and intermediate objectives should be significant enough to involve coalition members, the media, and the general public, but manageable enough for results to be reasonably expected (The Advocacy Institute, 2004). The potential for positive outcomes resulting from coalition intervention has already been demonstrated. However, we must refine our theories, implementation, and evaluation methods to ensure that we can detect change when it does occur. For example, equitable and reliable methods and measures are being developed to determine who is left out of community partnerships, how partners relate to their own organizations, and the extent that community-based organizations represent the actual community (Butterfoss, 2006). Coalitions are often frustrated when they end up recruiting less diverse partners than expected or desired. As Minkler and Wallerstein (2003a) suggest, we should shift our sights toward achieving *substantive* representation, where members are selected by and accountable to community interests, rather than *descriptive* representation, which mirrors the demographics of the community but has little accountability to it.

Signing on to a coalition should not have to be a lifelong commitment. A coalition does not have to exist forever. Partnerships should exist until they have reached their goals or find that they are not effective in doing so. Some coalitions have found the experience of working together collaboratively to be so desirable that they maintain their presence to address new or more complex issues. For these groups, the goal should be sustainability.

How do we know when a coalition is sustained or likely to be? Several broad indicators for program sustainability have been identified, including broad member participation; links to other organizations; demonstrated effectiveness in reaching clearly defined goals, including changes in knowledge and practices; integration of activities into other established institutional structures; significant levels of funding from national sources; and regular, effective training (Kegler, Twiss, and Look, 2000; Morgan, 2001).

Finally, perhaps the most compelling reason to encourage working in partnerships is that these organizations have proven themselves to accomplish some tasks very well. Namely, coalitions serve as catalysts to bring community issues to the forefront by connecting community members with diverse ideas and skills; collect data about health status and access to care from hard-to-reach populations; help community-based organizations develop feasible and integrated strategies; pilot promising and innovative strategies that may be adopted by invested community agencies; and advocate for critical health issues and priority populations.

REFERENCES

Abed, J., and others. "Comprehensive Cancer Control Initiative of the Centers for Disease Control and Prevention: An Example of Participatory Innovation Diffusion." *Journal of Public Health Management and Practice*, 2000, *6*(2), 79–92.

About Business & Finance. *Brochure Marketing: 12 Tips on How to Do It Effectively.* 2006. [http://marketing.about.com/od/directmarketin1/a/brochmktg_2.htm]. July 17, 2006.

Adams, J. D. "The Role of the Creative Outlook in Team Building." In W. B. Reddy and K. Jamison (eds.), *Team Building*. San Diego, Calif.: University Associates, 1988, pp. 98–106.

Addams, J. *Twenty Years at Hull-House with Autobiographical Notes*. New York: MacMillan, 1912.

Adler, M., and Ziglio, E. *Gazing into the Oracle: The Delphi Method and Its Application to Social Policy and Public Health*. Bristol, Penn.: Jessica Kingsley Publishers, 1996.

The Advocacy Institute. *Allocation of Tobacco Control Funds*. Washington, D.C.: The Advocacy Institute, 1998. [http://www.advocacy.org/publications/mtc/allocation.htm]. July 21, 2005.

The Advocacy Institute. *Tips for Making a Coalition Work*. Washington, D.C.: The Advocacy Institute, 2004. [http://www.advocacy.org/pdf/Building_a_Coalition.pdf]. Jan. 31, 2006.

The Advocacy Institute. *Basic Website Tips for Advocates.* Washington, D.C.: The Advocacy Institute, 2005a. [http://www.advocacy.org/communicate/basic_website_tips_for_advocates.pdf]. Jan. 31, 2006.

The Advocacy Institute. *Empower the Coalition: Making Partnerships and Collaborations That Work.* Washington, D.C.: The Advocacy Institute, 2005b. [http://www.advocacy.org/coalitions/]. Feb. 24, 2006.

The Advocacy Institute. *Leadership Roles Within an Advocacy Movement.* San Francisco: The Advocacy Institute, 2005c. [http://www.advocacy.org/pdf/Leadership_Taxonomy.pdf]. Feb. 1, 2006.

The Advocacy Institute. *Lobbying.* Washington, D.C.: The Advocacy Institute, 2005d. [http://www.advocacy.org/pdf/lobbying.pdf]. Jan. 31, 2006.

The Advocacy Institute. "Speak Your Truth: Creating Strategic Messages." *Advocacy.Org–The Advocacy Institute Newsletter,* Oct. 2005e. Washington, D.C.: The Advocacy Institute. [http://www.advocacy.org/enews/archive/05-10-Messaging.htm]. Feb. 2, 2006.

Agranoff, R., and McGuire, M. "Big Questions in Public Network Management." *Journal of Public Administration Research and Theory,* 2001, *11*(3), 295–326.

Alinsky, S. *Rules for Radicals.* New York: Random House, 1972.

Allensworth, D., and Patton, W. "Promoting School Health Through Coalition Building." *Eta Sigma Gamma Monograph Series,* 1990, 7.

Alter, C., and Hage, J. *Organizations Working Together: Coordination in Inter-Organizational Networks.* Newbury Park, Calif.: Sage, 1993.

Altschuld, J. W., and Witkin, B. R. (eds.). *From Needs Assessment to Action: Transforming Needs into Solution Strategies.* Thousand Oaks, Calif.: Sage Publications, 1999.

American Cancer Society National Advisory Group on Collaboration with Organizations. *1 + 1 = 3: A Collaboration Guidebook.* (2nd ed.) Code No. 5033. American Cancer Society National Distribution Center, 2000.

American Evaluation Association. *Guiding Principles for Evaluators.* 1994, revised 2004. [http://www.eval.org/Publications/GuidingPrinciples.asp]. Feb. 13, 2006.

Anderson, M., and Adams, S. *Key to Sustainability: A Diversified Funding Base.* Washington, D.C.: Academy for Educational Development Center for Community-Based Health Strategies, 2000. [http://coach.aed.org/pubs/factsheets/KeytoSustainability.pdf]. Jan. 19, 2005.

Andreasen, A. R. *Marketing Social Change: Changing Behavior to Promote Health, Social Development, and the Environment.* San Francisco: Jossey-Bass, 1995.

Andreasen, A. R. "Social Marketing: A New/Old Approach to Social Change." Nonprofit Marketing Summit Conference Report. Tampa, Fla.: Social Marketing Institute, 2000, p. 9.

Andrews, A. "Interdisciplinary and Interorganizational Collaboration." In A. Minnahan and others (eds.), *Encyclopedia of Social Work.* (18th ed.) Silver Spring, Md.: National Association of Social Workers, 1990.

Andringa, R., and Engstrom, T. *Nonprofit Board Answer Book: Size of the Board.* Washington, D.C.: BoardSource, 2001. [http://www.boardsource.org/FullAnswer.asp?ID=101]. Jan. 5, 2006.

Ansari, W., and Phillips, C. J. "The Costs and Benefits to Participation in Community Partnerships: A Paradox?" *Health Promotion Practice,* 2004, *5*(1), 35–48.

Ansari, W., and Weiss, E. S. "Quality of Research on Community Partnerships: Developing the Evidence Base." *Health Education Research,* 2006, *21*(2), 175–180.

Anspaugh, D. J., Dignan, M. B., and Anspaugh, S. L. *Developing Health Promotion Programs.* Boston: McGraw-Hill, 2000.

Archer, T. M., Cripe, R., and McCaslin, N. L. *Making a Difference: Needs Assessments for Building Coalitions.* Columbus: Ohio State University Agricultural Extension Fact Sheet CDFS-9, 1992. [http://ohioline.osu.bc-fact/0009.html]. Nov. 29, 2005.

Arkin, E. B. "Opportunities for Improving the Nation's Health Through Collaboration with the Mass Media." *Public Health Reports,* 1990, *105*(3), 219–223.

Arnstein, S. R. "A Ladder of Citizen Participation." *Journal of the American Institute of Planners,* 1969, *35*, 216–224.

Association for the Study and Development of Community. *Principles for Evaluating Comprehensive Community Initiatives.* Gaithersburg, Md.: Association for the Study and Development of Community, 2001. [www.capablecommunity.com]. Dec. 4, 2006.

Avolio, B. J. *Full Leadership Development: Building the Vital forces in Organizations.* Thousand Oaks, Calif.: Sage, 1999.

Bailey, C. A. *A Guide to Field Research.* Thousand Oaks, Calif.: Pine Forge Press, 1996.

Bailey, D., and Koney, K. M. "Interorganizational Community-Based Collaboratives: A Strategic Response to Shape the Social Work Agenda." *Social Work,* 1996, *41*(6), 602–611.

Balcazar, F., Seekins, T., Fawcett, S., and Hopkins, B. "Empowering People with Disabilities Thorough Advocacy Skills Training." *American Journal of Community Psychology,* 1990, *18*, 281–296.

Ballenger, B. *Membership Recruiting Manual.* Denver: Northern Rockies Action Group, 1981.

Bangs, D. H., Jr. *The Business Planning Guide: Creating a Plan for Success in Your Business.* (7th ed.) Chicago: Upstart Publishing Company, 1995.

Barry, C. A. "Choosing Qualitative Data Analysis Software: Atlas/ti and Nudist Compared." *Sociological Research Online,* 1998, *3*(3). [http://www.socresonline.org.uk/socresonline/3/3/4.html]. July 25, 2006.

Bartholomew, L. K., Parcel, G. S., Kok, G., and Gottlieb, N. H. *Intervention Mapping: Designing Theory- and Evidence-Based Health Promotion Programs.* Mountain View, Calif.: Mayfield, 2001.

Bartunek, J. M., Foster-Fishman, P. G., and Keys, C. B. "Using Collaborative Advocacy to Foster Intergroup Cooperation: A Joint Insider–Outsider Investigation." *Human Relations,* 1996, *49*(6), 701–731.

Bass, B. M. "Individual Capability, Team Performance and Team Productivity." In E. A. Fleischman and M. D. Dunnette (eds.), *Human Performance and Productivity.* Hillsdale, N.J.: Lawrence Erlbaum, 1980, pp. 179–232.

Bass, B. M. *Leadership and Performance Beyond Expectations.* New York: The Free Press, 1985.

Bauer, G. "Sample Community Health Indicators on the Neighborhood Level." In M. Minkler and N. Wallerstein (eds.), *Community-Based Participatory Research for Health.* San Francisco: Jossey-Bass, 2003, pp. 438–445.

Bazzoli, G., and others. "Public–Private Collaboration in Health and Human Service Delivery: Evidence from Community Partnerships." *The Milbank Quarterly,* 1997, *75*(4), 533–561.

Bazzoli, G. J., and others. "Collaborative Initiatives: Where the Rubber Meets the Road in Community Partnerships." *Medical Care Research and Review,* Supplement, 2003, *60*(4), 63S–94S.

Beckham, B., and King, J. *Communication in Coalitions.* Ohio State University Fact Sheet CDFS-6, 2005. [http://ohioline.osu.edu/bc-fact/0006.html]. Sept. 26, 2005.

Benard, B. "Working Together: Principles of Effective Collaboration." *Prevention Forum,* Oct. 1989, pp. 4–9.

Bennis, W. G., and Sheppard, H. A. "A Theory of Group Development." *Human Relations,* 1956, *9*, 415–437.

Berg, B. L. *Qualitative Research Methods for the Social Sciences.* Boston: Allyn and Bacon, 1998.

Berkowitz, B. "Studying the Outcomes of Community-Based Coalitions." *American Journal of Community Psychology,* 2001, *29*(2), 213–228.

Berkowitz, B. *Apply for a Grant: The General Approach.* Lawrence, Kans.: Community Tool Box, 2006a. [http://ctb.ku.edu/tools/EN/sub_section_main_1300.htm]. Jan. 4, 2006.

Berkowitz, B. *Creating a Business Plan.* Lawrence, Kans.: Community Tool Box, 2006b. [/EN/sub_section_main_1298.htm]. Jan. 4, 2006.

Berlin, X., Barnett, W., Mischke, G., and Ocasio W. "The Evolution of Collective Strategies Among Organizations." *Organization Studies,* 2000, *21*(2), 325–354.

Bernard, H. R. (ed.). *Handbook of Methods in Cultural Anthropology.* Walnut Creek, Calif.: AltaMira, 1998.

Besser, T. L. *Start with Community Strengths.* Ames: Community Connections, Iowa State University Extension, 1995.

Billings, W. *Jamestown and the Founding of the Nation.* Gettysburg, Penn.: Thomas Publications, 1990.

Birkby, B. "Community Coalitions: Questions, Controversy & Context." *Prevention Evaluation Perspectives,* 2003, *1*(1), 1–7.

Bishop, C., Earp, J. A., Eng, E., and Lynch, K. "Implementing a Natural Helper Lay Health Advisor Program: Lessons Learned from Unplanned Events." *Health Promotion Practice,* 2002, *3*(2), 217–232.

Black, T. "Coalition Building—Some Suggestions." *Child Welfare*, 1983, *62*, 263–268.

Block, P. *Flawless Consulting: A Guide to Getting Your Expertise Used.* San Diego, Calif.: University Associates, 1981.

BoardSource. *Board Essentials: Forming a Non-Profit Organization.* Washington, D.C.: BoardSource, 2002a. [http://www.boardsource.org/FullAnswer.asp?ID=101]. Jan. 5, 2006.

BoardSource. *Board Essentials: Should We Be a Membership Organization?* Washington, D.C.: BoardSource, 2002b. [http://www.boardsource.org/Knowledge.asp?ID=3.107] Jan. 5, 2006.

BoardSource. *Can Non-Profits Lobby?* Washington, D.C.: BoardSource, 2002c. [http://www.boardsource.org/FullAnswer.asp?ID=92]. Jan. 5, 2006.

BoardSource. *Diversity: Who Should Sit at Your Table?* Special Edition. Washington, D.C.: BoardSource, 2003. [http://www.boardsource.org/QnA.asp?Category=3]. Jan. 6, 2006.

Bobo, K., Kendall J., and Max, S. *Organizing for Social Change: Midwest Academy Manual for Activists.* (4th ed.) Santa Ana, Calif.: Seven Locks Press, 2001, pp. 4–28.

Bobowick, M. J., Hughes, S. R., and Lakey, B. M. *Transforming Board Structure.* Washington, D.C.: BoardSource, 2001. [http://www.boardsource.org/QnA.asp?Category=9]. Jan. 6, 2005.

Boissevain, J. *Friends of Friends—Networks, Manipulators, and Coalitions.* Oxford, England: Basil Blackwell, 1974.

Bonnet, D. G. *An Evaluation of Year One of the American Cancer Society's Collaborative Evaluation Fellows Project.* Indianapolis, Ind.: D. Bonnet Associates, 1999.

Borden, L. M., and Perkins, D. F. "Assessing Your Collaboration: A Self-Evaluation Tool." *Journal of Extension*, 1999, *37*(2), 1–3. [http://www.joe.org/joe/1999Apr./tt1.html]. Oct. 5, 2005.

Bornstein, D. *How to Change the World: Social Entrepreneurs and the Power of New Ideas.* Oxford: Oxford University Press, 2004.

Boydell, K. M. *Overview of the Current Literature on Coalition Development.* Toronto, Ontario, Canada: Canadian Coalition on Senior's Mental Health, 2003.

Bracht, N. (ed.). *Health Promotion at the Community Level.* Newbury Park, Calif.: Sage, 1990.

Bracht, N., Kingsbury, L., and Rissel, C. "A Five-Stage Community Organization Model for Health Promotion: Empowerment and Partnership Strategies." In N. Bracht (ed.), *Health Promotion at the Community Level: Empowerment and Partnership Strategies.* Thousand Oaks, Calif.: Sage, 1999, pp. 83–104.

Brager, G. A., Sprecht, H., and Torczyner, J. L. *Community Organizing.* (2nd ed.) New York: Columbia University Press, 1987.

Braithwaite, R. L., Bianchi C., and Taylor, S. E. "Ethnographic Approach to Community Organization and Health Empowerment." *Health Education Quarterly*, 1994, *21*(3), 407–416.

Braithwaite, R., Murphy, F., Lythcott, N., and Blumenthal, D. S. "Community Organization and Development for Health Promotion within an Urban Black Community: A Conceptual Model." *Health Education*, 1989, *20*(5), 56–60.

Braithwaite, R., Taylor, S., and Austin, J. *Building Health Coalitions in the Black Community.* Thousand Oaks: Sage, 2000.

Breckon, D. J., Harvey, J. R., and Lancaster, R. B. *Community Health Education: Settings, Roles, and Skills for the 21st Century.* (4th ed.) Gaithersburg, Md.: Aspen, 1998.

Brice, H. J. *Financial and Strategic Management for Nonprofit Organizations.* Englewood Cliffs, N.J.: Prentice-Hall, 1987.

Brieger, W. R., Salami, K. K., and Ogunlade, B. P. *Catchment Area Planning and Action: Documentation of the Community-Based Approach in Nigeria.* Arlington, Va.: BASICS II for the United States Agency for International Development, 2004.

Brieger, W. R., and others. "Community Partners for Health: Urban Health Coalitions in Lagos, Nigeria." *International Quarterly of Community Health Education*, 2000–2001, *20*(1), 59–81.

Brindis, C. *Adolescent Pregnancy Prevention: A Guidebook for Communities.* Palo Alto, Calif.: Stanford Center for Research in Disease Prevention, 1991.

Brinckerhoff, P. C. *Financial Empowerment: More Money for More Mission.* Dillon, Colo.: Alpine Guild, 1996.

Briss, P. A., Brownson, R. C., Fielding, J. E., and Zaza, S. "Developing and Using the Guide to Community Preventive Services: Lessons Learned About Evidence-Based Public Health." *Annual Reviews in Public Health*, 2004, *25*, 281–302.

Brogan, H. *Alexis de Tocqueville: A Life.* New Haven, Conn.: Yale University Press, 2005.

Brown, C. *The Art of Coalition Building.* New York: American Jewish Committee, 1984.

Brubach, A. *Coalition Ideas Corner: Utilizing Media Advocacy for Community Prevention.* Washington, D.C.: Community Anti-Drug Coalitions of America, [http://cadca.org/CoalitionsOnline/article.asp?id=809]. Jan. 26, 2006.

Bruner, C. *So You Think You Need Some Help? Making Effective Use of Technical Assistance.* Resource brief. New York: National Center for Service Integration Clearinghouse, National Center for Children in Poverty, Columbia University, 1993.

Bruner, C. "Rethinking the Evaluation of Family Strengthening Strategies: Beyond Traditional Program Evaluation Models." *The Evaluation Exchange*, 2004, *10*(2), Summer.

Bryson, J. *Strategic Planning for Public and Nonprofit Organizations: A Guide to Strengthening and Sustaining Organizational Achievement.* San Francisco: Jossey-Bass, 1989.

Buckley, J., and Mank, D. "New Perspectives on Training and Technical Assistance: Moving from Assumptions to Focus on Quality." *Journal of the Association for Persons with Severe Handicaps*, 1994, *19*(3), 223–232.

Burghardt, S. "Community-Based Social Action." In *Encyclopedia of Social Work*. (18th ed.) A. Minahan (Ed.) New York: National Association of Social Work, 1987.

Burns, J. M. *Leadership*. New York: HarperCollins, 1978.

Butler, L. M., and Howell, R. E. *Coping with Growth: Community Needs Assessment Techniques*. Corvallis, OR.: Western Regional Extension, 1980. [http://ext.usu.edu/crd/wrdcpub/]. Oct. 22, 2006.

Butterfoss, F. D. "Building Effective Coalitions with Consultation and Technical Assistance: Virginia's Healthy Start Initiative." *Health Promotion Practice*, 2004, *5*(2), 118–126.

Butterfoss, F. D. "Process Evaluation for Community Participation." *Annual Review of Public Health*, 2006, *27*, 323–340.

Butterfoss, F., Cashman, S., Foster-Fishman, P., and Kegler, M. "Roundtable Discussion of Berkowitz's Paper." *American Journal of Community Psychology*, 2001, *29*(2), 229–240.

Butterfoss, F. D., and Dunet, D. O. "State Plan Index: A Tool for Assessing the Quality of State Public Health Plans." *Preventing Chronic Disease*, 2005. Serial online. [http://www.cdc.gov/pcd/issues/2005/apr/04_0089.htm]. Nov. 15, 2006.

Butterfoss, F. D., and Francisco, V. T. "Culturally Competent Program Evaluation." *Health Promotion Practice*, 2000, *3*(2), 117–119.

Butterfoss, F. D., and Francisco, V. T. "Evaluating Community Partnerships and Coalitions with Practitioners in Mind." *Health Promotion Practice*, 2004, *5*(2), 108–114.

Butterfoss, F. D., Francisco, V. T., and Capwell, E. M. "Choosing Effective Evaluation Methods." *Health Promotion Practice*, 2000, *1*(4), 307–313.

Butterfoss, F. D., Francisco, V., and Capwell, E. "Stakeholder Participation in Evaluation." *Health Promotion Practice*, 2001, *2*(2), 114–119.

Butterfoss, F., Goodman, R., and Wandersman, A. "Community Coalitions for Prevention and Health Promotion." *Health Education Research*, 1993, *8*(3), 315–330.

Butterfoss, F., Goodman, R., and Wandersman, A. "Community Coalitions for Prevention and Health Promotion: Factors Predicting Satisfaction, Participation and Planning." *Health Education Quarterly*, 1996, *23*(1), 65–79.

Butterfoss, F. D., Goodman, R. M., and Wandersman, A. "Citizen Participation and Health: Toward a Psychology of Improving Health Through Individual, Organizational and Community Involvement." In A. Baum, T. A. Revenson, and J. E. Singer (eds.), *Handbook of Health Psychology*. Mahwah, N.J.: Lawrence Erlbaum Associates, 2001, pp. 613–626.

Butterfoss, F. D., Houseman, C., Morrow, A. L., and Rosenthal, J. "Use of focus group data for strategic planning by a community-based immunization coalition." *Family & Community Health*, 1997, *20*(3), 49–59.

Butterfoss, F. D., and Kegler, M. C. "Toward a Comprehensive Understanding of Community Coalitions: Moving from Practice to Theory." In R. J. DiClemente, R. A. Crosby, and M. C. Kegler (eds.), *Emerging Theories in Health Promotion Practice and Research: Strategies for Improving Public Health.* San Francisco: Jossey-Bass, 2002, pp. 157–193.

Butterfoss, F. D., Kelly, C. K., and Taylor-Fishwick, J. "Community Planning That Magnifies the Community's Voice: Allies Against Asthma." *Health Education and Behavior,* 2005, *32*(1), 113–128.

Butterfoss, F. D., Morrow, A. L., Webster, J. D., and Crews, C. "The Coalition Training Institute: Training for the Long Haul." *Journal of Public Health Management and Practice,* 2003, *9*(6), 522–529.

Butterfoss, F. D., Webster, J. D., Morrow, A. L., and Rosenthal, J. "Immunization Coalitions That Work: Training for Public Health Professionals." *Journal of Public Health Management and Practice,* 1998, 4(6), pp. 79–87.

Butterfoss, F. D., and others. "The Plan Quality Index: An Empowerment Research, Consultation and Feedback Tool." In D. Fetterman, S. Kafterian, and A. Wandersman (eds.), *Empowerment Evaluation: Knowledge and Tools for Self-Assessment and Accountability.* Thousand Oaks, Calif.: Sage, 1996, pp. 304–331.

Butterfoss, F. D., and others. "CINCH: An Urban Coalition for Empowerment and Action." *Health Education and Behavior,* 1998, *25*(2), 213–225.

Butterfoss, F. D., and others. "From Formation to Action: How the Allies Coalitions Are Getting the Job Done." *Health Promotion Practice,* Special Edition, 2006, *7*(2), 34–43S.

Cameron, R., and others. "Linking Science and Practice: Toward a System for Enabling Communities to Adopt Best Practices for Chronic Disease Prevention." *Health Promotion Practice,* 2001, *2*(1), 35–42.

Campbell, A., Divine, M., and Young, D. *A Sense of Mission.* London: Economist Books, 1990.

Capwell, E., Butterfoss, F. D., and Francisco, V. T. "Why Evaluate?" *Health Promotion Practice,* 2000, *1*(1), 15–20.

Carlaw, R., Mittelmark, M., Bracht, N., and Luepker, R. "Organization for a Community Cardiovascular Health Program: Experiences from the Minnesota Heart Health Program." *Health Education Quarterly,* 1984, *11*(2), 243–252.

Carnegie Corporation. *Turning Points: Preparing America's Youth for the 21st Century.* Washington, D.C.: Carnegie Council on Adolescent Development, 1989.

Carter, K. A., and Beaulieu, L. J. *Conducting a Community Needs Assessment: Primary Data Collection Techniques.* Gainesville: University of Florida Cooperative Extension Service CD-92, 1992.

Center for Prevention Research and Development. [http://www.coalitioninstitute.org/Evaluation-Research/CoalitionAssessmentTools/Checklist-of-PolicyIndicators.doc.]. Dec. 1, 2006.

Center for Prevention Research and Development. *Building Coalition Effectiveness for Sustainability: An Evaluation Rubric.* Urbana: University of Illinois, 1999. [http://www.cprd.uiuc.edu/sig/illinois/PDF%20files/coalition%20rubric.pdf]. Jan. 31, 2006.

Center for the Study and Prevention of Violence. *Blueprints for Violence Prevention Selection Criteria.* Boulder, Colo.: Institute of Behavioral Science at the University of Colorado at Boulder, 2005. [http://www.colorado.edu/cspv/blueprints/model/criteria.html]. Jan. 3, 2006.

Centers for Disease Control and Prevention, National Immunization Program. "U.S. Childhood Immunization Initiative Accelerates Goals." *Immunization Action News,* Dec. 7, 1993, pp. 1–2.

Centers for Disease Control and Prevention. "Core Elements of Health Education and Risk Reduction Activities." In *Guidelines for Health Education and Risk Reduction Activities,* 1995a. [http://wonder.cdc.gov/wonder/STD/RHER3704.PCW.html].

Centers for Disease Control and Prevention. "General Considerations Regarding Health Education and Risk Reduction Activities." In *Guidelines for Health Education and Risk Reduction Activities,* 1995b. [http://wonder.cdc.gov/wonder/STD/RHER3702.PCW.html].

Centers for Disease Control and Prevention. *Practical Evaluation of Public Health Programs.* PHTN course no. VC-0017. Atlanta: U.S. Department of Health and Human Services, Centers for Disease Control and Prevention, Public Health Training Network, 1998.

Centers for Disease Control and Prevention. "Framework for Program Evaluation in Public Health." *Morbidity and Mortality Weekly Report,* 1999, *48*(RR-11), updated 2001. Washington, D.C.: Superintendent of Documents, U.S. Government Printing Office, 1999. [http://www.cdc.gov/mmwr/preview/mmwrhtml]./rr4811a1.htm]. Aug. 15, 2005.

Centers for Disease Control and Prevention. *CDCynergy.* Atlanta: Centers for Disease Control and Prevention, 2000a. Reviewed Jan. 22, 2004; cited June 28, 2004. [http://www.cdc.gov/communication/cdcynergy.htm].

Centers for Disease Control and Prevention. *National Public Health Performance Standards Program.* Atlanta: Centers for Disease Control and Prevention, 2000b. [http://www.phppo.cdc.gov/nphpsp]. Aug. 2005.

Centers for Disease Control and Prevention. Adult Immunization Programs in Nontraditional Settings: Quality Standards and Guidance for Program Evaluation. *Morbidity and Mortality Weekly Report,* 2000c, *49*(RR01), 1–13.

Centers for Disease Control and Prevention. "Evaluation of HIV Prevention Community Planning." Unpublished report of the National Center for HIV, STD, TB Prevention, Division of HIV/AIDS Prevention, Program Evaluation Research Branch. Atlanta: Centers for Disease Control and Prevention, 2002.

Centers for Disease Control and Prevention. *CD-Cynergy 3.0: Your Guide to Effective Health Communication.* Atlanta: Centers for Disease Control and Prevention, 2003.

Centers for Disease Control and Prevention. *School Health Index.* Atlanta: Centers for Disease Control and Prevention, 2004. [http://apps.nccd.cdc.gov/shi/]. July 2005.

Centers for Disease Control and Prevention. *Racial and Ethnic Approaches to Community Health (REACH) 2010: Addressing Disparities in Health.* Atlanta: Centers for Disease

Control and Prevention, 2005. [http://www.cdc.gov/nccdphp/aag/aag_reach.htm]. July 20, 2005.

Centraide Canada Board Basics Kit Manual, United Way of Canada. [http://www.boarddevelopment.org/display_document.cfm?document_id=110]. Oct. 24, 2005.

Chavis, D. M. "The Paradoxes and Promise of Community Coalitions." *American Journal of Community Psychology,* 2001, *29*(2), 309–320.

Chavis, D., and Florin, P. *Community Development, Community Participation and Substance Abuse Prevention.* San Jose, Calif.: Prevention Office, Bureau of Drug Abuse Services, 1990.

Chavis, D., Florin, P., and Felix, M. "Nurturing Grassroots Initiatives for Community Development: The Role of Enabling Systems." In T. Mizrahi and J. Morrison (eds.), *Community Organization and Social Administration: Advances, Trends, and Emerging Principles.* Binghamton, N.Y.: Haworth Press, 1992.

Chavis, D. M., Florin, P., Rich, R., and Wandersman, A. *The Role of Block Associations in Crime Control and Community Development: The Block Booster Project.* Report to the Ford Foundation, 1987.

Cheadle, A., and others. "Conference Report: Community-Based Health Promotion—State of the Art and Recommendations for the Future." *American Journal of Preventive Medicine,* 1997, *13*(4), 240–243.

Checkoway, B. "Six Strategies of Community Change," *Community Development Journal,* 1989, *30*(1), 2–20.

Chen, H. *Theory-Driven Evaluations.* Thousand Oaks, Calif.: Sage, 1990.

Chinman, M. J., and others. "The Perceptions of Costs and Benefits of High Active Versus Low Active Groups in Community Coalitions at Different Stages in Coalition Development." *Journal of Community Psychology,* 1996, *24*, 263–274.

Chinman, M., and others. "Using the Getting To Outcomes (GTO) Model in a Statewide Prevention Initiative." *Health Promotion Practice,* 2001, *2*(4), 204–209.

Chinman, M., Imm, P., and Wandersman, A. *Getting to Outcomes: Promoting Accountability Through Methods and Tools for Planning, Implementation and Evaluation.* Washington, D.C.: Rand Corporation, 2004; Report TR-101-CDC. [http://www.rand.org/publications/TR/TR101/]. Feb. 1, 2007.

Chrislip, D., and Larson, C. *Collaborative Leadership.* San Francisco: Jossey-Bass, 1994.

Civicus. *Promoting Your Organization.* 2005. [http://www.civicus.org/new/media/Promoting%20your%20organisation.doc]. Jan. 31, 2006.

Cividin, T. M., and Ottoson, J. M. "Linking Reasons for Continuing Professional Education Participation with Post-Program Application." *Journal of Continuing Education in the Health Professions,* 1997, *17*, 46–55.

Clark, N., Baker, E., and Chawla, A. "Sustaining Collaborative Problem-Solving: Strategies from a Study in Six Asian Countries." *Health Education Research,* 1993, *8*(3), 385–402.

Clark, N. M., Friedman, A. R., and Lachance, L. L. "Summing It Up: Collective Lessons from the Experience of Seven Coalitions." *Health Promotion Practice,* Supplement, 2006, *7*(2), 149–152S.

Clark, N. M., Malveaux, F., and Friedman, A. R. "An Introduction to Allies Against Asthma." *Health Promotion Practice,* Supplement, 2006, *7*(2), 8–12S.

Clark, N., and others. "Community Coalitions to Control Chronic Disease: Allies Against Asthma as a Model and Case Study." *Health Promotion Practice,* Supplement, 2006, *7*(2), 14–22S.

Clark, P., and Wilson, J. "Incentive Systems: A Theory of Organizations." *Administrative Science Quarterly,* 1961, *6,* 129–166.

Coe, B. A. "Open Focus: Implementing Projects in Multi-Organizational Settings." *International Journal of Public Administration,* 1988, *11*(4), 503–526.

Cohen, D. "Collaboration: What Works?" *Education Week,* 1989, *13.*

Cohen, L., Baer, N., and Satterwhite, P. "Developing Effective Coalitions: An Eight-Step Guide." In M. E. Wurzbach (ed.), *Community Health Education and Promotion: A Guide to Program Design and Evaluation.* (2nd ed.) Gaithersburg, Md.: Aspen, 2002, pp. 141–161. [http://www.opha.on.ca/resources/coalitions.pdf]. Sept. 15, 2005.

Cohen, L., and Gould, J. *The Tensions of Turf: Making It Work for the Coalition.* Oakland, Calif.: Prevention Institute, 2003.

Coley, S., and Scheinberg, C. *Proposal Writing.* Newbury Park, Calif.: Sage, 1990.

Collins, J. *Good to Great, Why Some Companies Make the Leap. . . , and Others Don't.* New York: HarperBusiness, 2001.

Collins, J. "Collins on Tough Calls." *Fortune, 75th Anniversary Special Issue,* June 27, 2005, pp. 89–94.

Community Catalyst, Inc. *Strength in Numbers: A Guide to Building Community Coalitions.* Boston: Community Catalyst, 2003. [http://communitycatalyst.org/resources]. Feb. 2, 2006.

Community Tool Box. *Developing an Organizational Structure for the Initiative: Writing Bylaws.* 2003. [http://ctb.ku.edu/tools/en/sub_section_main_1098.htm]. Apr. 6, 2006.

Community Tool Box. *Developing a Strategic Plan.* 2005a. [http://ctb.ku.edu/tools/en/section_1085.htm]. Jan. 15, 2006.

Community Tool Box. *Ethical Considerations in Community Interventions.* 2006. [http://ctb.ku.edu/tools/en/sub_section_main_1165.htm]. July 17, 2006.

Conone, R. M., Brown, D., and Willis, R. *Understanding the Problem Solving Process.* Fact Sheet CDFS-13. Columbus: Ohio State University Extension Service, 2005.

Connell, J. P., and Kubisch, A. C. "Applying a Theory of Change Approach to the Evaluation of Comprehensive Community Initiatives: Progress, Prospects, and Problems." In K. Fulbright-Anderson, A. C. Kubisch, and J. P. Connell (eds.), *New Approaches to Evaluating Community Initiatives: Theory, Measurement, and Analysis.* Washington, D.C.: Aspen Institute, 1998.

Connell, J. P., Kubisch, A. C., Schorr, L. B., and Weiss, C. H. *New Approaches to Evaluating Communities Initiatives: Concepts, Methods, and Contexts.* Washington, D.C.: Aspen Institute, 1995.

Cook, R., Roehl, J., Oros, C., and Trudeau, J. "Conceptual and Methodological Issues in the Evaluation of Community-Based Substance Abuse Prevention Coalitions: Lessons Learned from the National Evaluation of the Community Partnership Program." *American Journal of Community Psychology,* Special Issue, 1994, pp. 155–169.

Coombe, C. M. "Using Empowerment Evaluation in Community Organizing and Community-Based Health Initiatives. In M. Minkler (ed.), *Community Organizing and Community Building for Health.* New Brunswick, N.J.: Rutgers University Press, 1997.

Cosentino, A. J. *A Passion for Liberty: Alexis de Tocqueville on Democracy and Revolution.* Washington, D.C.: Library of Congress, 1989.

Cottrell, L. S., Jr. "The Competent Community." In R. Warren and L. Lyon (eds.), *New Perspectives on the American Community.* Homewood, Ill.: Dorsey, 1983, pp. 398–432.

Cousins, J. B., and Whitmore, E. "Framing Participatory Evaluation." In E. Whitmore (ed.), *Understanding and Practicing Participatory Evaluation,* 1998, vol. 80. San Francisco: Jossey-Bass, pp. 5–24.

Couto, R. A. "Social Capital and Leadership." In *Kellogg Leadership Studies Project: Transformational Leadership, Working Papers.* College Park, Md.: Academy of Leadership Press, 1997.

Couto, R., Simpson, N., and Harris, G. *Sowing Seeds in the Mountains: Community-Based Coalitions for Cancer Prevention and Control.* NIH Monograph No. 94-3779. Bethesda, Md.: National Institutes of Health, National Cancer Institute, 1994.

Covey, S. R. *Principle-Centered Leadership.* New York: Fireside Books, Simon and Schuster, 1990.

Cox, T. "The Multicultural Organization." *Academy of Management Executive,* 1991, 5(2), 34–47.

Crisp, B., Swerissen, H., and Duckett, S. "Four Approaches to Capacity Building in Health: Consequences for Measurement and Accountability." *Health Promotion International,* 2000, 15(2), 99–107.

Croan, G., and Lees, J. *Building Effective Coalitions: Some Planning Considerations.* Arlington, Va.: Westinghouse National Issues Center, 1979.

David, F. *Concepts of Strategic Management/Cases in Strategic Management,* 5th ed., 1995. Paramus, NJ: Prentice-Hall.

David, F. *Strategic Management: Concepts and Cases.* Indianapolis Prentice-Hall, 2001.

Delbecq, A. L., Van de Ven, A. H., and Gustafson, D. H. *Group Techniques for Program Planning: A Guide to Nominal Group Technique and Delphi Processes.* Glenview, Ill.: Scott Foresman, 1975.

Delgado, G. *From the Ground Up: Problems and Prospects for Community Organizing*. Applied Research Center Report. Oakland, Calif.: Ford Foundation, 1993.

DeLizia, J. S. "A Bumper Crop." *Component Relations*. Washington, D.C.: American Society of Association Executives, Sept. 2002.

The Democracy Center. *Citizen Action Series: Developing an Advocacy Strategy*. San Francisco: The Democracy Center, 2002. [http://www.democracyctr.org/resources/manual/curricula/doc1.htm]. Feb. 1, 2006.

Dill, A. "Institutional Environments and Organizational Responses to AIDS." *Journal of Health and Social Behavior*, 1994, *35*, 349–369.

Doble, J., and Johnson, J. *Science and the Public*. New York: The Public Agenda Foundation, 1991.

Dowling, J., O'Donnell, H., and Wellington Consulting Group. *A Development Manual for Asthma Coalitions*. Northbrook, Ill.: The CHEST Foundation and the American College of Chest Physicians, 2000.

Downs, A. "Up and Down with Ecology." *Public Interest*, Summer 1972, *28*, 38–50.

Downton, J. V. *Rebel Leadership: Commitment and Charisma Is a Revolutionary Process*. New York: Free Press, 1973.

Drinka, T. J. "Development and Maintenance of an Interdisciplinary Health Care Team: A Case Study." *Gerontology and Geriatrics Education*, 1991, *12*, 111–125.

Drucker Foundation. *Meeting the Collaboration Challenge*. San Francisco: Jossey-Bass, 2002.

DrugStrategies. *Assessing Community Coalitions*. Washington, D.C.: DrugStrategies, 2001.

Dryfoos, J. *Adolescents at Risk: Prevalence and Prevention*. New York: Oxford University Press, 1990.

Dugan, M. A. "Participatory and Empowerment Evaluation." In D. M. Fetterman, S. J. Kafterian, and A. Wandersman (eds.), *Empowerment Evaluation: Knowledge and Tools for Self-Assessment and Accountability*. Thousand Oaks, Calif.: Sage, 1996, pp. 277–303.

Dukes, E. Franklin. *Reaching Higher Ground: A Guide for Preventing, Preparing for, and Transforming Conflict for Tobacco Control Coalitions*. San Francisco: Tobacco Technical Assistance Consortium, 2000, pp. K1–K2. [http://www.cme.hsc.usf.edu/coph/immcoal/Duke%20Manual.pdf]. Sept. 23, 2006.

Dukes, E. F., Piscolish, M. A., and Stephens, J. B. *Reaching for Higher Ground in Conflict Resolution: Tools for Powerful Groups and Communities*. San Francisco: Jossey-Bass, 2000.

Dunet, D. O., Butterfoss, F. D., Hamre, R., and Kuester, S. "Using the State Plan Index to Evaluate the Quality of State Plans to Prevent Obesity and Other Chronic Diseases." *Preventing Chronic Diseases*. 2005. [http://www.cdc.gov/pcd/issues/2005/apr/04_0090.htm]. Jan. 12, 2007.

Edwards, S. L., and Stern, R. F. *Building and Sustaining Community Partnerships for Teen Pregnancy Prevention*. Houston, Tex.: Cornerstone Consulting Group, Inc., 1998.

Ellis, T. M., and Lenczner, S. J. "Lessons from the Field: A Report to the Annie E. Casey Foundation." Alexandria, Va.: Community Anti-Drug Coalitions of America, 2000.

Eng, E., and Blanchard, L. "Action-Oriented Community Diagnosis: A Health Education Tool." *International Quarterly of Community Health Education,* 1991, *11*(2), 93–110.

Eng, E., and Parker, E. "Measuring Community Competence in the Mississippi Delta: The Interface Between Program Evaluation and Empowerment." *Health Education Quarterly,* 1994, *21*, 199–220.

Eng, E., and Parker, E. "Natural Helper Models to Enhance a Community's Health and Competence." In R. DiClemente, R. Crosby, and M. C. Kegler (eds.), *Emerging Theories in Health Promotion Research and Practice,* San Francisco: Jossey-Bass, 2002, pp. 126–156.

Erfurt, J. C., Foote, A., Heirich, M. A., and Gregg, W. "Improving Participation in Worksite Wellness: Comparing Health Education Classes, a Menu Approach, and Follow-Up Counseling." *American Journal of Health Promotion,* 4(4), 1990, 270–278.

Every Child By Two. *News for Every Child.* Washington, D.C.: Every Child By Two, Aug. 1997. [http://www.ecbt.org/newsltr/local.htm]. Feb. 10, 2006.

Every Child By Two. *The Birth of Every Child By Two.* 2005. [http://www.ecbt.org/background.htm]. July 20, 2005.

Farquhar, J., and others. "Effects of Community-Wide Education on Cardiovascular Disease Risk Factors: The Five-City Project." *Journal of the American Medical Association,* 1990, *264*(3), 359–365.

Farrelly, M. C., Pechacek, T. R., and Chaloupka, F. J. The *Impact of Tobacco Control Programs on Aggregate Cigarette Sales, 1991–1998.* NBER Working Paper No. w8691. Cambridge, Mass.: National Bureau of Economic Research, Dec. 2001.

Fawcett, S., Francisco, V., Paine-Andrews, A., and Schultz, J. "Working Together for Healthier Communities: A Research-Based Memorandum of Collaboration." *Public Health Reports,* 2000, *115*(2/3), 174–179.

Fawcett. S., Paine, A., Francisco, V., and Vliet, M. "Promotion Health Through Community Development." In D. Glenwick and L. A. Jason (eds.), *Promoting Health and Mental Health in Children, Youth and Families.* New York: Springer, 1993, pp. 233–255.

Fawcett, S., and others. *Work Group Evaluation Handbook: Evaluating and Supporting Community Initiatives for Health and Development.* Lawrence, Kans.: Work Group on Health Promotion and Community Development, University of Kansas, 1993.

Fawcett, S. B., and others. *Preventing Adolescent Substance Abuse: An Action Planning Guide for Community-Based Initiatives.* Lawrence, Kans.: Work Group for Community Health and Development, University of Kansas, 1994.

Fawcett, S. B., and others. In collaboration with J. Johnston. *Reducing Risk for Chronic Disease: An Action Planning Guide for Community-Based Initiatives.* Lawrence, Kans.: University of Kansas, 1995.

Fawcett, S., and others. "Evaluating Community Coalitions for Prevention of Substance Abuse: The Case of Project Freedom." *Health Education and Behavior,* 1997, *24*(6), 812–828.

Fawcett, S. B., and others. "Evaluating Community Initiatives for Health and Development. In I. Rootman and others (eds.), *Evaluation in Health Promotion: Principles and Perspectives.* Copenhagen: World Health Organization—Europe, 2001.

Fawcett, S., and others. "Building Capacity for Participatory Evaluation Within Community Initiatives." *Journal of Prevention and Intervention in Community,* 2003, *26*(2), 21–36.

Federal Register, Superintendent of Documents, U.S., Washington, D.C.: Government Printing Office. [http://grants.gov]. Oct. 5, 2005.

Feighery, E., and Rogers, T. *Building and Maintaining Effective Coalitions.* Guide No. 12 in the series *How-to Guides on Community Health Promotion.* Palo Alto, Calif.: Health Promotion Resource Center, Stanford Center for Research in Disease Prevention, 1990.

Fetterman, D. M., Kaftarian, S. J., and Wandersman, A. (eds.). *Empowerment Evaluation: Knowledge and Tools for Self-Assessment and Accountability,* Thousand Oaks, Calif.: Sage, 1996.

Fetterman, D. M., and Wandersman, A. (eds.). *Empowerment Evaluation Principles in Practice.* New York: The Guilford Press, 2005.

Finklestein, E., French, S., Variyam, J. A., and Haines, P. S. "Pros and Cons of Proposed Interventions to Promote Healthy Eating." *American Journal of Preventive Medicine,* 2004, *27*(3s), 163–170.

Fisher, R. *Let the People Decide: Neighborhood Organizing in America.* New York: Twayne Publishers, 1994.

Fisher, R. "Social Action Community Organizing: Proliferation, Persistence, Roots and Prospects." In M. Minkler (ed.), *Community Organizing and Community Building for Health.* (2nd ed.) New Brunswick, N.J.: Rutgers University Press, 2005, pp. 51–65.

Fisher, R., and Romanofsky, P. (eds.). *Community Organization for Social Change.* Westport, Conn.: Greenwood Press, 1981.

Fisher, R., and Ury, W. *Getting to Yes: Negotiating Agreement Without Giving In.* (2nd ed.) New York: Penguin Books, 1991.

Florin, P., Mitchell, R., and Stevenson, J. "Identifying Training and Technical Assistance Needs in Community Coalitions: A Developmental Approach." *Health Education Research,* 1993, *8*(3), 417–432.

Florin, P., Mitchell, R., Stevenson, J., and Klein, I. "Predicting Intermediate Outcomes for Prevention Coalitions: A Developmental Perspective." *Evaluation and Program Planning,* 2000, *23*, 341–346.

Florin, P., and Wandersman, A. "An Introduction to Citizen Participation, Voluntary Organizations, and Community Development: Insights for Empowerment Research." *American Journal of Community Psychology,* 1990, *18*(1), 41–54.

Flynn, B. S. "Measuring Community Leaders' Perceived Ownership of Health Education Programs: Initial Tests of Reliability and Validity." *Health Education Research,* 1995, *10,* 27–36.

Forsythe, J. *A Guide to Coalition Building.* Canada: Cypress Consulting, 1997. [http://cypresscon.com/coaltion.html]. July 8, 2005.

Foster-Fishman P. G., and others. "Building Collaborative Capacity in Community Coalitions: A Review and Integrative Framework." *American Journal of Community Psychology,* 2001, *29*(2), 241–261.

Francisco, V. T., Butterfoss, F. D., and Capwell, E. M. "Key Issues in Evaluation: Quantitative and Qualitative Methods and Research Design." *Health Promotion Practice,* 2001, *2*(1), 20–23.

Francisco, V. T., Capwell, E. M., and Butterfoss, F. D., "Getting Off to a Good Start with Your Evaluation." *Health Promotion Practice,* 2000, *1*(2), 126–131.

Francisco, V., Fawcett, S., Schultz, J., and Paine-Andrews, A. "A Model of Health Promotion and Community Development." In F. B. Balcazar, M. Montero, and J. R. Newbrough (eds.), *Health Promotion in the Americas: Theory and Practice.* Washington, D.C.: Pan American Health Organization, 2000, pp. 17–34.

Francisco, V. T., Paine, A. L., and Fawcett, S. B. "A Methodology for Monitoring and Evaluating Community Health Coalitions." *Health Education Research,* 1993, *8*(3), 403–416.

Franklin, B. *Benjamin Franklin: His Autobiography 1706–1757.* First published in Philadelphia: J. B. Lippincott and Co., 1868. [http://etext.lib.virginia.edu/ benjaminfranklinhisautobiography/]. Mar. 17, 2005.

Friere, P. *Education for the Critical Consciousness.* New York: Seabury, 1973.

Friedman, A. R., and Wicklund, K. "Allies Against Asthma: A Midstream Comment on Sustainability." *Health Promotion Practice,* Supplement, 2006, *7*(2), 140–148.

Gabriel, R. "Methodological Challenges in Evaluating Community Partnerships and Coalitions: Still Crazy After All These Years." *Journal of Community Psychology,* 2000, *28*(3), 339–352.

Gallagher, K., and Drisko, J. *Building Community Capacity for Teen Pregnancy Prevention.* Denver: The Colorado Trust, 2000.

Gallegos, B. *Chasing the Frogs and Camels out of Los Angeles: The Movement to Limit Alcohol and Tobacco Billboards.* San Rafael, Calif.: Marin Institute for the Prevention of Alcohol and Other Drug Problems, 1999.

Garza, H. "Evaluating Partnerships: Seven Success Factors." *The Evaluation Exchange,* 2005, *10*(1), 18–19.

Gastil, J. *Common Problems in Small Group Decision Making.* Rome: United Nations' Food and Agriculture Organization, 1997. [http://www.fao.org/sd]. Nov. 15, 2005.

Giamartino, G., and Wandersman, A. "Organizational Climate Correlates of Viable Urban Block Organizations." *American Journal of Community Psychology,* 1983, *11*(5), 529–541.

Gilbert, G., and Sawyer, R. *Health Education: Creating Strategies for School and Community Health.* (2nd ed.) Boston: Jones and Bartlett, 2000.

Glidewell, J., Kelly, J., Bagby, M., and Dickerson, A. "Natural Development of Community Leadership." In R. S. Tindale and others (eds.), *Theory and Research on Small Groups.* New York: Plenum Press, 1998a.

Glidewell, J. C., Kelly, J. G., Bagby, M., and Dickerson, A. *Community Leadership: Theory and Practice.* In R. S. Tindale and others (eds.), *Applications of Theory and Research on Groups to Social Issues.* New York: Plenum, 1998b, pp. 61–86.

Goeppinger, J., and Baglioni, A. J., Jr. "Community Competence: A Positive Approach to Needs Assessment." *American Journal of Community Psychology,* 1985, *13,* 507–523.

Goldberg, M. E., Fishbein, M., and Middlestat, S. E. (eds.). *Social Marketing: Theoretical and Practical Perspectives.* Washington, D.C.: The Academy for Educational Development, 1997.

Goldman, K. D., and Schmalz, K. J. (eds.). "Media Do's and Don'ts." *Health Education Tools of the Trade.* Washington, D.C.: Society for Public Health Education, 2005.

Goldstein, S. "Community Coalitions: A Self-Assessment Tool." *American Journal of Health Promotion,* 1997, *11,* 430–435.

Goodman, R. M. "Principles and Tools for Evaluating Community-Based Prevention and Health Promotion Programs." *Journal of Public Health Management Practice,* 1998, *4*(2), 37–47.

Goodman, R. M., McLeroy, K. R., Steckler, A. B., and Hoyle, R. H. "Development of Level of Institutionalization Scales for Health Promotion Programs." *Health Education Quarterly,* 1993, *20,* 161–178.

Goodman, R. M., and Steckler, A. "A Model for Institutionalization of Health Promotion Programs." *Family and Community Health,* 1989, *11,* 63–78.

Goodman, R. M., Steckler, A., Hoover, S., and Schwartz, R. "A Critique of Contemporary Community Health Promotion Approaches: Based on a Qualitative Review of Six Programs in Maine." *American Journal of Health Promotion,* 1993, *7*(3), 208–220.

Goodman, R. M., and Wandersman, A. "FORECAST: A Formative Approach to Evaluating Community Coalitions and Community-Based Initiatives." *Journal of Community Psychology,* CSAP Special Issue, 1994, pp. 6–25.

Goodman, R. M., Wheeler, F. C., and Lee, P. R. "Evaluation of the Heart to Heart Project: Lessons from a Community-Based Chronic Disease Prevention Project." *American Journal of Health Promotion,* 1995, *9*(6), 443–455.

Goodman, R. M., and others. "An Ecological Assessment of Community-Based Interventions for Prevention and Health Promotion: Approaches to Measuring Community Coalitions." *American Journal of Community Psychology,* 1996, *24,* 33–61.

Goodman, R. M., and others. "Identifying and Defining the Dimensions of Community Capacity to Provide a Basis for Measurement." *Health Education and Behavior,* 1998, *25*(3), 258–278.

Gottlieb, N. H., Brink, S. G., and Gingiss, P. L. "Correlates of Coalition Effectiveness: The Smoke Free Class of 2000 Program." *Health Education Research*, 1993, *8*(3), 375–384.

Granner, M. L., and Sharpe, P. A. "Evaluating Community Coalition Characteristics and Functioning: A Summary of Measurement Tools." *Health Education Research*, 2004, *19*(5), 514–532. [http://prevention.sph.sc.edu/tools/CoalitonEvalInvent/pdf]. Jan. 12, 2006.

Gray, B. *Collaborating: Finding Common Ground for Multiparity Problems.* San Francisco: Jossey-Bass, 1989.

Gray, B. "Cross-Sectoral Partners: Collaborative Alliances Among Business, Government and Communities." In C. Huxham (ed.), *Creating Collaborative Advantage.* London: Sage, 1996.

Gray, B., and Wood, D. "Collaborative Alliances: Moving from Practice to Theory." *Journal of Applied Behavioral Science*, 1991, *27*(1), 3–22.

Green, L. "Caveats on Coalitions: In Praise of Partnerships." *Health Promotion Practice*, 2000, *1*(1), 64–65.

Green, L., George, M., Frankish, C., Herbert, C., Bowie, W., and O'Neil, M. *Study of Participatory Research in Health Promotion: Review and Recommendations for the Development of Participatory Research in Health Promotion in Canada.* Ottawa: Royal Society of Canada, 1995.

Green, L., and Kreuter, M. "CDC's Planned Approach to Community Health as an Application of PRECEDE and an Inspiration for PROCEED." *Journal of Health Education*, 1992, *23*(3), 140–147.

Green, L., and Kreuter, M. *Health Promotion Planning: An Educational and Ecological Approach.* (3rd ed.) Mountain View, Calif.: Mayfield, 1999, pp. 32–43.

Green, L., and Kreuter, M. "Fighting Back or Fighting Themselves? Community Coalitions Against Substance Abuse and Their Use of Best Practices." *American Journal of Preventive Medicine*, 2003, *23*(4), 303–306.

Green, L., Richard, L., and Potvin, L. "Ecological Foundations of Health Promotion." *American Journal of Health Promotion*, 1996, *10*, 270–81.

Greene, J. C. "Qualitative Program Evaluation: Practice and Promise." In N. K. Denzin and Y. S. Lincoln (eds.), *Handbook of Qualitative Research.* Thousand Oaks, Calif.: Sage, 1994.

Greene, J. C., and Caracelli, V. (eds.). *Advances in Mixed-Method Evaluation: The Challenges and Benefits of Integrating Diverse Paradigms: New Directions for Evaluation, No. 74.* San Francisco: Jossey-Bass, 1997.

Greene, J. C., and others. "Advantages and Challenges of Using Inclusive Evaluation Approaches in Evaluation Practice." *American Journal of Evaluation*, 1998, *19*(1), 101–122.

Griffin, S. F., and others. "Development of Multidimensional Scales to Measure Key Leaders' Perceptions of Community Capacity and Organizational Capacity for Teen Pregnancy Prevention." *Family and Community Health*, 2005, *28*(4), 307–319.

Grohol, J. *Community Organizing.* 2005. [http://psychcentral.com/psypsych/Community_organizing/]. July 14, 2005.

Grove Consultants International. *The Five Bold Steps Vision Plan.* San Francisco: Grove Consultants International. [http://www.grove.com/store/gg_fiveboldsteps.html]. Oct. 11, 2005.

Guetzkow, H., and Gyr, J. "An Analysis of Conflict in Decision-Making Groups." *Human Relations,* 1954, *7,* 367–382.

Gulati, R. "Social Structure and Alliance Formation Patterns: A Longitudinal Analysis." *Administrative Science Quarterly,* 1995, *40,* 619–652.

Habana-Hafner, S., Reed, H. B., and Associates. *Partnerships for Community Development: Resources for Practitioners and Trainers.* Amherst: University of Massachusetts Center for Organizational and Community Development, 1989.

Hall, R., and others. "Patterns of Interorganizational Relationships." *Administrative Science Quarterly,* 1977, *22,* 457–473.

Hall-Ellis, S. D., and others. In F. W. Hoffman (ed.), *Grantsmanship for Small Libraries and School Media Centers.* Englewood, Colo.: Libraries Unlimited, 1999.

Hallfors, D., Cho, H., Livert, D., and Kadushin, C. "'Fighting Back' Against Substance Abuse: Are Community Coalitions Winning?" *American Journal of Preventive Medicine,* 2002, *23*(4), 237–245.

Hancock, T. "The Evolution, Impact and Significance of the Healthy Cities/Healthy Communities Movement." *Journal of Public Health Policy,* 1993, *14*(1), 5–18.

Hancock, T., and Duhl, L. *Healthy Cities: Promoting Health in the Urban Context.* Copenhagen: World Health Organization, 1986.

Hancock, T., LaBonte, R., and Edwards, R. "Indicators That Count! Measuring Population Health at the Community Level." *Canadian Journal of Public Health,* Supplement, 1999, *90*(1), 22–26.

Hancock, T., and Minkler, M. "Community Health Assessment or Healthy Community Assessment?" In M. Minkler (ed.), *Community Organizing and Community Building for Health.* (2nd ed.) New Brunswick, N.J.: Rutgers University Press, 2005, pp. 138–157.

Harvey, T. B., and Drolet, B. *Building Teams, Building People: Expanding the Fifth Resource.* (2nd ed.) Lanham, Md.: Rowman & Littlefield, 2004.

Hawkins, C. *First Aid for Meetings: Quick Fixes and Major Repairs for Running Effective Meetings.* Wilsonville, Oreg.: BookPartners, 1998.

Hawkins, J. D., Miller, J. Y., and Catalano, R. J., Jr. *Communities That Care: Action for Drug Abuse Prevention.* San Francisco: Jossey-Bass, 1992.

Hays, C. E., Hays, S. P., DeVille, J. O., and Mulhall, P. F. "Capacity for Effectiveness: The Relationship Between Coalition Structure and Community Impact." *Evaluation and Program Planning,* 2000, *23,* 373–379.

Heffner, R. D. (ed.). *Democracy in America.* Translation of Alexis de Toqueville's *Democracy in America,* vol. I (1835) and vol. II (1840). New York: Penguin Putnam, 2001.

Heider, J. *The Tao of Leadership*. Atlanta: Humanics–New Age, 1985.

Heim P. and Chapman, E. N. *Learning to Lead, An Action Plan for Success,* 1990. Menlo Park, CA: Crisp Publication, Inc.

Heimlich, J. E., and Dresbach, S. H. *Written Documents for Community Groups: Bylaws and Standard Operating Procedures. Fact Sheet on Community Development.* Columbus: Ohio University, 2004. [http://ohioline.osu.edu/cd-fact/co-bl.html]. Oct. 18, 2005.

Henderson, N., Bernard, B., and Sharp-Light, N. (eds.). "Resiliency in Action: Practical Ideas for Overcoming Risks and Building Strengths in Youth, Families, and Communities." San Diego, Calif.: Resiliency in Action, 1999.

Herman, K., Wolfson, M., and Forster, J. "The Evolution, Operation, and Future of Minnesota SAFEPLAN: A Coalition for Family Planning." *Health Education Research,* 1993, *8*(3), 331–344.

Herron, D. B. *Marketing Nonprofit Programs and Services: Proven and Practical Strategies to Get More Customers, Members, and Donors.* San Francisco: Jossey-Bass, 1997.

Hersey, P. *The Situational Leader,* New York: Warner, 1984.

Hersey, P., Blanchard, K. H., and Johnson, D. E. *Management of Organizational Behavior.* (8th ed.) Englewood Cliffs, N.J.: Prentice-Hall, 2005.

Himmelman, A. *Communities Working Collaboratively for a Change.* Monograph. Minneapolis, Minn.: Himmelman Consulting Group, 1992.

Himmelman, A. "Communities Working Collaboratively for a Change." In M. S. Herrman (ed.), *Resolving Conflict: Strategies for Local Government.* Washington, D.C.: International City/County Management Association, 1994, pp. 27–47.

Himmelman, A. *Collaboration for a Change.* Minneapolis, Minn.: Himmelman Consulting, 2001. [http://www.aacpi.org/meeting/present_05/Roundtble/Petty.org]. Oct. 12, 2005.

Hingson, R., and others. "Reducing Alcohol-Impaired Driving in Massachusetts: The Impact of the Saving Lives Program." *American Journal of Public Health,* 1996, *86,* 791–797.

Holden, D., Pendergast, K., and Austin, D. *Literature Review for American Legacy Foundation's Statewide Youth Movement Against Tobacco Use—Draft Report.* Research Triangle Park, N.C.: Research Triangle Institute, 2000.

Holder, H. D., and Reynolds, R. I. "Application of Local Policy to Prevent Alcohol Problems: Experiences from a Community Trial." *Addiction,* 1997, *92,* 285–292.

Holli, B. B., and Calabrese, R. J. *Communication and Education Skills for Dietetics Professionals.* (3rd ed.) Baltimore, Md.: Williams and Wilkins, 1998.

Hord, S. "A Synthesis of Research on Organizational Collaboration." *Educational Leadership,* Feb. 1986, 22–26.

Huxham, C. "Theorizing Collaboration Practice." *Public Management Review,* 2003, *5*(3), 401–423.

Huxham, C., and Vangen, S. "What Makes Partnerships Work?" In S. Osborne (ed.), *Public-Private Partnerships: Theory and Practice in International Perspective.* London: Routledge, 2000.

ImpactTeen. *Tracking the Media and Policy Impacts of State-Level to Control: Smokeless States Evaluation.* Chicago, Ill.: ImpactTeen, 2005. [http://www.impactteen.org/states/aboutus.htm].

Independence Hall Association. *The Electric Franklin.* Philadelphia: Independence Hall Association. [http://www.ushistory.org/franklin/facts/index.htm/1995–2005]. July 12, 2005.

Institute of Medicine. *The Future of Public Health.* Washington, D.C.: The National Academies Press, 1988.

Institute of Medicine. In *The Future of the Public's Health in the 21st Century.* Washington, D.C.: The National Academies Press, 2002a.

Institute of Medicine. "The CHIP Model." In *The Future of the Public's Health in the 21st Century.* Washington, D.C.: National Academies Press, 2002b.

IRS Publication 557: Tax Exempt Status for Your Organization. 1997. [http://www.muridae.com/nporegulation/documents/exempt_orgs.html]. July 18, 2006.

Israel, B. A. "Special Networks and Health Status: Linking Theory, Research and Practice." *Patient Counseling and Health Education,* 1982, *4*(2), 65–79.

Israel, B. A., Checkoway, B., Schultz, A., and Zimmerman, M. "Health Education and Community Cmpowerment: Conceptualizing and Measuring Perceptions of Individual, Organizational and Community Control." *Health Education Quarterly,* 1994, *21*(2), 149–170.

Israel, B. A., Schultz, A. J., Parker, E. A., and Becker, A. B. "Review of Community-Based Research: Assessing Partnership Approaches to Improve Public Health." *Annual Review of Public Health,* 1998, *19*, 173–202.

Israel, B. A., and others. "Critical Issues in Developing and Following Community-Based Participatory Research Principles." In M. Minkler and N. Wallerstein (eds.), *Community-Based Participatory Research for Health.* San Francisco: Jossey-Bass, 2003, pp. 53–76.

Jackson, D., and Maddy, W. *Introduction to Coalitions.* Ohio State University Fact Sheet CDFS-1. Columbus: Ohio Center for Action on Coalitions, 2001. [http://ohioline.osu.edu/bc-fact/0001.html]. Sept. 26, 2005.

Jasuja, G. K., and others. "Using Structural Characteristics of Community Coalitions to Predict Progress in Adopting Evidence-Based Prevention Programs." *Evaluation and Program Planning,* 2005, *28*, 173–184.

Joffres, C., and others. "Facilitators and Challenges to Organizational Capacity Building in Heart Health Promotion." *Qualitative Health Research,* 2004, *14*(1), 39–60.

Join Together. *How Do We Know We Are Making a Difference?: A Community Alcohol, Tobacco, and Drug Indicators Handbook.* Boston: Join Together, 2005. [http://indicatorshandbook.org/indicators/]. Feb. 12, 2006.

Joint Committee on Standards for Educational Evaluation. *Program Evaluation Standards: How to Assess Evaluations of Educational Programs.* (2nd ed.) Thousand Oaks, Calif.: Sage, 1994.

Josephson Institute on Ethics. *Making Ethical Decisions.* Marina del Ray, Calif.: Josephson Institute on Ethics, 2003. [http://www.josephsoninstitute.org/MED/ MED-intro + toc.htm]. Nov. 14, 2005.

Julian, D. "Utilization of the Logic Model as a System Level Planning and Evaluation Device." *Evaluation and Program Planning,* 1997, *20*(3), 251–257.

Justice, T. I. *A Readers' Digest of the State of the Art in Organizational Development, Part One: On Being a Consultant: What Works.* Santa Monica, Calif.: T. I. Justice, 1993.

Kagan, S. L. *United We Stand: Collaboration for Child Care and Early Education Services.* New York: Columbia University Teachers College Press, 1991, pp. 1–3.

Kanter, R. M. "Collaborative Advantage: The Art of Alliances." *Harvard Business Review,* 1994, *72*(4), pp. 96–108.

Kanter, R. M. "The Enduring Skills of Change Leaders." *Leader to Leader,* 1999, *13*. [http://www.pfdf.org/leaderbooks/L2L/summer99/kanter.html]. Oct. 1, 2005.

Kaplan, M. "Cooperation and Coalition Development Among Neighborhood Organizations: A Case Study." *Nonprofit and Voluntary Sector Quarterly,* 1986, *15*(4), 23–34.

Katz, D., and Kahn, R. L. *The Social Psychology of Organizations.* (2nd ed.) New York: Wiley, 1978.

Katzenbach, J. R., and Smith, D. K. *The Wisdom of Teams: Creating the High Performance Organization.* Boston: Harvard Business School Press, 1993.

Kaye, G. "Grassroots Involvement." *American Journal of Community Psychology,* 2001, *29*(2), 269–275.

Kaye, G., and Wolff, T. (eds.). *From the Ground Up: A Workbook on Coalition Building and Community Development.* Amherst, Mass.: Area Health Education Center/ Community Partners, 1995.

Kaye, G., and Wolff, T. *American Lung Association Handbook.* 2000. New York: ALA.

Kayser, T. A. *Mining Group Gold: How to Cash in on the Collaborative Power of a Group.* San Diego, Calif.: Pfeiffer, 1990.

Kegler, M. C., Norton, B. L., and Aronson, R. E. *Evaluation of the Five-Year Expansion Program of California Healthy Cities and Communities, 1998–2003.* Sacramento, Calif.: Center for Civic Partnerships, 2003. [http://www.civicpartnerships.org/files/ TCEFinalReport9-2003.pdf]. Feb. 27, 2006.

Kegler, M., Steckler, A., Malek, S., and McLeroy, K. "A Multiple Case Study of Implementation in 10 Local Project ASSIST Coalitions in North Carolina." *Health Education Research,* 1998a, *13*(2), 225–238.

Kegler, M., Steckler, A., McLeroy, K., and Malek, S. "Factors That Contribute to Effective Community Health Promotion Coalitions: A Study of 10 Project ASSIST Coalitions in North Carolina." *Health Education and Behavior,* 1998b, *25*(3), 338–353.

Kegler, M., Twiss, J., and Look, V. "Assessing Community Change at Multiple Levels: The Genesis of an Evaluation Framework for the California Healthy Cities and Communities Project." *Health Education and Behavior,* 2000, *27*(6), 760–779.

Kegler, M. C., Wyatt, V. H., and Rodine, S. "Process Evaluation of an Asset-Based Teen Pregnancy Prevention Project: Healthy, Empowered, and Responsible Teens of Oklahoma City." In A. Steckler and L. Linnan (eds.), *Process Evaluation for Public Health Interventions and Research.* San Francisco: Jossey-Bass, 2005, pp. 31–57.

Kelly, C. S., Butterfoss, F. D., and Taylor-Fishwick, J. C. *CINCH Allies Against Asthma Planning.* Unpublished document. Norfolk, Va.: Center for Pediatric Research at Eastern Virginia Medical School, 2004.

Kelly, C. S., and others. "Engaging Health Care Providers in Coalition Activities." *Health Promotion Practice,* Supplement, 2006, *7*(2), 66–75S.

Keyser, B. B., and others. *Practicing the Application of Health Education Skills and Competencies.* Boston: Jones and Bartlett Publishers, 1997.

Kickert, W., Klijn, E. H., and Koopenjan, J. "Managing Networks in the Public Sector: Findings and Reflections." In W. Kickert, E. H. Klijn, and J. Koopenjan (eds.), *Managing Complex Networks.* London: Sage, 1997.

Kieffer, G. D. *The Strategy of Meetings.* New York: Simon and Schuster, 1998.

Kitzinger, J. "The Methodology of Focus Groups: The Importance of Interaction Between Research Participants." *Sociology of Health,* 1994, *16*(1), 103–121.

Kitzinger, J. "Introducing Focus Groups." *British Medical Journal,* 1995, *311,* 299–302.

Klijn, E. H., and Teisman, G. R. "Governing Public-Private Partnerships: Analyzing and Managing the Processes and Institutional Characteristics of Public-Private Partnerships." In S. Osborne (ed.), *Public-Private Partnerships: Theory and Practice in International Perspective.* London: Routledge, 2000.

Kline, M. V., and Huff, R. M. "Tips for the Practitioner." In R. M. Huff and M. V. Kline (eds.), *Promoting Health in Multicultural Populations.* Thousand Oaks, Calif.: Sage, 1999, pp. 103–111.

Klitzman, S., Kass, D., and Freudenberg, N. "Coalition Building to Prevent Childhood Lead Poisoning: A Case Study from New York City." In M. Minkler (ed.), *Community Organizing and Community Building for Health.* (2nd ed.) New Brunswick, N.J.: Rutgers University Press, 2005, pp. 314–327.

Klitzner, M. *National Evaluation Plan for Fighting Back.* Bethesda, Md.: Robert Wood Johnson Foundation, 1991.

Knoke, D., and Wright-Isak, C. "Individual Motives and Organizational Incentive Systems." *Research in the Sociology of Organizations,* 1982, *1,* pp. 209–254.

Kotler, P., Roberto, N., and. Lee, N. *Social Marketing: Improving the Quality of Life.* Thousand Oaks, Calif.: Sage, 2002.

Kotter, J. P. *The New Rules: How to Succeed in Today's Post-Corporate World.* New York: The Free Press, a Division of Simon and Schuster, 1995.

Kouzes, J. M., and Posner, B. Z. *The Leadership Challenge.* San Francisco: Jossey-Bass, 1987.

Kretzmann, J., and McKnight, J. *Building Communities from the Inside Out: A Path Toward Finding and Mobilizing a Community's Assets.* Evanston, Ill.: Center for Urban Affairs and Policy Research, Northwestern University, 1993.

Kretzmann, J., and McKnight, J. "Mapping Community Capacity." In M. Minkler (ed), *Community Organizing and Community Building for Health.* (2nd ed.) New Brunswick, N.J.: Rutgers University Press, 2005, pp. 158–172.

Kreuter, M. "PATCH: Its Origins, Basic Concepts, and Links to Contemporary Public Health Policy." *Journal of Health Education,* 1992, *23*(3), 135–139.

Kreuter, M., Lezin, N., and Young, L. "Evaluating Community-Based Collaborative Mechanisms: Implications for Practitioners." *Health Promotion Practice,* 2000, *1*(1), 49–63.

Kreuter, M. W., Nelson, C. F., Stoddard, R. P., and Watkins, N. B. *Planned Approach to Community Health.* Atlanta: Centers for Disease Control and Prevention, 1985.

Krieger, J. W., and others. "Integrating Asthma Prevention and Control: The Role of the Coalition." *Health Promotion Practice,* Supplement, 2006, *7*(2), 127–138S.

Kumpher, K., Turner, C., Hopkins, R., and Librett, J. "Leadership and Team Effectiveness in Community Coalitions for the Prevention of Alcohol and Other Drug Abuse." *Health Education Research,* 1993, *8*(3), 359–374.

LaBonte, R. *Health Promotion and Empowerment: Practice Frameworks.* Toronto, Ontario: Canada: Centre for Health Promotion, University of Toronto, 1993.

LaBonte, R. "Health Promotion and Empowerment: Reflections on Professional Practice." *Health Education Quarterly,* 1994, *21*(2), 253–268.

Langmeyer, D. B. "Sticky Figures: Using a Needs Assessment." Fact Sheet No. 27. Chapel Hill, N.C.: Action Research and Community Health and Development, 1993.

Lara, M., and others. "Improving Quality of Care and Promoting Health Care System Change: The Role of Community-Based Coalitions." *Health Promotion Practice,* Supplement, 2006, *7*(2), 87–95S.

Lasker, R. D., and Weiss, E. S. "Broadening Participation in Community Problem Solving: A Multidisciplinary Model to Support Collaborative Practice and Research." *Journal of Urban Health,* 2003, *80*(1), 14–48.

Lasker, R., Weiss, E., and Miller, R. *Promoting Collaborations That Improve Health.* Paper commissioned for the 4th Annual Community-Campus Partnerships for Health Conference, Apr. 29, 2000–May 2, 2000, Arlington, Va.

Lasker, R. D., Weiss, E. S., and Miller, R. "Partnership Synergy: A Practical Framework for Studying and Strengthening the Collaborative Advantage." *Milbank Quarterly,* 2001, *79*(2),179–205.

Lee, J., and Jackson, S. F. *Community-Based Coalitions and Intersectoral Partnerships: A Literature Review.* New York Community Health Promotion Research Unit Report Series 97-02, 1997.

Lefebvre, R., Lasater, T., Carleton, R., and Petersen, G. "Theory and Delivery of Health Programming in the Community: The Pawtucket Heart Health Program." *Preventive Medicine,* 1987, *16,* 80–95.

Levine, S., and White, P. "Exchange as a Conceptual Framework for the Study of Inter-Organizational Relationships." *Administrative Science Quarterly,* 1961, *5,* 583–601.

Lin, N. "Building a Network Theory of Social Capital." *Connections,* 1999, *22*(1), 28–51.

Lindsay, G., and Edwards, G. "Creating Effective Health Coalitions." *Health Education,* Aug./Sept. 1988, 35–36.

Linder and Ledlow, Five Issues to Be Considered in Teambuilding, 2005. [http://www.public.asu.edu/ledlow/sledlow/teambuilding.htm]. Oct. 22, 2005.

Linnan, L., and Steckler, A. (eds). *Process Evaluation for Public Health Interventions and Research.* San Francisco: Jossey-Bass, 2002.

Linney, J., and Wandersman, A. *Prevention Plus III: Assessing Alcohol and Other Drug Prevention Programs at the School and Community Level: A Four-Step Guide to Useful Program Assessment.* Rockville, Md.: U.S. Department of Health and Human Services, Center for Substance Abuse Prevention, 1991.

Lippincott, S. *Meetings: Do's, Don'ts, and Donuts.* Pittsburgh, Penn.: Lighthouse Point Press, 1994.

Loden, M., and Rosener, J. B. *Workforce America: Managing Diversity as a Vital Resource.* Homewood, Ill.: Business One Irwin Publishers, 1991.

Lofquist, W. A. *Discovering the Meaning of Prevention: A Practical Approach to Positive Change.* Tucson, Ariz.: AYD Publications, 1983.

Lolly, E. *Transformational Leadership.* Ohio Literacy Resource Center Leadership Institute, 1996. [http://literacy.kent.edu/Oasis/leadership/over2.htm]. Aug., 31, 2005.

Lynch, P. J., and Horton, S. *Web Style Guide: Basic Design Principles for Creating Web Sites.* (2nd ed.) New Haven, Conn.: Yale University Press, 2001. [http://www.webstyleguide.com/process/plan.html]. July 21, 2006.

Madison, A., Hung, R., and Jean-Louis, E. "The Boston Haitian HIV Prevention Coalition Formative Evaluation: A Participatory Approach to Community Self-Assessment." *Ethnicity and Disease,* 2004, *14,* S20-6.

Mannino, D. M., Homa, D. M., Pertowski, C. A., and others. "Surveillance for Asthma—United States, 1960–1998." *Morbidity and Mortality Weekly Report,* 1998, *47,* 1–28.

Mansergh, G., and others. "Process Evaluation of Community Coalitions for Alcohol and Other Drug Abuse: A Case Study Comparison of Researcher- and Community-Initiated Models." *Journal of Community Psychology,* 1996, *24,* 118–135.

Marmot, M., and Wilkinson, R. G. *Social Determinants of Health.* Oxford, England: Oxford University Press, 1999.

Marrett, C. "On the Specification of Interorganizational Dimensions." *Sociology and Social Research,* 1971, *56,* 83–99.

Martin, G., and Pear, J. *Behavior Modification: What It Is and How To Do It.* Englewood Cliffs, N.J.: Prentice-Hall, 1992.

Mattesich, P., Murray-Close, M., and Monsey, B. *Collaboration: What Makes It Work—A Review of the Research Literature on Factors Influencing Successful Collaboration.* (2nd ed.) St. Paul, Minn.: Amherst H. Wilder Foundation, 2001.

Mattesich, P., and Monsey, B. *Community Building: What Makes It Work—A Review of Factors Influencing Successful Community Building.* (2nd ed.) St. Paul, Minn.: Amherst H. Wilder Foundation, 2005.

Matthews, D. *The Promise of Democracy.* Dayton, Ohio: Kettering Foundation, 1994.

Maxwell, J. A., and Lincoln, Y. S. "Methodology and Epistemology: A Dialogue." *Harvard Educational Review,* 1990, *60*(4), 497–512.

Mayer, J., and others. "Practices of Successful Community Coalitions: A Multiple Case Study." *American Journal of Health Behavior,* 1998, *22*(5), 368–377.

McClelland, D. C. *Human Motivation.* New York: Cambridge University Press, 1988.

McConnell, R. "Minutes." *Parliamentary Internet Newsletter,* 1996, *2*(4). Robert McConnell Productions. [http://www.parli.com/newsletter/news697.htm]. Nov. 14, 2005.

McConnell, R. "Bylaws." *Parliamentary Internet Newsletter,* 1997a, *3*(3). Robert McConnell Productions. [http://www.parli.com/newsletter/news697.htm]. Nov. 14, 2005.

McConnell, R. "Parliamentary Procedure in a Community Group from a Communication Perspective." *Parliamentary Internet Newsletter,* 1997b, *3*(5). Robert McConnell Productions. [http://www.parli.com/newsletter/news697.htm]. Nov. 14, 2005.

McDermott, R. J., and Sarvela, P. D. *Health Education Evaluation and Measurement: A Practitioner's Perspective.* (2nd ed.) New York: McGraw-Hill, 1999.

McDonald, M., Sarche, J., and Wang, C. C. "Using the Arts in Community Organizing and Community Building." In M. Minkler (ed.), *Community Organizing and Community Building for Health.* (2nd ed.) New Brunswick, N.J.: Rutgers University Press, 2005, pp. 346–364.

McEwan, K. L., and Bigelow, D. A. "Using a Logic Model to Focus Health Services on Population Health Goals." *Canadian Journal of Program Evaluation,* 1997, *12*(1), 167–174.

McGinnis, J. M. "With Both Eyes Open: The Guide to Community Preventive Services." *American Journal of Preventive Medicine,* 2005, *28*(5S), 223–225.

McKenzie, J. F., Neiger, B. L., and Smeltzer, J. L. *Planning, Implementing and Evaluating Health Promotion Programs.* (4th ed.) San Francisco: Pearson/Benjamin Cummings, 2005.

McKinlay, J. "A Case for Refocusing Upstream: The Political Economy of Illness." In P. Conrad (ed.), *The Sociology of Health and Illness.* (6th ed.) London: Worth Publishers, 2000, pp. 551–564.

McKnight, J. *The Careless Society: Community and Its Counterfeits.* New York: Basic Books, 1995.

McKnight, J., and Kretzmann, J. "Community Organizing in the 80s: Toward a Post-Alinsky Agenda." *Social Policy,* Winter 1984, pp. 145–147.

McLaughlin, J. A., and Jordan, G. B. "Logic Models: A Tool for Telling Your Program's Performance Story." *Evaluation and Program Planning,* 1999, *22*(1), 65–72.

McLeroy, K., Bibeau, D., Steckler, A., and Glanz, K. "An Ecological Perspective on Health Promotion Programs." *Health Education Quarterly,* 1988, *15*(4), 351–377.

McLeroy, K., and others. "Community Coalitions for Health Promotion: Summary and Further Reflections." *Health Education Research,* 1994, *9*(1), 1–11.

McMillan, B., and others. "Empowerment Praxis in Community Coalitions." *American Journal of Community Psychology,* 1995, *23*(5), 699–727.

McNamara, C. *Evaluation Pitfalls to Avoid.* 2006. [http://www.mapnp.org/library/evaluatn/fnl_eval.htm].#anchor1586742]. Oct. 29, 2005.

McNeese, I. C. *Communication: Model and Types, Family Community Leadership Program.* Columbus: The Ohio State University Cooperative Extension Service, 1991.

McQueen, D. V., and Anderson, L. M. "What Counts as Evidence? Issues and Debates on Evidence Relevant to the Evaluation of Community Health Promotion Programs." In I. Rootman, M. Goodstadt, and B. Hyndman (eds.), *Evaluation in Health Promotion: Principles and Perspectives.* Copenhagen: World Health Organization, 1999.

Meek, J. *Goals and Objectives.* Columbus: Ohio State University CRD 4, 1993. [http://www.extension.iastate.edu/Publications/PM1486C.pdf]. Nov. 10, 2005.

Merzel, C., and D'Affliti, J. "Reconsidering Community Based Health Promotion: Promise, Performance and Potential." *American Journal of Public Health,* 2003, *93*(4), 557–574.

Milio, N. *Promoting Health Through Public Policy.* Ottawa: Canadian Public Health Association, 1989.

Miles, M. B., and Huberman, A. M. *Qualitative Data Analysis: An Expanded Sourcebook.* (2nd ed.) Thousand Oaks, Calif.: Sage, 1994.

Miller, L. C., Rossing, B. E., and Steel, S. M. *Partnerships: Shared Leadership Among Stakeholders.* Madison: University of Wisconsin, 1992.

Millstein, B., Wetterhall, S., and the Centers for Disease Control and Prevention Evaluation Working Group. "Developing a Process-Evaluation Plan for Assessing Health Promotion Program Implementation: A How-To Guide." *Health Promotion Practice,* 2000, *1*(3), 221–228.

Minkler, M. (ed.). *Community Organizing and Community Building for Health.* (2nd ed.) New Brunswick, N.J.: Rutgers University Press, 2005.

Minkler, M. "Using Participatory Action Research to Build Healthy Communities." *Public Health Reports,* 2000, *115,* 191–197.

Minkler, M., and Wallerstein, N. "Improving Health Through Community Organization and Community Building: A Health Education Perspective." In M. Minkler (ed.), *Community Organizing and Community Building for Health.* (2nd ed.) New Brunswick, N.J.: Rutgers University Press, 2005, p. 26.

Mitchell, S. M., and Shortell, S. M. "The Governance and Management of Effective Community Health Partnerships: A Typology for Research, Policy and Practice." *The Milbank Quarterly,* 2000, *78*(2), 241–289.

Mittelmark, M. "Health Promotion at the Community Level: Lessons from Diverse Perspectives." In N. Bracht (ed.), *Health Promotion at the Community Level*. Thousand Oaks: Sage, 1999.

Mittelmark, M. B., Hunt, M. K., Heath, G. W., and Schmidt, T. L. "Realistic Outcomes: Lessons from Community-Based Research and Demonstration Programs for the Prevention of Cardiovascular Diseases." *Journal of Public Health Policy*, 1993, *14*, 437–462.

Mittelmark, M., and others. "Community-Wide Prevention of Cardiovascular Disease: Education Strategies of the Minnesota Heart Health Program." *Preventive Medicine*, 1986, *15*(1), 1–17.

Mizrahi, T., and Rosenthal, B. "Managing Dynamic Tensions in Social Change Coalitions." In T. Mizrahi and J. Morrison (eds.), *Community Organization and Social Administration Trends and Emerging Principles*. New York: Haworth Press, 1993, pp. 11–35.

Mizrahi, T., and Rosenthal, B. S. "Complexities of Coalition Building: Leaders' Successes, Strategies, Struggles and Solutions." *Social Work*, 2001, *46*(1), 63–78.

Mizruchi, M., and Galaskiewicz, J. "Networks of Interorganizational Relations." In S. Wasserman and J. Galaskiewicz (eds.), *Advances in Social Network Analysis: Research in the Social and Behavioral Sciences*. Thousand Oaks, Calif.: Sage, 1994.

Mojkowski, C. "Systemic School Restructuring: Implications for Helping Organizations." *Journal of Staff Development*, 1995, *16*(2), 50–54.

Moore, C. *Group Techniques for Idea Building*. Applied Social Research Methods Series, vol. 9. Thousand Oaks, Calif.: Sage, 1990.

Moore, K. A., Sugland, B. W., and others. *Adolescent Pregnancy Prevention Programs: Interventions and Evaluations*. Washington, D.C.: Child Trends, Inc., 1995.

Moos, R. *Group Environment Scale Manual*. (2nd ed.) Palo Alto, Calif.: Consulting Psychologists Press, 1986.

Moos, R. H., Insel, P. M., and Humphrey, B. *Preliminary Manual for Family Environment Scale, Work Environment Scale, and Group Environment Scale*. Palo Alto, Calif.: Consulting Psychologists Press, 1974.

Morgan, D. L. *Focus Groups as Qualitative Research*. (2nd ed.) London: Sage, 1997.

Morgan, L. M. "Community Participation in Health: Perpetual Allure, Persistent Challenge." *Health Policy and Planning*, 2001, *16*(3), 221–230.

Morgan, D. L., and Krueger, R. A. "When to Use Focus Groups and Why." In D. L. Morgan (ed.), *Successful Focus Groups*. London: Sage, 1993.

Morrow, A. L., and others. "A Population-Based Study of Risk Factors for Under-Immunization Among Urban Virginia Children Served by Public, Private and Military Health Care Systems." *Pediatrics*, 1998, *101*(2), E5.

Mosaica. *Boards of Directors and Private-Sector Fundraising: Getting Started*. Washington, D.C.: Mosaica, 2005a. [http://mosaica.coure-tech.com/resources/brdfdr.pdf]. Jan. 5, 2005.

Mosaica. *Developing an Effective Organizational Message.* Washington, D.C.: Mosaica, 2005b. [http://mosaica.coure-tech.com/resources/mess.pdf]. Jan. 6, 2006.

Mosaica. *From Concept to Funded Program: Practical Steps in Program Development.* Washington, D.C.: Mosaica, 2005c. [http://mosaica.coure-tech.com/resources/con2des.pdf]. Jan. 6, 2006.

Mosaica. *Preparing Effective, Competitive Grant Applications.* Washington, D.C.: Mosaica, 2005d. [http://mosaica.coure-tech.com/preapps.pdf]. Jan. 5, 2005.

Mosaica. *Sustainability.* Washington, D.C.: Mosaica, 2005e.

Mulroy, E. A. "Building a Neighborhood Network: Interorganizational Collaboration to Prevent Child Abuse and Neglect." *Social Work,* 1997, *42*(3), 255–264.

Munodawafa, D., Gwede, C., and Mubayira, C. "Using Focus Groups to Develop HIV Education Among Adolescent Females in Zimbabwe." *Health Promotion,* 1995, *10*(2), 85–92.

Nagy, J. "Developing a Plan for Financial Sustainability." In T. Wolff and P. Rabinowitz (eds.), *Community Tool Box.* Lawrence, Kans.: Community Tool Box, 2006. [http://ctb.ku.edu/tools/EN/sub_section_main_1297.htm]. Jan. 4, 2006.

National Assembly of National Voluntary Health and Social Welfare Organizations. *The Community Collaboration Manual.* Washington, D.C.: National Assembly of National Voluntary Health and Social Welfare Organizations, 1993.

The National Campaign to Prevent Teen Pregnancy. *Breaking Ground: Lessons Learned from the Centers for Disease Control and Prevention's Community Coalition Partnership Programs for the Prevention of Teen Pregnancy.* Washington, D.C.: The National Campaign to Prevent Teen Pregnancy, 2003. [http://www.dhs.state.or.us/children/publications/tpp/breakingground.pdf]. Dec. 19, 2005.

National Cancer Institute. *Making Health Communications Work.* 2002. [http://www.cancer.gov]. July 20, 2005.

National Cancer Institute. *Study Shows Strong Tobacco Control Programs and Policies Lower Smoking Rates.* 2003. [http://www.cancer.gov/newscenter/pressreleases/ASSIST]. July 20, 2005.

National Cancer Institute. *NCI ASSIST: Shaping the Future of Tobacco Prevention and Control.* Monograph No. 16. Bethesda, Md.: U.S. Department of Health and Human Services, National Institutes of Health, National Cancer Institute. 2005. [http://dccps.nci.nih.gov/tcrb/monographs/16/m16_11.pdf]. Feb. 7, 2006.

National Network for Collaboration. *Collaboration Framework . . . Addressing Community Capacity.* Fargo, N.D.: National Network for Collaboration, 1996.

National Network for Health. *Collaboration Checklist.* 2004. [http://www.nnh.org/tobacco/appe-18-2.htm]. Feb. 23, 2006.

Nelson, G. "The Development of a Mental Health Coalition: A Case Study." *American Journal of Community Psychology,* 1994, *22*(2), 229–255.

Nelson, R. B., and Economy, P. *Better Business Meetings.* Burr Ridge, Ill.: Irwin, 1995, p. 5.

Nezlek, J., and Galano, J. "Developing and Maintaining State-Wide Adolescent Pregnancy Prevention Coalitions: A Preliminary Investigation." *Health Education Research*, 1993, *8*(3), 433–447.

Nicholas, E. A., and others. "Coalition-Based Approaches for Addressing Environmental Issues in Childhood Asthma." *Health Promotion Practice*, Supplement, 2006, *7*(2), 108–116S.

Northouse, P. G. *Leadership.* (2nd ed.) Thousand Oaks, Calif.: Sage, 2001.

Norton, B., and others. "Community Capacity: Concept, Theory, and Methods." In R. DiClemente, R. Crosby, M. Kegler (eds.), *Emerging Theories in Health Promotion Practice and Research.* San Francisco: Jossey-Bass/Wiley, 2002, pp. 194–227.

Norton, B., Kegler, M., and Aronson, R. *Evaluation of the Five-Year Expansion Program of California Healthy Cities and Communities (1998–2003).* Sacramento, Calif.: Center for Civic Partnerships, 2003. [http://www.civicpartnerships.org/files/ExecSummary.pdf]. Feb. 15, 2006.

Novelli, W. D. "Marketing Health and Social Issues: What Works?" In R. Dunmire (ed.), *Social Marketing: Accepting the Challenge in Public Health.* Atlanta: Centers for Disease Control and Prevention, 1988.

O'Donnell, J., and others. "Partners for Change: Community Residents and Agencies." *Journal of Sociology and Social Welfare*, 1998, *25*(1), 133–151.

Office of Minority Health. *Minority Community Health Coalition Demonstration Program, HIV/AIDS.* 2003. [http://www.omhrc.gov/omh/aids/2k3/2937_3C8.htm]. July 20, 2005.

Office of Quality Improvement. *Composite Checklist for Responsibilities of Meeting Chair.* Madison: University of Wisconsin System Board of Regents, 2002.

Ogden, L., Shepherd, M., and Smith, W. A. *Applying Prevention Marketing.* Atlanta: Centers for Disease Control and Prevention, Public Health Service, 1996.

Ohio State University. *Tapping Private Resources.* Ohio State University Fact Sheet CDFS-16. Columbus: Ohio State University, 2002. [http://ohioline.osu.edu/bc-fact/0016.html]. Dec. 20, 2005.

Ohio State University. *Working with Diverse Cultures.* Ohio State University Extension Fact Sheet CDFS-14. Columbus: Ohio State University, 2005. [http://ohioline.osu.edu/bc-fact/0014.html]. Sept. 9, 2005.

Online PR and Marketing. *How to Create a Brochure.* [http://onlinepr.gbwatch.com/?p=25]. July 17, 2006.

Ontario Healthy Communities Coalition, "Is a Coalition Right for you?" *From the Ground Up: An Organizing Handbook for Healthy Communities.* Toronto, Ontario: Author, 2003. [http://www.healthycommunities.on.ca/publications/ground/Ground-Section4.pdf.]. Feb. 10, 2007.

Opubor, A., Egero, B., and Mensah-Kumah, O. Strategic *Options for HIV/AIDS Advocacy in Africa: Report of the Joint UNFPA, UNAIDS, HIV/AIDS Advocacy Mission to Africa.* New York: Joint United Nations Programme on HIV/AIDS, 2000.

Oral Health America. *Coalition Best Practices White Paper.* Chicago: Oral Health America, 2001.

Ottoson, J. M. "After the Applause: Exploring Multiple Influences on Application Following an Adult Education Program." *Adult Education Quarterly*, 1997, *47*(2), 92–107.

Parachini, L., and Covington, S. *Community Organizing Toolbox: A Funder's Guide to Community Organizing.* Neighborhood Funders Group. 2001. [http://www.nfg.org/cotb/09historyco.htm]. July 14, 2005.

Paris, C. A., Salas, E., and Cannon-Bowers, J. A. "Teamwork in Multi-Person Systems: A Review and Analysis." *Ergonomics*, 2000, *43*(8), 1052–1075.

Partnership for Prevention. *Comprehensive and Integrated Chronic Disease Prevention Action Planning Handbook for States and Communities*, version 1.0. Washington, D.C.: Partnership for Prevention, 2004.

Patton, M. Q. *Utilization-Focused Evaluation: The New Century Text.* (3rd ed.) Thousand Oaks, Calif.: Sage, 1997a.

Patton, M. Q. "Toward Distinguishing Empowerment Evaluation and Placing It in a Larger Context." *Evaluation Practice*, 1997b, *18*(2), 147–163.

Peck, G. P., and Hague, C. E. *Turf Issues.* Fact Sheet CDFS-12. Columbus: Ohio State University Extension, 2005. [http://ohioline.osu.edu/bc-fact/0012.html]. Sept. 26, 2005.

Penner, S. "A Study of Coalitions Among HIV/AIDS Service Organizations." *Sociological Perspectives*, 1995, *38*(2), 217–239.

Pepper, S. K., Herrera, C., and Leviton, L. *Faith in Action: Using Interfaith Coalitions to Support Voluntary Care Giving Efforts.* 2003. [http://www.religionandsocialpolicy.org/docs/events/2003_spring_research_conference/pepper.pdf]. Nov. 17, 2005.

Perkins, D. D., Brown, B. B., and Taylor, R. B. "The Ecology of Empowerment: Predicting Participation in Community Organizations." *Journal of Social Issues*, 1996, *52*(1), 85–110.

Perkins, D., and others. "Participation and the Social and Physical Environment of Residential Blocks: Crime and Community Context." *American Journal of Community Psychology*, 1990, *18*(1), 83–115.

Peterson, J. W., and others. "Engaging the Community in Coalition Efforts to Address Childhood Asthma." *Health Promotion Practice*, Supplement, 2006, *7*(2), 56–65S.

Phillips, J. J. *Handbook of Training, Evaluation and Measurement Methods.* (3rd ed.) Houston, TX: Gulf Publishing Company, 1997.

Pickeral, T. "Coalition Building and Democratic Principles." *Service Learning Network Newsletter*, 2005, *11*(1), 1–2.

Pickett, G. E., and Hanlon, J. J. *Public Health Administration and Practice.* St. Louis, Mo.: Moseby–Year Book, McGraw-Hill, 1990.

Porteous, N. L., Sheldrick, B. J., & Stewart, P. J. "Enhancing Manager's Evaluation Capacity: A Case Study from Ontario Public Health." *The Canadian Journal of Program Evaluation*, 1999, Special Issue, 137–154.

Prestby, J., and Wandersman, A. "An Empirical Exploration of a Framework of Organizational Viability: Maintaining Block Organizations." *The Journal of Applied Behavioral Science*, 1985, *21*(3), 287–305.

Prestby, J., and others. "Benefits, Costs, Incentive Management and Participation in Voluntary Organizations: A Means to Understanding and Promoting Empowerment." *American Journal of Community Psychology,* 1990, *18*(1), 117–149.

Prochaska, J. O., DiClemente, C. C., and Norcross, J. C. "In Search of How People Change: Applications to Addictive Behaviors." *American Psychologist,* 1992, *47*(9), 1102–1114.

Promising Practices Network on Children, Families and Communities. *Programs That Work.* 2005. [http://www.promisingpractices.net/research.asp]. Jan. 3, 2005.

Provan, K. and Milward, H. "A Preliminary Theory of Interorganizational Network Effectiveness: A Comparative Study of Four Community Mental Health Systems." *Administrative Science Quarterly,* 1995, *40,* 1–33.

Provan, K. G., and Milward, H. B. "Do Networks Really Work? A Framework for Evaluating Public-Sector Organizational Networks." *Public Administration Review,* 2001, *61*(4), 414–424.

Putnam, R. *Making Democracy Work.* Princeton, N.J.: Princeton University Press, 1993.

Putnam, R. D. "Bowling Alone: America's Declining Social Capital." *Journal of Democracy,* 1995, *6*(1), 65–78.

Quinn, S. C. "Teaching Community Diagnosis: Integrating Community Experience with Meeting Graduate Standards for Health Educators." *Health Education Research,* 1999, *14*(5), 685–696.

Quinn, S. C. "Professional Development of Health Educators Through a Community Diagnosis Training Experience: Observations and Perspectives." *Health Promotion Practice,* 2000, *1*(2), pp. 159–167.

Rabinowitz, P. "Criteria for Choosing Promising Practices and Community Interventions." In J. Schultz and V. Renault (eds.), *Community Tool Box.* Lawrence, Kans.: Community Tool Box, 2003a. [http://ctb.ku.edu/tools/EN/sub_section_main_1152.htm]. Jan. 15, 2006.

Rabinowitz, P. "Building Teams: Broadening the Base for Leadership." In B. Berkowitz (ed.), *Community Tool Box.* Lawrence, Kans.: Community Tool Box, 2003b. [http://ctb.ku.edu/tools/en/sub_section_main_1123.htm]. Jan. 18, 2006.

Rabinowitz, P. "Planning and Writing an Annual Budget." In B. Berkowitz and T. Brownlee (eds.), *Community Tool Box.* Lawrence, Kans.: Community Tool Box, 2006. [http://ctb.ku.edu/tools/EN/sub_section_main_1303.htm]. Jan. 12, 2006.

Ramirez, C. "The Power of Branding." *The Virginian Pilot,* Sept. 25, 2005, p. B2.

Rappaport, J. "Studies in Empowerment: Introduction to the Issue." *Prevention in Human Services,* 1984, *3*(2–3), 1–7.

Rebori, M. "Two Techniques to Foster Collaboration Within a Group." *Journal of Extension,* 2000, *38*(4). [http://www.joe.org/joe/2000August/tt4.html.] Jan. 18, 2007.

Reichardt, C. S., and Rallis, S. F. (eds.). "The Qualitative-Quantitative Debate: New Perspectives." In W. R. Shaddish (ed.), *New Directions for Program Evaluation,* vol. 61. San Francisco: Jossey-Bass, 1994, pp. 1–98.

Reinheimer R., and Jenkins, S. *Southern Appalachia Leadership Initiative on Cancer Coalition Manual.* Athens, Ga.: Institute of Community and Area Development, 1994.

Reininger, B., Dinh-Zarr, T., Sinicrope, P., and Martin, D. "Dimensions of Participation and Leadership: Implications for Community-Based Health Promotion for Youth." *Family and Community Health,* 1999, *22*(2), 72–82.

Rich, R. "The Dynamics of Leadership in Neighborhood Organizations." *Social Science Quarterly,* 1980, *60*(4), 570–587.

Riker, W. "The Theory of Political Coalitions." In E. Weisner (ed.), *Notes on Policy and Practice.* New Haven, Conn.: Yale University Press, 1962.

Robert Wood Johnson Foundation. *The Fighting Back National Program Report.* 2002. [http://www/rwjf.org/reports/npreports/fighting back.htm]. July 19, 2005.

Robert Wood Johnson Foundation. *Back to School Campaign Promotes Uninsured Kids' Enrollment in SCHIP and Medicaid.* Princeton, N.J.: Robert Wood Johnson Foundation, 2005a. [http://www.rwjf.org/newsroom/activitydetail.jsp?id=10151andtype=2]. Aug. 2, 2005.

Robert Wood Johnson Foundation. *SmokeLess States National Tobacco Policy Initiative.* Princeton, N.J.: Robert Wood Johnson Foundation, 2005b. [http://www.rwjf.org/reports/npreports/smokeless.htm]. Feb. 24, 2006.

Robert, H. M., III, Evans, W. J., Honemann, D. H., and Balch, T. J. *Robert's Rules of Order.* (10th ed.) Cambridge, Mass.: Perseus Books Group, 2000.

Roberts-DeGennaro, M. "Factors Contributing to Coalition Maintenance." *Journal of Sociology and Social Welfare,* 1986, *13,* 248–264.

Robinson, L. "The Seven Doors Social Marketing Approach." *Enabling Change,* 2006. [http://www.enabling-change.com.au/]. Nov. 29, 2006.

Rogers, E. M. *Diffusion of Innovations.* (4th ed.) New York: Free Press, 1995.

Rogers, T., and others. "Characteristics and Participant Perceptions of Tobacco Control Coalitions in California." *Health Education Research,* 1993, *8*(3), 345–357.

Rosenthal, B. "Multicultural Issues in Coalitions." In G. Kaye and T. Wolff (eds.), *From the Ground Up: A Workbook on Coalition Building and Community Development.* Amherst, Mass.: AHEC/Community Partners, 1995, pp. 51–73.

Rosenthal, B. *1 + 1 = 3: A Collaboration Guidebook.* (2nd ed.) Code No. 5033. Atlanta: American Cancer Society National Advisory Group on Collaboration with Organizations, 2000.

Rosenthal, B., and Rubel, D. *How to Conduct a Needs Assessment Study in Your Community: A Training Manual for Community Board and Area Policy Members.* Prepared for the New York City Community Development Agency, 1991.

Ross, R. S. "Conflict." In R. Ross and J. Ross (eds.), *Small Groups in Organizational Settings.* Englewood Cliffs, N.J.: Prentice-Hall, 1989, pp. 139–178.

Rothschild, M. L. "Carrots, Sticks and Promises: A Conceptual Framework for the Management of Public Health and Social Issue Behaviors." *Journal of Marketing,* 1999, *63*(3), 24–37.

Rothman, J. "Approaches to Community Intervention." In J. Rothman, L. Erlich, and J. E. Tropman (eds.), *Strategies of Community Intervention.* (5th ed.) Itasca, Ill.: Peacock, 1995, pp. 27–64.

Roussos, S., and Fawcett, S. "A Review of Collaborative Partnerships as a Strategy for Improving Community Health." *Annual Review of Public Health,* 2000, *21,* 369–402.

Rowitz, L. "The Mystery of Public Health Workforce Development." *Journal of Public Health Management and Practice,* 1999, *5*(3), 101–104.

Russell, W. *High Quality Technical Assistance. Benchmarks.* Washington, D.C.: The National Clearinghouse for Comprehensive School Reform, 2002. [http://www.goodschools.gwu.edu.]. Nov. 23, 2005.

Safe Kids. *National Safe Kids Campaign Becomes Safe Kids Worldwide.* Washington, D.C.: Safe Kids, 2005. [http://www.safekids.org/news/news_press070105.html]. July 20, 2005.

Salas, E., Dickinson, T. L., Converse, S., and Tannenbaum, S. I. "Toward an Understanding of Team Performance and Training." In R. W. Swezey and E. Salas (eds.), *Teams: Their Training and Performance.* Norwood, Mass.: Ablex, 1992, pp. 3–29.

Sanchez, V. "Reflections on Community Coalition Staff: Research Directions from Practice." *Health Promotion Practice,* 2000, *1*(4), 320–322.

Santelli, J., and Beilenson, P. 1992. "Risk Factors for Adolescent Sexual Behavior, Fertility, and Sexually Transmitted Diseases." *Journal of School Health,* 1992, *62*(7), 271–279.

Schermerhorn, J. "Determinants of Interorganizational Cooperation." *Academy of Management Journal,* 1975, *18*(4), 846–856.

Schermerhorn, J. "Open Questions Limiting the Practice of Interorganizational Development." *Group and Organization Studies,* 1981, *6,* 83–95.

Schmidt, F. "Citizen Development: Program Outcomes for Communities." *Evaluating the National Outcomes.* Tempe, Ariz.: Arizona Cooperative Extension, 1998. [http://ag.arizona.edu/fcs/cyfernet/nowg/cd_essay.html]. Oct. 18, 2005.

Schooler, C., Farquhar, J. W., Fortmann, S. P., and Flora, J. A. "Synthesis of Findings and Issues from Community Prevention Trials." *Annals of Epidemiology,* Supplement, 1997, *7,* 54–68.

Schorr, L. B. *Common Purpose: Strengthening Families and Neighborhoods to Rebuild America.* New York: Doubleday, Anchor Books, 1997.

Schultz, J. *Key Questions for Developing an Advocacy Strategy.* San Francisco: The Democracy Center, 2002. [http://www.democracyctr.org/resources/strategy.html]. Feb. 1, 2006.

Scott, J. *Network Analysis: A Handbook.* (2nd ed.) Newbury Park, Calif.: Sage Publications, 2000.

Senge, P. M. *The Fifth Discipline: The Art and Practice of the Learning Organization.* New York: Doubleday/Currency, 1990.

Search Engine Marketing. *How to Write Effective Newsletters.* [http://www.lsfnetwork.com/write-eff-newsletters.html]. July 22, 2006.

Shadish, W. R., Jr., Cook, T. D., and Leviton, L. C. *Foundations of Program Evaluation: Theories of Practice,* Newbury Park, Calif.: Sage, 1991.

Shaffer, R. *Beyond the Dispensary.* Nairobi, Kenya: African Medical and Research Foundation, 1983.

Sharfman, M., Gray, B., and Yan, A. "The Context of Interorganizational Collaboration in the Garment Industry: An Institutional Perspective." *Journal of Applied Behavioral Science,* 1991, *27*(2), 181–208.

Shaw, R. A., and others. "Effects on Adolescent ATOD Behaviors and Attitudes of a 5-year Community Partnership." *Evaluation and Program Planning,* 1997, *20,* 307–313.

Shea, S., and Basch, C. "A Review of Five Major Community-Based Cardiovascular Disease Prevention Programs. Part 1: Rationale, Design and Theoretical Framework." *American Journal of Health Promotion,* 1990, *4*(3), 203–213.

Shediak-Rizkallah, M. C., and Bone, L. R. "Planning for the Sustainability of Community-Based Health Programs: Conceptual Frameworks and Future Directions for Research, Practice and Policy." *Health Education Research,* 1998, *13*(1), 87–108.

Shinn, R., and Williams, M. (eds.). "Team Building—What It Is and How Do You Do It?" *Across the Board,* Fall Newsletter, 2005, *10*(2). Richmond, Va.: Virginia Primary Care Association.

Shortell, S. M., and others. "Evaluating Partnerships for Community Health Improvement: Tracking the Footprints." *Journal of Health Politics, Policy and Law,* 2002, *27*(1), pp. 49–92.

Siegel, M., and Doner, L. *Marketing Public Health: Strategies to Promote Social Change.* New York: Aspen, 1998.

Simons-Morton, D. G., Simons-Morton, B. G., Parcel, G. S., and Bunker, J. F. "Influencing Personal and Environmental Conditions for Community Health: A Multilevel Intervention Model." *Family and Community Health,* 1988, *11*(2), 25–35.

Sink, D., and Stowers, G. "Coalitions and Their Effect on the Urban Policy Agenda." *Administration in Social Work,* 1989, *13,* 83–98.

Smith, N. L. "The Context of Investigations in Cross-Cultural Evaluations." *Studies in Educational Evaluation,* 1991, *17,* 3–21.

Smith, P., and Siek, G. *Notes on Fundraising and Grant-Writing.* Ohio State University Fact Sheet #8: Extra Resources for a Coalition. Columbus: The Ohio State University Agricultural Extension, 2002. [http://ohioline.osu.edu/bc-fact/0008.html]. Dec. 20, 2005.

Social Enterprise Magazine Online. *What Is Social Enterprise?* 2003. [http://www.socialenterprisemagazine.org/]. Nov. 28, 2006.

Social Marketing Institute. *Branding in the Non-Profit Environment: Promises and Limits.* Report on the Nonprofit Marketing Summit Conference, Mar. 16–17, 2000a. Tampa, Fla. Sponsored by the Social Marketing Institute, David and Lucile Packard Foundation, and McDonough School of Business, Georgetown University.

Social Marketing Institute. *Marketing on the Internet: The Advent of E-Everything.* Report on the Nonprofit Marketing Summit Conference, Mar. 16–17, 2000b. Tampa, Fla. Sponsored by the Social Marketing Institute, David and Lucile Packard Foundation, and McDonough School of Business, Georgetown University.

Social Marketing Institute. *Spreading Marketing Thinking in Your Organization: What Marketing Needs in Order to Flourish. Report on the Nonprofit Marketing Summit Conference,* Mar. 16–17, 2000c. Tampa, Fla. Sponsored by the Social Marketing Institute, David and Lucile Packard Foundation, and McDonough School of Business, Georgetown University. [http://www.social-marketing.org/papers/NMS-report.pdf]. Nov. 15, 2005.

Social Marketing National Excellence Collaborative. *The Basics of Social Marketing.* Seattle, Wash.: Turning Point, 2005.

Soet, J. E., and Basch, C. E. "The Telephone as a Communication Medium for Health Education." *Health Education and Behavior,* 1997, *24*(6), 759–772.

Sofaer, S. *Working Together, Moving Ahead: A Manual to Support Effective Community Health Coalitions.* New York: City University of New York, 2001.

Solomon, R., Davidson, N., and Solomon, E. *The Handbook for the Fourth R: Relationship Activities for Cooperative and Collegial Learning.* Columbia, Md.: Institute for Relationship Training, 1993.

Soriano, F. I. *Conducting Needs Assessments. A Multidisciplinary Approach.* Thousand Oaks, Calif.: Sage, 1995.

Steckler, A. B., Goodman, R. M., Alciati, M. H. "The Impact of the National Cancer Institute's Data-Based Intervention Research Program on State Health Agencies." *Health Education Research,* 1997, *12*(2), 199–211.

Steckler, A., Orville, K., Eng, E., and Dawson, L. "Summary of a Formative Evaluation of PATCH." *Journal of Health Education,* 1992, *23,* 174–178.

Steckler, A., and others. "Toward Integrating Qualitative and Quantitative Methods: An Introduction." *Health Education Quarterly,* 1992, *19*(1), 191–198.

Steckler, A., and others. "Health Education Intervention Strategies: Recommendations for Future Research." *Health Education Quarterly,* 1995, *22*(3), 307–328.

Steuart, G. W. "Health Behavior and Planned Change: An Approach to the Professional Preparation of the Health Education Specialist." In A. B. Steckler, B. A. Israel, L. Dawson, and E. Eng (eds.), "Community Health Development: An Anthology of the Works of Guy W. Steuart." *Health Education Quarterly,* Supplement, 1993, *1,* S49–70.

Stevens, G. L., and Lodl, K. A. "Community Coalitions: Identifying Changes in Coalition Members as a Result of Training." *Journal of Extension,* 1999, *37*(2), pp. 1–9.

Stevenson, W., Pearce, J., and Porter, L. "The Concept of Coalition in Organizational Theory and Research." *Academy of Management Review,* 1985, *10,* 256–268.

StockLayouts LLC. *Brochure Writing Tips.* [http://www.stocklayouts.com/downloads/Brochure-Writing-Tips.pdf]. July 17, 2006.

Stokols, D. "Establishing and Maintaining Healthy Environments: Toward a Social Ecology of Health Promotion." *American Psychologist,* 1992, *47*(1), 6–22.

Strawn, H. B., Sumners, J., and Easterwood, M. "Strategic Planning for Local Communities and Government." *Action Newsletter*, Fall edition. Auburn, Ala.: Alabama Cooperative Extension Service, 1999. [http://www.aces.edu/crd/publications/action/Action-fall-99.html]. Oct. 17, 2005.

Suarez, T. M., and Montgomery, D. L. *What Is Technical Assistance?* Paper presented at the annual meeting of the American Educational Research Association. San Francisco: American Educational Research Association, 1989.

Substance Abuse and Mental Health Services Administration. *The Community Partnership Program, 1990–96: The 48 Community Study.* DHHS Publication No. 00-3373. Rockville, Md.: Substance Abuse and Mental Health Services Administration, 2000.

Sullivan Mort, G., Weerawardena, J., and Carnegie, K. "Social Entrepreneurship: Toward Conceptualization." *International Journal of Nonprofit and Voluntary Sector Marketing*, 2003, *8*(1), 76–88.

Susskind, L. "A Short Guide to Consensus Building." In L. Susskind, S. McKearnan, and J. Thomas-Larmer (eds.), *The Consensus Building Handbook: A Comprehensive Guide to Reaching Agreement.* Thousand Oaks, Calif.: Sage, 1999.

Sussman, S. "The Six-Step Program Development Chain Model." In S. Sussman (ed.), *Handbook of Program Development for Health Behavior Research and Practice.* Thousand Oaks, Calif.: Sage, 2001.

Tagliere, D. *How to Meet, Think, and Work to Consensus.* San Francisco: Jossey-Bass, 1993.

Taylor-Powell, E., Rossing, B., Geran, J. *Evaluating Collaboratives: Reaching the Potential.* Madison: University of Wisconsin-Extension, 1998. [http://s142412519.onlinehome.us/uw/pdfs/G3658_8.pdf]. Feb. 12, 2006.

The Teal Trust. Team Process. 2002. [http://www.teal.org.uk/EasyPrint/epteamldr.htm]. Sept. 1, 2005.

Tesh, S. *Hidden Arguments: Political Ideology and Disease Prevention Policy.* New Brunswick, N.J.: Rutgers University Press, 1988.

Thompson, B., and Kinney, S. "Social Change Theory: Applications to Community Health." In N. Bracht (ed.), *Health Promotion at the Community Level.* Newbury Park, Calif.: Sage, 1999, pp. 45–65.

Thompson, B. R., Spickard, A., and Dixon, G. L. *Fighting Back the First Eight Years: Mobilizing People and Communities in the Fight Against Substance Abuse.* Nashville, Tenn.: Vanderbilt University Press, 2001.

Timmreck, T. *Planning, Program Development and Evaluation.* (2nd ed.) Boston: Jones and Bartlett, 2003.

Torres, R. T., Preskill, H. S., and Piontek, M. E. *Evaluation Strategies for Communicating and Reporting: Enhancing Learning in Organizations.* Thousand Oaks, Calif.: Sage, 1996.

Trohanis, P. *Background Information and Planning Materials on Designing State Technical Assistance Systems.* Chapel Hill: Frank Porter Graham Child Development Center, University of North Carolina, 1998.

Tuckman, B. W., and Jenson, M. A. "Stages of Small Group Development Revisited." *Group and Organization Studies,* 1977, *2,* 419–427.

Turning Point. *Collaborative Leadership and Health: A Review of the Literature.* Seattle, Wash.: Robert Wood Johnson Foundation, 2001a.

Turning Point. *Collaborative Leadership: Fundamental Concepts.* Seattle, WA: Robert Wood Johnson Foundation, 2001b.

Turning Point Social Marketing National Excellence Collaborative. *Social Marketing and Public Health: Lessons from the Field.* Seattle, Wash.: Turning Point, 2003.

Turning Point Social Marketing National Excellence Collaborative. *The Basics of Social Marketing.* Seattle, Wash.: Turning Point, 2005.

Twin Cities Public Television. *Benjamin Franklin.* [http://www.pbs.org/benfranklin/12_citizen.html]./2002. July 12, 2005.

Tyler Norris Associates. *The Community Indicators Handbook: Measuring Progress Toward Healthy and Sustainable Communities.* Boulder, Colo.: Tyler Norris Associates, 1997. [http://www.rprogress.org/publications/ciguide.pdf]. Feb. 13, 2006.

United Nations Association of the United States of America. *UNA-USA Advocacy Guide.* 2005. [http://www.unausa.org/site/pp.asp?c=fvKRI8MPJpFandb=363105]. Aug. 22, 2005.

United States Department of Education. *Identifying and Implementing Educational Practices Supported by Rigorous Evidence: A User Friendly Guide.* [http://www.ed.gov/rschstat/research/pubs/rigorousevid/guide_pg3.html.#purpose%20and%20executive%20summary]. Jan. 3, 2006.

United States Department of Health and Human Services. *Healthy People 2010.* (2nd ed.) With *Understanding and Improving Health and Objectives for Improving Health,* 2 vols. Washington, D.C.: U.S. Government Printing Office, 2000a.

United States Department of Health and Human Services. *Planned Approach to Community Health (PATCH): Guide for the Local Coordinator.* Atlanta: Centers for Disease Control and Prevention, 2000b.

United States Department of Health and Human Services. *Reducing Tobacco Use: A Report of the Surgeon General.* Atlanta: Centers for Disease Control and Prevention, National Center for Disease Prevention and Health Promotion, Office on Smoking and Health, 2000c.

United States Department of Health and Human Services, Office of Disease Prevention and Health Promotion. *Healthy People in Healthy Communities: A Community Planning Guide Using Healthy People 2010.* Washington, D.C.: United States Department of Health and Human Services, 2001. [http://www.healthypeople.gov/Publications/HealthyCommunities2001/default.htm]. July 20, 2005.

United States Department of Transportation, National Highway Traffic Safety Administration. *Community How-to Guide on Needs Assessment and Strategic Planning.* 2001. [http://www.nhtsa.dot.gov/people/injury/alcohol/Community%20Guides%20HTML]./Book2_NeedsAssess.html#strategic%20plan]. Dec. 16, 2005.

United States Office of Management and Budget. *What Constitutes Strong Evidence of a Program's Effectiveness?* Washington, D.C.: United States Office of Management and Budget, 2004. [http://www.whitehouse.gov/omb/part/2004_prgram_eval.pdf]. Jan. 3, 2006.

United Way of America. *Measuring Program Outcomes.* Alexandria, Va.: United Way of America, 1996.

University of Florida Extension. *Community How-To Guide on Coalition Building.* Gainesville: University of Florida Extension, 2002.

University of Michigan, National Program Office. *Allies Against Asthma.* 2004. [http://www.asthma.umich.edu/about_us/program_overview.html]. Aug. 3, 2005.

University of Nevada Cooperative Extension. *Community Leader Guide (Communication).* 2005a. [http://www.unce.unr.edu/publications/ebpubs/eb0103/communication3.htm]. Nov. 9, 2005.

University of Nevada Cooperative Extension. *Community Leader Guide (Grantwriting).* 2005b. [http://www.unce.unr.edu/publications/EBPubs/EB0103/fundraising5.htm]. Nov. 10, 2005.

University of Nevada Cooperative Extension. *Community Leader Guide (Team Building).* 2005c. [http://www.unce.unr.edu/publications/ebpubs/eb0103/teambuilding.htm]. Oct. 25, 2005.

University of Wisconsin—Cooperative Extension. *Evaluating Collaboratives.* Madison, Wisc.: Cooperative Extension Publications, 1998.

University of Wisconsin Office of Quality Improvement. *Facilitator Tool Kit.* 2001. [http://www.wisc.edu/improve/factoolkit.pdf] Nov. 1, 2005.

Useem, J. "Decisions, Decisions." *Fortune,* 75th Anniversary Special Issue, June 27, 2005, pp. 55–56.

Valdiserri, R. O., Aultman, T. V., and Curran, J. W. "Community Planning: A National Strategy to Improve HIV Prevention Programs." *Journal of Community Health,* 1995, *20*(2), 87–100.

Valdiserri, R. O., and others. "Applying the Criteria for the Development of Health Promotion and Education Programs to AIDS Risk Reduction Programs for Gay Men." *Journal of Community Health,* 1987, *12,* 4.

Valente, T. W. *Network Models of the Diffusion of Innovations*, 1995. Cresskill, NJ: Hampton Press.

Vangen, S., and Huxham, C. "Enacting Leadership for Collaborative Advantage: Dilemmas of Ideology and Pragmatism in the Activities of Partnership Managers." *British Journal of Management,* 2004, *15*(1), 39–56.

Wallack, L. "Media Advocacy: A Strategy for Empowering People and Communities." In M. Minkler (ed.), *Community Organizing and Community Building for Health.* (2nd ed.) New Brunswick, N.J.: Rutgers University Press, 2005, pp. 419–432.

Wallack, L., Dorfman, L., Jernigan, D., and Themba, M. *Media Advocacy and Public Health: Power for Prevention.* Newbury Park, Calif.: Sage, 1993.

Wallack L., Woodruff, K., Dorfman, L., and Diaz, I. *News for a Change: An Advocate's Guide to Working with the Media.* Thousand Oaks, Calif.: Sage, 1999.

Wandersman, A., and Alderman, J. "Incentives, Barriers and Training of Volunteers for the American Cancer Society: A Staff Perspective." *Review of Public Personnel Administration,* 1993, *13*(1), 67–76.

Wandersman A., and Florin, P. "Community Interventions and Effective Prevention." *American Psychologist,* 2003, *58,* 441–448.

Wandersman, A., Florin, P., Friedmann, R., and Meier, R. "Who Participates, Who Does Not, and Why? An Analysis of Voluntary Neighborhood Associations in the United States and Israel." *Sociological Forum,* 1987, *2*(3), 534–555.

Wandersman, A., and Goodman, R. M. "Community Partnerships for Alcohol and Other Drug Abuse Prevention." *Family Resource Coalition,* 1991, *10,* 8–9.

Wandersman, A., and others. "Toward a Social Ecology of Community Coalitions." *American Journal of Health Promotion,* 1996, *10*(4), 299–307.

Wang, E., and Burris, M. "Empowerment Through Photo Novella: Portraits of Participation." *Health Education Quarterly,* 1994, *21*(2), 171–186.

Wang, E., and Burris, M. "Photovoice: Concept, Methodology and Use for Participatory Needs Assessment." *Health Education and Behavior,* 1997, *24*(3), 369–387.

Waterman, R. H., Jr. *The Renewal Factor.* New York: Bantam Books, 1987.

Weiner, B. J., Alexander, J. A., and Shortell, S. M. "Management and Governance Process in Community Health Coalitions: A Procedural Justice Perspective." *Health Education and Behavior,* 2002, *29*(2), 737–754.

Weinrich, N. K. *Hands-On Social Marketing.* Thousand Oaks, Calif.: Sage, 1999.

Weiss, C. H. "Nothing as Practical as a Good Theory: Exploring Theory-Based Evaluation for Comprehensive Community Initiatives for Families and Children." In J. P. Connell, A. C. Kubisch, L. B. Schorr, and C. H. Weiss (eds.), *New Approaches to Evaluating Community Initiatives: Concepts, Methods, and Contexts.* Washington, D.C.: Aspen Institute, 1995, pp. 65–92.

Weiss, C. H. *Evaluation: Methods for Studying Programs and Policies.* (2nd ed.) Upper Saddle River, N.J.: Prentice Hall, 1998a.

Weiss, C. H. "Have We Learned Anything New About the Use of Evaluation?" *American Journal of Evaluation,* 1998b, *19*(1), 21–33.

Weitzel, A., and Geist, P. "Parliamentary Procedure in a Community Group: Communication and Vigilant Decision Making." *Communication Monographs,* Sept. 1998.

Whetten, D. "Interorganizational Relations: A Review of the Field." *Journal of Higher Education,* 1981, *I*(1), 1–28.

Whitt, M. *Fighting Tobacco: A Coalition Approach to Improving Your Community's Health.* Lansing: Michigan Department of Public Health, 1993.

Wing, S. "Whose Epidemiology, Whose Health?" *International Journal of Health Services,* 1998, *28,* 241–252.

Wilkins, C., Tremethick, M., Walker, K. and Meier, P. "Community Coalitions: Founda-tions for Success in Health Promotion for Older Adults." *Journal of Family and Consumer Sciences,* 1999, *91*(4), 83–87.

Wilkins, C. and Walker, K. *A 10-Step Decision Making Model for Choosing Between Right and Right.* Fact Sheet FCS9203. Gainesville: University of Florida Institute of Food and Agricultural Sciences, 1993. [http://edis.ifas.ufl.edu/FY664]. Nov. 14, 2005.

Windsor, R. A., Baranowski, T., Clark, N., and Cutter, G. *Evaluation of Health Promo-tion and Education Programs.* Palo Alto, Calif.: Mayfield, 1994.

Winer, M., and Ray, K. *Collaboration Handbook: Creating, Sustaining, and Enjoying the Journey.* St. Paul, Minn.: Amherst H. Wilder Foundation, 1994.

Wischnowski, M. W., and McCollum, J. A. "Managing Conflict on Local Interagency Coordinating Councils." *Topics in Early Childhood Special Education,* 1995, *15*(3), 281–295.

Witkin, B. R., and Altschuld, J. W. (eds.). *Planning and Conducting Needs Assessments: A Practical Guide.* Thousand Oaks, Calif.: Sage, 1995.

W. K. Kellogg Foundation. *Developing Community Capacity—Module One.* Battle Creek, MI., W. K. Kellogg Foundation, 1994.

W. K. Kellogg Foundation. *Sustaining Community-Based Initiatives: Community and Economic Development: Module One: Developing Community Capacity.* Battle Creek, MI: W. K. Kellogg. Foundation, 1995. [http://www.wkkf.org/DesktopModules/ WKF.00_DmaSupport/Viewdoc.aspx?fld=PDFFile&CID=287&ListID=28&ItemID= 10658&LanguageID=0] Dec. 18, 2006.

W. K. Kellogg Foundation. *W. K. Kellogg Foundation Evaluation Handbook.* Battle Creek, MI.: W. K. Kellogg Foundation, 1998. [http://www.wkkf.org/Pubs/Tools/ Evaluation/Pub770.pdf]. Feb. 6, 2006.

Wolff, T. "Community Coalition Building—Contemporary Practice and Research: Intro-duction." *American Journal of Community Psychology,* 2001a, *29*(2), 165–172.

Wolff, T. "A Practitioner's Guide to Successful Coalitions." *American Journal of Community Psychology,* 2001b, *29*(2), 173–191.

Wolff, T. "The Future of Community Building." *American Journal of Community Psychology,* 2001c, *29*(2), 263–268.

Wolff, T. "A Practical Approach to Evaluating Coalitions." In T. Backer (ed.), *Evaluating Community Collaborations.* New York: Springer Publishing, 2002, pp. 57–112.

Wolff, T., and Kaye, G. "Collaborative Leadership." *Collaborative News: Newsletter of the National Funding Collaborative on Violence Prevention,* 1998, *3.* 3–4.

Wood, D. and Gray, B. "Toward a Comprehensive Theory of Collaboration." *Journal of Applied Behavioral Science,* 1991, *27*(2), 139–162.

Worthen, B. R., Sanders, J. R., and Fitzpatrick, J. L. *Program Evaluation: Alternative Approaches and Practical Guidelines.* (2nd ed.) White Plains, N.Y.: Longman, 1996.

Yin, R. K. *Case Study Research: Design and Methods. (2nd ed.)* Newbury Park, Calif.: Sage, 1994.

Yin, R. K., Kafterian, S. J., Yu, P., and Jansen, M. A. "Outcomes from CSAP's Community Partnership Program: Findings from the National Cross-Site Evaluation." *Evaluation and Program Planning,* 1997, *20,* 345–355.

Yin, R. K., and Ware, A. J. "Using Outcome Data to Evaluate Community Drug Prevention Initiatives: Pushing the State of the Art." *Journal of Community Psychology,* 2000, *28*(3), 323–338.

Yin, R. K., and White, J. L. *Federal Technical Assistance Efforts: Lessons and Improvement in Education for 1984 and Beyond.* Washington, D.C.: Cosmos, 1984.

Yukl, G. *Leadership in Organizations.* (6th ed.) New York: Prentice Hall, 2005.

Zakocs, R. C., and Edwards, E. M. "What Explains Community Coalition Effectiveness? A Review of the Literature." *American Journal of Preventive Medicine,* 2006, *30*(4), 351–361.

Zald, M. N. "Organizations as Politics: An Analysis of Community Organization Agencies." In R. M. Kramer and H. Sprecht (eds.), *Readings in Community Organization Practice.* Englewood Cliffs, N.J.: Prentice Hall, 1969.

Zapka, J., and others. "Inter-Organizational Responses to AIDS: A Case Study of the Worcester AIDS Consortium." *Health Education Research,* 1992, *8*(3), 31–46.

Zimmerman, M. "Empowerment Theory: Psychological, Organizational, and Community Levels of Analysis." In J. Rappaport and E. Seidman (eds.), *Handbook of Community Psychology.* New York: Kluwer Academic/Plenum, 2000, pp. 43–63.

Zimmerman, M. A., and Rappaport, J. "Citizen Participation, Perceived Control, and Psychological Empowerment." *American Journal of Community,* 1988, *16,* 725–750.

Zook, L. *Getting Beyond Communication Roadblocks.* Nov. Newsletter. Carlsbad, Calif.: Buffini and Company, 2005. [http://www.provcom.com/(z5fzby45rlzw1hfm0z4yi255)/providence/newsletter/200511/thereferraldialog.aspx]. Nov. 24, 2005.

NAME INDEX

A

Abed, J., 359
Adams, J. D., 167
Adams, S., 278, 279, 294, 302
Addams, J., 6
Adler, M., 343
Agranoff, R., 181
Alciati, M. H., 95
Alderman, J., 54, 55, 56, 98
Alexander, J. A., 111
Alinsky, S., 7, 8, 9
Allensworth, D., 32
Alter, C., 29, 55, 56
Altschuld, J. W., 331, 339, 353, 355
Anderson, L. M., 463, 486
Anderson, M., 278, 279, 294, 300
Andreasen, A. R., 407
Andrews, A., 122, 127, 182, 223, 240
Andringa, R., 163
Ansari, W., 55, 467
Anspaugh, D. J., 307
Anspaugh, S. L., 307
Anthony, S. B., 6
Archer, T. M., 330, 331, 350, 371

Arkin, E. B., 404
Arnstein, S. R., 13
Aronson, R., 491
Aronson, R. E., 326, 358, 502, 503, 505, 508, 509
Aultman, T. V., 371, 431
Austin, D., 76
Austin, J., 63, 80, 82, 108
Avolio, B. J., 111, 115

B

Baer, N., 127, 241, 490
Bagby, M., 80, 108
Baglioni, A. J. Jr., 475
Bailey, C. A., 54, 56, 340
Bailey, D., 122
Baker, E., 51
Balcazar, F., 130
Ballenger, B., 146
Bangs, D. H., Jr., 277
Baranowski, T., 348
Barnett, W., 14
Bartholomew, L. K., 359
Bartunek, J. M., 141
Basch, C. E., 16, 401, 404
Bass, B. M., 112, 115, 163
Bauer, G., 335
Bazzoli, G. J., 14, 55, 222, 223

Beaulieu, L. J., 340, 341, 344, 346, 347, 354
Becker, A. B., 148
Beckham, B., 182, 185
Beilenson, P., 20
Benard, B., 54
Bennis, W. G., 165
Berg, B. L., 346
Bergstrom, A., 68
Berkowitz, B., 84, 90, 265, 299, 301, 302, 309, 310, 313, 470, 487, 488, 489, 490
Berlin, X., 14
Bernard, B., 400
Bernard, H. R., 337, 460
Besser, T. L., 328, 329
Bibeau, D., 32, 50, 83
Bigelow, D. A., 454
Billings, W., 4
Birkby, B., 17, 487, 489
Bishop, C., 449
Black, T., 32, 33
Blanchard, K. H., 168
Blanchard, L., 338
Block, P., 129
Blumenthal, D. S., 62
Bobo, K., 5, 7, 324
Bobowick, M. J., 230

Boissevain, J., 32, 33
Bonaparte, N., 195
Bone, L. R., 261
Bonnet, D. G., 448
Borden, L. M., 46, 472
Bornstein, D., 281
Boydell, K. M., 55
Bracht, N., 10, 16, 62
Brager, G. A., 8, 12, 78, 139
Braithwaite, R. L., 62, 63, 80, 82, 108
Breckon, D. J., 433
Brice, H. J., 319
Brieger, W. R., 502, 503, 505
Brinckerhoff, P. C., 279
Brindis, C., 20
Brink, S. G., 99, 223, 472, 473, 474
Briss, P. A., 397
Brodin, B., 95
Brogan, H., 5
Brown, B. B., 13
Brown, C., 31, 33, 104, 108, 122, 327, 474, 490, 507
Brown, D., 192
Brownson, R. C., 397
Brubach, A., 414, 415
Bruner, C., 128, 130, 400
Bryson, J., 224
Buckley, J., 129
Bumpers, B., 19
Bunker, J. F., 357
Burghardt, S., 7
Burns, J. M., 112, 113
Burris, M., 339
Butler, L. M., 333, 353
Butterfoss, F. D., 8, 31, 32, 33, 34, 49, 51, 55, 61, 65, 66, 71, 72, 76, 77, 78, 79, 80, 81, 82, 86, 87, 89, 90, 95, 97, 98, 108, 109, 130, 131, 132, 134, 140, 141, 158, 176, 182, 183, 196, 223, 327, 328, 334, 343, 345, 356, 357, 361, 371, 373, 378, 379, 434, 436, 442, 449, 456, 459, 460, 463, 468, 470, 471, 472, 473, 474, 489, 490, 493, 505, 509

C
Calabrese, R. J., 183
Cameron, R., 397

Campbell, A., 224
Cannon-Bowers, J. A., 163, 166
Capwell, E. M., 334, 343, 449, 456, 459, 460, 468, 493
Caracelli, V., 460
Carlaw, R., 16
Carleton, R., 16
Carnegie, K., 280
Carter, K. A., 340, 341, 344, 346, 347, 354
Carter, R., 19
Cashman, S., 90, 490
Catalano, R. J., Jr., 429
Chaloupka, F. J., 18
Chavez, C., 7, 9
Chavis, D. M., 14, 17, 30, 62, 82, 131, 132, 223, 470, 487, 505
Chawla, A., 51
Cheadle, A., 470
Checkoway, B., 13, 475
Chen, H., 435
Chinman, M., 54, 55, 79, 141, 359, 471, 487
Cho, H., 488
Choate, E., 318
Chrislip, D., 112
Cividin, T. M., 130
Clark, N. M., 22, 34, 51, 53, 58, 77, 99, 348, 502, 503, 505
Clark, P., 54
Clark, R., 68
Clinton, B., 19
Coe, B. A., 176
Cohen, D., 122
Cohen, L., 127, 146, 182, 213, 214, 241, 242, 490
Collins, J., 144, 145, 196
Connell, J. P., 435, 448, 486, 487
Conone, R. M., 192
Converse, S., 163
Cook, R., 471, 472, 473, 474
Cook, T. D., 460
Coombe, C. M., 435
Cosentino, A. J., 5
Cottrell, L. S., Jr., 13
Cousins, J. B., 436, 437
Couto, R. A., 113
Covey, S. R., 121
Covington, S., 7, 9, 10
Cox, T., 153

Cresswell, 459
Crews, C., 130
Cripe, R., 330, 331, 350, 371
Crisp, B., 15, 84
Croan, G., 33, 98, 122
Curran, J. W., 371, 431
Cutter, G., 348

D
D'Affliti, J., 488
David, F., 224
Davidson, N., 167
Dawson, L., 392
Debs, W., 7
Delbecq, A. L., 343, 344
Delgado, G., 6, 9
DeLizia, J. S., 109, 111
DeVille, J. O., 471, 472, 474
Diaz, I., 431
Dickerson, A., 80, 108
Dickinson, T. L., 163
Dignan, M. B., 307
Dill, A., 51, 77
Dinh-Zarr, T., 51, 100
Divine, M., 224
Dixon, G. L., 17
Doble, J., 127
Doner, L., 277
Dorfman, L., 406, 407, 412, 414, 416, 431
Douglass, F., 6
Dowling, J., 55, 58, 77, 79, 99, 119, 122, 139, 140, 141, 145, 147, 183, 262
Downs, A., 413
Downton, J. V., 112
Dresbach, S. H., 231
Drinka, T. J., 165
Drisko, J., 20
Drucker, P., 321
Dryfoos, J., 20
Duckett, S., 84
Dugan, M. A., 437
Duhl, L., 330
Dukes, E. F., 140, 186, 198, 203, 204, 208, 212, 213, 256, 198, 206, 256
Dunet, D. O., 356, 361, 378, 379

E
Earp, J. A., 449
Easterwood, M., 361, 362, 371
Economy, P., 240, 241

Edwards, E. M., 487, 489, 490
Edwards, G., 122
Edwards, R., 335
Edwards, S. L., 20, 98, 222
Egero, B., 21
Ellis, T. M., 97
Eng, E., 15, 117, 338, 392, 449, 475
Engstrom, T., 163
Epictetius, 181
Erfurt, J. C., 401

F

Farquahr, J., 16
Farquahr, J. W., 470
Farrelly, M. C., 18
Fawcett, S. B., 66, 67, 76, 84, 95, 99, 108, 109, 113, 122, 130, 176, 223, 224, 278, 347, 354, 356, 379, 429, 442, 443, 468, 470, 471, 473, 474, 475, 487, 488, 490, 499, 505
Feighery, E., 31, 32, 34, 98, 100, 122
Felix, M., 131, 132
Fetterman, D. M., 436
Fielding, J. E., 397
Finklestein, E., 393
Fishbein, M., 429
Fisher, R., 6, 7, 8, 9, 10, 208
Fitzpatrick, J. L., 449, 453, 469
Flora, J. A., 16, 470
Florin, P., 13, 30, 55, 76, 79, 82, 95, 127, 131, 132, 141, 223, 470, 471, 473, 474, 488, 489
Flynn, B. S., 472
Foote, A., 401
Forster, J., 78, 223
Forsythe, J., 33
Fortmann, S. P., 16, 470
Foster-Fishman, P. G., 14, 15, 76, 90, 109, 141, 153, 176, 223, 278, 356, 391, 490
Francisco, V. T., 67, 76, 334, 343, 347, 354, 393, 434, 442, 443, 449, 456, 459, 460, 468, 470, 489, 493, 505
Franklin, B., 4, 24, 278
Freeman, H. E., 499
French, S., 393

Freudenberg, N., 488
Friedman, A. R., 22, 58, 261, 502, 503, 505
Friedmann, R., 55, 79, 141
Friere, P., 63, 255

G

Gabriel, R., 433, 489, 490
Galano, J., 78, 223
Galaskiewicz, J., 14
Gallagher, K., 20
Gallegos, B., 419, 420
Garrison, L., 6
Garza, H., 222
Gastil, J., 196
Geist, P., 255
Geran, J., 332, 448, 471, 472, 473, 474
Ghandi, M., 112
Giamartino, G., 141, 471, 472, 473, 475
Gilbert, G., 404
Gingiss, P. L., 99, 223, 472, 473, 474
Glanz, K., 32, 50, 83
Glidewell, J., 80, 108
Goeppinger, J., 475
Goethe, J. von, 356
Goldberg, M. E., 429
Goldman, K. D., 416, 417
Goldstein, S., 472, 473
Goodman, R. M., 14, 31, 32, 33, 54, 55, 62, 65, 66, 71, 76, 81, 83, 84, 85, 86, 95, 97, 98, 108, 109, 130, 140, 141, 176, 182, 183, 196, 223, 358, 361, 373, 379, 392, 434, 470, 475, 487, 491
Gottlieb, N. H., 99, 223, 359, 472, 473, 474
Gould, J., 146, 213, 214
Granner, M. L., 470
Gray, B., 14, 27, 29, 51, 53, 54, 55, 77, 140
Green, L., 16, 50, 67, 90, 349, 357, 358, 408, 436, 438, 488
Greene, J. C., 438, 439, 448, 460
Gregg, W., 401
Griffin, S. F., 108
Grohol, J., 10
Guetzkow, H., 214

Gulati, R., 14, 55
Gustafson, D. H., 343, 344
Gwede, C., 345
Gyr, J., 214

H

Habana-Hafner, S., 27, 28, 29, 51, 63, 64
Hage, J., 29, 55, 56
Hague, C. E., 212, 214
Haines, P. S., 393
Hakuta, K., 278
Hall, R., 140, 182
Hallfors, D., 488
Hamre, R., 361, 379
Hancock, T., 329, 330, 334, 335, 358
Hanlon, J. J., 349
Harvey, J. R., 433
Hawkins, C., 245
Hawkins, J. D., 429
Hays, C. E., 471, 472, 474
Hays, S. P., 471, 472, 474
Heath, G. W., 470
Heffner, R. D., 3
Heider, J., 122
Heimlich, J. E., 231
Heirich, M. A., 401
Henderson, N., 400
Herman, K., 78, 223
Herrera, C., 127
Herron, D. B., 277
Hersey, P., 168
Himmelman, A., 11, 27, 29, 139, 144
Hingson, R., 488
Hogue, T., 68
Holden, D., 76
Holder, H. D., 223
Holli, B. B., 183
Hoover, S., 358, 392
Hopkins, B., 130
Hopkins, R., 78, 82, 109, 118, 183, 357, 361, 472, 474
Hord, S., 32, 54, 122, 490
Horton, S., 273, 274, 275, 277
Houseman, C., 87, 345
Howell, R. E., 333, 353
Hoyle, R. H., 475
Hsieh, T., 61
Huff, R. M., 408
Hughes, S. R., 230
Humphrey, B., 473
Hung, R., 352

Hunt, M. K., 470
Huxham, C., 138, 162, 181

I

Imm, P., 359, 487
Insel, P. M., 473
Israel, B. A., 13, 78, 148, 183, 436, 472, 475

J

Jackson, D., 54, 56
Jackson, S. F., 98
Jansen, M. A., 488, 502, 504
Jasuja, G. K., 183
Jean-Louis, E., 352
Jenkins, S., 146
Jenson, M. A., 164, 165
Jernigan, D., 406, 407, 412, 414, 416
Joffres, C., 122, 470
Johnson, 223
Johnson, D. E., 168, 354
Johnson, J., 127
Joly, 469
Jordan, G. B., 454
Julian, D., 454
Justice, T. I., 129

K

Kadushin, C., 488
Kafterian, S. J., 436, 488, 502, 504
Kagan, S. L., 27, 28, 487
Kahn, R. L., 64, 323
Kanter, R. M., 129, 162
Kaplan, M., 54
Kass, D., 488
Katz, D., 64
Katzenbach, J. R., 166, 167
Kaye, G., 11, 56, 77, 79, 86, 120, 141, 147, 160, 162, 175, 183, 325, 484
Kayser, T. A., 240
Kegler, M. C., 8, 14, 17, 51, 54, 61, 62, 72, 77, 79, 80, 81, 82, 83, 90, 91, 95, 98, 99, 104, 107, 108–109, 109, 141, 163, 183, 203, 326, 356, 357, 358, 361, 442, 470, 471, 472, 473, 474, 475, 487, 488, 490, 491, 502, 503, 505, 508, 509
Kelley, F., 6
Kelly, C. K., 327, 328, 345

Kelly, C. S., 148, 463
Kelly, J., 80, 108
Kendall, J., 5, 7, 324
Keys, C. B., 141
Keyser, B. B., 392
Kickert, W., 181
Kieffer, G. D., 240
King, J., 182, 185
King, M. L., 26
Kingsbury, L., 10
Kinney, S., 16, 32, 62
Kitzinger, J., 345
Klein, I., 471, 473, 474
Klijn, E. H., 162, 181
Kline, M. V., 408
Klitzman, S., 488
Klitzner, M., 488
Knoke, D., 141
Kok, G., 359
Koney, K. M., 122
Koopenjan, J., 181
Kotter, J. P., 126
Kretzmann, J. P., 5, 138, 214, 322, 328, 329, 339, 354
Kreuter, M., 67, 77, 82, 83, 84, 95, 349, 357, 358, 361, 408, 487, 488, 490, 508
Kreuter, M. W., 16, 358
Krieger, J. W., 506
Krueger, R. A., 344, 345, 346
Kubisch, A. C., 435, 441, 448, 486, 487
Kuester, S., 361, 379
Kumpher, K., 78, 80, 82, 109, 118, 183, 357, 361, 472, 474

L

LaBonte, R., 11, 14, 31, 335
Lachance, L. L., 58, 502, 503, 505
Lakey, B. M., 230
Lancaster, R. B., 433
Langmeyer, D. B., 354
Lao Tzu, 222
Lara, M., 488, 506
Larson, C., 112
Lasater, T., 16
Lasker, R., 69, 76, 77, 81
Lasker, R. D., 51, 54, 70, 81, 90, 109, 223, 328
Lathrop, J., 6
Ledlow, S., 166
Lee, J., 98
Lee, P. R., 95

Lees, J., 33, 98, 122
Lefebvre, R., 16
Lenczner, S. J., 97
Levine, S., 212, 213
Leviton, L., 127
Leviton, L. C., 460
Lewin, K., 9
Lezin, N., 77, 82, 83, 84, 95, 357, 487, 490, 508
Librett, J., 78, 82, 109, 118, 183, 357, 361, 472, 474
Lin, N., 176
Lincoln, Y. S., 435
Linder, D., 166
Lindsay, G., 122
Linnan, L., 438
Linney, J., 371, 499
Lippincott, S., 243, 244
Lipsey, M. W., 499
Livert, D., 488
Loden, M., 153, 154
Lodl, K. A., 127
Lofquist, W. A., 9, 322
Lolly, E., 120, 121
Look, V., 83, 513
Luepker, R., 16
Lynch, K., 449
Lynch, P. J., 273, 274, 275, 277
Lythcott, N., 62

M

Mabely, M., 391
McCaslin, N. L., 330, 331, 350, 371
McClelland, D. C., 145
McClintock, H. D., 500
McCollum, J. A., 141
McConnell, R., 250, 251, 255
McDermott, R. J., 307
McDonald, M., 339
McEwan, K. L., 454
McGinnis, J. M., 397
McGuire, M., 181
McKenzie, J. F., 332, 348, 392, 401, 403, 404, 405, 406, 410, 439
McKnight, J. L., 5, 138, 214, 322, 328, 329, 339, 354, 421
McLaughlin, J. A., 454
McLeroy, K., 14, 16, 17, 32, 50, 51, 54, 62, 77, 79, 80, 81, 82, 83, 95, 98, 99, 104,

107, 108–109, 109, 141, 163, 183, 203, 356, 357, 361, 471, 472, 473, 474, 475, 487
McLeroy, K. R., 475
McMillan, B., 141, 183, 471, 472, 473, 474, 475
McNeese, I. C., 184, 190
McQueen, D. V., 463, 486
Maddy, W., 54, 56
Madison, A., 352
Malek, S., 14, 17, 54, 62, 77, 79, 80, 81, 82, 95, 98, 99, 104, 107, 108–109, 109, 141, 163, 183, 203, 356, 357, 361, 471, 472, 473, 474, 475, 487
Malveaux, F., 22
Mank, D., 129
Mannino, D. M., 22
Mansergh, G., 77
Marrett, C., 223
Martin, D., 51, 100
Martin, G., 337
Mattesich, P., 26, 27, 51, 52, 323, 325
Matthews, D., 127
Max, S., 5, 7, 324
Maxwell, J. A., 435
Mayer, J., 79, 82, 141, 183, 196, 204
Meade, M., 49
Meek, J., 363
Meier, P., 203
Meier, R., 55, 79, 141
Mensah-Kumah, O., 21
Merzel, C., 488
Middlestat, S. E., 429
Milio, N., 16, 62
Miller, J. Y., 429
Miller, L. C., 130
Miller, R., 51, 54, 69, 76, 81, 90, 109, 223
Millstein, B., 442, 443, 444
Milward, H. B., 14, 437
Minkler, M., 10, 11, 12, 13, 14, 15, 65, 69, 329, 334, 354, 405, 406, 436, 508, 509
Mischke, G., 14
Mitchell, R., 76, 82, 95, 127, 223, 470, 471, 473, 474
Mitchell, S. M., 222
Mittelmark, M. B., 16, 84, 470, 486, 490
Mizrahi, T., 76, 79, 108, 122, 153, 203, 206, 213, 437

Mizruchi, T., 14
Mojkowski, C., 128
Monsey, B., 26, 27, 51, 52, 323, 325
Montgomery, D. L., 128, 129
Moore, C., 191
Moore, K. A., 20
Moos, R. H., 79, 141, 183, 473
Morgan, D. L., 345
Morgan, L. M., 510
Morrisey, E., 487
Morrow, A. L., 87, 89, 130, 345, 487, 488
Mott, L., 6
Mouden, L. D., 315
Mubayira, C., 345
Mulhall, P. F., 471, 472, 474
Mulroy, E. A., 98
Munodawafa, D., 345
Murphy, F., 62
Murray, K., 321
Murray-Close, M., 26, 27, 51
Mutz, J., 321

N
Nagy, J., 293, 294
Neiger, B. L., 332, 348, 392, 401, 403, 404, 405, 406, 410, 439
Nelson, C. F., 358
Nelson, G., 51, 77
Nelson, R. B., 240, 241
Nezlek, J., 78, 223
Nicholas, E. A., 488
Northouse, P. G., 112, 113, 115
Norton, B. L., 54, 84, 326, 358, 491, 502, 503, 505, 508, 509
Novelli, W. D., 262

O
Ocasio, W., 14
O'Donnell, H., 55, 58, 77, 79, 99, 119, 122, 139, 140, 141, 145, 147, 176, 183, 262
O'Donnell, J., 172
Ogden, L., 430
Ogunlade, B. P., 502
Opubor, A., 21
Oros, C., 471, 472, 473
Orville, K., 392
Orwell, G., 507
Osborn, A., 191
Ottoson, J. M., 130

P
Paine, A. L., 76, 347, 354, 470
Paine-Andrews, A., 67, 442, 443, 468, 505
Parachini, L., 7, 9, 10
Parcel, G. S., 357, 359
Paris, C. A., 163, 166
Parker, E. A., 15, 117, 148, 475
Patton, M. Q., 437, 449, 468
Patton, W., 32
Pear, J., 337
Pearce, J., 32
Pechacek, T. R., 18
Peck, G. P., 212, 214
Pendergast, K., 76
Penner, S., 55
Pepper, S. K., 127
Perkins, D. D., 13
Perkins, D. F., 46, 68, 472
Peterson, G., 16
Peterson, J. W., 175
Phillips, J. J., 332
Phillips, C. J., 55
Pickeral, T., 57
Pickett, G. E., 349
Piontek, M. E., 468
Piscolish, M. A., 140, 186, 198, 203, 204, 208, 213
Poreteous, N. L., 448
Porter, L., 32
Potvin, L., 50
Preskill, H. S., 468
Prestby, J., 13, 54, 55, 64, 65, 79, 82, 87, 122, 140, 141, 471, 472
Provan, K. G., 14, 437
Putnam, R., 15, 16, 78, 183, 323

Q
Quinn, S. C., 338, 459

R
Rabinowitz, P., 285, 287, 393, 394, 395, 398, 396, 399, 400, 402
Rallis, S. F., 460
Ramirez, C., 267
Rappaport, J., 13, 14
Ray, K., 27, 29, 149, 175
Rebori, M., 190, 191, 192, 195, 199, 207, 208, 210
Reed, H. B., 27, 29, 51, 63

Reichardt, C. S., 460
Reinheimer, R., 146
Reininger, B., 51, 77, 80, 100, 108, 109, 491
Reynolds, R. I., 223
Rich, R., 54, 56, 82, 122, 223
Richard, L., 50
Riker, W., 162
Rissel, C., 10
Roberts-DeGennaro, M., 33, 54, 82
Rodine, S., 488
Roehl, J., 471, 472, 473
Rogers, E. M., 399
Rogers, K., 59
Rogers, T., 31, 32, 34, 79, 80, 81, 82, 98, 99, 100, 109, 122, 183, 223, 471, 472, 473, 474
Romanofsky, P., 6, 9
Roosevelt, E., 504
Rosener, J. B., 153, 154
Rosenthal, B. S., 27, 30, 33, 48, 76, 79, 87, 108, 119, 122, 153, 154, 155, 203, 206, 213, 289, 345, 355, 437
Rosenthal, J., 89, 130
Ross, F., 7
Ross, R. S., 212, 213
Rossi, P. H., 499
Rossing, B. E., 130, 332, 448, 471, 472, 473, 474
Rothman, J., 7, 10
Rothschild, M. L., 404
Roussos, S., 76, 84, 99, 108, 109, 113, 122, 176, 223, 224, 278, 356, 487, 488, 490, 505
Rowitz, L., 95
Rubel, D., 355
Russell, W., 128, 129, 135

S
Salami, K. K., 502
Salas, E., 163, 166
Samuels, B., 355
Sanchez, V., 80, 99
Sanders, J. R., 449, 453, 469
Santelli, J., 20
Sarche, J., 339
Sarvela, P. D., 307
Satterwhite, P., 127, 241, 490
Sawyer, R., 404

Schermerhorn, J., 56, 223
Schmalz, K. J., 416, 417
Schmidt, F., 323
Schmidt, T. L., 470
Schooler, C., 470
Schorr, L. B., 399, 400, 402, 403, 441, 486, 487
Schultz, A., 13, 475
Schultz, A. J., 148
Schultz, J., 66, 417, 442, 443, 505
Schwartz, R., 358, 392
Scott, J., 183
Seekins, T., 130
Senge, P. M., 126, 128
Shadish, W. R. Jr., 460
Shaffer, R., 339
Sharfman, M., 14
Sharp-Light, N., 400
Sharpe, P. A., 470
Shaw, R. A., 488
Shea, S., 16, 401
Shediak-Rizkallah, M. C., 261
Sheldrick, B. J., 448
Shepherd, M., 430
Sheppard, H. A., 165
Shinn, R., 164
Shortell, S. M., 111, 181, 222
Siegel, M., 277
Siek, G., 279, 292, 293, 294, 299
Simons-Morton, B. G., 357
Simons-Morton, D. G., 357
Sinicrope, P., 51, 100
Sink, D., 32, 487
Slinski, M., 68
Smeltzer, J. L., 332, 348, 392, 401, 403, 404, 405, 406, 410, 439
Smith, D. K., 166, 167
Smith, N. L., 448
Smith, P., 279, 292, 293, 294, 299
Smith, W. A., 430
Soet, J. E., 404
Sofaer, S., 37, 50, 51, 52, 53, 69, 96, 97, 99, 118, 122, 139, 158, 229
Solomon, E., 167
Solomon, R., 167
Soriano, F. I., 355
Spickard, A., 17
Sprecht, H., 8, 12, 78, 139

Steckler, A., 14, 17, 32, 50, 54, 62, 77, 79, 80, 81, 82, 83, 95, 98, 99, 104, 107, 108-109, 109, 141, 159, 183, 203, 223, 356, 357, 358, 361, 392, 438, 460, 471, 472, 473, 474, 475, 487
Steckler, A. B., 95, 475
Steel, S. M., 130
Stephens, J. B., 140, 186, 198, 203, 204, 208, 213
Stern, R. F., 20, 98, 222
Steuart, G. W., 392
Stevens, G. L., 127
Stevenson, J., 76, 82, 95, 127, 223, 470, 471, 473, 474
Stevenson, W., 32
Stewart, P. J., 448
Stoddard, R. P., 358
Stokols, D., 16, 62
Stowers, G., 32, 487
Strawn, H. B., 361, 362, 371
Suarez, T. M., 128, 129
Sullivan Mort, G., 280
Sumners, J., 361, 362, 371
Susskind, L., 200, 244
Sussman, S., 358
Swerissen, H., 84

T
Tagliere, D., 190
Tannenbaum, S. I., 163
Taylor, R. B., 13
Taylor, S., 63, 80, 82, 108
Taylor-Fishwick, J. C., 327, 328, 345, 463
Taylor-Powell, E., 332, 448, 471, 472, 473, 474
Teisman, G. R., 162
Tesh, S., 16, 62
Themba, M., 406, 407, 412, 414, 416
Thompson, B. R., 16, 17, 32, 62
Thompson, N. J., 500
Thoreau, H. D., 261
Timmreck, T., 307, 392
Tocqueville, A. de, 3, 4–5, 24
Torczyner, J. L., 8, 12, 78, 139
Torres, R. T., 468
Tremethick, M., 203
Trohanis, P., 128

Tropman, J. E., 7
Trudeau, J., 471, 472, 473
Truth, S., 6
Tubman, H., 6
Tuckman, B. W., 164, 165
Turner, C., 78, 82, 109, 118, 183, 357, 361, 472, 474
Twiss, J., 83, 510

U
Ury, W., 208
Useem, J., 196

V
Valdiserri, R. O., 371, 431
Valente, 183
Van de Ven, A. H., 343, 344
Vangen, S., 162, 181
Variyam, J. A., 393
Vliet, M., 76

W
Walker, K., 202, 203
Wallack, L., 406, 407, 412, 413, 414, 416, 431
Wallerstein, N., 11, 12, 13, 14, 15, 69, 405, 406, 508, 509
Wandersman, A., 13, 31, 32, 33, 54, 55, 56, 64, 65, 66, 71, 76, 79, 82, 85, 86, 87, 95, 97, 98, 108, 109, 122, 140, 141, 176, 182, 183, 196, 223, 359, 361, 371,

373, 379, 436, 470, 471, 472, 473, 475, 488, 489, 499
Wang, C. C., 339
Wang, E., 339
Ware, A. J., 489
Waterman, R. H. Jr., 166
Watkins, N. B, 358
Webster, J. D., 89, 130
Weerawardena, J., 280
Weiner, B. J., 111
Weinrich, N. K., 431
Weiss, C. H., 435, 486, 487, 489
Weiss, E. S., 51, 54, 69, 70, 76, 81, 90, 109, 223, 328, 467
Weitzel, A., 255
Wetterhall, S., 442, 444
Wheeler, F. C., 95
Whetten, D., 54, 55
White, J. L., 129
White, P., 212, 213
Whitmore, E., 436, 437
Whitt, M., 50, 53, 71
Wicklund, K., 261
Wilkins, C., 202, 203
Williams, M., 164
Willis, R., 192
Wilson, J., 54
Windsor, R. A., 348
Winer, M., 27, 29, 149, 175
Wing, S., 436
Wischnowski, M. W., 141

Witkin, B. R., 331, 339, 353, 355
Wolff, T., 11, 50, 52, 55, 56, 77, 79, 86, 98, 108, 120, 141, 153, 154, 162, 183, 278, 325, 351, 356, 491, 505
Wolfson, M., 78, 223
Wood, D., 14, 53
Woodruff, K., 431
Worthen, B. R., 449, 453, 469
Wright-Isak, C., 141
Wyatt, V. H., 488

Y
Yan, A., 14
Yin, R. K., 129, 460, 488, 489, 502, 504
Young, D., 224
Young, L., 77, 82, 83, 84, 95, 357, 487, 490, 508
Yu, P., 488, 502, 504
Yukl, G., 163

Z
Zakocs, R. C., 487, 489, 490
Zald, M. N., 204, 213
Zapka, J., 54, 55
Zaza, S., 397
Ziglio, E., 343
Zimmerman, M., 13, 14, 475
Zook, L., 189

SUBJECT INDEX

A

About Business and Finance, 268
Accommodating conflict style, 210e
Accommodating strategy, 208
Accountability: autonomy versus, 207; principle of, 57; staff, 100
Action networks, 29
Action Planning Guide (Fawcett and others), 379
Action plans, 370–371, 474
Action-set coalitions, 34
Active listening, 187, 208, 211
Active members, 139
Activities. See Coalition programs
Administration on Aging, 24
Administrative assistants, 103e–104e
Advising communication roadblock, 189e
Advisory committee, 29
Advocacy: media, 411–419; strategies for community, 406–407
The Advocacy Institute,

18, 189, 213–214, 413, 417, 418, 501, 502, 505, 509
Advocacy Project, 428
Advocate, 144
Agenda (meeting), 249–250
AIDS Action, 21
AIDS Alliance for Children, Youth and Families, 21
AIDS NGO Network of East Africa (ANNEA), 21
AIDS Treatment Activists Coalition, 21
AIDS Vaccine Advocacy Coalition, 21
Alcohol prevention, 17–18, 65
Alcohol, tobacco, and other drug abuse (ATOD), 65
Alliance, 30
Alliance for Justice, 428
Allies Against Asthma Initiative, 22, 490, 502
Allstate Foundation, 426
Alternative members, 140
Altruistic recruitment approach, 146–147
American Cancer Society, 18, 22

American Dental Association, 19
American Dental Hygienists Association, 19
American Evaluation Association Task Force, 449
American Heart Association, 22, 300
American Legacy Foundation, 428
American Lung Association, 300
American Philosophical Society, 4
American Psychological Association, 433
American Public Health Association (APHA), 300, 433
American Stop Smoking Intervention Study (ASSIST), 18
American Trauma Society, 425
Annie E. Casey Foundation, 20, 300
APEX-PH (Assessment Protocol for Excellence in Public Health), 358, 360t

Appalachia Leadership Initiative on Cancer (ALIC), 36
Appalachian Partnership for Welfare Reform, 409
Archdiocese of Chicago, 7
Are Your a Transformational Leader?, 114e–115e
Arkansas Office of Oral Health, 315–316
The Art of Coalition Building (Brown), 507
Assessment/planning: CCAT proposition on, 82; CINCH application of CCAT on, 87–88; community assessment, 321–355; needs, 133e, 328; public health planning, 356–390; resource development, 293–298t; self-assessment for promising coalition practices, 398e; social marketing planning, 10, 409–411t; strategic planning process, 361–363, 370–379. *See also* Evaluation
Asset mapping, 338–339
Association for Conflict Resolution (ACR), 219
Association for the Study and Development of Community (ASCD), 433
Associations, 4–5
Asthma: CINCH goals and objectives regarding, 365e; coalitions involved in prevention of, 22–23
AtHealth, 433
ATLAS/ti program, 466
Audience segmentation, 408
Autonomy versus accountability, 207
Avoiding conflict style, 209e
Avoiding strategy, 208

B

Back of the Yards Neighborhood Council (BYNC), 7
Behavior: description of, 187; ground rules for meeting, 243–244; "higher ground" metaphor for, 204
Behavioral Risk Factor Surveillance Survey, 340
Benchmarking, 371

BikeWise in West Philadelphia project, 425–426
Binding responses, 187
Black Panthers, 8
Black Women's Health Imperative, 22
Blind vote, 199
Block Booster Project (NYC), 13
BoardSource: Building Effective NonProfit Boards, 177, 256–257, 283
Body orientation, 184
Bowling Alone: America's Declining Social Capital (Putnam), 15
Box leadership approach, 119
Brain pool method, 191
Brainstorming, 191, 193e, 201, 244
Branding, 267
"Breaking Barriers to Success in Your Coalition" (Kaye and Wolfe), 56
Brochure Content Worksheet, 269e
Brochures, 268–270
Buckle Up America!, 428
"Buddy System" recruitment, 159
Budget request, 308
Budgeting steps: 1: estimating coalition expenses, 287; 2: estimating coalition income, 288; 3: creating budget spreadsheet, 288–289; 4: creating budget document, 289
Budgets: Coalition for a Health Future (fiscal 2010), 290t; developing the coalition, 285, 287, 291e; evaluation, 451, 453; grant application information on, 308; managing the coalition, 291e; preparing data collection, 347; steps in creating, 287–290t
Built to Last (Collins), 196
Business partnerships, 280
Business plan, 265–266
Bylaws, 231–240
Bylines (or slogans), 225
BYNC (Back of the Yards Neighborhood Council), 7

C

CADCA (Community Anti-Drug Coalitions of America), 17, 97, 132133, 219, 415, 480e
California Coalition for Childhood Immunization, 492–493
California Endowment, 22
California Healthy Cities and Communities Program, 326, 358, 502, 509
California Wellness Foundation, 20
Camera Club project, 426
Campaigns, 10
Cancer prevention, 21–22
Capacity builder, 144
Capacity building typology, 11fig–12
CAQDAS (computer-assisted qualitative data analysis software), 466
Cardiovascular disease prevention, 21–22
Case studies design, 459
Catalog of Federal Domestic Assistance, 317
Catalyst, 144
Catch a Kid Doing the Right Thing campaign, 426
Catchment Area Planning and Action (CAPA), 502
Cause and effect (or fishbone), 191
CCAT. *See* Community Coalition Action Theory (CCAT)
CCPPA (Community Coalition Partnerships Programs for the Prevention of Teen Pregnancy) [CDC], 325, 327
CDCynergy model, 358, 410, 433
Center for Community Change, 177–178
Center for Creative Leadership (CCL), 135
Center for the Study and Prevention of Violence, 399
Center for Substance Abuse Prevention (CSAP), 17, 130, 502
Centers for Disease Control and Prevention (CDC): Arkansas Office of Oral

Health support by, 315; childhood asthma reports by, 22; childhood immunization promoted by, 19; Choose Your Cover program of, 428; Community Coalition Partnerships Programs for the Prevention of Teen Pregnancy (CCPPA) of, 325, 327; Comprehensive Cancer Control program of, 22; Diabetes and Control Program of, 22; on evaluations, 433, 454, 455; Framework for Program evaluation in Public Health by, 444–445*fig*; grant funding by, 300; on health engineering strategies, 405; HIV/AIDS prevention funding by, 20; National Asthma Control Program of, 22; National Immunization Program of, 84; National Program to Promote Diabetes Education Strategies in Minority Communities of, 22; Oral Health Division of, 19; REACH 2010 program of, 23–24; School Health Index, 371; *Standards for Effective Evaluation* by, 445; teen pregnancy prevention efforts by, 20; training and technical-assistance aid by, 130; Youth Media Campaign of, 428

Centers for Substance Abuse Prevention (CASP), 65

Chair/vice-chair positions, 105*e*

Challenger explosion (1986), 196

Chamber of Commerce, 341

Change leadership approach, 119

Channels (communication), 408

Charisma (or idealized influence), 112

Checklists: Checklist for Choosing Coalition Problems or Issues, 324*e*; Checklist of Policy Indicators for Alcohol, Tobacco, and Other Drugs, 477*e*–479*e*; Checklist for Selecting an Evaluator, 452*e*; Collaboration Checklist, 45*e*–46*e*; Collaboration Readiness Checklist, 47*e*–48*e*; for developing bylaws, 231–232; 501(c)(3) Charitable Organization, 284*e*; Inclusivity Checklist, 155*e*; Team Effectiveness Checklist, 173*e*

Cheerleader role, 125

Children: CDC reports on asthma in, 22; health insurance for, 365*e*

Children's National Medical Center, 20

CHIs (community health indicators), 335

Choose Your Cover (CDC), 428

Chronicle of Philanthropy, 317

CINCH (Consortium for Infant and Child Health), 37–38, 364*e*–365*e*

Citizen participation: defining, 25; early development of, 12–13

Citizen power, 13

Civic participation principle, 57

CIVICUS, 277

Civil rights movement, 8

Civil society, 4–5

Clarifer (or summarizer), 175

Coach leadership role, 108, 125

Coaching (or selling) leadership, 169*e*

Coalition approach: benefits of working using a, 53–55; challenges associated with, 55–57; issues to consider before using, 58–59

Coalition building: applying democratic principles to, 57; definition of, 10

Coalition for a Health Future, 290*t*

Coalition infrastructure: bylaws and guidelines for operation, 231–240; coalition vision and mission statements, 223–225; evaluation of, 440–441; formalized rules and procedures, 223; importance and variety of, 222–223; meetings and, 240–256; organizational charts of, 227*fig*–229*fig*; resources on, 256–258; roles and job descriptions, 225–226; steering committee and governance, 226*e*, 229–230. *See also* Coalition structures; Work groups

The Coalition Institute, 494

Coalition intervention strategies: community mobilization strategies, 405–407; health communication, 403–404; health education, 404; health engineering, 405; health-policy and enforcement, 404–405; health-related community service, 405

Coalition interventions: assessing promising, 395–398; characteristics of successful, 399–400; effectiveness, plausibility, and practicality criteria for, 397; ethical guidelines for community, 421*e*; evaluation of, 441–442; implementing community-based strategies for, 401; Injury Free Coalition for Kids (IFCK) of Philadelphia example of, 425–426; legal and ethical issues in, 421*e*–425; levels of, 401–402; proven, 396; reinvented innovations as, 399; replicating community-based strategies for, 402–403; resources on, 428–432; self-assessment for promising, 398*e*; types of strategies used for, 403–407

Coalition measures: described, 470; level 1 measures of infrastructure, function, and processes,

Coalition: *(continued)* 470–474; level 2 measures of programs and interventions, 474–475; level 3 measures of health status/community change outcomes, 475–476. *See also* Evaluation

Coalition member engagement: CCAT proposition on, 87; CINCH application of CCAT on, 87

Coalition membership: building community ownership in, 175–176; building diversity in, 149, 153–155, 156e–158e; building effective teams/work groups, 163–175e; categories of, 139–140; CCAT on engagement of, 87; CCAT proposition on, 77–78; characteristics, capacities, and skills, 140–141; CINCH application of CCAT, 85; convening versus participating, 139, 140, 144; evaluation of, 471–472; Inclusivity Checklist for, 155e; member organizations versus individual, 138–139; Model Commitment Letter for, 143e; recruitment of, 144–149; resources on, 177–179; responsibilities of, 142–143; retention of, 158, 158–159; roles of, 144; "The Six 'R's' of Participation" for, 160, 160e–162e; size of, 162–163

Coalition models: Collaboration Framework, 67–69; Community Coalition Action Theory (CCAT), 61, 62, 71–91, 442; Community Coalition Model, 65–66fig; Community Organization and Development Model (COD), 62–63; The Conceptual Framework for Coalition Assessment, 69; Framework of Organizational Viability, 64–65fig; Framework for Partnerships for Community

Development (The Framework), 63–64fig; Model of Community Health Governance, 69–71; PRECEDE-PROCEED, 67, 264t, 357, 358, 408; Typology of Community Organization and Community Building, 10–12, 69; Work Group on Health Promotion and Community Development, 66–67fig

Coalition operations/processes: CCAT proposition on, 78–79; CINCH application of CCAT, 86

Coalition processes: effective decision solving, 195–203; evaluation of, 440–441; internal communication, 182–190t; problem solving, 190–195; resolving conflict, 203–216; resources on, 219–221; Virginians for a Healthy Future example of, 216–217. *See also* Inward work; Outward work

Coalition programs: assessing promising practices/interventions of, 395–398; effectiveness, plausibility, and practicality criteria for, 397; evaluation of, 441–442; Los Angeles County Alcohol, Tobacco, and Drug Policy Coalition example of, 419–420; media advocacy of, 411–419; phases of implementation of, 392; practical steps in development of, 393e; project team for, 394–395; replicating community-based strategies for, 402–403; resources on, 428–432; selecting and implementing, 392–407; social marketing through, 407–411; as social-capital builders, 400

Coalition spokespersons, 175, 275–276

Coalition structures: CCAT proposition on, 81; CINCH application of CCAT, 87;

impact on coalition staff, 98–99. *See also* Coalition infrastructure

Coalition Technical Assistance and Training (CTAT), 130

Coalitions: as "action sets," 32; building community ownership of, 175–176; building competent communities through, 16–17; CINCH (Consortium for Infant and Child Health) example of, 37–38, 364e–365e; comparing community coalitions to other types of, 34–36; competing, 36–37; contemporary roots of health promotion, 12–16; criteria for defining, 31–32; definition of, 30, 31; factors promoting success of, 505–507; future research on, 507–510; importance of community context for, 51–53; influence levels of, 50–51; issues to consider before establishing, 58–59; lifespan of, 59; needs assessment of, 133e; resources on partnerships and, 135–137; situations promoting establishment of, 49–51; technical assistance/training report made to, 132e; technical assistance/training responsibilities of, 129, 131e; types of, 32–34; unique accomplishments of, 501. *See also* Health issues

Coalitions types: action-set, 34; community-based, 32–33; grassroots, 32; organization-set, 33; professional (agency-based), 32

Collaborating: as conflict resolution strategy, 208; as conflict style, 209e; definition of, 28

Collaboration: comprehensive, 31; conflict resolution, 31; contextual factors affecting, 51–52; continuum for building relationships/ doing work in, 28*fig*; defining, 26–27; definitions for each partnering relationships of, 29–30; factors influencing the success of, 39*e*–40*e*; intensity and levels of, 27–29; models of, 30–31; risk factors for participation in, 41*e*–44*e*; steps of, 27. *See also* Partnerships

Collaboration and Change, LLC, 178

Collaboration Checklist, 45*e*–46*e*

Collaboration Framework, 68–69

Collaboration models: service integration efforts, 31; strategic partnerships, 30–31

Collaboration Readiness Checklist, 47*e*–48*e*

Collaborative leadership. *See* Transformational leadership

Colorado's Storm King Mountain disaster (1994), 196

Commanding (or ordering) communication, 187*e*–188*e*

Commission, 30

Commitment Letter, 143*e*

Communication: channels of, 185–187; characteristics of internal, 182–183; coalition intervention strategies related to, 403–404; comparing productive/less productive group, 190*t*; of evaluation findings, 468–470; factors increasing group cohesiveness and, 183; features of effective group, 186–189, 189; getting past roadblocks to, 187*e*–188*e*; *Healthy People 2010* objectives for health, 370*e*; Internet and e-mail, 186; miscommunication during, 185; process of effective, 183–185; social marketing channels of, 408

Communities Advocating Emergency AIDS Relief Coalition (CAEAR), 21

Community: choosing issues that resonate with, 322–323; cultural climate of, 52–53; empowerment of, 13–14; evaluating change outcomes of, 442; *Healthy People 2010* objectives for health in, 367*e*–368*e*; importance of coalitions in context of, 51–53; profiles of, 334

Community Action to Fight Asthma (CAFA), 22

Community advocacy, 406–407

Community Anti-Drug Coalitions of America (CADCA), 17, 97, 132–133, 219, 415, 480*e*

Community assessment: asset-based approach to, 328–330; benefits and challenges of conducting, 330–331; Checklist for Choosing Coalition Problems or Issues, 324*e*; choosing issues that resonate with community, 322–323; conducting the, 331–350; in context of a coalition, 328; framing issue to build support, 323, 325–326; impact of issue on the coalition, 326; lessons learned about issues and, 351–352; Metropolitan Boston Haitian HIV Prevention Coalition's experience with, 352; need for, 321; of priority populations, 326–328; resources on conducting, 353–355

Community assessment steps: 1: determining assessment's purpose and scope, 332; 2: defining the assessment's goals and objectives, 332; 3: selecting approach and methods for collecting data, 332–347; 4: designing and pilot-testing instruments and procedures, 347; 5: preparing timeline and budget, 348; 6: collecting the data, 348; 7: analyzing the data, 348–349; 8: preparing

and disseminating findings, 349–350; 9: evaluating assessment's merit and worth, 351

Community building: coalition interventions through, 405; typology of, 11*fig*–12

Community Building Institute (CBI), 219–220

Community capacity: CCAT proposition on, 84; CINCH application of CCAT on, 88; definition of, 14–15; evaluation measuring outcome of, 475

Community Catalyst, Inc., 178, 415, 502

Community change outcomes. *See* Outcomes

Community Coalition Action Theory (CCAT): assessment and planning proposition of, 82; CINCH application of, 84–88; coalition membership proposition of, 78; coalition operations and processes proposition of, 78–79; coalition structures proposition of, 81; community capacity proposition of, 84; community change outcomes proposition of, 83; community context proposition of, 77; empirical support for the, 76–77; as evaluation framework, 442; future directions of, 90–91; health and social outcomes proposition of, 83–84; implementation of strategies proposition of, 83; introduction to, 61; lead agency or convener group proposition of, 77; leadership and staffing propositions of, 80; member engagement proposition of, 82; origin and roots of, 62; other coalition frameworks/ models contributing to, 62–71; outline of propositions, 71–75*fig*; pooled member and external resources propositions of, 81; stages of development

Community: *(continued)*
proposition of, 76–77;
strengths and limitations of,
88–90
Community Coalition Model,
65–66*fig*
Community Coalition Partnerships Programs for the Prevention of Teen Pregnancy
(CCPPA) [CDC], 325, 327
Community coalitions:
building competent
communities through,
16–17; compared to
regional or national coalitions, 36; compared to state
coalitions, 34–36; definition
of, 32–33; functions of, 34;
historic rise and applications of, 17–23
Community competence, 15
Community context: CCAT
proposition on, 76–77;
CINCH application of CCAT
on, 85; importance of, 51–53
Community foundations, 300
Community Guide, 396–397
Community health assessment, 329
Community health communication, 404
Community Health Improvement Program (CHIP), 358
Community health indicators
(CHIs), 335
Community Health Ventures
Program (Pfizer Foundation), 303
Community HIV/AIDS Mobilization Project Office of
Minority Health, 21
Community Intervention Trial
for Smoking Cessation
(COMMIT), 18
Community Leader Guide
(University of Nevada
Cooperative Extension), 159
Community Leadership
Guide, 219
Community level influence, 51
Community meeting
recruitment, 148
Community mobilization
strategies, 405–406

Community (or systems)
outcomes, 440
Community Organization and
Development Model (COD),
62–63
Community organizer, 144
Community organizing, 405
*Community Organizing and
Community Building for
Health* (Minkler), 10
Community outreach, 406
Community ownership,
175–176
Community participation:
defining, 25; risk propositions for collaborative,
41*e*–44*e*
Community Resources, 354
Community Service Organization for Mexican American
Workers in California, 7
Community Tool Box (CTB),
232, 257, 296, 304, 354,
390, 400, 402, 407, 421, 422
Community-based initiative
evaluations, 486–487
Community-based participatory research (CBPR), 436
Community-development (or
neighborhood-maintenance)
approach: citizen participation element of, 12–13;
community capacity
building element of, 14–15;
community competence element of, 15; contemporary
roots of, 12–16; empowerment element of, 13–14;
four historical periods of, 9;
origins of, 12; social capital
element of, 15–16; social
change through, 8–9; typology of, 11*fig*–12; United
Nations design for, 12
Community-organizing movements: early history (1800s)
of, 5–6; neighborhood-maintenance or community-development approach to,
8–9; political activist
approach to, 7–8; social
work approach to, 6–7;
typology of community-building and, 11*fig*

Competence issue, 424
Competing strategy, 208
Comprehensive Cancer
Control program (CDC),
22, 359
Comprehensive Cancer Prevention and Control, 356
Comprehensive
collaboration, 31
Compromising conflict
style, 209*e*
Compromising strategy, 208
Computer-assisted qualitative
data analysis software
(CAQDAS), 466
The Conceptual Framework
for Coalition Assessment, 69
Conduit, 144
Conference (or training)
recruitment, 147
Confidentiality issues,
422–423
Conflict: A Continuum of
Approaches to Conflict,
210*e*–211*e*; evaluation findings on coalition, 473; turfism, 212–216; types of,
204, 206–207; understanding differing styles of,
209*e*–210*e*
Conflict of interest, 424–425
Conflict management: continuum of approaches to,
210*e*–211*e*; skills for, 208,
211–212
Conflict resolution: collaborations for, 31; Conflict Resolution Capacity Inventory,
205*e*–206*e*; continuum of
approaches to, 210*e*–211*e*;
general strategies used for,
208; importance of developing effective, 203–204
Conflict Resolution Capacity
Inventory, 205*e*–206*e*
The Conflict Resolution
Information Source
(CR Info), 220
Congress of Industrial
Organizations (CIO), 7
Conscience/imagination
traits, 121
Consensus: as decision making style, 198; levels of,

200; techniques for building, 199–200
Consensus builder leader, 125
Consensus log, 200
Consortium: definition of, 30; service integration efforts of, 31
Constitutional Convention, 4
Constructivist (or interpretivist) evaluation, 435
Contextual factors: affecting collaboration, 51–52; CCAT community, 77; definition of, 68; social capital as coalition, 52
Continuous improvement/self-renewal, 121
Continuum for Building Relationships/Doing Work, 28*fig*
Controlling abuse of power principle, 57
Controlling Asthma in America, 22
Convening members, 139, 140, 144
Cooperation ideology: birth of, 3; definition of, 28; early American, 3–4
Coordinating, 28
Coordinators: duties/responsibilities of, 100*e*–102*e*; as leadership role, 108; qualifications of, 102*e*
Core foundation, 68
Courage-consideration balance, 121
Critical incident technique, 339
Criticizing communication roadblock, 187*e*–188*e*
CSAP (Center for Substance Abuse Prevention), 17, 130, 502
Cultural miscommunication, 185

D

Data analysis: described, 348–349*t*; evaluation, 466–467
Data collection: conducting the, 348; designing and pilot-testing instruments

for, 347; evaluation, 459–461*fig*, 463–465; preparing and disseminating findings from, 349–351; preparing timeline and budget for, 348; selecting approach and methods for, 332–347
Data collection methods: asset mapping, 338–339; community health indicators (CHIs) development, 335; critical incident technique, 339; Delphi Technique, 344; document review, 335–336*t*; evaluation, 459–460, 461*fig* 463–465; focus groups, 342*t*, 343*t*, 344–446; interviews, 340–342*t*; neighborhood and community profiles, 334; Nominal Group Technique (NGT), 191, 194*e*, 343–344; observations, 336–337; Photovoice, 339; public forums, 339–340; selecting the approach and, 332–334; self-completed diaries or logs, 347; standardized tests, 334; types listed, 333; windshield tours or surveys, 338, 342*t*, 346–347
DAWN (Disability Advocates/Wisconsin Network), 431
Decision making: importance of effective, 195–196; majority-rule, 198, 199; during meetings, 246; principles of, 57; prioritizing tools for, 200–203; Robert's Rules of Order used in, 200–201; styles of, 196, 198–199; What's Your Coalition's Participant Involvement Score?, 197*e*–198*e*
Decision making prioritizing tools: ethical decision making, 202–203; multi-voting, 201; zero to ten rating, 201–202
Declaration of Independence, 4
Delegating leadership, 169*e*

Deliberation principle, 57
Delphi Technique, 344
Delta Dental, 19, 315, 316
Democracy in America (de Tocqueville), 3, 4, 24
The Democracy Center, 418
Democracy Center Advocacy Training and Resources, 429
Democracy expansion, 5
Devil's advocate (or skeptic): as decision making technique, 199; taking role of, 175
Diabetes and Control Program (CDC), 22
Diabetes prevention, 21–22
Diagnosing the Health of Your Coalition Assessment Instrument, 481*e*–484*e*
Diagnosing the Health of Your Coalition Score Sheet, 484*e*
Diaries (or logs), 347
Direct action strategies, 406
Directing (or telling) leadership, 169*e*
Director leadership role, 108
Disclosure issues, 424
Discussion principle, 57
Disease prevention, 21–22
Disseminating: community assessment, 349–351; evaluation reports, 469–470
Distilling concerns, 200
Diverse coalition membership, 149, 153–155, 156*e*–158*e*
Diverting communication roadblock, 189*e*
Do We Need a Promotion Plan for Our Coalition?, 263*t*
Document review, 335–336*t*
Doer role, 108
Door-to-door recruitment, 147
Dots (decision making technique), 199
Drug abuse prevention, 17–18
Drug Free Communities Act, 17
Drug Strategies, 17, 489, 505

E

E-mail: communication through, 186; newsletters sent through, 270

Earned income businesses, 280
Educational Technology Grants and Grant-Writing, 316
EffectiveMeetings.com, 220
Effectiveness criteria, 397
Empowerment: health definition of, 13; *Transformation for Health* approach to meeting, 255–256
Empowerment evaluation, 436
Enabler leader role, 122
Energy level, 185
Enforcement (legal or legislative), 210e–211e
Engaging Potential Partners Worksheet, 152e
Environmental health objectives, 367e
Equality principle, 57
Ethical issues: competence, 424; confidentiality, 422–423; conflict of interest, 424–425; for decision making, 202–203; disclosure, 424; guidelines for community interventions, 421e; informed consent, 423–424; liability, 422; websites resources on, 431–432
Ethnograph software, 466
Evaluation: California Coalition for Childhood Immunization experience with, 492–493; challenges of coalition, 487–490; community assessment, 351; of community-based initiatives, 486–487; designs of, 458–459; frameworks and models of, 442–447; instruments used in, 476–477, 480e–486e; key concepts and levels of, 437–442; lessons learned from coalition, 502–505; overall strength of health plan, 378e; planning the, 447–449, 451, 453, 462e–465e; promoting self-reflection and improvement, 436–437; reporting, 469–470; resources on,

494–500; solving the dilemma of coalition, 490–492; steps in, 447–449, 451, 453–455, 458, 459, 461–470; strategic health planning process, 371–379; ten principles to guide coalition, 433–434; timeline of, 458. *See also* Assessment/planning; Coalition measures
Evaluation instruments: Community Anti-Drug Coalitions of America Coalition self-assessment, 480e; Diagnosing the Health of Your Coalition Assessment Instrument, 481e–484e; Diagnosing the Health of Your Coalition Score Sheet, 484e; overview of, 476–477; Plan Quality Assessment Tool: Plan Quality Index (PQI) for, 372e–378e; policy indictors for alcohol, tobacco, and other drugs, 477e–479e; resources on, 494–497; State Plan Index (SPI) for, 371, 378–379, 380e–389e; Tobacco-Free Youth Coalition Self-Evaluation Instrument, 485e–486e
Evaluation models: CCAT, 442; CDC's Framework for Program Evaluation in Public Health, 444–445fig; Kansas University Work Group's Framework for Participatory Evaluation of Community Initiatives, 443–444; Kellogg Foundation's Steps to Program Evaluation, 446–447; summary of, 443t
Evaluation plan, 307
Evaluation steps: 1: planning the evaluation, 447–449, 451, 453, 462e–463e; 2: describing the program and developing questions, 453–455, 460e; 3: focusing the evaluation design, 458–459; 4: deciding on data collection methods, 459, 461fig, 464–465;

5: analyzing and interpreting the data, 466–467; 6: communicating and ensuring use of evaluation findings, 468–470
Evaluators: Checklist for Selecting an Evaluator, 452e; guiding principles for, 450e–451e; hiring professional, 448–449; skills of effective, 449
Every Child by Two (ECBT), 19, 492
Exchange networks, 29
Executive boards (or committees), 30
Experimental evaluation design, 459
Expertise leadership, 119
Eye contact, 184

F
Face-to-face discussion, 210e–211e
Face-to-face recruitment, 147
Facilitator (or leader): described, 140, 144; meeting guidelines for, 245; team and work group roles of, 174–175
Family Resource Center, 426
Federation, 30
Feedback communication, 184
Field Notes on Fund-Raising, 291–292
Fighting Back, 17, 488, 494
Fishbone (or cause and effect) diagram, 191
Five City Projects, 16
501(c)(3) tax status, 283–285e, 286e
501(c)(4) tax status, 283–285e, 286e
501(c)(6) tax status, 283–285e, 286e
Flyer recruitment approach, 148
Focus groups, 342t, 343t, 344–346
Forcing conflict style, 209e
Ford Foundation,
Formal leaders, 117
Formative evaluation, 439
Forming team development stage, 164

Fortune magazine, 195

Foundation Center, 316–317

"4 Ps" of Marketing, 408–409

Framework of Organizational Viability, 64–65*fig*

Framework for Partnerships for Community Development (The Framework), 63–64*fig*

Framework for Program Evaluation in Public Health (CDC), 444–445*fig*

Freeing responses, 187

FTEs (full time equivalents), 308

Full (or voting) members, 140

Full participation communication, 186

Fund-raising: Arkansas Office of Oral Health experience with, 315–316; characteristics of coalition, 281–282; description of, 278–279; field notes on, 291–292; nonprofit organization status and, 282–285*e*, 286*e*; roles involved in, 290; setting objectives of, 295–296; social enterprise, 280; social entrepreneurs role in, 281; through grants, 298–314

Funder, 144

Fundraising for Dummies (Mutz and Murray), 318

Funds: developing budget to manage, 285, 287–290*t*; using grants for additional, 298–314; resource development plan regarding, 292–298*t*; sources of coalition, 279; sustainability through, 279. *See also* Resources (coalition)

Future of Public Health report (IOM), 358

Future Smiles, 315–316

G

Geographical conflict, 206

Getting to Outcomes (GTO), 359, 361

Goals: CINCH objectives and, 364*e*–365*e*; conflict over, 204; defining community

assessment, 332; means versus model conflict and, 207; public health strategic planning, 363; setting fundraising, 295–296. *See also* Objectives

Good to Great (Collins), 144, 196

Governance, 229–230

Grant applications: common mistakes in, 311*e*–312*e*; dealing with rejection of, 309–310; improving competitive, 310, 312–314, 310, 312–314; letters of intent (LOI), 305; sections of, 305–309

Grant funders: contacting, 301; identifying and researching, 299–301; RFPs (request for proposals), 302–303, 304, 306, 310, 312–314

Grant proposals: building support for, 301–302; elements of award-winning, 310*e*; letters of intent (LOI), 305; reviewing process for competitive applications, 304–305; RFPs (request for proposals), 302–303, 304, 306, 310, 312–314

Grants: advantages of applying for, 298–299; contacting the funder, 301; identifying and researching sources of, 299–301; timing of applications, 298–299

Grantsmanship Center, 317

Grass tips organizing, 10

Grassroots coalitions, 32

Grassroots organizing: definition of, 10; "The Six 'R's' of Participation" of, 160, 160*e*–162*e*

Ground rules, 243–244

Grounding, 68

Group cohesiveness factors, 183

Group communication: comparing productive/less productive, 190*t*; features of effective, 186; guide to getting past roadblocks of, 187*e*–188*e*

The Grove Consultants International, 257

GTO (Getting to Outcomes), 359, 361

Guiding Principles for Evaluators (AEA), 449

H

Health care access objectives, 369*e*

Health Care and Finance Administration (HCFA), 130

Health Care Trust Fund, 217

Health communication: as coalition intervention strategy, 403–404; objectives of, 370*e*

Health community assessment, 329–330

Health disparities goals, 365*e*

Health education strategies, 404

Health engineering strategies, 405

Health insurance: CINCH goals for child, 365*e*; coalitions promoting, 21

Health issues: checklist for choosing, 324*e*; CINCH goals and objectives regarding, 368*e*–365*e*; framing to build support, 323, 325–326; impact on the coalition, 326; lessons learned about community assessment and, 351–352; priority populations and, 326–328; that resonate with the community, 322–323. *See also* Coalitions

Health Resources and Services Administration (HRSA), 24, 130, 300, 428

Health status change evaluation, 442

Health-policy/enforcement strategies, 404–405

Health-related community service strategies, 405

HealthierUS, 24

Healthy Cities and Healthy People in Healthy Communities, 326, 358, 502, 509

Healthy Communities, 356, 360e
Healthy People 2010, 356, 367e–370e
Healthy People in Healthy Communities (UDDHHS), 358, 366
Hepatitis B Coalition, 19
"Higher ground" metaphor, 204
HIV Prevention Community Planning, 356
HIV/AIDS prevention, 20–21
Home Safety Project, 426
Honest communication, 186
Horizontal organizational charts, 227fig
Human assets leadership, 119
Human rights principle, 57

I

"I" messages, 187
Idea bin (or parking lot), 244
Identifying Potential Collaboration Partners worksheet, 149e–151e
Identity conflicts, 206
IFCK (Injury Free Coalition for Kids), 425–426
Image vision, 224
Imagination/conscience traits, 121
Immunization: CINCH goals for, 364e; coalitions promoting, 19; evaluating coalition program promoting, 492–493; Tracker the hound mascot promoting, 267; Tracker Talk newsletter on, 271e–272e
Immunization Action Coalition, 19
Impact evaluation, 438
Impact vision, 225
Impacts, 69
Implementation of strategies: CCAT proposition on, 83; CINCH application of CCAT on, 88
Inactive members, 139
Inclusivity Checklist, 155e
Independence Hall Association, 4
Independent foundations, 300

Independent Task Force on Community Preventive Services, 397
Indicators (evaluation), 464
Individual outcomes, 439
Individualized consideration, 112
Informal conciliation, 210e–211e
Informal leaders, 117
Informed consent, 423–424
Initiators, 174
Injury Free Coalition for Kids (IFCK), 425–426
Injury prevention: CINCH goals and objectives for, 365e; history of coalitions involved in, 20
Innovation Network, 245
Innovator leader role, 122
Inspirational motivation, 112
Institute of Medicine (IOM), 356, 358
Insurance. *See* Health insurance
Intellectual stimulation, 112
Inter-organizational outcomes, 440
International Association of Facilitators, 244–245
International Association for Public Participation (IAP2), 219
International Leadership Association (ILA), 136
Internet communication, 186
Internet Nonprofit Center, 317
Internet recruitment, 148
Interpersonal health communication, 404
Interpersonal level influence, 51
Interpretivist (or constructivist) evaluation, 435
Intervention Mapping, 358
Interviews: advantages and disadvantages of, 342t; data collection using, 340; individual or key informant, 341, 343; media advocacy, 416–417
Intrapersonal health communication, 403

Intrapersonal level influence, 51
Inward work: bylaws and guidelines for, 231–240; coalition rules and procedures, 223; conducting meetings, 240–256; description of, 181; funding and resource development, 278–318; marketing the coalition, 261–277; organizational charts for, 227fig–229fig; roles and job descriptions, 225–226; steering committee, 226e, 229–230, 292; vision and mission statements, 223–225. *See also* Coalition processes; Outward work; Work groups
Issues. *See* Health issues

J

Jicarilla Apache, 379
John S. and James L. Night Foundation, 17
Join Together, 476
Joseph and Edna Josephson Institute on Ethics, 219
Judging communication roadblock, 187e–188e
Just Associates (JASS), 136

K

Kansas University Work Group's Framework for Participatory Evaluation of Community Initiatives, 443–444
Kellogg Foundation's Steps to Program Evaluation, 446–447
Khmer Health Advocates (Cambodian), 22
Kiwanis Club, 341
The Knowing Your Community, Showing Your Community Method and Handbook (Community Resources), 354

L

Labeling communication roadblock, 187e–188e

Language Line
Services, 315
Lead agency (or convener
group): CCAT proposition
on, 77; characteristics of
good, 97–98; CINCH appli-
cation of CCAT, 85; description of, 96; role of, 97;
types of, 96–97
Leader Mentor Program
(CADCA), 133, 134
Leaders: categories of, 117;
characteristics of ideal
coalition, 131e; innovator,
linker, enabler roles of, 122;
recruitment of, 117–118;
technical assistance to,
128–130, 131e; training,
126–128, 129, 130–134;
traits, skills, and roles of,
121–122, 122, 125, 126;
transformational, 109,
111–113fig, 114e–115e,
115e–116e, 120t–121
Leadership: CCAT proposition
regarding, 80; description of
different roles of, 108–109;
developing quality volun-
teer, 110e–111e; Manage-
ment and Leader
Assessment Scale,
122e–124e; styles of,
118–119; sustainability of
coalition dependence on,
95; team and work group,
126, 167–168, 169e, 170e;
ten commitments of, 125t.
See also Staff
Leadership (Burns), 112
Leadership Learning Community (LLC), 136–137
Leadership style: comparing
collaborative versus traditional, 120t–121; described,
118; five types of, 119;
team, 169e; ten collaborative characteristics of,
119–120; transformational,
109, 111–113fig, 114e–115e,
115e–116e, 120t–121
Leadership training: coalition
role/responsibilities for,
129; overview of, 126–127;
recommendations for,

127–128; reports made to
coalitions on, 132e; roles,
responsibilities, characteris-
tics of, 129; venues of,
130–134
League, 30
Legal (or legislative) enforce-
ment, 210e–211e
Legislation: Drug Free Com-
munities Act, 17; Ryan
White Care Act, 20; Social
Security Act, 7
Less active members, 139
Less formal meeting recruit-
ment, 147
Letters of intent (LOI), 305
Liability issues, 422
Liaison (or
spokesperson), 175
The Library Company, 4
Linker leader role, 122
Linking agent role, 108
Locality development
model, 10
Logic models, 454–455,
456e–457e
Logo, 267
Long-term outcomes, 438
Los Angeles City Council,
419–420
Los Angeles City Department
of Building and
Safety, 420
Los Angeles County Alcohol,
Tobacco, and Drug Policy
Coalition, 419–420
Los Angeles Unified School
District, 420
Loyalty conflicts, 207

M
Majority-rule decisions,
198, 199
Management and Leader
Assessment Scale,
122e–124e
MAPP (Mobilizing Action
through Planning and Partnership), 357–358, 360t
Marketing Campaign Devel-
opment Tool, 411t
Marketing coalitions: business plan development,
265–266; coalition branding

with logo and name, 267;
need for, 262; promotion
plan for, 263t; promotional
materials used for, 267–276;
resources for, 277. See also
Social marketing
Marshall Fields, 7
Mascots, 267
Mass media: advocacy strategies by, 411–419, 428–431;
evaluation of coalition coverage by, 474; health communication through, 404;
outlets of, 416t
Master Settlement Agreement
(MSA), 18, 504
MATCH (Multilevel Approach
to Community Health),
357, 360t
MCI Conferencing White
Paper, 240
Means versus model, 207
Media advocacy: advocacy
team roles in, 418–419;
described, 411–412; developing a strategy for,
417–418; interview basics
for, 416–417; resources on,
428–431; steps in developing, 412–413; strategies of,
413–416
Media Advocacy and Public
Health (Wallack and col-
leagues), 413
Mediation Information and
Resource Center, 220
Meetings: agenda for,
249–250; chair's or facilitator's guidelines for, 245;
common challenges of,
245–249; ground rules for,
243–244; importance of
effective, 240–241; minutes
of, 250–254e; parliamentary
procedure during, 255;
process and roles during,
244–245; seven tips for
chairing effective, 241–242;
timing of, 242–243; Transformation for Health
approach to empowered,
255–256
Membership. See Coalition
membership

Messages: communication channels for, 185–186; description of, 184; developing organizational, 262, 264e–265; "I," 187
Methodology conflicts, 206
Metropolitan Boston Haitian HIV Prevention Coalition, 352
Minimum winning coalition, 162
Minnesota Heart Health Program, 16
Minority Community Health Coalition Demonstration Program, 20–21
Minority HIV/AIDS Initiative, 21
Minority rule decision, 196, 198
Minutes (meeting), 250–251e
Miscommunication, 185
Mission statements, 223–224, 225, 363, 364e
Mixed loyalty conflicts, 207
Model Commitment Letter, 143e
Model of Community Health Governance, 69–71
Moralizing communication roadblock, 187e–188e
Mosaica, 264e, 293, 294, 303, 304, 305, 310, 317–318, 453
Mourning (or re-forming) development stage, 165
Multi-voting, 201
Multicultural coalition building, 149, 153–155, 156e–158e
Multijurisdictional Counterdrug Task Force Training Program (MCTFT), 132

N
Name branding, 267
Naming communication roadblock, 187e–188e
NASA (National Aeronautic and Space Administration), 196
National Alliance for Hispanic Health, 22
National Alliance of State Prostate Cancer Coalitions (NASPCC), 22

National Assembly of National Voluntary Health, 122
National Association of City and County Health Officials (NACCHO), 357, 358
National Asthma Control Program (CDC), 22
The National Campaign to Prevent Teen Pregnancy, 325, 351, 390, 503, 504
National Cancer Institute (NCI), 18
National Center on Minority Health and Health Disparities (NCMHHD), 23
National Center for Nonprofit Boards, 256
National Coalition Academy (CADCA), 133–134
National Coalition Institute (CADCA), 134
National Coalition for Tobacco-Free Older Persons, 35
National coalitions, 36
National Folic Acid Coalition, 36
National Guard Bureau (NGB), 132, 134
National Highway Traffic Safety Administration, 330, 428
National Immunization Program (CDC), 84
National Institutes of Health (NIH), 24
National Medical Association, 22
National Network for Collaboration, 178–179
National Partnership for Immunization, 19
National Program to Promote Diabetes Education Strategies in Minority Communities (CDC), 22
National Public Health Performance Standards, 371
National SAFE KIDS USA, 20
National Science Foundation (NSF), 318
National Speakers Association, 245
Natural helpers, 117

Needs assessments, 133e, 328
Neighborhood Participation Project (Nashville), 12–13
Neighborhood profiles, 334
Neighborhood-maintenance. See Community-development (or neighborhood-maintenance) approach
Networking, 27
Networks: action, 29; definition of, 29; exchange, 29; service integration efforts of, 31
New Deal Programs, 7
Newsletters, 270–272e
No decision style, 196
Nominal Group Technique (NGT), 191, 194e, 343–344
Non-Governmental Coalition Against Tobacco, 35
Nonprofit Online News, 318
Nonprofit tax status, 282–285, 286e
Nonverbal communication, 184–185
Norming team development stage, 165
NUD*IST program, 466

O
Obesity prevention goals, 364e
Objectives: CINCH goals and, 364e–365e; Healthy People 2010, 367e–370e; setting public health goal, 363, 366; seven categories of, 366; SMART, 366. See also Goals
Observation data collection, 336–337
Observers, 140
Office of Minority Health (OMH) [USDHHS], 21, 300
Office of Quality Improvement, 241
Ohio Literacy Resource Center, 318
Ohio State University, 301
OhioLine, 318
On the Use Which the Americans Make of Associations in Civil Life (de Tocqueville), 4
OnLine PR and Marketing, 268

Openness, 186
Operation guidelines
 (bylaws), 231–240
Optimist, 175
Oral Health America, 19
Oral Health Call to Action
 (2003), 19
Oral health promotion:
 Arkansas Office of Oral
 Health fund-raising for,
 315–316; history of coali-
 tions in, 19
Ordering (or commanding)
 communication, 187e–188e
Organization-set
 coalitions, 33
Organizational charts, 141,
 227fig–229fig
Organizational climate, 141
Organizational health communication, 404
Organizational level influence, 51
Organizational outcomes,
 439–440
Organizations: climate of,
 141; developing effective
 message of, 262, 264e–265;
 "personality" of, 183
Organizer leader role, 125
Outcome evaluation, 307,
 438–439
Outcomes: CCAT proposition
 on, 83–84; CINCH
 application of CCAT, 88;
 community change, 136,
 440; definition of, 71; ecological levels of, 439–440;
 focusing efforts on measurable, 491; long-term community, 438
Outward work: description of,
 181, 182. See also Coalition
 processes; Inward work

P
Papa Ola Lokani (Asian
 Pacific Islander group), 22
Paraphrasing, 187
Parking lot (or idea bin), 244
Parliamentary Internet
 Newsletter (Robert
 McConnell
 Productions), 258
Parliamentary procedure, 255

Participating members, 139
Participating (or supporting)
 leadership, 169e
Participation (social market-
 ing "Ps"), 409
Participatory evaluation,
 435–436
Partner, 144
Partnership Self-Assessment
 Tool, 179
Partnership (social marketing
 "Ps"), 409
Partnership Tool Kit: Public
 Health Excellence Through
 Partnership, 257–258
Partnerships: benchmarks of
 empowered community,
 491; business, 280; defini-
 tion of, 30; Engaging Poten-
 tial Partners Worksheet,
 152e; Identifying Potential
 Collaboration Partners
 worksheet, 149e–151e;
 reflections on power of
 working in, 501–502;
 resources on coalitions and,
 135–137; strategic, 30–31.
 See also Collaboration
PATCH (Planned Approach to
 Community Health),
 358, 360t
Pawtucket Heart Health
 Program, 16
Pennsylvania Hospital, 4
Perception checking, 187
Performing team development
 stage, 165
Personal contact
 recruitment, 147
Personal costs, 55
Personality conflicts, 206–207
Persons Living with
 HIV/AIDS (PLWHA), 21
Pfizer Foundation, 303
Philanthropy Journal
 Online, 318
Philanthropy Links, 318
Photovoice, 339
Place (4 Ps of marketing), 408
Plan Quality Assessment
 Tool: Plan Quality Index
 (PQI), 372e–378e
Planned Action toward Com-
 munity Health (PATCH)
 initiative, 10

Planning. See Public health
 planning
Plausibility criteria, 397
Policy (social marketing
 "Ps"), 409
Political activists approach,
 7–8
Politics (social marketing
 "Ps"), 409
Pooled member/external
 resources: CCAT proposi-
 tion on, 81; CINCH applica-
 tion of CCAT on, 87
Positive confrontation,
 210e–211e
Practicality criteria, 397
PRECEDE-PROCEED model,
 67, 357, 358, 360t, 408
Preinatal health goals, 364
Prevent and Control
 Tobacco Use (IMPACT)
 program, 18
Price (4 Ps of marketing), 408
Principle-Centered Leadership
 (Covey), 121
"Principled negotiation," 208
Priority populations: description of, 326–327; developing community ownership
 of issue by, 327–328; target
 versus, 326
Proactiveness trait, 121
Problem solving: step 1:
 defining problem, 190;
 step 2: identifying and defining root causes, 190–192,
 194e; step 3: generating
 alternative solutions, 192;
 step 4: evaluating alternatives, 192; step 5: selecting
 best solution, 192; step 6:
 implementing the solution,
 192; step 7: evaluating the
 solution, 195
Process evaluation, 307, 438
Process factors, 69
Product (4 Ps of
 marketing), 408
Professional (agency-based)
 coalitions, 32
Programs. See Coalition
 programs
Project Immunize
 Virginia, 267
Project team, 394–395

Promising interventions/ practices: assessing, 395–398; definition of, 396; self-assessment to find, 398e

Promising Practices Network on Children, Families, and Communities, 396

Promotion: 4 Ps of marketing, 409; materials used in, 267–276; planning, 263t

Promotional materials: brochures, 268–270; coalition spokespersons as part of, 275–276; described, 267–268; newsletters, 270–272e; websites, 273–275

Proven interventions, 396

Public forums, 339–340

Public health planning: Decade of Hope Coalition experience with, 379, 387e, 389; evaluating the process of, 371–379; GTO (Getting to Outcomes), 359, 361; as key to addressing complex health issues, 356–357; models used for, 357–359, 360t; process of strategic, 361–363, 370–371; resources on, 390

Public leader, 122

Public perception conflicts, 206

Public policy level influence, 51

Q

Quasi experimental pre-post-test design, 459

Quirks.Com, 429

R

Racial and Ethnic Approaches to Community Health (REACH 2010), 23–24

Re-forming (or mourning) development stage, 165

Reaching for Higher Ground in Conflict Resolution (Dukes, Piscolish, and Stephens), 203

Receiver (communication), 183, 184

Recorder (or secretary), 175

Recruiting: coalition leadership, 117; coalition members, 144–148; investing in membership, 148–149

Reflector, 175

Reframing, 212

Regional coalitions, 36

ResearchInfo.com, 429

Resource development plan: activities of, 297t–298t; deciding available funding possibilities/strategies, 296, 297; described, 293–294; drafting the, 297, 298; evaluating coalition's current financial status, 295; examining organization and resources, 294–295; setting fund-raising objectives, 295–296

Resource development team, 292–293

Resource information: on coalition infrastructure, 256–258; on coalition membership, 177–179; on coalition processes, 219–221; on coalition programs/interventions, 428–432; on community assessments, 353–355; on evaluation, 494–500; on marketing coalitions, 277; on partnerships and coalitions, 135–137; on public health planning, 390. See also Websites

Resource members, 140

Resources (coalition): CCAT on pooled member/external, 8182, 87; conflict over, 204; evaluation findings on, 473–474. See also Funds

RFPs (request for proposals), 302–303, 304, 306, 310, 312–314

Robert F. Greenleaf Center for Servant Leadership, 136–137

Robert McConnell Productions, 255, 258

Robert Wood Johnson Allies Against Asthma initiative, 50

Robert Wood Johnson Foundation (RWJF), 17, 18, 21, 22, 23, 300, 303, 428, 488, 490, 502, 503, 504, 505

Robert's Rules of Order, 201

Robert's Rules of Order, Revised, 1990, 258

Ronald McDonald House Charities, 425

Rule of law principle, 57

Ryan White Care Act, 20

S

Safe KIDS International, 36

Safe Kids movement, 20

Safe Kids USA, 20

Safe Kids Worldwide, 20

SAMHSA (Substance Abuse and Mental Health Services Administration), 502–503, 504, 505

SCHIP (state-sponsored child health insurance program), 37–38

School Health Index (CDC), 371

School health objectives, 368e

Search Engine Marketing, 270

Secretary (or recorder), 175

Secretary-treasurer position, 106e

Self-appointed decision maker, 196

Self-Assessment to Find or Choose Promising Practices, 398e

Self-completed diaries (or logs), 347

Self-interest recruitment approach, 146

Self-renewal/continuous improvement, 121

Selling (or coaching) leadership, 169e

Sender (communication), 183

Service Corps of Retired Executives (SCORE), 277

Service linkages, 31

70/30 vote, 199, 200

Shared members, 139–140

Show Your Love, Put Your Child in a Car Seat workshop, 426

"Silver bullet" solutions, 400

"Six Pillars of Characters," 202

"The Six 'R's' of Participation," 160, 160e–162e

Six-Step Program Development Chain Model, 358

Skeptic (or Devil's advocate), 175

Slogans (or bylines), 225

SMART objectives, 366

SmartDraw, 228

SmokeLess States: National Tobacco Policy Initiative, 18, 488, 502

SmokeLess States National Program Office (NOP), 18

Snowball technique, 341, 343

Social action model, 10

Social action organizing: definition of, 7; overview of contemporary efforts and models of, 10–12; typology of community organization and, 11fig

Social capital: as coalition contextual factor, 52; definition of, 15–16

Social change: community organizing for, 5–9; neighborhood-maintenance or community-development approach to, 8–9; political activist approach to, 7–8; social work approach to, 6–7

Social enterprise, 280

Social Enterprise Magazine Online, 297

Social entrepreneurs, 281

Social marketing: coalition branding through, 267; definition of, 407; essential elements of, 407; features of, 408–409; four additional "Ps" of, 409; resources on, 428–431; six-step model of, 410–411. See also Marketing coalitions

Social Marketing Institute, 429

Social Marketing Place, 429

Social marketing plan: creating a, 409–411; Marketing Campaign Development Tool for, 411t; model of, 10

Social Marketing in Public Health Conference, 429

Social purpose businesses, 280

Social Security Act, 7

Social Welfare Organizations, 122

Social work approach, 6–7

Social-capital builders, 400

Social-needs recruitment approach, 147

Social-organizational costs, 55

Society of Women Against AIDS in Africa (SWAA), 21

Spokesperson (or liaison), 175, 275–276

Staff: accountability of, 100; administrative assistant, 103e–104e; chair and vice-chair, 105e; coordinator, 100e–102e; evaluation of, 472–473; FTEs (full time equivalents), 308; leadership and structure impact on, 98–99; roles of coalition, 99–100, 104, 107–108; secretary-treasurer, 106e; work group chair and vice-chair, 106e–107e. See also Leadership

Stages of development: CCAT on, 76–77; CINCH application of CCAT, 84–85

Standardized tests, 334

Standards for Effective Evaluation (CDC), 445

Stanford Health Programs, 16

Staock Layouts, LLC, 268

State Children's Health Insurance Program (SCHIP), 21

State coalitions, 34–36

State Plan Index (SPI), 371, 378–379, 380e–389e

Steering committee: coalition governance by, 226e, 229–230; resource development team subgroup of, 292–293

Steps to Program Evaluation (Kellogg Foundation), 446–447

Storm King Mountain disaster (1994), 196

Storming team development stage, 164–165

Strategic leadership approach, 119

Strategic partnerships, 30–31

Strategic planning process: elements of, 361–363, 370–371; evaluating the, 371–379

The Strategy of Meetings (Kieffer), 240

Straw man technique, 200

Street outreach: community mobilization through, 406; recruitment through, 148

Student movements, 8

Students for a Democratic Society, 8

Substance Abuse and Mental Health Services Administration (SAMHSA), 502–503, 504, 505

Summarizer (or clarifier), 175

Summative evaluation, 439

Supporting (or participating) leadership, 169e

Surveys (or windshield tours): advantages and disadvantages of, 342t; described, 338, 346–347

Sustainability: definition of, 316; evaluation of, 447; fund-raising to maintain, 279; grant application plans for, 309

SWOT analysis, 224, 358, 362, 389

Symbolic communication, 184

Synergy trait, 121

Systems (or community) outcomes, 440

T

The Tao of Leadership (Heider), 122

Target populations, 326

Task force, 30

Tax issues: nonprofit organization status, 282–285e, 286e; Tax-Exempt Organization Reference Chart, 286e

The Teal Trust, 168

Team building: importance of effective, 163–164; integration of theories on, 166t; stages of development, 164–165

Team Effectiveness Checklist, 173e

Team Effectiveness Critique, 173e–174e

Team Effectiveness Questionnaire, 171e–172

Team leadership, 126

TeamBonding, 179

Teambuilding, Inc., 179

Teams: competencies of effective, 166–167; group communication in, 186–190t; leadership of, 126, 167–168, 169e, 170e; membership of, 168–169; roles within, 174, 175; Team Effectiveness Checklist, 173e; Team Effectiveness Critique, 173e–174e; Team Effectiveness Questionnaire on, 171e–172e; traits of, 165–167

Technical assistance: building and sustaining, 129–130; coalition role/responsibilities for, 129, 131e; member providers of, 144; overview of, 128–129; recommendations for, 127–128; reports made to coalitions on, 132e; roles, responsibilities, characteristics of, 129; venues of, 130–134

Teen pregnancy prevention, 20

Teeth on the Go, 315

Telling (or directing) leadership, 169e

Texas Oral Health Coalition bylaws, 233e–240

Theory-based evaluation, 435

Third-party mediation, 210e–211e

Time series design, 459

Timekeeper, 175

Tobacco prevention: early history of coalitions in, 17–18; Health Care Trust Fund for, 217; Master Settlement

Agreement (MSA) and, 18, 504; Virginians for a Healthy Future for, 59, 216–217

Tobacco-Free Youth Coalition Self-Evaluation Instrument, 485e–486e

Tolerance principle, 57

Tools of Change, 429

Town meeting recruitment, 147

Tracker the hound (mascot), 267

Tracker Talk newsletter, 271e–272e

Training (or conference) recruitment, 147

Transactional recruitment approach, 146

Transformation for Health meeting approach, 255

Transformational leadership: characteristics of, 109, 111–113fig; comparing traditional and, 120t–121; self-assessment questionnaire on, 114e–115e; ten traits of, 115e–116e

Transparency principle, 57

Treaty of Paris (1783), 4

Trusted communication, 186

Turf management tips, 215–216

Turfism: avoiding and resolving battles over, 213–215; described, 212–213; types of, 213–214

Turning Point Social Marketing National Excellence Collaborative, 23, 111, 356, 408, 409, 429

Twin Cities Public Television, 4

Typology of Community Organization and Community Building, 10–12, 69

U

United Farm Workers Union, 7

United Nations, 12

Unity versus diversity, 207

University of Florida Extension, 142

University of Kansas (KU Work Group), 379

University of Nevada Cooperative Extension, 159, 189

University of Arkansas College of Dentistry Scholarships, 315

Urban Car Seat Initiative, 426

U.S. Census Bureau, 340

U.S. Department of Health and Human Services (USDHHS), 18, 19, 20, 21, 358, 390, 461, 465

U.S. Department of Transportation, 330, 390, 429

U.S. Forest Service, 196

U.S. Office of Management and Budget, 396

U.S. Surgeon General, Oral Health Call to Action (2003) called by, 19

V

Vaccines for Children, 35

Venture philanthropy, 296–297

Verbal communication, 184

Verbal quality, 184–185

Vertical organizational charts, 227fig

Virginians for a Healthy Future, 59, 216–217, 229fig

Virtual Foundation, 318

Vision statements, 224–225, 362, 364e

Visual chart, 225

Voluntary arbitration, 210e–211e

Volunteer leaders: described, 117; developing quality, 110e–111e

Voting (or full) members, 140

W

Websites: on ethics, 431–432; as promotional material, 273–275; questions guiding development of, 273; on social marketing and media advocacy, 428–431. See also Resource information

Wellington Consulting Group, 119, 122, 139, 140, 141, 145, 147, 183, 262

What's Your Coalition's Participant Involvement Score?, 197e–198e

White House Office of National Drug Control Policy's National Youth Anti-drug Media Campaign, 428

Wilder Research Center, 27

Win-win mindset, 121

Windshield tours (or surveys), 338, 342t, 346–347

Wisconsin Council on Developmental Disabilities, 431

W.K. Kellogg Foundation, 23, 122, 136, 300, 303, 340, 446, 454, 458, 460, 464, 466, 467, 468

Work group chair/vice-chair, 106e–107e

Work Group on Health Promotion and Community Development, 66–67fig

Work groups: coalition infrastructure position of, 230; competencies of effective, 166–167; group communication in, 186–190t; importance of effective, 163–164; integration of theories on, 166t; leadership of, 167–168; roles within, 174, 175; stages of development, 164–165; Team Effectiveness Checklist, 173e; Team Effectiveness Questionnaire on, 171e–172e; traits of, 165–167. See also Coalition infrastructure; Inward work

Worksheets: Brochure Content Worksheet, 269e; Engaging Potential Partners Worksheet, 152e; Identifying Potential Collaboration Partners, 149e–151e; Worksite health objectives, 369e

World Health Organization, 358

Y

Youth Media Campaign (CDC), 428

Z

Zero to ten rating, 201–202